☞ P9-BZO-985

CRC handbook series in zoonoses /
James H. Steele, editor-in-chief.
-- Boca Raton, Fla. : CRC Press,
c1979-<c1982 >
  v. <1-3 > in <6 > : ill. ;
26 cm. Library has: sec. C, v.1-3
  Contents: section A: Bacterial, rickettsial,
and mycotic diseases / section editors,
Herbert Stoenner, William Kaplan, Michael
orten (2 v.) -- section B. Viral zoonoses <v.
  > -- section C. Parasitic zoonoses (3 v.)
  Includes bibliographies and indexes.
  ISBN 0-8493-2900-0 (set)
  1. Zoonoses. 2. Bacterial diseases. 3.
ickettsial diseases. 4. Mycoses. 5.
ommunicable diseases in animals. I. Steele,

(continued)

WaOE   78-10696//r81

CRC Handbook
Series in Zoonoses

James H. Steele, Editor-in-Chief

Assistant Surgeon General (Retired)
U.S. Public Health Service
Professor of Environmental Health
School of Public Health
University of Texas at Houston

Section C: Parasitic Zoonoses
Volume I

The Editor, Part 1

Leon Jacobs, Ph.D.
Scientist Emeritus
Laboratory of Parasitic Diseases
National Institute of Allergy and Infectious Diseases
National Institutes of Health
Bethesda, Maryland

The Editor, Part 2

Primo Arambulo, III, DVM, CPH, DAP&E, MPH, Dr.P.H.
Regional Advisor in Veterinary Medicine
Pan American Health Organization
World Health Organization
Washington, D.C.

CRC Press, Inc.
Boca Raton, Florida

Library of Congress Cataloging in Publication Data
Main entry under title:

Parasitic zoonoses.

   (CRC handbook series in zoonoses;
section C)

   Bibliography: p.
   Includes index.
   1. Parasitic diseases. 2. Zoonoses.
I. Jacobs, Leon. II. Series.
RC113.5.C72 Sect. C [RC119] 616.9'59s   81-18127
ISBN 0-8493-2915-9 (set)   [616.9'6]   AACR2

   Direct all inquiries to CRC Press, Inc., 2000 Corporate Blvd., N.W., Boca Raton, Florida, 33431.

© 1982 by CRC Press, Inc.

International Standard Book Number 0-8493-2900-0 (Set)
International Standard Book Number 0-8493-2915-9 (Section C)
International Standard Book Number 0-8493-2916-7 (Volume I)
International Standard Book Number 0-8493-2917-5 (Volume II)
International Standard Book Number 0-8493-2918-3 (Volume III)

Library of Congress Card Number 81-18127
Printed in the United States

PREFACE
CRC HANDBOOK SERIES IN ZOONOSES

The biological adventurousness of animal diseases is exceeded only by the insatiable adventuresomeness of man. The struggle of the infectious diseases of lower forms of life to adapt themselves to more highly developed hosts is unending. As these disease agents insure their continued existence by adapting themselves to a broader host spectrum, they become a greater threat to man's well-being. Man, in his most tenuous position on this earth, has been able to protect himself from this biological onslaught by his skill in developing the preventive medical practices that are the foundation of our present public health practices.

In this century, man has made greater progress in holding back or eliminating infectious diseases than he has since he appeared on earth. Progress in the control of host-specific human diseases, such as smallpox, diphtheria, cholera, poliomyelitis, and syphilis, has brought to the fore animal disease problems which in many areas of the world are major challenges to human health. The eradication of smallpox is one of the major health achievements of our times. One reason this was possible was that there is no animal reservoir of smallpox. The control of diphtheria, cholera, poliomyelitis, and other childhood diseases was possible because none of these diseases have an animal reservoir.

Animal diseases threaten man's health and well-being in many ways. To examine the importance of animal health to human health, it is well for us to consider the World Health Organization (WHO) definition of health as a guide. "Health is not the mere absence of disease or injury . . . it is a state of complete physical, mental, and social well-being." The contributions that veterinary medicine can make to reach the WHO objective are succinctly presented in the definition of veterinary public health:
. . . "comprises all the community efforts influencing and influenced by the veterinary medical arts and science applied to the prevention of disease, protection of life, and promotion of the well-being and efficiency of man." The present epidemic of Rift Valley Fever in the Nile Valley is an example of how serious some zoonoses can be. The 1978 epidemic has effected thousands of persons and tens of thousands of cattle, sheep, and goats. Why Rift Valley Fever became so wide spread and virulent is unknown.

The definition of health, as established by WHO, provides a very broad framework upon which to develop our theme. How veterinary medicine will participate in protecting the public health and welfare is well expressed in the broad definition of veterinary public health, and the inter-relationship of disease and health in man and animals provides a challenge that tests the imagination, ingenuity, and knowledge of man.

James H. Steele
Editor-in-Chief

JAMES H. STEELE, EDITOR-IN-CHIEF
CRC HANDBOOK SERIES IN ZOONOSES

Dr. James H. Steele has held a broad and rewarding experience in veterinary medicine and public health. He entered the Michigan State Veterinary College in 1938 and completed his veterinary training in 1941 when he was awarded the D.V.M. degree. After an internship in veterinary medicine and the Michigan Public Health Laboratory, he was sent to Harvard School of Public Health on a U.S. Public Health Service Fellowship. On the completion of the M.P.H. degree in 1942, he was assigned to the Ohio Health Department as a sanitarian. In 1943, he was commissioned in the U.S. Public Health Service and assigned to Puerto Rico where he had his first opportunity to become acquainted with animal diseases in the tropics and received encouragement to develop a national and international program.

After world War II, he was called to the U.S. Public Health Service, Washington, D.C. to plan a program to deal with the zoonoses and veterinary public health. This was to be a part of the Communicable Disease Center in Atlanta, Georgia where it grew into a national program with an international influence. In addition to directing the CDC veterinary public health program, Dr. Steele was a consultant to U.S. government agencies and international organizations relating to the health of man and animals.

After the inauguration of the veterinary public health program in 1947, a category for veterinary officers was approved by the Surgeon General in 1948. In 1950 Dr. Steele was made veterinary consultant to the Surgeon General and liaison to a professional health organization. Later in 1967 he was to become the Assistant Surgeon General for Veterinary Affairs in the Public Health Service and Department of Health Education and Welfare. The first veterinary officer to be named to this post. He remained in this position until his retirement in 1971. During 1969 he was designated advisor to the White House office on Consumer Affairs.

Dr. Steele was a technical advisor to Surgeon General Thomas Parran when the United Nations organized the World Health Organization in 1946. Later he was appointed to the WHO Expert Committee on Zoonoses and served in varying roles. In 1966 he was elected Chairman. During 1946 the Food Agriculture Organization was having technical meetings at which he represented the United States. He has served as a consultant to the FAO on many occasions since. The Pan American Sanitary Bureau was the first to request his services in disease outbreaks in the Carribean and Panama during and after World War II. He has been a consultant to the Pan American Health Organization since 1945 and served as chairman of their Scientific Advisory Committee in 1970. In addition to serving as a consultant to international agencies, he has been an advisor to a number of countries and universities in developing veterinary public health programs.

He has received national and international recognition from numerous governments, agencies, and societies. The U.S. Public Health Service awarded him the Medal of Merit in 1963 and the Distinguished Service plaque on his retirement in 1971. The American Public Health Service presented Dr. Steele the prestigous Bronfman Award in 1971 and the Centennial medal in 1972. In 1966 the Conference of Public Health Veterinarians honored him with the K. F. Meyer Gold Headed Cane Award. These Handbooks of the Zoonoses are dedicated to K. F. Meyer. Dr. Steele has been made an honorary member of various scientific organizations in the Americas, Europe and Asia. In 1965 he was named president of the American Veterinary Epidemiology Society. He was instrumental in the establishment of the World Veterinary Epidemiology Society in 1972 which is affiliated with the World Veterinary Association. An award was established in his name by the WVES in 1976 which is presented to a young leader in international veterinary public health. He has been described by many of his colleagues as *Mister Veterinary Public Health.*

His publications span a period of almost 40 years and cover various subjects, especially the zoonoses of which there are more than 100 titles. He is a man of many interests.

PARASITIC ZOONOSES

INTRODUCTION

"THE WORMY WORLD"

"It is not given to any one man, however endowed, to rise spontaneously into intellectual splendor without the parentage of antecedent thought."

John Tyndall (1820-1893)

The dispersion of biological knowledge is in accord with the Tyndall light phenomenon — light is dispersed by suspended particles, knowledge by people. In parasitology, facts have been painstakingly accumulated to be dispersed into related fields — medicine and veterinary medicine, public health, animal science, food processing, and hygiene. The Parasitic Zoonoses were written by authors who are highly regarded by their colleagues in their special fields. We are all indebted to them for their contributions, and to the Section Editors, Leon Jacobs, Myron Schultz, George Hillyer, Primo Arambulo, and Cluff Hopla. I am especially grateful for their recommendations in selecting the most qualified individuals in their respective areas. It is with much appreciation and humility that I write this introduction.

To put these volumes into perspective I have turned to an old colleague who is one of the respected parasitologits of our times, Norman Stoll, who when President of the American Society of Parasitologists in 1946, presented a memorable address entitled *The Wormy World* [1] in which he described the status, importance, and distribution of parasites affecting the public health of the world at the end of the great war — World War II. In the following, his address will be paraphrased and a present day commentary based on our present knowledge gathered by the contributors to these volumes.

One cannot have experienced the war without having been impressed anew, and depressed by the amount of parasitism in the world. Speaking helminthologically, it may be referred to as the grave host role which the lives of men play in the lives of worms. [1]

One could add the role of all other animals in the lives of worms — some definitive hosts, others intermediate hosts, and in some instances either/or both man and animals as accidental hosts.

Or, think of it the other way about, for there is likewise the great parasitic role the lives of worms play in the lives of men. Back from the Pacific come a thousand-odd Americans with schistosomiasis, and a few times that many with filariasis, and several multiples more with ancylostomiasis (*sensu strictu*). To homes widely dispersed throughout the land go these ex-service men, to live a lifetime in familiarity with the strangely sounding names of their distantly-acquired helminthiases.

Just how much human helminthiasis is there in the world?

The bare mention of the question will make those of you with helminthogeographical interests — warily scratch a mental ear . . . I need scarcely remind you of what some of these hurdles are; so many parasitological surveys of small numbers of people frequently of other design than to represent fair samples of an area, done by workers of varying aims and by techniques of even more variable efficiency in relation to the task at hand . . .

One cannot change this state of affairs at the moment. Instead, one takes the data as they are and does the best one can. The information presented today is from the same kind of data we all have had of necessity, to employ in putting together the impressions we currently possess of the extensiveness of the problem to be discussed. In substance, . . . I have restated such adjectival generalizations of the reference books as "rare", "common", "prevalent" into the best quantitative terms which searching of the records and epidemiological insight have permitted.

The census bases used vary in date from 1920 to 1942, more than half of the censuses occurring between 1935-1940. An approximate statement as to the dates applies to the helminthic infection figures, although publications in 1946 have been consulted.[1]

The world census cited is 2166 million for 1940. The sources were the Office of Population Research, Princeton University, and the League of Nations Statistical Yearbook, the latter total was 2170 million. By 1980 these figures had doubled, and continued to increase by almost 100 million annually even with efforts to control world population. The prediction is that the world population will pass 5 billion (5000 million) before 1990.

Stoll started his analysis of specific infections with *Trichinella spiralis,* a parasite which has been known since the 1830s and an infection about which good epidemiological data was available. In 1942 Augustine reported it as the "most serious parasitic disease in New England".[2]

Trichinella is almost completely absent in man in a major portion of the world. East of Suez, all the way to San Francisco, as well as in Australia, Africa, and the torrid zone, it is substantially nonexistent as a human infection. In these regions live about 2/3 of the earth's inhabitants, but few cases of record suggest an infection rate there of the order of <.01 percent (1/10,000) in man.

The classic zones of infection have been in Central Europe and those parts of temperate America to which emigrants and their eating habits have gone. In Europe, the reports in the pre-war years of infection in man, as well as officially inspected pork have suggested exceedingly low rates. During the war years, however, outbreaks occurred in nearly all European countries. Recurrent episodes were reported after the war in German troops, especially in Poland and Russia. If we assume the diaphragm infection rate throughout Europe to be as low as one percent, much higher than pre-war indices, that would mean about 5 million cases.[1]

Post-war Poland and old Poland, annexed by Russia in 1939, had large outbreaks in the 1950s. Otherwise the incidence of trichinosis is low in northern and western Europe. The disease likewise, is sporadic in southern Europe. The U.S.S.R. reports an incidence of less than 1/10 of 1% (<0.1). Surveys in northern Russia and Siberia reveal the disease is present in many wild animals. These studies are presented in the Trichinosis chapter.

In South America, recent rates reported from Chile slightly exceeded 10 percent, and from Uruguay 3 percent with the probability that the latter may reflect the situation in Argentina. A rate of 12 percent, is cited for Mexico City. These 4 areas of Middle and South America possess then, by extrapolation, about one million cases.[1]

Surveys in the 1950s to 1970s indicate that trichinosis is widespread in Chile. Uruguay and Argentina have sporadic outbreaks. Mexico D.F. has a high incidence according to serological surveys. The disease has been recognized in most of Latin America but it would be difficult to find evidence to support extrapolation of a million cases.

In Canada, according to examinations in the early 1940s, there is a trifling infection rate of about 1 percent — perhaps 100,000 in all Canada — which is not so trifling but that clinical outbreaks occasionally develop. This low rate, and trichinosis outbreaks nonetheless occurring in Canada without the exigencies of famine, may be taken as a pointer toward how low the index must become before complete control of trichina is accomplished.[1]

Canada has been thought to be free of pig trichinosis since the inauguration of garbage cooking to control hog cholera in the early 1920s. The first recognition of the disease was in rats, later in bears and marine mammals in the far north. There have been sporadic outbreaks among Indians and Eskimos due to the ingestions of bear meat — polar or ice bears have the greatest incidence of infection.

In the U.S.A. we have trichinosis in a bigger way. Thanks to nearly 12,000 necropsy examinations in recent years, nearly half of them by the National Institute of Health workers, who combined microscopic and digestive techniques, we have now what must be considered a rather good perspective of the situation throughout this country. It's overall finding is about 1 in 6 Americans infected. On the basis of the 1940 census of 131 million people, there are 21 million Americans who have ingested *Trichinella spiralis*. Proportionately, in certain parts of the country it would be higher.

Trichinella incidence obtained at necropsies has the advantage of being a figure which indicates total exposure, inasmuch as most infected individuals would appear to retain evidence of calcified larvae throughout life. It is further of interest, therefore, that the NIH data show 4½ pecent of positives with counts of 50 or more larvae per gram of muscle, infections of an order "capable of causing pronounced clinical symptoms." These individuals, if adults, would, I calculate, be carrying muscle loads in excess of one million trichina larvae.

Hall and Collins (1937) emphasized that the United States "has the greatest problem of trichinosis of any country in the world".[3] The figures adduced indicate that also it should be said: we have in this country more than 3 times as much trichinosis as is known in all the rest of the world put together.

Because the problem is thus predominantly our own, one is tempted to digress and to muse a little about such a record, which, of course, is a preventable one, and maintained primarily through allowing hogs to be fed uncooked garbage containing meat scraps harboring live Trichinella. Those of you who travel the Pennsylvania R.R. into New York become aware that we maintain, in the Jersey meadows at Secaucus, a malodorous demonstration for every traveler to observe how it is done. When we Americans manifest an unbecoming impatience at how slothful other people are, in undertaking the necessary and obvious steps to free themselves from this, that or the other endemic helminthiasis, let us pause a moment with ourselves. We can ruminate with profit on the extraordinary slowness demonstrated by a supposedly widely educated people, in failing to protect itself against trichinosis, when it can do so by the simple device of eating pork only when the trichinae in it have been cooked, say, to the consistency of medium boiled eggs. Such a simple protective measure has been propagandized in this country widely for well-nigh a half-century. We can also ruminate on the extraordinary inertia of public officials, legislative and other, in their odd failure to adequately control the feeding of uncooked trichinae in raw garbage to hogs.

One is given to wonder, considering that our scientific analysis of the subject is now competent, and the road to control thus clear, whether we are dealing here not with a mercenary, but with a psychological block against effective action. Perhaps "trichinosis" is a word of too little odium. Would Americans be equally comfortable in realizing that each 6th among them is harboring garbage worms? And that one in 150 persons dying from other causes takes to the grave a million or more garbage worm larvae? What wasted "blind alley" effort from the standpoint of Trichinella demography![1]

Stoll truly illuminated the trichinella problem that Wright, Jacobs, and Kerr[4,4a] uncovered in the 1940s, and Hall and Collins in the 1930s.[3] Their findings and description received attention throughout the world. In 1963, when I was a guest of the U.S.S.R. along with other American veterinary scientists: Carl Brandly, Howard Dunn, Eugene Papp, and Herbert Stoenner, we were regularly asked why the U.S. had so much trichinosis. It embarassed us. We knew the incidence in swine and persons was much lower due to the education of the American consumer, the elimination of much of the garbage feeding of swine around metropolitan areas, which was enforced to control vesicular exanthema, a virus disease spread by pork meat scraps, and good epidemiological investigations identifying sources such as home made ethnic sausages. All these circumstances made us realize that a national survey of swine and human beings was needed to bring the disease in focus in the 1960s. Such was the genesis of national surveys of Zimmerman, Steele, Kagen[5] and Zinter[6] in those years, 1966 to 1970. These studies included almost 8000 human cadavers and a like number of hog carcasses. The results speak for the success of the efforts to reduce, control and eliminate trichinosis in the U.S. The human cadaver had an adjusted infection rate of 2.2% (22/1000) or 1 in 44 persons.

Even this low figure would result in an estimated 506,000 infections if we use 1980 census data. This figure of estimated infections should decline with the passing of older persons who were exposed in an earlier era when garbage fed and home fed pigs were more widely consumed.

The pig infection rate of the late 1960s was less than 1/1000, and even the infected pigs had low levels of cysts, usually being less than five cysts per gram of flesh, compared to hundreds or thousands of larva per gram found in surveys 50 years ago or earlier. But the low infection rate should not deceive us. The market swine population of the U.S. approaches 100 million annually of which possibly 100,000 pigs may be carriers of low grade infection, some of which may have a heavier larva load. This no doubt accounts for most of the clinical trichinosis cases reported annually — that number has remained low at between 100 and 200 cases, with one death or less annually.

The high incidence of sylatic trichinosis adds a new dimension. Trichinosis is truly a circumpolar disease with the highest incidence in the polar bears and arctic mammals declining into the temperate zones and not frequently found in the subtropics or the tropical regions (see discussion of Africa and Latin America). Most of the human infections reported in the U.S.S.R., Canada, and Alaska are from wild game. The human incidence in continental U.S. from game is estimated to be about 5% of the total cases reported.

> If time permitted considering the helminths of man, species by species, in relation to their incidence and the populations of individual countries or other geographical units, it would be as illuminating an experience to you, I think, as it has been to me. It is a sort of new perspective in helminthology, or at least a new emphasis — this view of the worms man lives with, not primarily in their taxonomic relations, nor in the accident of historical or local interest, but in terms of the over-all number of his fellows that are burdened with them. Omitting many of the steps by which the factual statements are made, we come out like this at the world level for some familiar forms:
> *Taenia saginata,* the beef tapeworm, 39 million infections, most ascribed to Africa and to the U.S.S.R., but *Taenia solium,* the pork tapeworm, less than 3 million with nearly a half in Asia. Cysticercosis manifestly makes up only a small part of these.[1]

The experienced Taeniasis experts of the WHO Expert Committee of Parasitic Zoonoses and the Pan American Health Organization believe the prevalence of these infections are much greater today than 40 years ago.[7] The taeniasis cases treated in the U.S. are few in number as reported to CDC, a hundred at the most. A reasonable estimate of human cases of *T. saginata* can be determined by the number of cattle feed lot outbreaks and those identified on post-mortem inspection — the respective numbers being less than 100 feed lots or farms with bovine cysticercosis, and about 10,000 retained carcasses with cysticercosis. But there may be severe complications with porcine cysticercosis *T. solium* in man which is seen in south Texas, and along the U.S./Mexico border. The infection in pigs is very rare in those inspected.

In Latin America, the meat borne tapeworms are widely prevalent. It is difficult to obtain rates but the Mexico D.F. public health authorities, epidemiologists and physicians related that *T. saginata* is common among rural Indian populations as well as those moving into urban areas. Complications are minimal, but with *T. solium* a much more serious problem exists. Cysticercosis is frequent among the Indians, especially in children where it is the most common cause of neurological disorders requiring brain surgery. Pathology specimens are shown to visitors at the Children's Hospital. A similar situation exists among Peruvian Indians where the infection rate is reported in excess of 100 percent per annum — some persons will have more than one infection yearly. The same exists further south in Chilean Indians. The constant movement of these people northward carry tapeworm and cysticercosis into the western U.S.

Tapeworms in Africa and Asia are common. In Nigeria, veterinary public health scientists state cysticercosis affects more animals than any other recognizable disease. In East Africa, human tapeworm disease is one of the most common parasitic diseases, especially in children,[7] one of the reasons being the scarcity of fuel — wood or oil for cooking fires. Southeast Asia and India both have *T. saginata* and *T. solium* in tens of thousands of the millions of cattle and swine in that region. The problem is well recognized in cattle and pigs coming to the Hong Kong market. How many millions of human infections occur in Africa and Asia is unknown.

The Philippines have an interesting problem with both tapeworms, which is discussed by Primo Arambulo. On the basis of reported infection of animals in the U.S.S.R. and neighboring countries the disease has declined. The estimates of Stoll may be low for the world, with more cases in Latin America, Africa, and Asia then 40 years ago — possibly, 60 million cases.

> Further, one is surprised to discover that the best estimates for hydatid disease....come to less than 100,000 cases, with South America leading.[1]

This is truly surprising according to present day reporting and estimates. Southern South America has inaugurated control activity in Uruguay, Argentina, and Chile with good results. The Pan American Health Organization has provided research support for these programs in the southern region. Hydatid disease is rare or sporadic in the northern hemisphere. Peter Schantz, who writes on hydatid disease, has had much experience with the infection in the Americas, the Middle East and North Africa. The highest incidence of hydatid disease is in North Africa and the Middle East. The most successful control program has been carried out by K. Polydorou, the director of veterinary services in Cyprus.[8,8a] This is a model for the world where dogs are the reservoir. Australia and New Zealand have greatly reduced human and animal infection in the past decades. No doubt there is more disease than Stoll reported, but how much is difficult to estimate — maybe a million or more.

> For *Hymenolepis nana* there are about 20 million currently indicated infections, 2/3 of them in Asia. This species seems rare in Oceania. On Guam we did not encounter it or any other tapeworm in natives, although infections were found in 0.5 percent of service men, which they had evidently brought to the area from homeside.[1]

No doubt *H. nana* is widespread, but where the millions of human cases are in Asia or elsewhere cannot be answered or guesstimated intelligently.

> *Diphyllobothrium latum,* the broad or fish tapeworm, shows about 3 million cases each in the Baltic littoral, northern Russia, the U.S.S.R., and in Asia, and a world total of 10 million. Thus, the cestodes altogether represent 72 million infected individuals.[1]

The author of the chapter on the *D. latum,* Goran Bylund, points out that the infection has declined precipitiously in the Scandinavian countries, and dropped in the Baltic states: Estonia, Latvia, and Lithuania, as well as Poland and Germany. Likewise, the infection has declined across the U.S.S.R. with improved hygiene and health education. Fish tapeworms are not unknown in North America, where they were reported in Canada and the northern U.S. but have almost disappeared in regions where they previously were not uncommon. One would be hard pressed to think that there may be 10 million cases in the world. It is very doubtful there are a million cases, possibly a lesser decimal (100,000) at the most. As to the total of cestodes, the taenias infect many millions and probably exceed the earlier estimates.

> Of fish-transmitted trematodes, *Clonorchis sinensis,* the human liver fluke, confined to Asia, seems not to be in excess of 19 million infections, about half of which are in Chekiang endemic center. The related *Opisthorchis felineus,* confined to fisherfolk in East Prussia, the Dneiper river basin, and norther Sverdlovsk in Asiatic U.S.S.R., has indications of one million.[1]

The human liver fluke remains a big problem in Eastern Asia as has been written by Han-Jong Rim in this series. How big is unknown, but hopefully the cases are less than 19 million estimated in the 1940s.

Opisthorchis felineus extends across Asia to Thailand and Indochina. *O. viverrini* is endemic in southeast Asia, especially among the hill people of Thailand. The estimate of 1 million may be low because of poor sanitation in the war disturbed areas.

> Of the fishborne small intestinal flukes, Metagonimus and Heterophyes, I have been unable to find evidence of more than a few hundred thousand probable infections. A similar statement holds for Echinostoma and Gastrodiscoides.[1]

It is difficult to guesstimate how prevalent the intestinal flukes are in Asia. They are widespread but reported in no orderly manner to base an estimate.

> The large intestinal fluke, *Fasciplopsis buski,* again a form confined to Asia, totals 10 million infections, about half of which are in the Chekiang endemic center. The related form, *Fasciola hepatica* of the ruminant liver passages, has been reported with increasing frequency in man and from all continents, but there is no indication that more than 100,000 cases are involved. *Dicrocoelium dendriticum,* also normally in ruminants, has been found (including confirmations at necropsy) especially in the Stalingrad and Transcaucas regions, where it occurs in sufficient degree to indicate several hundred thousand cases.[1]

F. buski is recognized as being common in Southeast Asia. The population in the endemic areas has increased 100 to 200 % in the past 40 years; add revolution and war, the conditions for spread are augmented. Ten million human infections may be low, a 1980 estimate would be 30 million or more.

F. hepatica and *F. gigantica* are worldwide in sheep, cattle, water buffalo, and other large ruminants. The economic loss is great because it interferes with growth and production, and loss of millions of pounds of liver that is unfit for human use. Human infection has been diagnosed in most countries of the world. In some areas, i.e., the Peruvian altoplano, the infection is common in school children.

Dicrocoelium dendriticum, another fluke of ruminants, is reported in regions of Eurasia and other countries. There are few reports of the infection in human beings.

> *Paragonimum westermani* incidence has not been easy to define, but with the aid of some relatively recent surveys it is possible to place the limiting value of about 3 million cases of lung fluke infection in Asia and a few thousand in West Africa.[1]

P. westermani, the lung fluke, has become a much more complicated problem in recent years with the new species being reported. The excellent chapters by Miyazaki and Yokogawa review the new diseases and their epidemiology in Asia including Siberia, Africa, Central and South America. The disease is also seen in North America among refugees from southeast Asia. The diagnosis in areas where the disease is unknown has been confused with lung cancer.

The several trematode infections of man mentioned infected millions of persons. Stoll estimates the several trematodes, liver, intestinal, and lung flukes to cause infection in about 34 million individuals. To update that estimate is difficult but it is generally believed these infections are fairly common. An estimate of two or three times higher is a probable figure today, 1982.

> The Schistosomes represent more than three times as many additional trematode infections, with S. japonicum the most numerous. For the six major centers of S. japonicum endemicity in the Yangtze valley, an average incidence is given of about 7 percent microscopic positives, barring some heavily infected villages (Faust and Meleney, 1925). If for present purposes and to include non-egg-passing cases, one takes 20 percent of the entire populations of such other Chinese provinces and Japanese prefectures as are known to have foci, and includes for the Philippines 30 percent of the population of the islands of Leyte, Samar, Mindoro, and Mindianao — the total infected with S. japanicum represents 46 million people. The anamalous Dutch East Indies focus in the Celebes presumably contains only a few thousand infections.[1]

The statement that Schistosomes are three times more prevalent than the other trematodes infections is certainly true today. The doubling or possible tripling of the population in eastern Asia provides even greater opportunities for S. japonicum infection in the 1980s. Japan is the only country in which S. Japonicum has been controlled and possibly eradicated in many prefects. There has been a continuous effort in the Philippines and China as well as Taiwan but the number of infected persons past and present may exceed 100,000,000.

> For S. haematobium, some regons as in East Africa, suggest a 50 percent incidence, others grade down to 10 percent as in North Africa, and for Egypt we have the estimate of Scott (1937)[9] of 6 million infected. The African areas free of infection are in general of low population. To the millions carrying S. haemotobium in Africa are to be added only an approximate 200,000 in the Near East and a few thousands in Europe, for a world total of 39 million bilharzia-infected individuals.[1]

S. hematobium has become an enormous problem across Africa, as well as the Middle East. The ten-fold increase in regions, with new dams and water irrigation projects, has created a specter of an unmanageable disease. The 6 million cases estimated in Egypt more than 40 years ago has grown to many millions — possibly 12 million or more. Much of northeast Africa is an epidemic region.

> S. mansoni is the most dispersed of the three schistosomes of man (if we include intercalatum with haematobium). Besides the equatorial zone in Africa there is a band of infection from northern Nigeria westward. These with Scott's 3 million cases in Egypt total 23 million for Africa. Whether establishment of our western hemisphere endemic areas is to be ascribed exclusively to the slave trade, seems to be a matter to question. But foci on this side of the Atlantic appear to account for about a third of a million cases in the West Indies, 30,000 in Venezuela according to Scott,[9] and nearly 6 million in the spreading infective zones in northeastern Brazil. All told this gives 29 million persons infected with S. mansoni, and 114 million for the 3 schistosome species combined.[1]

S. mansoni has increased in all areas of Africa, especially in northern Nigeria and countries to the west, where blood in the urine is considered normal for young men and boys; it being readily noticed. George Hillyer states that the foci in tropical America have been reduced in the West Indies, i.e. Puerto Rico, and eradicated in St. Kitts.

The foci in Venezuela may also have been reduced. Brazil has a large problem in the northeast which has been augmented by water development projects. The 29 million estimated by Stoll have increased proportionately to some 60 million or more.

The total Stoll gave for all three Schistosomes, 114 million people infected, is low by all current estimates. Weller estimated 200 million ten years ago, which no doubt can be close to 300 million today. The chronicity of these diseases increases the number of people affected annually. The only hope is to reduce the number of new cases reported, which is difficult in the regions with the high infection rates because of limited resources, poverty, and culture including little education.

In the absence of comprehensive surveys for parasites such as guinea worm and the filarids, a device of limiting values has been employed. The areas in India from which *Dracunculus medinesis* has been reported — which having small rainfall are in general the low hookworm zones in India — have about 110 million inhabitants. If as high as 25 percent is used for the guinea worm incidence, there are 27½ million infections indicated. A similar tactic applied to Afghan, Iran, Arabia, and southwestern U.S.S.R. in Asia, yields slightly over 5 million more cases as "the fiery serprent". Similarly the African endemic areas would contribute another 15 million infected, but the single focus on this continent, in northern Bahia, Brazil, involves only a few thousand. Figured by this method, which may be too generous, the world has 48 million guinea worm cases.[1]

Guinea worms — dracunculus infection — is coming under a world attack led by parasitologists such as O. O. Kale of Nigeria and public health administrators such as William Foege of the U.S. Centers for Disease Control. The numbers used in the 1940s are out of date. Current estimates of human infection range from 100 to 200 million cases in the endemic areas where epidemics occur with the change of seasons. The foci in southwestern U.S.S.R. and Asia probably has disappeared as well as the foci in Brazil.

Onchocerca in Central America is localized on the Pacific slopes of 3 states in Guatemala, and 2 (not 3) departments of Mexico. (Both Dampf (1942), and Bartter (1945) have taken occasion to insist that the department of Guerrero is free from the disease). These 5 political subdivisions have a combined population of 2 1/3 million. In Africa, the zone from Sierra Leone eastward through the infected regions contains 57 million inhabitants. If a third of all these are involved with the infection, the world total for Onchocerca would not exceed 20 million.[1]

The report by the authors Engelkirk, Williams, Schmidt, and Leid indicate *Onchocerca spp.* are widespread in Mexico, Central America, West Africa, and northeast Africa. The WHO and the World Bank have given these infections and disabling diseases a high priority, and much support has been forthcoming for control. But the disease incidence remains high in the endemic areas. Some authorities estimate that river blindness, the sequellae to chronic disease, may be the most serious problem in some endemic areas. To complicate the problem, there is much to be learned about the natural history of the carriers.

Mansonella ozzardi is confined to regions of Middle and South America with a population of 21 million. If a third are infected, there are 7 million with Mansonella.

Acanthocheilonema perstans occupies the Onchocerca regions in Africa, supplemented by foci in North America; and in South America overlaps, in part, the Mansonella areas. It is also found in Dutch New Guinea in the Pacific. These regions have a combined population of about 81 million and if a third are infected, there are 27 million Acanthocheilonema cases.

Loa Loa is strictly an African filarid of the west and west central regions where dwell 39 million people. If a third of these have loaiasis, there are 13 million.

These four filarid forms, conveyed respectively by Simuliu, by Culicoides, and by Chrysops, parasitize then 67 million people. Despite the simplified method of approximating this total, it may have considerable validity, the estimate for Onchocerca is possibly too high, and that for Acanthocheilonema too low.[1]

These filarid diseases are not zoonoses although some have been recognized in animals, i.e., subhuman primates. Of greater interest today are the zoonotic filaria found in animals and affecting man, i.e., *Dirofilaria ssp.* These infections are generally rare in man, although widespread in animals. The following Stoll paragraphs are concerned with Wuchereri infections of which *Malayan filariasis, Brugia malayi* is a true zoonoses.

The same general method can be used for orientation of Wuchereria, although it cannot be applied so simply. In the following analysis *W. bancrofti* and *W. malayi* have not been distinguished. One, the other, or both, are at home in human beings and appropriate mosquitoes pretty much throughout the tropical part of the world. Wuchereria is endemic in Oceania, with the notable exception of New Zealand, most of Australia, and some of the lesser Islands; it is in the Dutch East Indies, with Java's 40 millions surprisingly free, however; it is in the Philippines, Formosa, and southern Japan; in the coastal area of Asia — broadly interpreted — from northern Kiangsu province in China clear around the eastern, southeastern, and southern fringe of the continent, almost to Suez; it is in the broad equatorial belt across Africa, together with Madagascar off the southeast coast, and North Africa; it is in South America, especially in an area around Belem, Brazil (Causey et al. 1945), and a coastal belt from the Guianas to Columbia; and in the West Indies.

How many in this broad tropical territory shall we define as having filariasi? Only those who show microfilariae in the blood? If so, the marines garrisoned near Samoan villages and later invalided home with tell-tale symptoms could not be said to have had this infection, for the number showing microgilaremia, even up to now, is of the order of much less than one percent. But if these servicemen were properly diagnosed as having filariasis after endemic residence measured in months, is there reasonable probability that anyone fails to receive infection who grows up from babyhood in a filariated area? The simplest assumption then would be to say that all the population in endemic regions is filariated, and put the responsibility on any disputant to prove how many were not. That would mean 758 million people, about 1/3 of the population of the globe.[1]

Fortunately, most of these filarial disease can be controlled by insecticides and human therapy — the animal reservoir is only a small component.

Filarial infections have been greatly reduced and even eradicated in many islands and some continental districts. The number of infected and diseased individuals is no longer 1/3 of the world's population. With modern insect control and good medication, the disease should not be a major problem where governments assume their responsibility to protect the health and well-being of their people.

Stoll discussed Enterobius infections in the next paragraph — a disease of children that affects millions, even today. The animal pinworms do not infect man nor can human infection spread to animals.

Hookworms also received attention as it was a serious disease in the early decades of this century in most of the world. Anti-hookworm was one of the first community health programs funded by philantropic foundations (Rockefeller). Stoll's estimate was almost 500 million cases. There is no animal reservoir of human hookworms but the dog and cat hookworm larva cause cutaneous dermatitis in human beings — which is uncomfortable but not as serious as hookworm.

Ascaris were discussed later and estimated to cause 644 million human cases. That is a reasonable figure and probably a close guess for the 1980s. No animal reservoir is recognized for the human disease.

Trichuriasis, whipworms, were likewise common with a total of 355 million infected persons. These human whipworms are unknown in animals, nor do animal whipworms affect man.

Strongloides were estimated by Stoll to cause some 35 million infections, which may have increased with population growth. These helminths are found both in man and animals, and are thought to move freely between these hosts.

Of recent years another small-intestine-inhabiting nematode has obtruded itself more and more in surveys for human helminths, namely Trichostrongulus. Usually thought of as a parasite of ruminants, or perhaps better of herbivores, a half-dozen species have now been reported from man. The data suggest about 3 million infections in Japan and Korea, and an additional 1½ million in India, with a million more in the U.S.S.R., mostly in Transcaucasus and the Ural region. The foci in Africa appear to involve no more than a few thousand cases, but even so the world total is 5½ million.[1]

The distribution of trichostrongylus is widespread today in cattle and sheep. Human cases are not commonly reported but may be a problem. Most likely the foci in Japan has been reduced or eradicated, likewise in Korea. The same may be true in the U.S.S.R. African infections probably have risen with population growth.

All told we have noted just over 2200 million helminthic infections assigned to just under 2200 million people on the planet. If you have gained the impression that it must be scientifically labelled a "tentative" statement, you may also have gained the impression that it was by no means lightly arrived at. Both impressions are correct.

The Chinese have a saying, "If you do not scale the mountain, you cannot view the plain." Once population totals of the helminthically infected are available, certain generalizations immediately emerge.

First, a host view. Some people in the U.S.A. and Canada — Northern America in our classification — have a way of feeling that we are a relatively helminth-free people — it is the rest of the world that is really parasitized. Well, part of such a statement is partly true. Actually Northern America shares with Oceania and Europe, exclusive of the U.S.S.R., a status of about 1/3 as many helminthiases as people; for the U.S.S.R. in both Europe and Asia this rises to 2/3; for Asia and Middle and South America it is not far from 4/3; for Africa over 6/3.[1]

We would not be amiss in agreeing in general that the western world, (Europe, northern and southern America, Australia, and New Zealand) are relatively free of helminths. The 1/3 ratio, infections among the population is most likely lower, probability 1/5 or 1/6. For the U.S.S.R. the status is lower likewise, down from 2/3 to 1/3. For Asia, the incidence is about the same 4/3 with great improvement in Japan and more infections in southern Asia and the Middle East. In South and Middle America, the 4/3 ratio would vary from south to north, with improvements in the south, higher in the tropical areas and about the same in urban areas. Africa had the highest infection rate, 6/3, and continues with probably a higher ratio because so many more people are exposed.

Second, a worm view. The relative survival ability of different parasitic groups is thrown into sharp relief in terms of the number of parasitized human hosts. There are only 72 million cestode and 148 million trematode infections in our totals, but over 200 million nematode infections. This is doubtless a tribute to the variety and comparative biological efficiency of nematode life cycles. All cestodes reach man by the host's own act, albeit at times not consciously, through ingestion by man or egg or larval forms; trematodes similarly reach him passively, through ingestion of larval forms, but in addition actively though the parasite's own efforts, as witness schistosome cercariae. It is, however, the nematodes that exhibit the most varied methods. They reach man by his own act of ingesting ova that have been recently passed, and ova that have had to ripen externally for days or weeks; by his own act of ingesting larval forms in water, and larval forms in food. They also reach him not through his own act but on the initiative of the parasites themselves, infective larvae actively penetrating his bare skin in contact with moist soil, and actively penetrating his skin in contact with the mouthparts of blood sucking insects which reached him by air-borne tactics. Each of five helminthic species, illustrating four of these nemic life-history styles, registers more human infections than either all the cestodiases or all the trematodiases. Only two in the classification, namely Dracunculus and Trichinella, which come in by water and food, show so few parasitisms as do the food-transported flatworm species.[1]

The worm view has changed. The availability of cheap medication has reduced the incidence rates in developing countries, although this improvement will vary according to social economic development, and the availability of state medical services. Current information would show that Dracunculus is probably more widespread than ever in Africa and Asia, while Trichinella has declined worldwide. The tapeworms probably infected more people today than ever before.

Third, a sanative view (which might, less provocatively, be called a sanitary view). If we bar hydatid and garbage worms from consideration (recall they represent only one percent of the total), all these helminthiases depend solely, or mainly, on man as the definitive host, not on the maintenance of reservoir hosts. In their ultimate cycle of man back to man, and cutting across the taxonomic fences, these helminthiases fall into two great categories. One in seven of the total helminthic infections of man can be classified as due to his ineffective insulation from his own excretory products. The one-seventh reach him via cyclops, or they reach him via mosquitoes (*sensu latu*). The other six-sevenths reach him immediately or eventually, by the method of *H. nana* and Enterobius, or by the method of Ascaris and Trichuris, or by the method of *T. saginata* and Clonorchis, or by the method of Ancylostoma and Necator, or by the method of the schistosomes. In all of these 6 out of 7 cases what comes back to him or to his fellows is, in fashion appropriate to each specific organism, something biologically nursed along a return journey, that began the moment a relaxing sphincter permitted the passing of waste products fom an infected person. Somewhere along the line between the time when an egg was lost from that human host and the time the specifically appropriate infective agent was ripe to return to him, somewhere along that line a different brand of sanitation, broadly interpreted, would have broken the biological chain and spared new human hosts.[1]

The sanitary view has advanced in the western world, China, and the U.S.S.R. and the European socialist countries. But for the other 3 billion persons, sanitation development is only beginning, or has been set back by population pressure and lack of capital. To break the biological chain calls for unlimited resources for the development of water distribution and removal of human waste; much more than the military budgets of the countries that need sanitary capital improvements.

My analysis has concerned itself with helminthic infections over-all, ot alone those with the most serious worm burdens, for it is the whole pattern of infection of helminths in the world of man we are aiming to grasp. Tactically it may require that we concentrate attack for amelioration and control on persons and communities most severely affected. Strategically, at the world level, we need to know of the enemy wherever he rears his head, in order that over-all planning omit no favorable opportunity for neutralizing him. Helminthiases do not have the journalistic value of great pandemics like flu or plague, although they may have an as yet unrecognized relation to them; they do not, for the most part, present dramatic clinical cases, but to make up for their lack of drama, they are unremittingly corrosive. If you were aroused by the sufferings of say, ten thousand service men with filariasis and schistosomiasis, what can your imagination do with ten thousand upon ten thousand natives in endemic areas — who have no homeside relatives to write letters to their congressmen?[1]

The analysis is correct today as when written almost 40 years ago. One seldom ever sees or hears reports about parasitic epidemics, in the daily media fare, or even in the usual public health literature. It is difficult to get a legislative body to support worm control unless there is an economic motive, such as tourism or the export of agriculture products (meat).

> The world population, according to informed prediction, may reach 3300 million by the end of the century, an increase of 50 percent (Notestein, 1945).[10] The parasitoses, by extrapolation may grow even more, for some of the areas marked for most population growth are among those with higher helminthic indices.[1]

The world population passed 3300 million in the 1960s, passed 4000 million in 1976 and in the 1980s will pass 5000 million. The end of the century offers no relief — the 6000 million will be passed before then. Parasitoses by extrapolation will surely keep pace and even out perform in some regions of the highest population growth. The control of population is important to all biologists, and should receive our support everywhere and at all times.

> Are there ways paraitologists can help reduce the prospect of having the world forge ahead to more than 3000 million human helminthiases by the year 2000?[1]

The point of no return was passed in the last decade, and will fade further with little hope of improvement with the lack of human concern. If we could encourage the shift of capital outlay from destruction to construction there would be hope.

> It seems to me there are possibilities.
> I. Certainly we can widely uphold, and strengthen the teaching of, the nuclear principles that apply in our field. They obviously should be known by intelligent world citizens, and we should make it popular that they are. Certainly we should assist the firm establishment of competently taught parasitology in medical schools, which the war has fostered.[1]

The teaching of parasitology has advanced worldwide, in the biological sciences, in agriculture, in medicine and veterinary medical education, but is inadequate in human medicine according to W.H.O. expert consultants.

> There are some red entries in our own ledger of the war because such knowledge was not more freely dispensed earlier. For instance, soon after Pearl Harbor, training centers for marines were established in the South Pacific, including Samoa, where American forces had been for decades. Somewhere in the higher echelons there must have been a medical officer in a position of advice, or decision, as to how close to native huts and villages it was prudent to barrack the men. Evidently that medical officer never heard of bancroftian filariasis being present where men in uniform saw it with dismay, or else he did not know that filariasis is transmitted by mosquitoes. In the name of Manson, it is for us all to blush at that hiatus.
> II. We can encourage by precept and example a shortening of the usual lag period there is in getting acceptable improvements in ideas through to where they will do the most good, and be less tolerant when the lag seems unnecessarily long. I have two illustrations.
> The Health Section of the League of Nations recently published a valuable "Handbook of Infectious Diseases" (1945 III 1, Ch 1454), up-to-date enough to include "new chapters on the sulphonamides, penicillin, etc.," but with serious omissions concerning anti-helminth drugs. For instance, the recommended treatment for ascaris is merely santonin and chenopodium, and for hookworm thymol, chenopodium or carbon tetrachloride. This handbook had the admirable aim of noting "every recent addition to scientific knowledge concerning methods of combating these diseases." Why under a League imprint, should it miss being up-to-date about such antihelmintics as tetrachlorethylene and hexylresorcinol which have been valuable and accepted for more than a decade and a half?[1]

The World Health Organization, the Food and Agriculture Organization, Pan American Sanitary Bureau, and other international agencies, and international assistance programs have fulfilled these needs to a considerable degree. Implementation with drugs and chemicals are the next step.

III. Besides the possibilities mentioned, of encouraging wider dissemination of the central ideas in our field, and their application, there is another side of the problem which is a challenge specifically to us. The question is legitimately raised whether the tools furnished for attacking the helminthiases of man are not in need of sharpening. Against the intestinal helminths we think of them as education, sanitation, and treatment. Stiles (1932) wisely observed in an article on hookworm disease, that among important factors in public health advancement of the South were "the automobile filling stations with the practical demonstration in public health connected with their comfort rooms." Perhaps he was saying obliquely what is all too true. Logically necessary as is the pit latrine to combat soil pollution, the esthetic affront it gives to those who are supposed to use it, vitiates its virtues and drives adults as well as children back to the out-of-doors where the air is free. That is true even in this latitude, and the closer to the tropics the truer it is. No wonder latrine construction and use is hard to establish there. Vaeger's bored hole substitute is praiseworthy, but makes slow advances. What we need to do is find a "convenience of civilization", and excusado, as attractive in its way as is the filling station comfort room.[1]

The latrine has moved across the world but soil contamination is still with us. Again capital outlays are essentials — more than is spent on hospitals or sick houses.

In another direction, methods of soil sterilization, in which progress is being made against plant parasitic nematodes, could be profitably exploited to determine whether they might not protect man against the consequences of his using unconfined defecation sites. Have we too easily shrugged off improvements here, continuing to make and recommend Model T ideas, when the demand is for less bumpy riding?[1]

Soil alteration and sterilization is still being investigated to determine cost benefit ratios, environmental impact, and ecological alteration. Certainly it is well known that too many bodies, human or animal, will mess up an area but how does one keep the young people down on the farm. Sport shoes or running shoes have probably put shoes on more people than ever before. Peer review — good muster.

New chemo-therapeutic preparations are desirable, to encourage more widely the breaking of parasitic life cycles within man himself. Against hookworm our best present bet is tetrachlorethylene, against ascaris in children hexylresorcinol, against pinworm gentian violet. But all these leave something to be desired, and against trichuris and other forms we are in worse case. What we need are worm treatments as effective and well-tolerated as phenothiazine in sheep, and from the greatness of the need we ought to have a hundred workers seeking them, instead of a handful in desultory effort. For our familiar intestinal fauna, as well as parenteral forms, one of the goals could well be something of less drastic action in individual dose, but potent cumulatively, and thus applicable to population groups, as are vitamins in bread, iodine in salt, and fluorides in water.[1]

The developments in parasitic disease therapy and prevention are just as great as the antibiotics in bacterial disease therapy. The problem is getting medication to the field at a reasonable cost. The advances are discussed by the many authors in their chapters. It is a good record. Twenty years ago, 1966, the late Karl F. Meyer to whom these books are dedicated, sat with me at a meeting with representatives of the leading pharmaceutical houses of Switzerland and discussed where they should place their research efforts. We agreed the major problem was parasitic disease medication and prevention. Similar meetings followed in other countries and continue to emphasize the need to control parasitic diseases in man and animals.

And here, deliberately on a note of unfinished business, I prefer to interrupt consideration of the problem of human helminthiases at the world level. We need to leave it in a mood of work still to be done.

In March, with the Society becoming of age, my distinguished predecessor told you of the making of a parasitologist. If by chance he had ended wih the line "Bring me men to match my mountains", it would have been allowed me to say: "Here are some of the mountains."[1]

The unfinished business is a challenge to all biologists and those concerned with human well being and humaneness to all creatures great and small. May we have the opportunity to disperse the knowledge of mankind and put it to use for all — man and animals. May we climb the mountain and look out and say, well done in our time.

REFERENCES

1. **Stoll, R.**, This wormy world, *J. Parasitol.,* 33, 1, 1947.
2. **Augustine, D.** (1942) Cited by Stoll,[1] 1947.
3. **Hall, M. and Collins,** Studies on trichinosis, I. The incidence of trichinosis as indicated by postmortem examination of 200 diaphragms, *Public Health Reports,* 52, 468, 1937. Cited by Stoll,[1] 1947.
4. **Wright, W. H., Kerr, K. B., and Jacobs, L.,** Studies on trichinosis XV. Summary of the findings of Trichinella Spiralis in a random sampling and other samplings of the population of the United States, *Public Health Reports,* 58, 1293, 1943. Cited by Stoll,[1] 1947.
4a. **Wright, W. H., Jacobs, L., and Walton, A. C.,** Studies on Trichinosis XVI. Epidemiological considerations based on the examination for trichinae of 5313 diaphragms from 189 hospitals in 37 states and the District of Columbia, *Public Health Reports,* 59, 669, 1944. Cited by Stoll,[1] 1947.
5. **Zimmerman, W. J., Steele, J. H., and Kagan, I. G.,** The changing status of trichinosis in the United States population, *Public Health Reports,* 83, 957, 1968.
6. **Zimmerman, W. J. and Zinter, D. C.,** The prevalence of trichinosis in swine in the United States, 1966-1970, *Public Health Reports,* 86, 937, 1971.
7. Parasitic Zoonoses, Report of a WHO Expert Committee with the participation of FAO, Technical Report Series 637, World Health Organization, Geneva, 1979.
8. **Polydorou, K.,** Control of Echinococcosis in Cyprus XI. International Congress of Hydatidosis, Athens, 1977.
8a. **Polydorou, K.,** Antiechinococcosis campaign, 52-66 Annual Report of the Dept. of Veterinary Services, Nicosia, Cyprus, 1978.
9. **Scott, J. A.,** The incidence and distribution of the human Schistosomiasis in Egypt, *Am. J. Hygiene,* 25, 566, 1937. Cited by Stoll,[1] 1947.
9a. **Scott, J. A.,** The epidemiology of Schistosomiasis in Venezuela, *Am. J. Hygiene,* 35, 337, 1942. Cited by Stoll,[1] 1947.
10. **Notestein, F.,** Office of Population Research, Princeton University, 1947. Cited by Stoll (1) 1947.

FOREWORD

With the publication of Section C of the CRC handbook series on the parasitic zoonoses another important milestone has been achieved in the field of Veterinary Public Health. These volumes focus on a wide range of parasitic infections affecting man and the lower animals. Notable examples are: protozoal diseases like simian malaria and toxoplasmosis, which have received considerable attention, but, nevertheless, many problems concerning transmission have yet to be resolved; taeniasis and cysticercosis are still widespread and there is evidence of their increasing prevalence; echinococcosis or hydatidosis remain public health problems in sheep-raising areas in South America, the Mediterranean region, parts of Africa and in the Western Pacific region, particularly in New Zealand and Australia; zoonotic schistosomiasis and filariasis continue to pose potential risks to infection in resettlement areas.

I congratulate Dr. James H. Steele and his colleagues who have dedicated many years in the preparation of the handbooks. Their collaborative efforts in bringing together all available information which was otherwise scattered in the literature are highly commendable. Equally praiseworthy is the orderly and systematic presentation of each subject and the inclusion of an extensive bibliography for further reference and source material.

These volumes will provide not only guidelines in the prevention, control and surveillance of parasitic zoonoses, but also basic information for further research that must be undertaken. I am therefore recommending them to public health workers and the specialists, and to many others who share the view that man's well-being and health are directly related to that of animals. In today's world where intensive campaigns and various measures to promote family planning have done little to arrest the steady growth of the human population, we are even more dependent on livestock management and production in order to cope with the ever-growing demand for a greater supply of animal protein foods to feed the world's hungry millions.

Francisco J. Dy

PREFACE

The parasitic zoonoses are represented by a motley array of forms commonly found in three large divisions of the Animal Kingdom, i.e., the Protozoa, the Helminths and the Arthropods. Within these groups are numerous parasites which occur both in lower animals and in man. Some parasites of the former are frequently transmitted to the human host — so frequently that they constitute important public health problems in various parts of the world. On the other hand, there are many more parasitic forms occurring in lower animals which are only occasionally, and others only rarely, found in man so that the occurrence in that host constitutes somewhat of a zoological curiosity. Then again, many of the parasites found in lower animals have never been reported from the human host.

It would seem that the transmission of parasites from lower animals to man and vice versa must occur more frequently than recognized, especially in regions in which medical, public health and veterinary services are inadequate. Distribution of the parasitic zoonoses is variable. Some are almost universally encountered; others are restricted in occurrence by climatic factors or by the presence or absence of suitable vectors or intermediate hosts. Distribution of many parasitic zoonoses is unknown. A pertinent illustration is provided by *Toxoplasma gondii*. Its occurrence was little recognized until the development of the Sabin-Feldman dye test. The widespread application of this test revealed an almost world-wide distribution of the parasite and contributed to the elucidation of its life cycle.

Parasite life cycles are extremely variable and constitute an important factor in the epizootiology and epidemiology of many species. Some parasites go through amazing transformations and utilize one or more intermediate hosts in order to reach another definitive host. Others require vectors in order to pass from one host to another. Certain protozoa and helminths, however, are transmitted directly through the medium of eggs, cysts, or larval forms.

Unlike some zoonotic bacterial, viral or rickettsial infections, zoonotic parasitic acquisitions are less responsible for epidemics or epizootics. Their role is more chronic in nature, although acute overwhelming infections may occur. Their pathogenesis is usually exerted over a long period of time and they damage the host in multiple ways. The extent of damage is usually related to the degree of infection. Because of their chronicity, parasitic infections in food-producing animals are frequently the cause of considerable economic loss.

Most parasitic invasions seldom provoke a solid immunity as do some bacterial, viral and rickettsial infections. However, some chronic unremitting intracellular protozoal infections do result in resistance to subsequent re-infection, a process known as premunition. Because of the external structure of most parasites, intimate contact of these parasites with the cellular components of the immune system is lacking. This may contribute to the lack of a solid immunity in many parasitic infections. In extracellular parasitism some resistance to re-infection may follow, especially when there is a heavy parasitic invasion. The low levels of immune response may be one of the answers to the relative chronicity of parasitic infections.

One of the curious things about zoonotic parasitisms is the extreme variation in the susceptibility of lower animals and man to certain species of parasites. For instance, the trematodes *Clonorchis sinensis* and *Fasciolopsis buski* are common in both groups of hosts in the Far East. Another example is *Trypanosoma cruzi*. On the other hand, man is markedly resistant to some parasites of lower animals. At the same time, some human parasites have never adapted themselves to existence in lower animals. *Schistosoma haematobium* and *Wuchereria bancrofti* are examples. These facts would seem to imply the existence of an inherent natural resistance. Such resistance is apparently not related to any immune process. Other factors may be involved. The physiology of the aberrant host may be inadequate to supply the needs of the parasite.

As a possible example of natural resistance, the tapeworm *Dipylidium caninum* occurs frequently in dogs and cats. Its intermediate hosts, the dog and cat fleas, are also common. Yet the close contact between household pets and children rarely leads to human infections in spite of the fact that children are notoriously prone to place foreign objects in the mouth.

In the Southern United States, *Dirofilaria immitis* occurs frequently in dogs and certain wild carnivores. Mosquito vectors are common and must frequently bite man. Yet the parasite is extremely rare in the human host, although cutaneous response to the migrating larvae may occur. Even more common is the invasion of the human skin by the larvae of *Ancylostoma braziliense*, the dog and cat hookworm. The condition is frequently encountered in the Gulf Coast States.

The extreme variability in life cycles of many parasites has already been noted. Some examples which will be elaborated upon in various chapters of these volumes are cited below.

Ascaris lumbricoides, which infects the human host by ingestion of the eggs, does not immediately settle down in the environmental locale in the upper small intestine. Rather the larvae hatched from the eggs undergo a series of molts while they invade the blood stream, the liver and the lungs and eventually arrive at the site of their adulthood in the intestine after their long passage.

The life cycle of various hookworms involves infection through the skin of the host and not through swallowing the larvae. After skin penetration the larvae follow the same migrating path as *Ascaris*. The ascarids and hookworms of lower animals have the same life cycle. When they enter into the wrong host, they cannot complete their life cycle and thus become aberrant wanderers. This accounts for cutaneous larva migrans due to the dog hookworm and for visceral larva migrans and ocular larva migrans due to dog (and possibly) cat ascarids.

Clearly, these phenomena are not manifestations of the immune processes of the hosts but probably reflect very subtle differences in the ability, biochemically and physiologically, of parasites to accommodate themselves to strange host environments. An even more bizarre case exists when the larvae of the rat lungworm, *Angiostrongylus cantonensis*, find their way into the human being either directly by the ingestion of snails or slugs which are their intermediate hosts, or indirectly on water plants on which the mollusks have deposited infective larvae. Ordinarily, *A. cantonensis* larvae have a brief sojourn in the rat brain before maturing in the blood vessels serving the lungs. Occasionally in the human being they do not succeed in evolving into adults in the lung blood vessels but persist in the brain, producing eosinophilic meningitis and infrequently severe encephalitis and death.

One can only anticipate that modern advances in the sciences of parasitology, pathology and immunology will be the means of elucidating reasons for the marked variations in zoonotic parasitic infections. There are glimmers of hope in these directions. However, the great public health and animal health importance of certain of these zoonoses indicates the need for much additional research into the abstruse problems involved.

Willard H. Wright
Died July 25, 1982
Washington, D. C.

PROLOGUE

During recent decades, advances in human knowledge have led to unprecedented accomplishments in the prevention, control, and successful treatment of infectious diseases, including many of the parasitic zoonoses. Medical achievements of comparable significance can be anticipated during the remaining years of the present century, although concurrently, factors of a seemingly uncontrollable nature can be expected to have increasingly adverse effects, to the extent that the potential benefits of recent and future accomplishments may not be fully realized. Ultimately, these factors are attributable to the magnitude of human populations and the ecological consequences of continued growth. To these elements are linked the importance of the parasitic zoonoses; these diseases are associated in occurrence and effect with both the numbers of people and the numbers of their domesticated animals.

The zoonoses only comparatively recently have come to represent serious medical problems. Before the development of agriculture, man subsisted as a hunter-gatherer, commonly living in small, nomadic or seminomadic groups, in size probably not exceeding a maximum of about 200, above which the ties of kinship were lost and emigration became necessary. Such a pattern of emigration and formation of new groups resembled that exhibited by populations of mammals of various other species. Under such conditions, the state of health of people was probably comparable to that of other natural mammalian populations well adapted to the biotope occupied. Very likely, the common diseases were natural-focal zoonoses, many of which are chronic in course and cause low mortality.

Aboriginal populations often were aware of the existence of natural foci of disease. Such people were excellent observers, able to recognize causal relationships, and their lack of understanding was manifested in taboos and superstition. Dietary taboos sometimes evolved in response to parasitic zoonoses, as with the Eskimos inhabiting the shores of the polar seas, who by tradition boiled the flesh of polar bears thoroughly, thereby avoiding infection by *Trichinella*. Natural foci of zoonoses also could be recognized and avoided, as were the highly endemic areas of Rocky Mountain spotted fever in western North America, or those of plague in Mongolia. Invading or immigrant populations unaware of the risks often suffered the consequences.

The importance of parasitic zoonoses as a cause of morbidity in human populations is partly a consequence of the domestication of animals, which began in Mesolithic time. Thereafter, animals of the same species were domesticated at different times under different cultural conditions, but the process itself began between 10,000 to 15,000 years ago. Dogs (derived from wolves), sheep, and goats appeared as early close associates of man. With their domestication, a synanthropic host-assemblage was completed, by which various parasitic zoonoses could be maintained. We can postulate that through the process of domestication, selective pressures associated with animal husbandry have led to adaptive changes in certain parasitic organisms, resulting in the formation of distinct biologic strains, or even species (e.g., *Taenia saginata*), which are restricted to the human host and synanthropic animals.

Patterns of distribution of parasitic zoonoses before early historical time are unknown, but presumably their spread continentally, and intercontinentally as well, was mediated by immigrations, commerce, and military expeditions, all of which involved considerable numbers of people and their domestic animals. Large-scale movements, such as the migrations of peoples into Europe beginning about 450 A.D. and the later Mongol invasions from Middle Asia, must have been potent forces in the dissemination of pathogens. Few specific details are known, but as one example, probably *Echinococcus granulosus*, and certainly other helminths, became established on Iceland prior to about the year 930, after which communication with Europe (mainly Norway) apparently ceased.

A process of change on a world-wide scale was initiated by Europeans at the end of the 15th century, with the beginning of the modern period of global colonization, when immigrants occupied and eventually populated lands formerly inhabited by small groups of people many of whom were nomadic. The cosmopolitan distribution of numerous zoonoses was brought about by the introduction of domestic animals from Europe to nearly all parts of the world. Specific details are available concerning some introductions into South America. Dogs were carried to the mouth of the Rio de la Plata in 1535 by De Mendoza, who founded colonies in that region. Herds of cattle and sheep were established there between the years 1536 and 1601. People from Spain also took dogs into western South America (Peru) in 1532, and they settled even earlier in the Panamanian region. In 1770, Cook noted the presence of various domestic animals on islands in the Indonesian region, apparently left there by earlier Dutch or Portuguese expeditions. Similarly, animals were taken to Australia in 1788, when a British penal colony was established at Port Jackson. It can be assumed that the presence of various pathogens dates from some of the earliest introductions of domestic animals from Europe, although diseases caused by them usually were not recognized until much later. An example is again *Echinococcus granulosus*, but now in South America, where prior to 1849, there appears to be no record of occurrence of hydatid disease. The presence of the same helminth in Australia became known only after the middle of the 19th century, by which time there, sheep-raising had become widespread.

The dispersal of pathogenic organisms with domestic animals is a continuing process, and not relevant only to the distant past. Very recently (1969), swine from Bali were given to the Ekari people in West New Guinea by Indonesian soldiers as part of an effort to induce them to accept Indonesian control. Unfortunately, the swine were infected by cysticerci of *Taenia solium*, and the human population became infected also, by both strobilar and larval stages of this helminth. The first indications of the magnitude of the resulting problem were noted in 1971, when many of the people suffered severe burns after falling into cooking-fires following epileptiform seizures caused by cerebral cysticercosis. Considering social factors, including the ritual significance of eating pigs, there appears to be little hope that this helminth soon can be controlled.

Concurrently with the dispersal of domestic animals and the pathogens associated with them, helminths and other host-specific organisms were directly introduced by man. The disastrous effects of communicable diseases on indigenous human populations following first contacts with Europeans are well known, but the origins of other, less spectacular infections were not so obvious. Introduced organisms having other than direct cycles were able to become established in different regions of the world where indigenous faunas included suitable hosts. In the Americas, etiologic agents of parasitic zoonoses were introduced from West Africa through the slave trade, but this did not become apparent for some time. Manson recognized in 1902 that *Schistosoma mansoni* is one of these. *Oncocerca volvulus* is another. The viral disease, yellow fever, seems certainly to have been of African origin and introduced with its vector, *Aedes aegypti*, on ships carrying slaves. It is now enzootic in tropical regions of South America, where it is transmitted among monkeys by indigenous mosquitoes that inhabit the forest canopy. Control of the introduced vector did not eliminate the disease, as had been initially hoped. Another example of an introduced helminth is *Diphyllobothrium latum*, which is now endemic in the lower Kuskokwim River region in western Alaska. In this case, its presence can be attributed to immigrants from western Russia during the early 19th century. Nematodes inhabiting the intestinal lumen of man probably owe their present nearly cosmopolitan distributions to repeated dispersals from southern Europe and Africa. It can be postulated that none, with the exception of *Enterobius vermicularis*, which occurs widely in indigenous populations of northern latitudes, could have accompanied Mongoloid immigrants into North America, and ultimately to South America, by way of Beringia millenia before colonizations by Europeans.

Very recently, social upheavals, particularly in southeastern Asia, have caused extensive emigrations of peoples from regions where numerous parasitic zoonoses are prevalent. We cannot yet assess the significance of these movements in introducing causative agents of such infections. Nor can we assess as yet the full significance of the intensive industralization and utilization of natural resources of the past century. As unprecedented as are the achievements in disease control, have been the recent worldwide disruptions of ecosystems following rapidly expanding agriculture and major alterations of lands and watercourses. Some effects of engineering projects have been severe. The changed prevalence of schistosomiasis in the region of the lower Nile River is a good example of predictable ecologic effects of a major modification of natural conditions. Prior to the extensive construction of canals, the habitat suitable for the intermediate host of *Schistosoma haematobium* was comparatively small in area, and rates of schistosomiasis in man were relatively low. Further changes favoring the completion of the cycle of this trematode resulted through the construction of Aswan Dam. The area has attracted and had the benefit of some of the world's best advisors in the field of health, if not in engineering, but little has been achieved in counteracting the ecological consequences of these developments. Comparable projects elsewhere, in progress or planned, may be expected to have comparable impacts, but these may not soon be detected where funds to support medical research are scarce.

As the present problems with schistosomiasis in the valley of the Nile River were predictable, so some of the consequences of our intensifying use of regions less populated, or uninhabited, can be foreseen. As people move into such regions, and encroach on naturally occurring parasite-host assemblages, the importance of parasitic zoonoses locally increases. Eventually, with disruption of ecosystems, components of such assemblages are eliminated, and transmission of natural-focal diseases occurs at a reduced level or not at all, but the indigenous zoonoses are replaced by those involving synanthropic animals. This pattern is typical of developing countries. At present, mainly in such countries, transmission of various parasitic zoonoses is enhanced in dense, urban populations existing under marginal conditions. Commensal rodents as well as dogs and cats are important sources of disease in such situations. The potential magnitude of the problem is suggested by credible predictions that some cities will have perhaps 30 million human inhabitants within the next 20 years.

For those involved in the prevention and control of parasitic zoonoses, these years will be a period of unprecedented change and unprecedented challenge. Continuing growth of human populations in combination with the destruction or severe alteration of ecosystems that we share with other living organisms will have effects that we probably cannot now comprehend. Nonetheless, these years can be perceived as a time of opportunity for those concerned with the prevention and control of parasitic zoonoses. Greater emphasis on biological control of pathogenic organisms, compatible with environmental considerations, could lead to major accomplishments. Reassessment of the possible utilization of other large ungulates, in place of the domesticated species, in regions where the latter do not thrive because of indigenous diseases, might lead to more efficient production of protein. Obviously, a greater understanding and awareness of the interactions of organisms should be a goal of those concerned with zoonotic disease. To this end, some modification of undergraduate and graduate curricula might be considered, particularly to provide a better background for contending with problems involving the complex ecosystems of tropical and subtropical regions. These are only a few of the approaches that might be contemplated. Much will depend on our ability to reassess and innovate, if we are to realize the potential benefits of recent and future accomplishments in the prevention and control of parasitic zoonoses.

Robert L. Rausch

THE EDITOR — PROTOZOAN ZOONOSES

Leon Jacobs, Ph.D., is now Scientist Emeritus at the National Institutes of Health, and Scientific Director of the National Society for Medical Research, Washington, D.C. Previously, he worked for 42 years at the National Institutes of Health, Bethesda, Md., as a bench scientist and then scientific administrator. His last positions were Associate Director for Collaborative Research, NIH, and Director of the Fogarty International Center, NIH. He had an interim assignment for 2 years, 1967 to 1969, as Deputy Assistant Secretary for Science, Department of Health, Education, and Welfare, Washington, D.C. He retired from Federal service in 1979.

Dr. Jacobs graduated from Brooklyn College in 1935 and obtained his Ph.D. in 1947 from George Washington University. He served in the Army of the United States from 1943 to 1946, mostly as Malaria Control Officer, South Atlantic Theater of Operations.

Dr. Jacobs is a member and past president of the American Society of Parasitologists, a member and past vice president of the American Society of Tropical Medicine and Hygiene, and a member and past president of the Helminthological Society of Washington. Other society memberships include the American Association of Immunologists, and the American Association for the Advancement of Science. He edited the *Journal of Parasitology* from 1956 through 1958.

Among other awards, Dr. Jacobs is the recipient of the Henry Baldwin Ward Medal of the American Society of Parasitologists, the Distinguished Service Medal of the U.S. Public Health Service, and the Arthur S. Flemming Award of the Junior Chamber of Commerce. He has been honored as a distinguished alumnus by both Brooklyn College and George Washington University. He has been a Fulbright scholar and a Guggenheim fellow.

Dr. Jacobs has authored over 100 papers and has lectured and taught laboratory classes at Johns Hopkins University School of Hygiene and Public Health, Case Western Reserve University School of Medicine, University of Arizona School of Medicine, University of South Florida School of Medicine, George Washington University, and Georgetown University. As Scientist Emeritus at NIH, he still has an ongoing research project on toxoplasmosis at the Laboratory of Parasitic Diseases, National Institute of Allergy and Infectious Diseases, and an active interest in amebiasis and other parasitic diseases.

THE EDITOR — CESTODE ZOONOSES

Dr. Primo V. Arambulo III is Regional Advisor in Veterinary Medicine, Pan American Health Organization, the Regional Office of World Health Organization for the Americas, Washington, D.C.

Dr. Arambulo was born in Manila, Philippines, on October 26, 1941. He obtained the degrees of Doctor of Veterinary Medicine (DVM, 1963) and Certificate in Public Health (CPH, 1964) from the University of the Philippines College of Veterinary Medicine at Diliman and Institute of Public Health at Manila, respectively; Diploma in Applied Parasitology and Entomology (DAP&E, 1971) from the Institute of Medical Research at Kuala Lumpur, Malaysia; and Master of Public Health (MPH, 1975) and Doctor of Public Health (DrPH, 1977) from the University of Texas Health Science Center, School of Public Health at Houston.

He has extensive postgraduate training at various institutions, including the Meat Hygiene Institute at Roskilde, Denmark (1968); Ateneo University Graduate School of Business Administration at Manila (1969 and 1970); Vanderbilt University School of Medicine at Nashville, Tennessee (1975); Harvard University School of Public

Health at Boston, Massachusetts (1976); U.S. Department of Agriculture at Hyattsville, Maryland (1975 and 1976); and the U.S. Centers for Disease Control at Atlanta, Georgia (1976 and 1977).

Dr. Arambulo has held various scientific, academic and administrative positions as Microbiologist, 5th Epidemiological Flight at USAF Clark Air Base Medical Center in the Philippines (1964 to 1966); Chief, Division of Research and Laboratory, Veterinary Inspection Board of the City of Manila (1966 to 1972); Assistant Professor of Medical Parasitology, Institute of Public Health, University of the Philippines (1972 to 1977); Assistant Professor of Veterinary Preventive Medicine and Public Health, Iowa State University College of Veterinary Medicine at Ames (1977 to 1978); and Chief Technical Advisor for Animal Health, Pan American Health Organization, World Health Organization at Kingston, Jamaica (1978 to 1980).

He has served as advisor and consultant in animal health and veterinary public health to the United Nations Development Program in Jamaica; external lecturer in parasitology and microbiology at the University of the West Indies Medical School in Jamaica; member of the Expert Advisory Panel in Food Hygiene and Zoonoses of the World Health Organization in Geneva; member of the scientific committees of the National Research Council and National Science Development Board of the Philippines.

Dr. Arambulo is the recipient of various honors and awards, among them are the Don Andres Soriano Research Award in Zoonoses of the Philippine Society of Animal Science; the Philippine Men of Science; the Abbott Research Award in Rural Medicine and Public Health of the Philippine Medical Association; the Jessie and William E. Strain Lecture in Veterinary Public Health, University of Phillipines; and election in the honor societies of Phi Zeta, Phi Kappa Phi, and Phi Sigma.

He has traveled and lectured extensively in Asia, Europe, the Caribbean, and the Americas in connection with his research on the epidemiology and control of the zoonoses and the organization of national veterinary public health services.

His extensive bibliographical listing includes over 150 publications. He is a member of several professional and scientific organizations all over the world.

CONTRIBUTORS

J. R. Baker, MA, Ph.D., D.Sc., F.I.
  Biol.
Head of Station
Culture Centre of Algae and Protozoa
Cambridge, England

Goran Bylund, FD.
Docent in Parasitology
University of Abo Akademi
Abo, Finland

William E. Collins, Ph.D.
Research Biologist
Parasitic Diseases Division
Center for Infectious Diseases
Centers for Disease Control
Atlanta, Georgia

James J. Daly, Ph.D.
Associate Professor of Microbiology
  and Immunology
University of Arkansas College of
  Medicine
Consulting Scientist
University Hospital
Little Rock, Arkansas

Francisco J. Dy
Regional Director Emeritus
WHO Western Pacific Region
Member, National Research Council of
  the Philippines
Manila, Philippines

R. Fayer, Ph.D.
Laboratory Chief
Animal Parasitology Institute
U.S. Department of Agriculture
Beltsville, Maryland

J. K. Frenkel, M.D.
Professor of Pathology
Universiity of Kansas School of
  Medicine
Kansas City, Kansas

George R. Healy, Ph.D.
Chief, Parasitology Division
Centers for Disease Control
Atlanta, Georgia

Edward L. Jarroll, Ph.D.
Senior Research Associate
Department of Preventive Medicine
New York State College of Veterinary
  Medicine
Cornell University
Ithaca, New York

Professor Nonette L. Jueco
Department of Parasitology
Institute of Public Health
University of the Philippines
Ermita, Manila, Philippines

Dennis D. Juranek, DVM
Deputy Cheif
Protozoal Diseases Branch
Parasitic Diseases Division
Center for Infectious Diseases

Ralph Lainson, FRS
Director, The Wellcome Parasitology
  Unit
Section of Parasitology
Instituto Evandro Chagas, Fundacao
  SESP
Belem, Para, Brazil
Associate Worker of the London
  School of Hygiene and Tropical
  Medicine

William B. Lushbaugh, Ph.D.
Assistant Professor of Medicine
Medical University of South Carolina,
  and Veterans Administration Medical
  Center
Charleston, South Carolina

Ernest A. Meyer, Sc.D.
Professor of Microbiology and
  Immunology
Oregon Health Sciences University
Portland, Oregon

Zbigniew S. Pawłowski
Clinic of Parasitic and Tropical
  Diseases
Medical Academy of Poznan
Poland

Fred E. Pittman, M.D., Ph.D.
Professor of Medicine
Medical University of South Carolina,
  and Veterans Administration Medical
  Center
Charleston, South Carolina

Robert L. Rausch
Professor of Animal Medicine, and
  Professor of Pathobiology
University of Washington
Seattle, Washington

Miodrag Ristic, DVM, MS, Ph.D.
Professor, Department of Veterinary
  Pathobiology
College of Veterinary Medicine
University of Illinois
Urbana, Illinois

Peter M. Schantz, VMD, Ph.D.
Deputy Chief
Helminthic Diseases Branch
Parasitic Diseases Division
Center for Infectious Diseases
Atlanta, Georgia

Peter D. Walzer, M.D.
Co-Chief
Division of Infectious Diseases
Veterans Administration Medical
  Center
Associate Professor of Medicine
University of Cincinnati College of
  Medicine
Cincinnati, Ohio

Robert G. Yaeger, Ph.D.
Professor of Tropical Medicine, and
  Professor of Medicine
Tulane Medical Center
New Orleans, Louisiana

Willard H. Wright, DVM, MS, Ph.D.
Veterinary Director
U.S. Public Health Service (Retired)
Washington, D.C.

ACKNOWLEDGMENTS

The *Handbook Series in Zoonoses* is indebted to many persons and institutions, as well as the U.S. Public Health Service which provided an intellectual environment for scientific exploration at the Communicable Disease Centers and the National Institutes of Health in the United States and abroad. The many persons who have influenced the editor in developing the *Handbook Series in Zoonoses* have been acknowledged in *The Bacterial, Rickettsial, and Mycotic Diseases Section A, Volumes I and II,* 1979 and 1980. *The Virus Zoonoses, Section B, Volumes I and II,* 1981, edited by George Beran, has enlarged upon those previously rendered acknowledgment.

Parasitic Zoonoses deals with a most important group of diseases world-wide, and required counsel and advice from scientists, educators, and government officials around the world. We remember those who had a positive influence in pointing to the parasitic diseases that affect the well-being of man and animals. At Michigan State College, the late Philip Hawkins, whose bright career was cut down by a paralytic disease in northern India in 1951, was a remarkable teacher and friend. He looked at world problems as a scientist and humanitarian who gave emphasis to the parasitic diseases by thought and action. At the Harvard School of Public Health, Tropical Medicine was an important field in preparing for problems of war and peace. The faculty was outstanding, including Shattock, Augustine, Tyzzer, and Geiman.

The war, years 1942 to 1945, gave many young Americans a first-hand experience with parasitic diseases. In Puerto Rico and the West Indies, academic problems came alive. There were schistosomiasis with aneurysms, filariasis with elephantiasis, hookworms and anemia, roundworms causing gross abdominal swelling — a place to observe and learn.

After the war, Washington was filled with men who had experienced all kinds of disease problems in their overseas assignments. As stated in an earlier acknowledgment (Section A), Drs. Joe Mountain and Joe Dean opened the door of the Public Health Service to new ideas and programs. Thus the conception of veterinary public health came into being. In describing the zoonoses in the first program proposal, Drs. Mountain and Dean were impressed with the number of animal diseases affecting man, especially the parasitic zoonoses. Dr. Willard Wright, who was Director of the NIH Tropical Medicine Laboratory, gave much-valued advice in those years and for many years after veterinary public health came into being.

In the fall of 1945 a conference was held, chaired by Dr. Charles Williams, Sr., Assistant Surgeon General, on quarantine measures to protect the United States against the importation of foreign diseases, vectors, and reservoir hosts. This was the first formal meeting where animal disease problems were discussed with the government authorities responsible for the repatriation of millions of men and women overseas. Dr. Wright was the source of fact and strength that carried the recommendations that were made to restrict the entry of animal pets from outside continental United States. Dr. Wright's knowledge was invaluable to the success of the quarantine measures adopted, and stimulated further investigation.

The Communicable Disease Center, where the Veterinary Public Health Division was established in 1947, offered contact with many persons who were interested in parasitic diseases. These included David Ruhe whom I had known at Michigan State, Marion Brook and Alan Donaldson in the Laboratory, and Justin Andrews, the Deputy Director and later Director of CDC; and later, Irving Kagan, George Healy, Ken Walls, the late Elvio Sadun, and many others who went on to be leaders in academia and international health agencies.

It is difficult to recall the lack of knowledge that existed about the parasitic zoonoses. Trichinosis and tapeworms were recognized indigenous public health problems, and even there the facts were few. This was dramatically brought to my attention in 1948 when Alan Donaldson asked if it would be possible to find some hydatid cysts, *Echinococcus granulosus* cysts. Authorities differed as to their presence in the United States. The late Benjamin Schwartz, the Director of the Parasitology Division, Bureau of Animal Industry, U.S. Department of Agriculture was quoted as saying the disease did not exist in the United States whereas Richard Turk, a veterinary parasitologist at Texas A&M College, would insist that hydatid disease was present in Texas. Both were proven to be wrong. To my great surprise, I learned that hydatid cysts were not uncommon in southern pigs from Georgia and Alabama. On the first occasion when fresh tissues with cysts were delivered to Dr. Donaldson he exclaimed that there was more than enough material to make an antigen (Casoni) and that laboratory demonstrations could be prepared. We were to learn more about hydatid disease in the South, but never identified the reservoir host although Dr. Tony Allen tried for two summers while a student at the University of Georgia Veterinary Medical College in the early 1950s. These occurrences of hydatid disease were to follow for some years and to date there is no explanation. But they did stimulate further investigation led by Calvin Schwabe and Peter Schantz.

Trichinosis was another important parasitic zoonosis which Willard Wright and Leon Jacobs had investigated in the late thirties and early forties. Data collected by them revealed that about 16% of the population that died during that period had evidence of trichinosis. This figure was to embarrass the United States for decades to come. In 1963, the U. S. Public Health Service sent a scientific delegation to the USSR to exchange knowledge on veterinary public health and prevention of disease. The members were Herbert Stoenner, Rocky Mountain Laboratory; Carl Brandly, then the Dean of the College of Veterinary Medicine, University of Illinois; Howard Dunn, Professor Veterinary Science, Pennsylvania State University; and myself as chief of delegation, along with Eugene Papp, Professor of Clinical Pathology, University of Georgia, who was our translator. Dr. Papp was skilled in all the eastern European languages and handled all events and situations skillfully. In the role of spokesman for the delegation I was asked to speak to conferences and meetings arranged by our hosts at the institutions and colleges we visited. A question period would follow each lecture, and invariably the question would be asked why the United States had so much trichinosis. There was a month of the same questions, including a round-table with the editors of *Veterinaryia*, the only Russian veterinary journal. They also examined me on the trichina problem and asked me to write an article for *Veterinaryia* on the U.S. epidemics. By then I realized that it was time to review the current status of trichinosis. On my return to CDC, I immediately reported the harassing that we had received. Drs. A. D. Langmuir, the Chief of Epidemiology, and James Goddard, the Director of the CDC, encouraged the reexamination of trichinosis. Within months, studies were organized with Dr. William Zimmerman, parasitologist at the Iowa Veterinary Research Institute, Ames, Iowa, to study the incidence of disease in swine and man. These studies, the largest ever undertaken, included a sampling of the human population of 50 states and New York City. The swine study included most of the swine-producing states. The study led to similar surveys in other countries, which are reviewed in the Trichinosis chapter. One must acknowledge the stimulus of these studies to be the encounter in the USSR.

Tapeworm investigations were prompted by outbreaks in Texas that received national attention because of the distribution of human infections across the U.S. Dr. Myron Schultz led these investigations which resulted in the establishment of a National Cysticercosis Study Group. Dr. Schultz also carried on an extensive study in Poland with Drs. M. Gerwel and Z. Pawlowski. Drs. Schultz and Pawlowski have reported their extensive work in many articles and a book. Their data appear in the *Taenia* chapter. With new reports of taeniasis in the western states the topic remains current and is reviewed annually by the National Cysticercosis Study Group.

Parasitic Zoonoses speaks to the world problem in Volumes I, II, and III. The chapters are a tribute to the men who wrote them. Most of these authors were found through the efforts of the section editors, Leon Jacobs, George Hillyer, Primo Arambulo, Myron Schultz, and Cluff Hopla, as well as the consultants and contributors. A brief word is included on their efforts that led to the successful culmination of these volumes.

Primo Arambulo, a public health veterinarian in Manila, had an unusual experience in the Philippines with cysticercosis in man and animals, which he describes. He was a teacher of parasitology at the University of the Philippines and was widely acquainted in southeast Asia; he helped prepare the outline of *Parasitic Zoonoses* when he was a graduate student at the University of Texas School of Public Health in 1974 to 1977. His knowledge of the leading parasitologists in southeast Asia and the western Pacific was a great help in seeking out authors who had clinical research experience with parasitic diseases enzootic and endemic in the Orient. The demands of his appointment in the Pan American Health Organization made it impossible for him to follow through as overall section editor, as he had hoped. He gave what time he had in editing the Cestode section, an area in which Myron Schultz, Director of the Parasitic Disease Division, CDC, has been an invaluable resource person.

Dr. Schultz then took over the editorship of the Nematodes. He and his staff associates, Dennis Juranek and Peter Schantz, gave much valuable counsel not only in editing the Nematode section but the Protozoa, Cestode and Trematode sections. They were always ready to give aid and assistance when called on.

George Hillyer, Professor of Biology, University of Puerto Rico, gave sound advice on revising the Trematode section and prepared an outstanding chapter on Schistosomiasis which he updated almost monthly during the past two years when new authors had to be sought for the Oriental parasitic diseases.

Leon Jacobs is a senior parasitologist and experienced public health administrator. He served as Deputy Assistant Secretary of Health in the Johnson administration, and later as an administrator of the National Institutes of Health and Director of the Fogarty Center. He was recruited rather late to organizing and editing the Protozoan Disease Section and to finding competent contributors to bring the section up to date. Leon's advice was always direct and to the problem at hand. His and Frenkel's chapter on Toxoplasmosis is excellent and current. George Healy also was of great help in getting the Protozoa Section together and contributed in the chapters on *Balantidium coli* and *Babesia* infections.

Cluff Hopla, Professor of Zoology at the University of Oklahoma and a renowned researcher, was able to bring together the wide-ranging section on arthropodiasis and allergy, which affect the well-being of man and animals. His chapter on arthropodiasis is of great merit and points to the problems of the future in the industrial and agricultural societies.

The consultants have all given generously of their experience and knowledge. Their contributions exceeded the usual and made the series that much better. To those who prepared manuscripts that could not be included, our deepest thanks for your generous contribution. Recognition is hereby made of the review of some of the protozoal infections by Drs. B. Rosicky, Director of the Academy of Science, Prague, Czechoslovakia; Hamed M. Khalil, Professor of Parasitology at Ain Shams University, Cairo, Egypt; and Ichiro Miyazaki, Professor of Parasitology, Fukuoka University, Japan. And a note of deep appreciation to Dario Cappucci who did so much to complete the series on short notice.

The authors of chapters have all been most patient. Unforeseen problems in completing the sections and editing have caused delays that have stretched out into months and years. We hope their patience is rewarded by the valuable information base that their chapters will give health officials and workers throughout the world. To all, thanks and peace be with you.

As always, there are the CRC editors and staff who have kept the processing of the contributions in order and moving toward completion. Sandy Pearlman, Joanne Del Mastro, Mary Kugler, and Janelle Sparks have been competent, diligent, and enjoyable to work with. The University of Texas administrators, President Roger Bolger and Dean Revel Stallones, have been most generous in their support of the project. Among the staff at the University of Texas School of Public Health special recognition goes to Mrs. Patricia McRoberts and Ms. Peggy Donnellan who helped finish the chapters; John Hubbard, artist, who prepared many illustrations and tables; and Ms. Marcia Willis for counsel; thanks for your help which made the series possible. Lastly, Brigitte, who calmed me with compassion and understanding when plans went asunder. Thank you all, and may your days be good.

James H. Steele
Editor-in-Chief

DEDICATION

Karl Friedrich Meyer was born May 19, 1884 in Basel, Switzerland, the son of Theodor and Sophie (Lichtenhahn) Meyer, and was educated at the University of Zurich. He received the D.V.M. degree from the University of Zurich in 1905. The recipient of nine honorary degrees, "K.F." was most proud of an Honorary M.D. from the University of Zurich in 1937. After working in South Africa, he came to the U.S. in 1910 and taught at the University of Pennsylvania. He was naturalized in 1922.

In 1913, K.F. married Mary Elizabeth Lindsay of Philadelphia. She died in 1958. Surviving is their daughter, Charlotte, and four grandchildren with two great-grandchildren. In 1960, K.F. married Marion Lewis who arranged his personal and professional papers.

K.F. came to the University of California in 1914 as Professor of Bacteriology and Experimental Pathology. He divided his time quite evenly between San Francisco, Berkeley, Davis, and the rest of the world. He became Director of the G. W. Hooper Foundation for Medical Research in 1924 and soon made it a center for study in world public health and epidemiology.

K.F. was a renwned and vigorous lecturer, sometimes lengthy, but never dull. His major contributions were in the control of botulism; the establishment of standards for the canning industry; the control of plague, encephalitis, and ornithosis; the development of public health standards and practices, and aid in many related research problems involving tropical diseases, mussel poisoning, dental caries, and disturbances of hearing. With over 300 publications, K.F. was the recipient of many honors. He was an avid philatelist with a unique collection of disinfected mail. The president of many scientific societies, K.F. was one of our most influential and distinguished scientific leaders.

K.F. was active until his 90th year. The May 1974 issue of *The Journal of Infectious Diseases* had a special supplement on plague that was dedicated to him. A longer biographical sketch is in the supplement. There are now plans for the editor and colleagues to edit his papers and publish a biography.

As that issue went to press, the Editors received the sad news of Dr. Meyer's death on April 27, 1974. The following is an excerpt form the lengthy obituary by Lawrence K. Altman that appeared in *The New York Times* on April 29:

Dr. Karl Friedrich Meyer was regarded as the most versatile microbe hunter since Louis Pasteur and a giant in public health.

As a youth in Basel, Switzerland, pictures of the Black Death, or plague, so fascinated him that he became an outdoor scientist instead of following in the aristocratic business world in which he grew up. He told friends that in choosing to become a veterinarian he could "be a universal man and study all diseases in all species."

Public health leaders yesterday called his contributions to medicine "monumental." His scientific work had such broad implications that it touched on virtually all fields of medicine.

Dr. Meyer is survived by his wife and daughter, to whom we extend our deep sympathy.

TABLE OF CONTENTS

PART 1. PROTOZOAN ZOONOSES

INTRODUCTION TO THE SECTION ON PROTOZOA

Leon Jacobs

The wide variety of structures within the protozoa, and the complexity of these organisms, both morphologically and physiologically, negate the idea that these are simple forms of life. They are really very remarkable creatures, and frequently are frustrating in our attempts to determine their biological relationships. As parasites, they have evolved as diverse organisms with a myriad of adaptations that ensure their survival and their transmission. They present remarkable capabilities for avoiding or counteracting the hosts' abilities to destroy them immunologically. Also, they remain capable of adapting to new host species and new environmental situations.

In dealing with the parasitic protozoa, therefore, it is important always to have one's mind prepared for new types of findings. In this section, for instance, we have a chapter on amebiasis, although the known epidemiology of infection with *Entamoeba histolytica* does not reveal any major animal source of human infection. It is well to remain aware of the possibility that *E. histolytica* may invade other hosts than man, and that under appropriate conditions such hosts may contaminate man's environment with infective amoeba cysts. While some may scoff at such a remote possibility, it can be pointed out that free-living amoebae such as *Naegleria fowleri* have, in recent years, been found to cause a fulminating meningo-encephalitis in human beings. It is hardly likely that this disease entity was entirely missed in the past; it is likely that recent changes in the organisms have occurred that provide them with the capabilities of assuming a parasitic existence. The fulminating nature of the disease is additional evidence that the association of amoebae and host is recent; sophisticated parasites do not so rapidly kill off their hosts. In regard to other intestinal protozoal pathogens, the ciliate *Balantidium coli* and the flagellate *Giardia lamblia* certainly seem capable of infecting man after residence in other hosts.

The hemoflagellates appear to be examples of continuing evolution over a long period of time. The two African trypanosomes of human beings, *Trypanosoma gambiense* and *T. rhodesiense*, are indistinguishable morphologically, but they are different in their host specifity and in their pathogenesis. *T. gambiense* is a human trypanosome. Its transmission is from man to fly to man. *T. rhodesiense* is an animal trypanosome. Its transmission is from animal to fly to animal except when man is present to receive the bite of the fly. *Rhodesiense* trypanosomiasis is more rapidly deadly than that produced by *T. gambiense*, although the latter is still highly pathogenic. These differences suggest the possibility that *T. rhodesiense* is more recently associated with man. The leishmanias present us with a perplexing series of human diseases, from cutaneous forms such as oriental sore to mucocutaneous ulcerations, and to highly fatal invasion of the reticulo-endothelial system in kala azar. These are all zoonoses, and the relations of the parasites to their multiple hosts must continue to be studied to understand their epidemiology and their pathogenesis. A recent report of canine leishmaniasis in Oklahoma, suggests that there is a possibility that more human cases may occur in the southern United States.[1]

The malaria parasites, while generally considered host-specific, are not always so, as is shown in the account of the simian malarias. Babesiosis in human beings, due to *Babesia microti*, is now a not uncommon infection in certain areas of New England, and will undoubtedly be found elsewhere by microscopists with prepared minds. Toxoplasmosis is a very common zoonosis, and while organisms related to *Toxoplasma* appear somewhat more restricted as to hosts, much more study is needed to complete knowledge of their epidemiology. *Sarcocystis* species, while exhibiting rather specific predator-prey cycles, occasionally appear in odd hosts. Man is usually involved as a predator in relation to *Sarcocystis* of beef and swine. It remains to be determined how specific the sexual stages of *Sarcocystis* species are for their various predator hosts. Occasional findings of sarcocysts in human beings and nonhuman primates indicate that there is certainly a zoonotic potential for these organisms. The relationships of the organisms in the Api-complexa, *Toxoplasma, Sarcocystis, Hammondia, Besnoitia, Frenkelia,* etc. are certain to be elucidated in coming years because the general features of their life cycles are now known and work with them is more easily accomplished. What does emerge clearly, from our present probings, is the realization that these protozoan parasites are highly versatile and can be expected to appear in a variety of "abnormal" hosts from time to time. It is only in man's mind that the idea of "species" exists, and similarly "host specificity" is our concept.

REFERENCE

1. MacVean, D., personal communication.

AMEBIASIS*

William B. Lushbaugh
and
Fred E. Pittman

Disease

Intestinal and extraintestinal amebiasis: defined as infection with the protozoan parasite, with or without the presence of clinical symptoms or pathology.

Etiologic Agent *Entamoeba histolytica* Schaudinn 1903 (Protozoa, Rhizopoda)

There are several genera of intestinal amoebae parasitic in man; of these, only *E. histolytica* is pathogenic. *E. histolytica* infections of man are endemic in most parts of the world[1] and may take a variety of forms. The most common form of amebiasis is infection without documented clinical or invasive disease. This asymptomatic carrier state is important epidemiologically since man is the only documented reservoir of infection, and the disease is usually transmitted from person to person. Naturally occurring infections of nonhuman primates by amoebae morphologically indistinguishable from *E. histolytica* are usually productive of cysts and could be a potential source of infection.

E. histolytica infection is usually acquired by ingestion of the cyst stage. Trophozoites are more easily destroyed in the external environment and thus usually do not play a role in transmission of the disease. The life cycle of *E. histolytica* is a direct one involving motile unicellular trophozoites in the bowel lumen or mucosa, and passage of the somewhat resistant cysts in normal stools. Patients with acute amoebic colitis, diarrhea, or dysentery may pass trophozoites in their stools, but these forms would ordinarily be quickly destroyed. A primary cutaneous form of amebiasis may be transmitted venereally.

Although popularly believed to be a "tropical disease" restricted in its distribution to temperate climes, amebiasis has a cosmopolitan distribution. The well-known centers for amoebic infection may parallel the distribution of the pathologists interested in the disease. The geographic distribution of *E. histolytica* was recently reviewed by Elsdon-Dew[2] and by the World Health Organization.[1] Mexico is certainly troubled by this disease, and has sponsored a semiannual symposium (published as an appendix to the *Archivos de Investigacion Medica* [Mexico]) and the First International Congress on Amebiasis.** The publications resulting from these meetings have served to bring together most of the workers in the field to discuss aspects of the epidemiology, pathogenesis, diagnosis, and treatment of amebiasis. They are one of the best sources for current information on amebiasis.

Historical Background

A complete review of the discovery and history of amebiasis is available in Elsdon-Dew's review[2] of the epidemiology of amebiasis. Highlights will be covered here. Lösch[3] provided the first description of severe dysentery from a patient he treated in St. Petersburg in 1875. The disease was caused by an amoeba present in the stools and in intestinal lesions at post-mortem. The amoeba was successfully transmitted to the dog producing a lasting infection. In this country, the description of amebiasis by Councilman and Lafleur[4] was the most complete. They described the chronic pro-

* Research supported by the The John A. Hartford Foundation, Inc., the Veterans Administration and the National Institutes of Health.
** Proceedings separately published, edited by B. Sepulveda and L. S. Diamond, 1979.

longed form of amebiasis, intermittent passage of cysts in stools of those infected, liver abscesses, and the histopathology of amebiasis in the intestines and liver. Few significant changes have since been made in our knowledge of amebiasis. At that time they called the etiologic agent *Amoeba dysenteriae.*

Schaudinn[5] distinguished the nonpathogenic *Entamoeba coli* from the pathogenic *E. histolytica* but also confused the issue by describing *E. tetragena,* a species from man with quadrinucleate cysts. After much dissent, the name now accepted as correct for the dysentery amoeba of man is *E. histolytica* Schaudinn, 1903. Dobell,[6] in his *Amoebae Living in Man* was probably most responsible for clarifying the life cycle of the amoeba after the more imaginative ramblings of other workers. He pointed out that all developmental stages were present in carriers as well as patients with disease. Cysts were passed in formed stools, although trophozoites, present at the mucosa and within the tissues, could be obtained by administration of a purgative. The question of what determines whether or not a certain infection will produce extensive pathogenic effects or a relatively uninvolved carrier state is still unanswered today.

Cultivation of amoebas and production of the disease in animal models has always been of interest. Dobell,[7] in his study of intestinal protozoa of monkeys and man, Hegner et al.[8] and Johnson[9] examined the role played by nonhuman primates in the epidemiology of amebiasis, and compared the severity of disease produced by human *E. histolytica* in primates and in kittens. Primates can carry a form of amebiasis that is usually milder than dysenteric amebiasis in man. The primate infection is usually asymptomatic. However, epidemics of amoebic dysentery can occur in crowded primate colonies and the attendant post-mortem pathology was first described by Eichhorn and Gallagher[10] in 1916. Frye and Meleney[11] studied the natural infections of domestic animals and peridomestic insects in a rural Tennessee community in 1932. They concluded that houseflies can be a factor in spread of *E. histolytica* in the community only in the presence of high incidence of infection and promiscuous defecation by the human population. The source of human infections in the community is man himself, through personal contact and poor hygiene aided to a lesser extent by the fly. In their survey of pigs, rats, mice, chickens, dogs, and cats, they found that only related nonpathogenic species of *Entamoeba* were present. None of the animals associated with man act as reservoir hosts in the transmission of *E. histolytica* to man.

Morphology and Transmission

Entamoeba histolytica is a unicellular protozoan with two stages in its life cycle. The trophozoite stage is the motile feeding ameboid stage found in the tissues or in loose stools. The trophozoite stage is delicate and easily killed. It usually plays no role in transmission of the disease. The cyst stage of *E. histolytica* is found only in formed stools, never in the tissues. Encystment takes place during passage from the body. Cysts have resistant walls not present in the trophozoite, and will remain viable for long periods of time if moist. Cysts and trophozoites are killed by complete drying.

Trophozoites of *E. histolytica* in tissue obtained at biopsy, proctoscopic scrapings of lesions, or in dysenteric stools must be differentiated from host cells, debris, and trophozoites of other intestinal protozoans. The size of the trophozoites, and the number or morphology of nuclei are the characteristics used in diagnosis. Careful training in the differentiation of these characteristics in unstained or stained preparations is necessary as the size ranges of other *Entamoeba* trophozoites (*E. coli, E. hartmani*) overlap with that of *E. histolytica.* Three other genera, *Endolimax, Iodamoeba,* and *Dientamoeba,* with a single nucleus in the trophozoite stage must also be distinguished. Nuclear morphology in stained fecal smears is the only way to distinguish between these with accuracy. The chromatin of *Entamoeba histolytica* is relatively evenly distributed in regular granules around the delicate nuclear envelope. The karyosome appears as a small centrally located dot. Detailed accounts of the morphology of these species and how to differentiate them are given by Swartzwelder,[12] Neal,[13] and Healy.[14]

Mature cysts of *E. histolytica* present in formed stools are usually quadrinucleate. Cysts of *E. coli* contain eight nuclei when mature and have a mean diameter twice that of *E. histolytica* (10 to 30 μm vs. 6 to 15 μm). Cysts of *E. nana* are oval and smaller than *E. histolytica* while those of *I. butchleii* are similar in size. Nuclear morphology again comes into play for differentiation between these organisms as they all may contain an intermediate number of nuclei at some stage in their development and may be distorted in size or shape by handling or fixation.

Electron Microscopy

The morphology of the tissue-dwelling trophozoites is well studied but remains somewhat enigmatic. This organism lacks many of the cytoplasmic organelles characteristic of mammalian eukaryotic cells or even more conventional protozoans; mitochondria and Golgi apparatus are not usually demonstrated. Golgi cisternae have been reported in a single instance from drug-treated trophozoites in vitro.[15] The surface morphology of the trophozoites has been believed to somehow participate in the production of cytopathic effects on host cells. Transmission electron microscopic studies of single thin sections demonstrated surface blebs that were interpreted as "surface-active lysosomes" because of their association in plane of section with acid phosphatase-positive vesicles.[16] Scanning electron microscopy of trophozoites revealed the presence of slender pseudopodia[17,18] that could account for the appearance of slender surface projections or detached vesicles in thin section.[19] Involvement of any surface structure(s) in the production of cytopathogenic effects by the amoeba has not been proven. The remainder of the trophozoite is relatively unremarkable, resembling that of other protozoa except for the absence of rough endoplasmic reticulum. This structure is functionally replaced in *E. histolytica* by short lengths of helical ribonucleoprotein bearing ribosomes.[20] Structures known as chromatoidal bars from light microscopy are formed by aggregation of the RNA helices bearing ribosomes. The chromatoidal material forms a crystalline lattice that could mediate temporary storage of the ribosomes during encystment.[21]

Diagnosis

Amebiasis is diagnosed on microscopic, serologic, and clinical criteria. The microscopic diagnosis of *E. histolytica* is based on the identification of the cysts and/or trophozoites in stool, or of the trophozoites in tissue samples. The clinical laboratory is usually involved in microscopic examination of stool specimens. A number of hospital laboratories have *overdiagnosed* amebiasis as a result of reporting macrophage in stools as *E. histolytica* trophozoites. True infections of *E. histolytica* may be *misdiagnosed* as a result of confusion with other intestinal protozoa or leukocytes. *Underdiagnosis* of amebiasis follows from misdiagnosis or from failure of physicians to consider *E. histolytica* as a possible pathogen in cases of dysentery in the U.S. The case histories of these instances are disclosed in Krogstad et al.,[22] "Amebiasis: Epidemiologic Studies in the United States, 1971—1974." These authors describe the currently accepted methods used to facilitate diagnosis of *E. histolytica* infections.

Serologic Diagnosis

Most patients with extraintestinal amebiasis will have a positive indirect hemagglutination titer (IHA) for amebiasis. The seropositivity of patients with intestinal disease is related to the amount of tissue involvement present. Clinically significant intestinal amebiasis is usually associated with a positive IHA.[23] Patients with asymptomatic amebiasis may not exhibit a positive titer. Although a positive titer may reflect recent experience with the disease rather than current infection, higher titers are suggestive of recent infection.[24]

Clinical Amebiasis

Amebiasis should be included in the differential diagnosis of ulcerative colitis, tourist diarrhea, dysentery, and lesions or masses in the large bowel. Extraintestinal amebiasis may present as a mass or abscess in any organ, although the liver is the most frequently involved extraintestinal site for amebiasis. Liver abscess may occasionally be diagnosed by aspiration, although trophozoites are not usually found in the content of the abscess. Their distribution is usually restricted to the inner aspect of the fibrous abscess wall. Amoebic liver abscess is usually odorless and bacterially sterile on the first aspiration. The absence of amoebae or of the once classical "anchovy paste color" from the aspirate should not exclude the diagnosis.[14]

Infections of *E. Histolytica* in Wild and Domestic Animals
Primates

The recent publication of Amyx et al.[25] calls attention to the fact that *E. histolytica* infections in primates can produce morbidity and mortality of epidemic proportions under the proper conditions. These authors reported that a colony of spider monkeys housed outdoors with rhesus, patas, and capuchin monkeys suffered a significant epidemic of amoebic dysentery often accompanied by amoebic liver abscess and high mortality. The autopsied animals had high IHA titers and extensive invasion of the liver parenchyma. The authors suggested that in their experience, spider monkeys are uniquely susceptible to *E. histolytica* infections. Vickers[26] reported that in his experience, tissue invasion is more common in new world monkeys (i.e., spider monkeys) than in old world monkeys. He suggested that rhesus are often quite resistant, perhaps as a result of harboring the infection in the wild. New world monkeys do not often come in contact with the ground or the parasite. *E. histolytica* infections in the chimpanzee appear to be quite similar to those of man. Miller and Bray[27] reported a similar epidemic of dysentery and liver abscess in a colony in Liberia. The intestinal and liver lesions had the same histopathologic appearance as that reported for human infections. Stool records of incoming chimps revealed that only 2 of 29 were infected on arrival and these had been in contact with human carriers of the disease prior to arrival. The usual infection rate in the colony was 10/24, all with asymptomatic infections. The authors concluded from their studies and the available literature that, like those of man, *E. histolytica* infections in chimpanzees may persist for long periods without producing symptomatology or tissue invasion. When the host-parasite relationship is modified from that of a commensal, the histopathologic changes observed resemble those found in humans.

Dobell[7] found naturally occurring infections in *Macacus rhesus, M. sinicus* and *M. nemestrueus* identical with *E. histolytica.* The rhesus *E. histolytica* produced infections in kittens identical with those produced by human *E. histolytica. M. rhesus* could be infected by *E. histolytica* from human cases and from cases in other species of *Macacus.* Although cysts were passed, no tissue invasion was observed in any infection of the monkeys. Dobell[7] concluded that macaques could harbor *E. histolytica*, but might have an *E. histolytica*-like *Entamoeba* species of their own. Accidental infection of man might occur with an *E. histolytica*-like amoeba from macaques.

The most extensive review of the historic literature to date was that of Miller.[28] He stated that the results of others and his own investigation showed that old world monkeys infected with human *E. histolytica* did not show evidence of invasion while Hegner et al.[8] described 12/16 new world monkeys with frank dysentery. Ratcliffe[29] reported an epidemic of amoebic dysentery among *Ateles* and *Lagothrix* initiated by contact with old world monkeys that were carriers of *E. histolytica.* Miller[28] also found that a more severe infection is produced by *E. histolytica* in new world monkeys than in old world monkeys. Old world monkeys have a naturally occurring infection with *E. histolytica* that mimics the infection in man. As such, the usual infections in old world primates were productive of cysts but usually not of clinical amebiasis. Clinical disease, when it occurs in old world monkeys, can be as severe as that occurring in man. The importance of nonhuman primates as reservoirs of infection for man is of the same magnitude as contact between humans and primates. While primates do not present a public health problem in the U.S., infections in these animals could be a source of infection in rural Africa. Their possible role has not been documented by field studies.

Other Animals

Although animals other than primates can be experimentally infected with properly administered human *E. histolytica,* these animals are not reservoirs of amebiasis in nature. Many animals have their own morphologically distinct species of *Entamoeba* with which they are naturally infected. Dr. Beaver prepared a review on this subject for the World Health Organization technical report series,[1] and Neal[13] had listed other species of the genus *Entamoeba* in his monograph on speciation. Pigs are naturally infected with *E. polecki,* and a human infection with *E. polecki* has been reported.[30] Frye and Meleney[11] reported a questionable infection of *E. histolytica* in the pig. The genus *Entamoeba* is well represented in rodents; in rats and mice it is called *E. muris,* in guinea pigs it is called *E. cobayae,* and in the rabbit it is *E. cunniculi.* Dogs and cats have been reported to occasionally carry an amoeba resembling *E. histolytica.*[31] *E. invadens* and *E. terrapinae* are found in snakes and turtles. Chickens have *E. galli-narum.* The presence of naturally occurring nonpathogenic *Entamoeba* in other animals has been a source of confusion, suggesting to some that domestic and wild reservoirs of *E. histolytica* might exist. At present there is no evidence to support this claim. The only significant reservoir host of amebiasis is man.

E. Histolytica Infection in Man

E. histolytica cysts are infective when passed in feces and require no extrinsic incubation period. Upon ingestion, the cysts are carried into the intestine where excystment occurs. The quadrinucleate metacystic amoeba escapes from the cyst and undergoes a complete series of nuclear and cytoplasmic divisions. During metacystic development, each of the nuclei divides followed by cytoplasmic division. Metacystic development results in the formation of eight uninucleate trophic amoebae per cyst.[6]

Intestinal Amebiasis

Infections of *E. histolytica* in the large bowel may be asymptomatic or symptomatic. Asymptomatic infections of *E. histolytica* in which little clinically detectable response is present may be the most frequent form of this disease. Tissue invasion by trophozoites may occur in asymptomatic amebiasis since extraintestinal forms of the disease may develop without any history of intestinal complaints.

Symptomatic intestinal amebiasis may be divided into two main clinical syndromes: nondysenteric amoebic colitis in which the patient complains of nonbloody diarrhea, and amoebic dysentery in which varying amounts of gross blood are seen in the diarrheal stool. In the older clinical descriptions of the appearance of colonic mucosa in the disease, the findings of focal ulceration were stressed. More recent descriptions have stressed the frequent finding on sigmoidoscopy or colonoscopy of a diffuse hermorrhagic mucosal inflammatory process which is difficult to differentiate from other types of infection or noninfectious colitis. Modern gastroenterologists hold the view that with few exceptions the gross appearance of the mucosa is not helpful in determining the type of colitis present. Histological examination of biopsy specimens from patients with well-documented amoebic colitis reveals amoebae in less than 50% of sections. When trophozoites are not demonstrated, the histopathological findings may be indistinguishable from other types of colitis. Diagnosis of amoebic colitis is best made by microscopic demonstration of motile trophozoites, preferably hematophagous, in exudate or stool obtained at initial sigmoidoscopy. Colonic amebiasis when chronic may show manifestations of ameboma, a mass of inflammatory tissue that intrudes into the lumen of the bowel giving the appearance of cancer or polyp of the colon. Ameboma is most common in the cecum, but may occur at any site in the large bowel.

Extraintestinal Amebiasis

Most extraintestinal amebiasis is secondary to intestinal infection and is the result of metastatic seeding of trophozoites through hematogenous and/or lymphatic spread.

The most common type of extraintestinal amebiasis is liver abscess. This condition is more frequent in men than women and usually involves the right lobe, producing characteristic elevation of the right hemidiaphragm. Pleural effusion and pulmonary abscess is an important complication of liver abscesses that rupture into the lung through the diaphragm or spread to the lung by the hematogenous route. Pericardial amebiasis can result by extension from an abscess in the left lobe of the liver. Other life-threatening metastatic infections include cerebellar and renal amoebic abscesses. Secondary cutaneous amebiasis can result from extension through the chest wall from an abscess or from frequent perianal irritation and ulceration in dysentery of prolonged duration. A primary form of cutaneous amebiasis presenting as balanitis (inflammation of the glans penis) has recently been described in homosexual males.[32,33]

Pathology of Amebiasis

The most recent extensive review of the pathology of human amebiasis was presented by Brandt and Tamayo.[34] Pathogenesis of amoebic disease is discussed by Biagi and Beltran,[35] Miller,[36] and Elsdon-Dew.[2] A classic description of the intestinal ulcerations and liver abscess was provided by Councilman and Lafleur in 1891.[4] A recent review of autopsy cases was published by Aikat et al.,[37] who also discussed the early lesion controversy and amoebic hepatitis.

Pathogenesis in amebiasis has been studied for some time. Councilman and Lafleur[4] suggested the effect of the amoebae was that of an enzyme, and the very name of the beast is suggestive of tissue lysis. Recent studies have included development of an in vitro system for studying the effects of living trophozoites on tissue culture cells. Eaton et al.[16] first proposed that surface structures of amoebae were responsible for producing cytopathic effects on mammalian cells. Bos and van der Griend[38] found a correlation between in vitro activity and liver abscess production. Lushbaugh et al.[39] described an enterotoxin/cytotoxin associated with virulent strains of *E. histolytica* from axenic cultures.[40] Bos[41] and Mattern et al.[42] have further characterized the toxic substance, but its actual participation in the production of cytopathic changes in vivo has not been demonstrated. There may be another toxin that is contact dependent and associated with the surface membrane rather than the cytosol of *Entamoeba.*[43]

Epidemiology of Amebiasis

A detailed account is given by Elsdon-Dew[2] and by Krogstad et al.[22] Man is the usual host of *Entamoeba histolytica* and the source of cysts that are the infective stage in transmission of this disease. Contamination of the diet with cysts of human origin is the usual method of transmission between persons. Cysts may be introduced into the mouth through hand-to-mouth contamination associated with poor personal hygiene among food handlers, family members, or hospital personnel. The studies of Frye and Meleney[11] showed that high infection rates among humans and unsafe disposal of human feces must be present before flies may play a role as mechanical agents of cyst dissemination. Some contact with soiled fingers of infected persons and the diet of the population at risk (uninfected susceptible persons) is the chief method of transmission among persons. Other factors that could be involved are community or dwelling sanitation, safety of water supplies, or distribution networks and institutional personnel who are unaware that they harbor asymptomatic *E. histolytica* infections (carriers or cyst passers). Crowded conditions and poor personal hygiene can contribute to higher rates of transmission among indigent and institutionalized persons. Young children are more susceptible than adults or older children to amebiasis, and in several cases were the only ones in the family with clinical disease. Other family members responsible for preparing food and feeding the children were carriers of *E. histolytica.*[44]

Although infections of nonhuman primates occur, these infections are usually not of epidemiologic importance as far as transmission of the disease to man is concerned. Few human populations are closely associated with nonhuman primates in such a way that fecal contamination of the other's diet occurs. Furthermore, the evidence for the natural occurrence of sylvatic amebiasis is not well documented. In several cases, reviewed above, there was indication that the animals had been in contact with human carriers of the disease prior to being brought to the laboratory for examination.

Prevention and Control of Amebiasis

Amebiasis can be prevented by avoidance of opportunities to ingest infective cysts of *E. histolytica.* This can be accomplished by treatment of all persons with a positive stool exam, proper disposal of human feces, chlorination, adequate uncontaminated dispersal of water, and attention to personal hygiene. Stool examinations should be performed on food handlers and institutional workers in endemic areas, as their involvement in contamination of the diet of others is the dominant form of transmission between persons. Sewage-contaminated water has played a significant role in the epidemiology of amebiasis in the past.[45]

Although amebiasis is a significant cause of tourist diarrhea, it is less common than bacterial diarrheas and must be differentially diagnosed. There are presently no drugs available in the U.S. that can be used in a prophylactic regimen against infection with *E. histolytica.*

Other Amoebic Infections of Man

Another disease called primary amoebic meningoencephalitis (PAM) is caused by otherwise free-living soil and water amoebae of the genera *Naegleria* and *Acanthamoeba.*[46] PAM is acquired (usually by young children) through swimming in organically rich lakes or pools resulting in the inoculation of the nasal mucosa with the ameboid trophozoites. The amoebae enter the frontal lobes to produce a meningitis that has usually led rapidly to coma and death. *Naegleria* sp. and *Acanthamoeba* sp. are morphologically distinct from *E. histolytica* and can be identified in cerebrospinal fluid and autopsy material by the presence of a large endosome (like that of *Iodamoeba*) within the nucleus of the trophozoites. *E. histolytica* trophozoites would probably not be found in the cerebrospinal fluid even if an amoebic (*E. histolytica*) brain abscess were present.

Conclusions

Although *E. histolytica* was estimated[1] to infect 10% of the world population in 1969 and probably 5% of the population of the U.S. about 20 years ago, it is now less prevalent.[45] *E. histolytica* has been the most frequently fatal intestinal protozoan of man in the U.S. up to present times, and as such is an important consideration in the differential diagnosis of diarrheal diseases. The most important mode of transmission is the passage of cysts between infected and uninfected persons through fecal contamination of the diet or water. Zoonotic infections, although apparently extant, probably are not often involved in transmission of the disease to humans from nonhuman primates.

REFERENCES

1. **Beaver, P.,** Amoebiasis: Report of a WHO Expert Committee, WHO Tech. Rep. Ser. No. 421, World Health Organization, Geneva, 1969.
2. **Elsdon-Dew, R.,** The epidemiology of amebiasis, in *Advances in Parasitology,* Vol. 6, Academic Press, New York, 1968, 1.
3. **Lösch, F.,** Massenhafte Entwickelung von Amöben in Diskdarm, *Virchows. Arch. Pathol. Anat. Physiol.,* 65, 196, 1875.
4. **Councilman, W. and Lafleur, H.,** Amoebic dysentery, *Johns Hopkins Hosp. Rep.,* 2, 395, 1891.
5. **Schaudinn, F.,** Untersuchungen ubun die Fortflanzung einiger Rizopoden, *Arb. Kais. Gesundheitsamte (Berlin),* 19, 547, 1903.
6. **Dobell, G.,** *Amoebae Living in Man: A Zoological Monograph,* John Bale Sons & Danielsson, London, 1919.
7. **Dobell, C.,** Researches on the intestinal protozoa of monkeys and man. IV. An experimental study of the *histolytica*-like species of *Entamoeba* living naturally in macaques, *Parasitology,* 23, 1, 1931.
8. **Hegner, R., Johnson, C. M., and Stabler, R. M.,** Host-parasite relations in experimental amoebiasis in monkeys in Panama, *Am. J. Hyg.,* 15, 394, 1932.
9. **Johnson, C. M.,** Observations on natural infections of *Entamoeba histolytica* in *Ateles* and *Rhesus* monkeys, *Am. J. Trop. Med. Hyg.,* 21, 49, 1941.
10. **Eichhorn, A. and Gallagher, B.,** Spontaneous amoebic dysentery in monkeys, *J. Infect. Dis.,* 19, 395, 1916.
11. **Frye, W. W. and Meleney, H. E.,** Investigations of *Entamoeba histolytica* and other intestinal protozoa in Tennessee. IV. A study of flies, rats, mice and some domestic animals as possible carriers of the intestinal protozoa of man in a rural community, *Am. J. Hyg.,* 16, 729, 1932.
12. **Swartzwelder, C.,** Laboratory diagnosis of amebiasis, *Am. J. Clin. Pathol.,* 22, 379, 1952.
13. **Neal, R. A.,** Experimental studies on *Entamoeba* with reference to speciation, in *Advances in Parasitology,* Vol. 4, Academic Press, New York, 1966, 1.
14. **Healy, G. R.,** Laboratory diagnosis of amebiasis, *Bull. N. Y. Acad. Med.,* 47, 478, 1971.
15. **Trevino, N. and Feria-Velasco, A.,** Golgi complex in trophozoites of *Entamoeba histolytica,* in *Proc. 29th Ann. E.M.S.A. Meetings,* Arcenaux, C. J., Ed., Claitor's Publishing Division, Baton Rouge, La., 1971.
16. **Eaton, R. D. P., Meerovitch, E., and Costerton, J. W.,** The functional morphology of pathogenicity in *Entamoeba histolytica, Ann. Trop. Med. Parasitol.,* 64, 299, 1970.
17. **McCaul, T. F. and Bird, R. G.,** Surface features of *Entamoeba histolytica* and rabbit kidney (RK₁₃) cell surface changes after trophozoite contact-observations by scanning electron microscopy, *Int. J. Parasitol.,* 7, 383, 1977.
18. **Lushbaugh, W. B. and Pittman, F. E.,** Microscopic observations on the filopodia of *Entamoeba histolytica, J. Protozool.,* 26, 186, 1979.
19. **Deas, J. E. and Miller, J. H.,** Plasmalemmal modifications of *Entamoeba histolytica* in vivo, *J. Parasitol.,* 63, 25, 1977.
20. **Barker, D. C.,** A ribonucleoprotein inclusion body in *Entamoeba invadens, Z. Zellforsch. Mikrosk. Anat.,* 58, 641, 1963.
21. **Barker, D. C. and Swales, L. S.,** Characteristics of ribosomes during differentiation from trophozoite to cyst in axenic *Entamoeba* sp., *Cell. Diff.,* 1, 297, 1972.
22. **Krogstad, D. J., Spencer, H. C., Jr., Healy, G. R., Gleason, N. N., Sexton, D. J., and Herron, C. A.,** Amebiasis: epidemiologic studies in the United States, 1971—1974, *Ann. Intern. Med.,* 88, 89, 1978.
23. **Krupp, I.,** Antibody response in intestinal and extraintestinal amebiasis, *Am. J. Trop. Med. Hyg.,* 19, 57, 1970.

24. Juniper, K., Worrell, C. L., Minshew, M. C., Roth, L. S., Cypert, H., and Uoyp, R. E., Serologic diagnosis of amebiasis, *Am. J. Trop. Med. Hyg.*, 21, 157, 1972.

25. Amyx, H. L., Asher, D. M., Nash, T. E., Gibbs, C. J., Jr., and Gajdusek, D. C., Hepatic amebiasis in spider monkeys, *Am. J. Trop. Med. Hyg.*, 27, 888, 1978.

26. Vickers, J. H., Gastrointestinal diseases of primates, in *Current Veterinary Therapy III. Small Animal Practice,* Kirk, R. W., Ed., W. B. Saunders, Philadelphia, 1968, 393.

27. Miller, M. J. and Bray, R. S., *Entamoeba histolytica* infections in the chimpanzee (*Pan satyrus*), *J. Parasitol.,* 52, 386, 1966.

28. Miller, M. J., The experimental infection of *Macaca mulatta* with human strains of *Entamoeba histolytica, Am. J. Trop. Med. Hyg.,* 1, 417, 1952.

29. Ratcliffe, H. L., A comparative study of amoebiasis in man, monkeys and cats, with special reference to the formation of the early lesions, *Am. J. Hyg.,* 14, 337, 1931.

30. Lawless, D. K. and Knight, V., Human infection with *Entamoeba polecki,* Report of four cases, *Am. J. Trop. Med. Hyg.,* 15, 701, 1966.

31. Jordan, H. E., Amebiasis (*Entamoeba histolytica*) in the dog, *Vet. Med.,* 62, 61, 1967.

32. William, D. C., Shookhoff, H. B., Felman, Y. M., and deRamos, S. W., High rates of enteric protozoal infections in selected homosexual men attending a veneral disease clinic, *Sex. Trans. Dis.,* 5, 155, 1978.

33. Schmerin, M. J., Gelston, A., and Jones, T. C., Amebiasis: an increasing problem among homosexuals in New York City, *JAMA,* 238, 1386, 1977.

34. Brandt, H. and Tamayo, R. P., Pathology of human amebiasis, *Human Pathol.,* 1, 351, 1970.

35. Biagi, F. F. and Beltran, F., The challenge of amebiasis: understanding pathogenic mechanisms, in *International Review of Tropical Medicine,* Vol. 3, Lincicome, D. R. and Woodrub, A. W., Eds., Academic Press, New York, 1969, 219.

36. Miller, M. J., Pathogenesis of amebic disease, *Prog. Drug Res.,* 18, 225, 1974.

37. Aikat, B. K., Bhusnurmath, S. R., Pal, A. K., Chhuttani, P. N., and Datta, D. V., The pathology and pathogenesis of fatal hepatic amoebiasis — a study based on 79 autopsy cases, *Trans. R. Soc. Trop. Med. Hyg.,* 73, 188, 1979.

38. Bos, H. J. and van de Griend, R. J., Virulence and toxicity of axenic *Entamoeba histolytica, Nature (London),* 265, 341, 1977.

39. Lushbaugh, W. B., Kairalla, A. B., Cantey, J. R., Hofbauer, A. F., and Pittman, F. E., Isolation of a cytotoxin-enterotoxin from *Entamoeba histolytica, J. Infect. Dis.,* 139, 9, 1979.

40. Lushbaugh, W. B., Hofbauer, A. F., Kairalla, A. B., Cantey, J. R., and Pittman, F. E., Relationship of cytotoxins of axenically cultivated *Entamoeba histolytica* to virulence, submitted.

41. Bos, H. J., *Entamoeba histolytica:* cytopathogenicity of intact amebae and cell-free extracts; isolation and characterization of an intracellular toxin, *Exp. Parasitol.,* 47, 369, 1979.

42. Mattern, C. F. T., Keister, D. B., and Natovitz, P. C., *Entamoeba histolytica* "toxin": fetuin neutralizable and lectin-like, *Am. J. Trop. Med. Hyg.,* 1980, in press.

43. Ravdin, J. I., Sullivan, J. A., Mandell, G. L., and Guerrant, R. L., Effect of *E. histolytica* on mammalian cells, *Clin. Res.,* 27, 788A, 1979.

44. Dykes, A. C., Ruebush, T. K., Gorelkin, L., Lushbaugh, W. B., Upshur, J. K., and Cherry, J. D., Extraintestinal amebiasis in infancy; report of 3 cases and epidemiologic investigations of their families, *Pediatrics,* 65, 799, 1980.

45. Krogstad, D. J., Spencer, H. C., Jr., and Healy, G. R., Current concepts in parasitology: amebiasis, *N. Engl. J. Med.,* 298, 262, 1978.

46. Carter, R. F., Primary amebic meningoencephalitis. An appraisal of present knowledge, *Trans. R. Soc. Trop. Med. Hyg.,* 66, 193, 1972.

47. Pittman, F. E., El-Hashimi, W. K., and Pittman, J. C., Studies of human amebiasis; I. Clinical and laboratory findings in eight cases of acute amebic colitis, *Gastroenterology,* 65, 581, 1973.

48. Pittman, F. E., El-Hashimi, W. K., and Pittman, J. C., Studies of human amebiasis; II. Light and electron-microscopic observations of colonic mucosa and exudate in acute amebic colitis, *Gastroenterology,* 65, 588, 1973.

49. Pittman, F. E., Pittman, J. C., and El-Hashimi, W. K., Studies of human amebiasis; III. Ameboma; A radiologic manifestation of amebic colitis, *Am. J. Dig. Dis.,* 18, 1025, 1973.

50. Pittman, F. E. and Hennigar, G. R., Sigmoidoscopic and colonic mucosal biopsy findings in amebic colitis, *Arch. Pathol.,* 97, 155, 1974.

51. Pittman, F. E., Intestinal Amebiasis, *Compr. Ther.,* 1, 61, 1975.

BALANTIDIASIS

Peter D. Walzer and George R. Healy

Disease

Balantidiasis, balantidosis, balantidial dysentery, ciliary dysentery.

Etiologic Agent

The genus *Balantidium* constitutes a group of ciliated protozoa which reside in the digestive tract of over 50 vertebrate and invertebrate hosts.[1,2] Of the several species of *Balantidium, B. coli* is the only one of medical importance.

B. coli was the first described by Malmstein in 1857 from diarrheal stools of patients; the organism was observed in pigs by Leuckart in 1861 and assigned to the genus *Balantidium* by Stain in 1862. *B. coli* is the largest protozoan parasite infecting man. The size range of the parasite varies somewhat according to different authors.[3] The *trophozoite* stage usually measures 50 to 70 μm (range 30 to 150 μm) in length and 40 to 50 μm (range 25 to 120 μm) in width, is ovoidal or sac-like in shape with narrow anterior and rounded posterior end.[1] Prominent morphologic features include at the anterior end a cone-shaped depression — the peristome which leads to the primitive mouth or cystome; two contractile and numerous food vacuoles; a large kidney-shaped macronucleus with small subspherical micronucleus lying along its inner curvature. The surface or pellicle is covered with oblique, longitudinal rows of cilia which propel the organism in synchronized motion. Encystation occurs when the trophozoite rounds up and secretes a double membrane wall.

The rounded or oval *cyst* measures 45 to 65 μm in diameter and shows the macronucleus and contractile vacuoles; the cilia can be seen beating, and there is some movement of the organism inside early in the cyst stage, but gradually the cilia degenerate and motion ceases.

The natural habitat of *B. coli* is the large intestine.[4] The trophozoite feeds on intestinal contents, blood and tissue cells, and other microorganisms (Figure 1). Waste materials are discharged through the cytopyge, an inconspicuous opening in the posterior end. Reproduction occurs only in the trophozoite stage and is mainly by transverse binary fission; conjugation has been observed in culture when two different strains are mixed but is of unknown significance.[5] Otherwise, *B. coli* is a facultative anaerobe but has been cultured on a variety of aerobic and anaerobic media.[6]

The cyst is thought to be the infective form of *B. coli*. After ingestion the cyst wall dissolves, liberating the trophozoite, which travels to the large intestine. The trophozoite is found in frankly diarrheal or dysenteric stools; the cyst is formed when the fecal specimen becomes dehydrated during passage down the intestine and is thus observed in formed or semiformed stools. The cyst is more resistant to adverse environmental conditions than the trophozoite. In a moist environment, the cyst survives for several weeks at 22°C, whereas the trophozoite survives for only 10 days.[7] The cyst, however, is quite sensitive to drying and direct sunlight.

True and Alternate Hosts

Although organisms morphologically indistinguishable from human *B. coli* have been found in the pig, peccary, chimpanzee, orangutan, macaque, dog, rat, guinea pig, and buffalo, it is unknown whether these organisms are truly the same.[8,9] The few comparative laboratory studies of different strains of *B. coli* have included susceptibility to changes in temperature, immunodiffusion, immunofluorescence, and immobilization.[5,10-12] Human and porcine *B. coli* have exhibited differences in sensitivity to

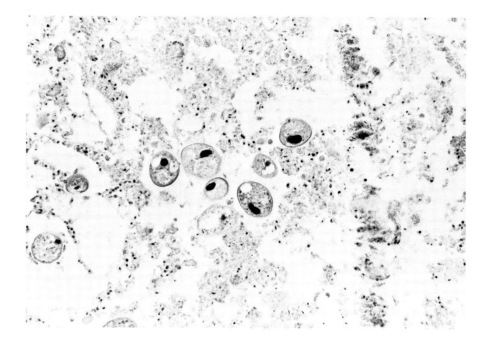

FIGURE 1.   *Balantidium coli* organisms in lumen of orangutan colon.

heating and cooling and in antigenic properties. Although Levine[1] concluded that *B. coli* of the pig, primate, etc. and *B. caviae* of the guinea pig were the same species, Westphal[13] concluded from morphologic and cross-infection experiments that *B. caviae* is a separate species found in the guinea pig.

In man, *B. coli* has a world-wide distribution but is an uncommon infection. Before 1960 there were only 722 patients described with balantidiasis.[14] Since that time most of the literature of *B. coli* has still consisted of case reports, suggesting that investigators continue to regard the organism as little more than a medical curiosity. Belding reviewed 12 surveys comprising 24,837 stool examinations and found an overall *B. coli* prevalence of 0.77%.[7] In many large series the frequency is only 0.02 to 0.1%; on the other hand, rates of 5.1% have been found when only fresh stool specimens were examined.[15,16] The freshness of the stool sample is important because the trophozoites may disintegrate within several hours after evacuation, particularly if not in a moist environment. Another problem contributing to the low frequency of *B. coli* reporting is lack of familiarity with the organism.[17] Both these factors are not unique to *B. coli*, but can also be applied to other intestinal protozoa.

The source of *B. coli* infection in man has been a subject of considerable controversy. The pig has been the prime suspect. Arean and Koppisch noted that over 50% of balantidiasis patients reported in the literature gave a history of contact with pigs, and cited an instance in which a family contracted the disease after eating raw pork sausage.[18] Epidemiologic studies in New Guinea, where people live in intimate contact with pigs, are of particular interest. Stool prevalence surveys of human populations from different areas of the country have revealed a frequency of *B. coli* as high as 29%.[19-22] Women, who have closer association with pigs than do men also have a higher frequency of *B. coli*. The infection in humans, as in pigs, was usually asymptomatic, suggesting a high degree of natural or acquired resistance.

On the other hand, *B. coli* has not been found in people who work closely with swine (for example, in abattoirs) even when poor sanitary conditions exist.[23,24] The difference in temperature susceptibility suggests that few strains of porcine *B. coli* can be transmitted among different experimental animals.[25] Attempts to infect human volunteers with either human or animal strains of the organism have failed.[26,27] Balantidiasis has occurred among Moslems and other persons who clearly had no contact with pigs.[28-30] Rats have been suggested as an alternative source of *B. coli*, and flies suggested as mechanical vectors.[31-37] The only two reported epidemics of balantidiasis have occurred in mental hospitals, where poor personal hygiene and coprophagy suggested person-to-person spread as the mode of transmission.[38,39]

Several years ago we had the opportunity to investigate a unique outbreak of balantidiasis on the islands of Truk, which may help clarify the epidemiology of this organism.[40] Situated among the Caroline Islands, Truk is part of the Trust Territory of the Pacific Islands, a United Nations trust territory administered by the U.S. The climate on Truk is tropical. The people live in close association with a variety of domestic animals, particularly pigs. Housing and sanitary facilities are rather primitive. Drinking water, which is not boiled or chlorinated before consumption, is obtained primarily by catchment from the roofs of houses. Alternative sources are springs or streams which are used for bathing and are contaminated by animals. Privies serve as toilet facilities, and children often defecate indiscriminately around their homes.

Medical care on Truk is provided at a central hospital and through a series of outlying dispensaries. The major public health problems are tuberculosis and infection with intestinal parasites. Although microbiology services are very limited, there is an active parasitology laboratory which examines approximately 100 stool specimens each week.

On May 1, 1971, a devastating typhoon swept through Truk with high winds and rainfall, causing extensive damage. Beginning in mid-May, the hospital laboratory reported a dramatic increase in the number of *B. coli* isolates, whereas the frequency of other intestinal parasites remained relatively constant (Figure 2). Analysis of laboratory records and procedures ruled out the possibility of a false epidemic. In fact, the laboratory reports of *B. coli* stool isolates represented the best source of epidemiologic information because of the language barrier (few Trukese people speak English) and primitive medical records and communications systems.

One hundred and ten persons developed proven *B. coli* infection for a crude overall attack rate of 11.8/1000. Cases occurred in all age groups with equal sex distribution and exhibited no geographic clustering. Clinical symptoms in *B. coli* patients were mild and nonspecific, and could not be distinguished from symptoms reported by a group of patients with intestinal parasites other than *B. coli* who served as controls.

The outbreak ended spontaneously by early July. The epidemic curve (Figure 3) suggested a common source of infection; secondary cases were not detected in the community at large or among family members of patients. Our stool surveys were performed during mid-June, well after the peak of the epidemic. No *B. coli* was detected in stools of 123 persons who were former *B. coli* patients, their household contacts, and other members of the community. The parasite was also not found in a few small water samples tested, although much of the damage to the catchment systems had been repaired by that time. By contrast *B. coli* was easily found in pig feces around the homes of several families.

We concluded that the epidemic probably resulted from widespread contamination of water supplies by pig feces. The typhoon caused extensive damage to the primitive catchment systems, forcing people to use the ground or surface facilities and thus promoting even closer contact with the pigs. Heavy rainstorms are relatively frequent on Truk, but typhoons are rare. There was little evidence for person-to-person transmission. The outbreak was multifocal in origin, with cases occurring simultaneously in widely separate geographic locations.

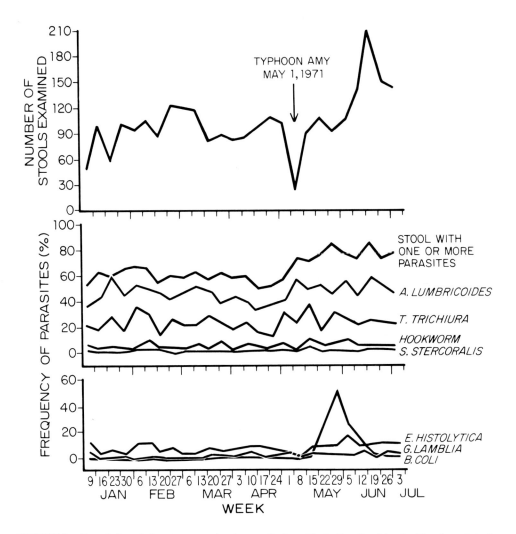

FIGURE 2.   Parasitology Laboratory examination results from Truk, Caroline Islands. (Number of stools examined, by week and frequency of parasites demonstrated, January 1 through July 1, 1971.)

The epidemic demonstrates that the Trukese people are normally quite resistant to porcine *B. coli* even when living in close association with pigs and under poor sanitary conditions. *B. coli* was found infrequently in the population before the outbreak and was absent in our stool survey afterward. Illness among infected persons was mild and self-limited. The brevity of the outbreak could reflect either this resistance of the population or the relatively rapid restoration of ecologic balance between people and the pigs.

This experience suggests fertile ground for future epidemiologic investigation. Further stool surveys of different geographic locations on Truk would be of interest. Studies comparing the population on Truk and New Guinea could be performed not only for *B. coli*, but also for other infections which can be acquired from pigs. Isolates of *B. coli* could be cultured in vitro for studies of antigenic properties and antibiotic sensitivities. The development of a reliable serologic test would provide valuable information about invasiveness of the organism.

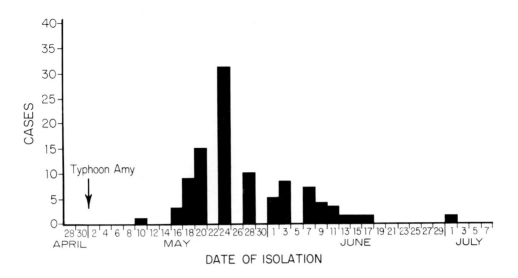

FIGURE 3. Epidemic curve balantidiasis outbreak on Truk, Caroline Islands. (Cases of balantidiasis, by date of laboratory isolation, April 28 through July 7, 1971.)

Pathology — Pathogenesis

B. coli is ordinarily a harmless commensal in pigs, but is a potential pathogen in man and other primates. The mechanism by which *B. coli* invades the intestinal mucosa in man is poorly understood. The organism produces a hyaluronidase-like substance which may aid the process once penetration is established.[41] As indicated previously, man is ordinarily quite resistant to *B. coli* infections. A number of host factors have been purported to enhance the development of *B. coli* infection: malnutrition (low protein, high carbohydrate diet); the status of the intestinal bacterial flora; concomitant helminthic infection, achlorhydria; alcoholism and other chronic, debilitating diseases.[7] These factors are nonspecific and could apply to infection with other intestinal protozoa as well.

The pathologic features of balantidiasis have been well described by Arean and Echevarria.[15] *B. coli* can invade anywhere along the colon, but most commonly involves the rectosigmoid area. Early lesions are small flask-shaped ulcers which, when more fully developed, resemble those produced by *Entamoeba histolytica.* The ulcers vary in number, and the mucosa surrounding them can be normal or inflamed. The ulcers have swollen, ragged borders, and are covered by friable, grayish, mucoid material. Ulcers may be superficial or penetrate completely through the intestinal wall.

Microscopically, *B. coli* may penetrate intact surface epithelium or epithelial crypts. At point of contact the epithelial cells shrink up and their cytoplasm becomes eosinophilic. The organism then invades the submucosa and the local lymphatic vessels. Lymphocytes, plasma cells, and eosinophils are produced as part of the host inflammatory response. With disruption of the epithelium, secondary bacterial infection presumably occurs, leading to an influx of neutrophils and the formation of submucosal abscesses. *B. coli* is often difficult to locate amidst this necrotic debris and is best seen at the leading edge or periphery of the ulcer.

B. coli occasionally involves the appendix, resulting in appendicitis; less commonly, the terminal ileum may be involved. Extraintestinal involvement is rare, and presumably results from direct extension from or perforation of the colon. Extraintestinal sites include the liver, lung, urinary tract, and vagina.[42,43] Whether this migration occurs before or after death is controversial. Of interest is the fact that Papanicolaou smears have demonstrated *B. coli* in peritoneal fluid of a patient with presumed peritonitis and on a routine cervicovaginal smear of another patient which probably resulted from fecal contamination.[44,45]

Clinical Features
Animals
   B. coli is considered to be a commensal organism of widespread distribution in pig populations. Rare occurrences of porcine clinical balantidiasis are manifested by mild to severe enteritis. Occasionally the parasite may invade the mucosa in pigs and cause deep ulcerations. Almejew reported acute infections in pigs.[46]

Balantidium is rarely reported from the dog, but Ewing and Bull cited a case of severe diarrhea in a dog associated with a *Balantidium-Trichuris vulpis* infection.[47] In other reported cases of canine balantidiasis cited by Ewing and Bull, access to hog carcasses or association with pigs was evident in the epidemiology of the dog infection.

In nonhuman primates, *B. coli* may cause clinical disease, especially among the great apes — chimpanzees, orangutans, and gorillas. A cause and effect relationship between *Balantidium* infection and diarrhea in apes is difficult to establish. The parasite has been recorded as a part of the "normal flora" of the primates in some cases, and in others has been determined to be the etiology of fatal infections.[48] Some idea of the prevalence of *B. coli* in primates has been furnished the authors by Dr. Harold McClure, Pathologist, Yerkes Primate Research Laboratory.[60] In an 11-year period, 49% (752 of 1521) of chimpanzee stools, 36% (333 of 928) of orangutan stools, 45% (89 of 198) of gorilla stools, and 26% (355 of 1367) of monkey stools were positive for *B. coli*. The results represent fecal samples examined, not individual animals, since over the 11-year period individual animals were examined a number of times. The specimens were submitted to the laboratory as part of the work on clinical diarrhea in animals.

Among lower animals, the guinea pig is universally infected with *B. caviae*, but clinical balantidiasis is virtually unknown. In the author's (GRH) laboratory, when guinea pigs are intracecally inoculated with pathogenic strains of *Entamoeba histolytica*, severe diarrhea and even death may occur in 10 to 14 days. Examination of the cecum shows myriads of *E. histolytica* and penetrating ulcers of the cecal wall, but the *B. caviae* are absent.

Man
   The clinical features of balantidiasis resemble those of intestinal amebiasis. Three types of *B. coli* infection have been described: asymptomatic, chronic (recurrent), and acute (dysenteric).[49] Asymptomatic *B. coli* infection is usually found in populations in which the parasite is endemic, such as among the people of New Guinea. The asymptomatic carrier is a public health threat as a potential source of infection to persons in certain occupations (for example, food handler), and in places such as mental institutions where there is crowding or poor sanitation and hygiene.

Chronic balantidiasis is characterized by recurrent episodes of diarrhea alternating with constipation. Symptoms include cramps, abdominal pain, and tenesmus. Bowel movements vary in number from a few to up to 15/day; stools are watery, contain mucus, but only rarely blood.[15] This condition may be protracted and can apparently last for years. Chronic weight loss, malnutrition, and debility can result.

Patients with acute balantidiasis complain of abdominal pain, nausea, vomiting, and tenesmus. As in the chronic form, fever is uncommon. Stools vary in number and are dysenteric (bloody). The peripheral blood leukocyte count is also variable, but marked leukocytosis is usually associated with secondary bacterial infection. A particularly fulminating form of acute *B. coli* infection occurs in patients with chronic debilitating diseases (such as cirrhosis). Here the onset is sudden, with severe toxic symptoms, fever of 38 to 38.5°C, and up to 25 bloody bowel movements a day. Frank intestinal hemorrhage can occur, with death resulting from exsanguination.

The prognosis of symptomatic balantidiasis depends on the balance between the intensity of the infection and status of host defenses. The chronic form is usually associated only with morbidity. Fulminating acute balantidiasis formerly had a case fatality of 30%. Death resulted from intestinal hemorrhage, perforation, or peritonitis. Appropriate antimicrobial and supportive treatment have considerably improved the prognosis, but deaths still occur. Correction of selected vitamin deficiencies (for example, administering ascorbic acid) has recently been suggested as an aid to treatment.[50] However, such studies are difficult to interpret without considering the entire nutritional status of the patient. *B. coli* patients are frequently infected with other intestinal protozoa, helminths, bacteria, viruses, as well as systemic diseases (for example, malaria, tuberculosis). These organisms complicate medical management and may well adversely affect recovery from *B. coli* infection.

Diagnosis

Infections with *B. coli* are usually easy to identify by applying standard, recommended procedures in examining stool specimens.[51] A portion of stool emulsified in 0.85% NaCl on a microscope slide is covered with a coverslip, and the preparation scanned at low power for the ciliated trophozoites which exhibit a rotary, boring motion. If motile trophozoites are not seen, cysts may be found. They are quite large and are often overlooked because of their size (45 to 65 μm in diameter). If fecal specimens are preserved in 10% formalin, the trophozoites may be mistaken for debris, artifacts, or eggs. The cytoplasm becomes coagulated, but the peripheral cilia and large kidney-shaped nucleus are usually visible. Since the organisms are so easily identifiable, use of stained slides or preservation in other than formalin is not necessary. If organisms are seen in freshly fixed-stained slides or PVA-fixed-stained slides, they may be overlooked because normal staining times generally overstain the cytoplasm, making internal differentiation difficult.

Treatment

The treatment of balantidiasis has been reviewed.[52] The infrequency of *B. coli* infection has made controlled clinical trials difficult. Of the many older homeopathic and toxic remedies, carbarsone emerged as the leading agent. Carbarsone has been replaced by tetracyclines, which are now generally considered to be the treatment of choice.[53] There is no convincing evidence that any one tetracycline preparation is superior. The usual dose of generic tetracycline is 500 mg qid × 10 days in adults and 10 mg/kg qid (max 2 g/day) in children.

Suitable alternative drugs include diiodohydroxyquin in adult dosage of 650 tid × 20 days and in pediatric dosage of 40 mg/kg/day (max 2 g/day) in three divided doses for 20 days; or paromomycin in adult or pediatric dosage of 25 to 35 mg/kg/day in three divided doses for 5 to 10 days.

Recent interest has focused on nitroimidazole derivatives. In vitro studies have shown that metronidazole and nitrimidazine are active against *B. coli*.[54-56] There is a possibility that human and porcine strains of *B. coli* may have different minimum inhibitory concentrations. Clinical studies have demonstrated the efficiency of nitroimidazoles in treating small numbers of patients with balantidiasis in several different parts of the world.[57-59] The largest study of metronidazole involved 20 patients divided among two treatment regimens: (1) children received 750 mg qd and adults 1.25 g qd for 10 days; (2) children received 500 mg qd and adults 1.0 g qd for 5 days. *B. coli* was eradicated in all instances.[53]

By contrast, metronidazole failed to cure three of five balantidiasis patients in the epidemic on Truk.[40] Two of these treatment failures were nonimmune Peace Corps volunteers. This limited experience raises the possibility that pathogenicity differs among different geographic strains of *B. coli,* and also suggests caution in using metronidazole. Further experience and controlled clinical trials are necessary before the place of metronidazole and related compounds in treating balantidiasis can be firmly established.

Prevention

Much more knowledge about *B. coli* and its public health importance is needed before appropriate preventive measures can be formulated. Application of modern techniques of in vitro culture, experimental transmission, and animal models would provide better data concerning the infectivity and pathogenicity of the organism. Comparative metabolic, immunologic, and drug sensitivity studies of human and animal strains of *B. coli* would be particularly valuable. Development of a serum antibody test for *B. coli* and further studies of populations living in contact with pigs would help clarify the epidemiologic role of the pig.

General preventive measures for *B. coli* are probably similar to those for *E. histolytica.* These include good personal hygiene and public sanitation (for example, properly disposing of feces and protecting drinking water from fecal contamination). Since the pig appears to be at least a potential source of human infection, abattoir workers and others who come in close contact with pigs should practice strict personal hygiene. This also applies to food handlers and patients and staff of mental institutions where the transmission of other parasites by the fecal-oral route has occurred. Travelers to countries endemic for *B. coli* or to tropical or developing nations where poor sanitary conditions exist should boil their drinking water and avoid uncooked fruit and vegetables.

REFERENCES

1. **Levine, N. D.**, *Protozoan Parasites of Domestic Animals and Man,* 2nd ed., Burgess Publishing, Minneapolis, 1973.
2. **Zaman, V.**, *Balatidium coli,* in *Parasitic Protozoa,* Vol. 2, Krier, J., Ed., Academic Press, New York, 1978, 633.
3. **Sargeant, P. C.**, The size range of *Balantidium coli, Trans. R. Soc. Med. Hyg.,* 65, 428, 1971.
4. **Faust, E. C., Russell, P. F., and Jung, R. C.**, The ciliate protozoa, *Craig and Faust's Clinical Parasitology,* 8th ed., Lea & Febiger, Philadelphia, 1970, 291.
5. **Svensson, R.**, On the resistance to heating and cooling of *Balantidium coli* in culture and some observations regarding conjugation, *Exp. Parasitol.,* 4, 507, 1955.
6. **Klaas, J.**, Two new gastric mucin cultivation media and a chemically defined maintenance medium for *Balantidium coli, J. Parasitol.,* 60, 907, 1974.
7. **Belding, D. L.**, The ciliata of man, in *Textbook of Parasitology,* 3rd ed., Appleton-Century-Crofts, New York, 1965.
8. **Levine, N. D.**, The ciliates, in *Protozoan Parasites of Domestic Animals and Man,* 2nd ed., Burgess Publ., Minneapolis, 1973, 351.
9. **Krishna, R. and Anjaneyulu, V.**, An outbreak of balantidiasis among buffaloes, *J. Commun. Dis.,* 6, 346, 1974.
10. **Krascheninnikow, S. and Jeska, E. L.**, Agar diffusion studies on the species specificity of *Balantidium coli, B. cariae* and *B. wenrichi, Immunology,* 4, 282, 1961.
11. **Zaman, V.**, The application of fluorescent antibody test to *Balantidium coli, Trans. R. Soc. Trop. Med. Hyg.,* 59, 79, 1965.
12. **Zaman, V.**, Studies on the immobilization reaction in the genus *Balantidium, Trans. R. Soc. Trop. Med. Hyg.,* 58, 255, 1964.
13. **Westphal, A.**, Experimentelle Infektion der Maus und des Meerschweinchens mig *Balantidium coli, Z. Tropenmed. Parasitol.,* 22, 138, 1971.

14. Woody, N. C. and Woody, H. B., Balantidiasis in infancy. Review of the literature and report of a case, *J. Pediatr.*, 56, 485, 1960.

15. Arean, V. M. and Echevarria, R., Balantidiasis, in *Pathology of Protozoal and Helminthic Diseases*, Marcial-Rojas, R. A., Ed., Wiliams & Wilkins, Baltimore, 1971, 234.

16. Stshensnovitsh, V., On the occurrence of *Balantidium coli* and other intestinal protozoa in man, *Med. Parazitol. (Mosk.)*, 10, 252, 1941.

17. Biagi, F., Unusual isolates from clinical material — *Balantidium coli*, *Ann. N.Y. Acad. Sci.*, 174, 1023, 1970.

18. Arean, V. C. and Koppisch, E., Balantidiasis. A review and report of cases, *Am. J. Pathol.*, 32, 1089, 1970.

19. van der Hoeven, J. A. and Rijpstra, A. C., Intestinal parasites in the Central Mountain District of Netherlands New-Guinea. An important focus of *Balantidium coli*, *Doc. Med. Geogr. Trop.*, 9, 225, 1957.

20. Couvee, L. M. J. and Rijpstra, A. C., The prevalence of *Balantidium coli* in the Central Highlands of Western New-Guinea, *Trop. Geogr. Med.*, 13, 284, 1961.

21. Vines, A. P. and Kelly, A., Highlands survey of intestinal parasites, *Med. J. Aust.*, 2, 635, 1966.

22. Radford, A., Balantidiasis in Papua, New Guinea, *Med. J. Aust.*, 1, 238, 1973.

23. Ostroumov, V. G., Materials on the problem of identity of *Balantidium suis* and *B. coli*, *Med. Parazitol. (Mosk.)*, 15, 43, 1946.

24. Dzbenski, T., In search for balantidiasis, *Bull. Inst. Mar. Med. Gdansk*, 15, 137, 1964.

25. Westphal, A., Experimental infection of guinea pig with *Balantidium coli.*, *Z. Tropenmed. Parasitol.*, 8, 288, 1957.

26. Knowles, R. and Gupta, B. M. D., Some observations on *Balantidium coli* and *Entamoeba histolytica* of macaques, *Ind. Med. Gaz.*, 69, 390, 1934.

27. Young, M. D., Attempts to transmit human *Balantidium coli*, *Am. J. Trop. Med.*, 30, 71, 1950.

28. Baskerville, L., Ahmed, Y., and Ramchand, S., Balantidium colitis, *Am. J. Dig. Dis.*, 15, 727, 1970.

29. McCarey, A. G., Balantidiasis in South Persia, *Br. Med. J.*, 1, 629, 1952.

30. Forsyth, D. M., Balantidiasis, *Lancet*, 1, 628, 1954.

31. Browne, S. G., Un cas mortel de dysenterie balantidienne, *Ann. Soc. Belg. Med. Trop.*, 37, 341, 1957.

32. Netik, J., Lariviere, M., and Quenum, G., Un cas de dysenterie balantidienne mortelle, *Bull. Med. AOF*, 3, 136, 1958.

33. Awakian, A., Studies on the intestinal protozoa of rats. II. Rats as carriers of Balantidium, *Trans. R. Soc. Trop. Med. Hyg.*, 31, 93, 1937.

34. Bogdanovich, V. V., Spontaneous balantidiasis in rats, *Med. Parazitol. (Mosk.)*, 24, 326, 1965.

35. Tsuchiya, T. and Kenamore, B., Report on a case of balantidiasis, *Am. J. Trop. Med.*, 25, 513, 1945.

36. Kennedy, C. C. and Stewart, R. C., Balantidial dysentery: a human case in Northern Ireland, *Trans. R. Soc. Trop. Med. Hyg.*, 51, 549, 1957.

37. Cockburn, T. A., Balantidium infection associated with diarrhoea in primates, *Trans. R. Soc. Trop. Med. Hyg.*, 42, 291, 1948.

38. Young, M. D., Balantidiasis, *JAMA*, 113, 580, 1939.

39. Ferri, L. V., Contribution to the epidemiology of balantidiasis, *Med. Parazitol., (Mosk.)*, 11, 108, 1942.

40. Walzer, P. D., Judson, F. N., Murphy, K. B., Healy, G. R., English, D. K., and Schultz, M. G., Balantidiasis outbreak in Truk, *Am. J. Trop. Med. Hyg.*, 22, 33, 1973.

41. Tempelis, C. H. and Lysenko, M. G., The production of hyaluronidase by *Balantidium coli*, *Exp. Parasitol.*, 6, 31, 1957.

42. Wegner, F., Abscesso hepatico producido por el *Balantidium coli*, *Kasmera*, 2, 433, 1967.

43. Cespedes, R., Rodrigues, D., Valverde, O., Fernandez, J., Gonzales, U. F., and Java, P., Balantidiosis: estudio de un caso anatomicoclinico marivo con lesiones y pustencia del parasito en el intestino delgado y pleuro, *Acta. Medica Costarricense*, 10, 35, 1967.

44. Lahiri, V. L., Elhence, B. R., and Agarual, B. M., Balantidium peritonitis diagnosed on cytologic material, *Acta Cytol.*, 21, 123, 1977.

45. Norman, J. G. and Jessop, P., *Balantidium coli* in a cervico-vaginal smear, *Med. J. Aust.*, 1, 694, 1973.

46. Almejew, C., Propagation of balantidium in the porcine intestine, *Mich. Vet. Med.*, 18, 250, 1963.

47. Ewing, S. and Bull, R., Severe chronic canine diarrhea associated with *Balantidium-Trichuris* infection, *J. Am. Vet. Med. Assoc.*, 149, 519, 1966.

48. Ruch, T. C., *Diseases of Laboratory Primates*, W. B. Saunders, Philadelphia, 1959.

49. Swartzwelder, J. C., Balantidiasis, *Am. J. Dig. Dis.*, 17, 173, 1950.

50. Khamstov, V. G., Disturbance of ascorbic acid and balance in patients with balantidiasis, *Med. Parazitol. (Mosk.)*, 42, 443, 1973.

51. **Melvin, D. and Brooke, M.,** Laboratory Procedures for the Diagnosis of Intestinal Parasites, Center for Disease Control, Atlanta, 1974.
52. **Steck, B. A.,** Chemotherapy of balantidiasis, in The Chemotherapy of Protozoan Diseases, Walter Reed Army Institute of Research, Washington, D.C., 1972.
53. **Anon.,** The Medical Letter on Drugs and Therapeutics Handbook of Antimicrobial Therapy, Medical Letter, New Rochelle, New York, 1978.
54. **Zaman, V. and Natarajan, P. N.,** *In vitro* trials of metronidazole against *Balantidium coli, Trans. R. Soc. Trop. Med. Hyg.,* 63, 152, 1969.
55. **Zrubec, J.,** Effect of metronidazole and paramomycin (Humatin) on *Balantidium coli* in in vitro and in vivo experiments, *Cas. Lek. Cesk.,* 110, 712, 1971.
56. **Carneri, I.,** Isolation of *Balantidium coli* in culture and speed of action of metrinidazine and metronidazole, *Rev. Inst. Med. Trop. S. Paulo,* 14, 321, 1972.
57. **Zrubec, J.,** Balantidiaza u deti ajej liecba metronidazolom, *Bratisl. Lek. Listy,* 47, 235, 1967.
58. **Delgado, Y., Garnica, R., and Britolugo, P.,** Balantidiacis in Mexico City, *Rev. Invest. Salud Pub.,* 31, 106, 1971.
59. **Biagi, F.,** Metronidazole in the treatment of balantidiasis., *Trans. R. Soc. Trop. Med. Hyg.,* 67, 43, 1972.
60. **McClure, H.,** unpublished information.

GIARDIASIS

Ernest A. Meyer and Edward L. Jarroll

Disease

In the Western hemisphere and in Western Europe, *giardiasis* and *Giardia enteritis* are names used to describe human disease caused by protozoa in the genus *Giardia*. In eastern Europe and the U.S.S.R., the disease is called *lambliasis*.[1] Hiker's diarrhea is the term employed to describe giardiasis acquired by ingestion of untreated water in unpopulated areas of western North America. *Traveler's diarrhea*[2,3] or *turista* is a clinical syndrome which can be caused by any of a number of organisms; although most frequently it is caused by enterotoxigenic strains of the bacterium *Escherichia coli*, some cases of this disease are caused by organisms in the genus *Giardia*.[3]

Giardiasis and *lambliasis* are the names commonly used to describe animal disease caused by members of this genus.

In this review, we shall use *giardiasis* to signify infection, whether symptomatic or asymptomatic, of the vertebrate host by organisms in the genus *Giardia*.

Etiologic Agent

All of the organisms in the genus *Giardia* are protozoan parasites of the intestine of vertebrate hosts; they occur in a trophozoite and a cyst form. All have a life cycle (Figure 1) in which the flagellated, binucleate trophozoites reside in the upper two thirds (the duodenum and jejunum) of the host's small intestine, where they attach by means of an adhesive disk to the epithelium and divide by binary fission. Encystation occurs as the organisms traverse the intestinal tract. Although the newly formed cyst contains two nuclei, each nucleus in the cyst undergoes one further division, so that the mature cyst contains four nuclei. The trophozoite to cyst transformation takes place in the intestinal tract; excreted trophozoites disintegrate. The cycle proceeds when the cyst, the transfer form of the organism, is ingested by a suitable vertebrate host. Passage through the stomach initiates the process of excystation, which is completed in the small intestine with the emergence from the cyst of a motile quadrinucleate organism which promptly completes the division process, yielding two binucleate trophozoites.

The genus and species nomenclature of these organisms is in a state of confusion. We will refer to these organisms here by the genus name *Giardia*, although the same organisms are frequently placed in the genus *Lamblia* in the literature of eastern Europe and the Soviet Union. Several investigators who have studied the genus status of these protozoa have concluded that the name *Giardia* has precedence.[4,5]

Giardia spp. nomenclature is confused because some of the criteria on which species designations are based have been shown to be invalid. The three principal criteria which have been used as the basis for *Giardia* speciation have been host specificity, various body dimensions, and variations in structure.[5]

Giardia are among the most widely distributed of the intestinal protozoan parasites of animals. Apparently on the assumption that these organisms were highly host specific, workers often assigned *Giardia* spp. status primarily on the basis of the animal host from which these parasites were recovered. There is evidence which indicates that at least some of the *Giardia* are capable of parasitizing more than one animal host species.[6-8]

Literature reports of new *Giardia* spp. often include, in addition to the species of the infected host, descriptions of the morphology and dimensions of the trophozoites and cysts. On the basis of such reports, at least 40 *Giardia* spp. have been proposed.[9,10]

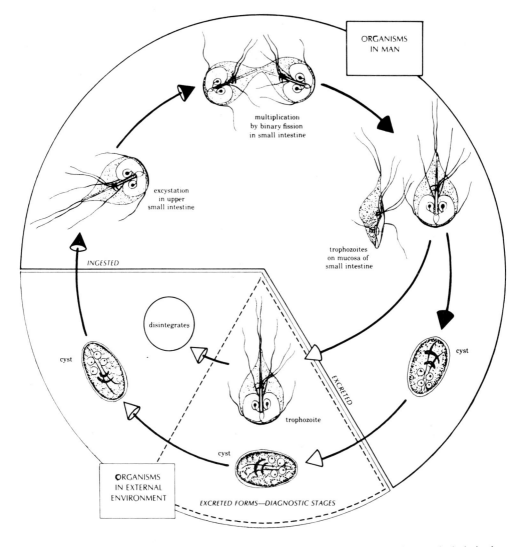

FIGURE 1.   Life cycle of *Giardia* in the human host. Note the double median bodies, particularly in the cyst form, which are typical of the *G. duodenalis* type and which resemble the claw of a claw hammer. Indistinguishable organisms parasitize a variety of vertebrate hosts and have the same type of life cycle. Some *Giardia* have been shown to be capable of parasitizing more than one vertebrate host species (see text). (Reproduced from E. A. Meyer, *Microorganisms and Human Disease,* Appleton-Century-Crofts, New York, 1974. With permission.)

Unfortunately, many of these organisms cannot be distinguished morphologically from *Giardia* described from other animal species. While the apparently unique dimensions of some of these organisms would seem to justify their being considered distinct, the observation that trophozoite size is subject to considerable variation, even during the course of a single infection[11] and under such influences as changes of diet,[12] casts doubt on the wisdom of using the dimensions of *Giardia* as a species criterion. Staining procedures are also known to affect the measured size of these organisms.[13]

Filice,[5] in a monograph published in 1952, addressed this problem by measuring, then statistically comparing, the body dimensions of *Giardia* trophozoites from different animal species. He concluded that the use of differences in body dimensions of these organisms and of host specificity were untrustworthy species criteria. Filice[5] then suggested a conservative approach to the problem; he proposed basing *Giardia* spp.

designations primarily on structural differences. The organelle which occurs in *Giardia* and which Filice proposed using as the basis for speciation is the median body, a microtubular structure, not bounded by a membrane, whose function is presently unknown. Filice proposed recognizing only three *Giardia* species, as follows:

1. *Giardia duodenalis,* whose single or double median body somewhat resembles the claw of a claw hammer. These organisms have been isolated from man, other mammals including rodents, and birds and reptiles.
2. *Giardia muris,* with two small rounded median bodies in the center of the organism. Rodents, birds, and reptiles have been shown to be hosts for this morphological type of *Giardia.*
3. *Giardia agilis,* with long, teardrop-shaped median bodies. Whereas the adhesive disk of the other two proposed species is of the order of half the trophozoite body length, the *Giardia agilis* adhesive disk approximates one fifth the body length of these organisms. Organisms of the *Giardia agilis* type have only been described from amphibian hosts.

Filice[5] also suggested assigning nontaxonomic status, such as race, to related forms of *Giardia* presently considered species on the basis of size or host. New *Giardia* species can be recognized when and if significant differences in the physiology or body dimensions of these organisms become evident.

Since by definition a zoonotic organism is one which can infect both man and vertebrate animals, it follows that the zoonotic *Giardia* are confined to those organisms classified as *Giardia duodenalis* by Filice.[5]

The *Giardia* described from humans may be found in the literature identified variously as *Giardia lamblia,*[14] *Giardia duodenalis,*[5] *Giardia intestinalis,*[10] and *Lamblia intestinalis.*[15] We will use the term *Giardia* hereafter in this review without species designation, to refer to those potentially zoonotic representatives of this genus (that is, *Giardia duodenalis,* as described by Filice[5]). Consensus regarding *Giardia* spp. nomenclature seems unlikely until further data are available.

True and Alternate Hosts

The list in Table 1 includes those described *Giardia* spp. which have been determined to belong to the same morphological group as the *Giardia* isolated from human infections. It is not known whether all of these organisms are capable of infecting man. However, the fact that at least some of them have been reported to be transmitted from animals to man or vice versa, or have been transmitted from one vertebrate species to another[8] suggests that none of these organisms can be excluded at this state of our knowledge from consideration as possible causes of human infection.

Given the presently known widespread occurrence of these protozoan flagellates among vertebrate species, it would not be surprising to find *Giardia* to be intestinal inhabitants of *any* vertebrate species whose parasites are studied in detail. Whether *Giardia* of this morphologic type should be classified as one, or as more than one, species remains an unresolved issue which can only be settled when more information becomes available. Until statistically valid differences can be demonstrated among these organisms, however, it would seem prudent to adopt Filice's view,[5] namely to consider all *Giardia* of this morphologic type as representatives of a single species and to consider host or size differences in these parasites as the basis for race designations.

Distribution

It is difficult to imagine that any global region is free from human or animal infections with *Giardia.* In humans such infections have been reported in countries from

Table 1
ANIMAL SPECIES REPORTED TO BE
HOSTS FOR *GIARDIA* OF THE
DUODENALIS TYPE

Animal host	*Giardia* spp.	Ref.
Man	*Giardia lamblia*	14
Monkeys	*Giardia duodenalis*	5
(14 different	*Giardia intestinalis*	9,10
species)	*Lamblia intestinalis*	15
Slendor loris	*Giardia wenyoni*	16
Ox	*Giardia bovis*	17
Goat, sheep	*Giardia caprae*	18
Three-toed sloth	*Giardia bradypi*	19
Dog	*Giardia canis*	20
Badger, raccoon		21
Cat, domestic &	*Giardia cati (Giardia felis)*	
wild, lion,		
& civet cat		22-24
Palm civet	*Giardia dasi*	16
Rabbit	*Giardia duodenalis*	25
Ground squirrel	*Giardia beckeri*	26
Guinea pig	*Giardia caviae*	27
Chinchilla	*Giardia chinchillae*	5
Vole	*Giardia microti*	28
Muskrat	*Giardia ondatrae*	29
Irara	*Giardia irarae*	30
Field vole	*Giardia pitymysi*	31
Norway rat	*Giardia simoni*	32
Viszcacha	*Giardia viscachae*	33
American bittern	*Giardia botauri*	29
Redbacked shrike	*Giardia marginalis*	9,34
Avocet	*Giardia recurvirostrae*	9,34
Varan	*Giardia varani*	33
Budgerigar	*Giardia duodenalis,* race psittaci	135

the tropics[35,36] to the arctic.[37] Many recent outbreaks have also been described from the U.S. and abroad.[3,38-44] Historic accounts of the distribution of *Giardia* in man can be found in reviews by Petersen[45] and Ansari.[46] In these reviews, the prevalence of human giardiasis in the world ranged from 1.1 to 12.5%; higher percentages were seen in some localities.

A recent report from the Centers for Disease Control (CDC, Atlanta, Ga.)[47] summarized the results of fecal examinations performed by state and territorial health departments in the U.S. This summary showed that as few as 1.1% of the human fecal specimens submitted in Virginia were positive for *Giardia* while as many as 16.7% of those submitted in Arkansas were positive. In the U.S., an average of 3.9% of 332,312 fecal specimens examined were positive for *Giardia*, and no state was free from infected individuals. Thus *Giardia* was the most commonly identified, pathogenic intestinal parasite in the U.S.[47] A similar report from the U.K.[48] dubbed *Giardia* the most commonly encountered intestinal parasite there as well.

Little literature exists regarding the endemicity of *Giardia* in lower animals. Perhaps this can be attributed to the belief that *Giardia* are host specific and, therefore, not likely to serve as reservoir hosts for human infections. Much recent evidence suggests that this view is changing.

One survey of giardiasis in chinchillas[49] was based on a population of caged, paired chinchillas in Georgia. It was found that about 21% of these pairs were positive for *Giardia*.

In other rodents, Haiba[50] stated that 26% of the brown rats in his studies were infected with *Giardia*, but that none of the black rats were infected. He also found that 22% of the wood mice harbored *Giardia* while no infections were detected among wild mice. In a more recent study, Grant and Woo[13] examined numerous laboratory and wild rodents in Ontario, Canada. In their study, they showed that 98.8% of the meadow voles and 99.0% of the deer mice were infected with *Giardia*. Grant and Woo[13] also found that all of their laboratory rats and golden hamsters were infected with *Giardia* when they arrived from the suppliers. These studies were based on examination of intestinal scrapings and may prove to be more accurate than studies based solely on the examination of fecal specimens. It should be emphasized that not all infected animals or humans shed cysts in their feces regularly[35,51-53] and occasionally *Giardia* infections may go undiagnosed because of undetectable numbers of cysts in the feces.

Burrows and Hunt[54] found that 2.5% of 757 stray domestic cats in central New Jersey were positive for *Giardia* cysts in their feces, and Davies and Hibler[7] found one of the four cats that they examined in Colorado had a *Giardia* infection.

Studies on the prevalence of *Giardia* in dogs have reported the parasite in as few as 0.5% of the German shepherds at a U.S. Army Dog Training Center in Colorado[55] to as many as 36% of the stray dogs in central New Jersey.[56] A recent review by Barlough[57] summarizes surveys of *Giardia* prevalence in dogs from the U.S., Canada, and Europe; the range of prevalences outside the U.S. is similar to those in the U.S.

Davies and Hibler[7] summarized an extensive survey of fecal specimens from a variety of wild and domestic animals in Colorado. They reported that 18% of the beavers, 6% of the coyotes, and 10% of the cattle were infected with *Giardia*.

Clearly, there exists a paucity of studies on the prevalence of *Giardia* in asymptomatic humans and animals. With the realization that at least some animals may serve as reservoir hosts for human giardiasis, more studies are required to assess accurately the endemicity of *Giardia* in animals generally and to determine the extent to which the cross-infection of *Giardia* among different species can occur.

Disease in Animals

Symptomatic giardiasis in both human and animal infections is often characterized by similar signs and symptoms. However, the course of the infection may vary greatly from one host species to another. Animals which have been reported to have symptomatic giardiasis include parakeets, chinchillas, mice, rats, oxen, goats, sheep, cats, dogs, monkeys, and man.[10] Rodents, which frequently exhibit symptomatic giardiasis, may be parasitized by either *Giardia duodenalis* or *G. muris* type organisms. Inasmuch as many of these reports fail to include a description of the *Giardia* type, we have included a discussion of this disease in rats and mice.

In parakeets giardiasis has been associated with high morbidity and mortality.[58] Infected birds may exhibit diarrhea, decreased food and water intake, and debility. Mortality among such parakeets may range from 20 to 50%. In fatal cases, Panigrahy et al.[58] examined smears from the intestinal mucosa of the birds and found a heavy *Giardia* trophozoite burden with mortality occurring even in the absence of bacterial, chlamydial, or viral infections.

In chinchillas Sachs[59] found *Giardia* trophozoites in the blood of an infected animal at autopsy. Shelton[49] observed signs similar to those found in parakeets when he infected chinchillas with *Giardia*. He noted that not all of the chinchillas became symptomatic, but that three of the four that did become symptomatic died. Among the symptoms, he observed diarrhea, anorexia and occasionally cessation of fecal elimination. In the three fatal cases, necrotic foci in the large bowel, fatty changes in the liver, hemorrhagic gastritis, and emaciation were evident; and, in two of these animals, *Pseudomonas* was isolated from the heart and kidneys. In the third case the tapeworm, *Hymenolepis,* was found in the intestine. Finding these other potential pathogens in addition to *Giardia* masks the identity of the etiological agent(s) in these cases. However, the possibilities must include *Giardia, Pseudomonas, Hymenolepis* viruses or some combination of these acting synergistically.

Most of the information presently available regarding *Giardia*-induced pathology in animals is based on studies of this infection in mice. Schneider[60] found that *Giardia muris* (synonym *Lamblia muris*) infections were more prevalent in younger mice than in older ones. He was, however, unable to find evidence of pathology even in mice heavily infected with *Giardia.* These findings are in direct opposition to those of a number of other workers.[61-63] Sebesteny[62] described mice infected with *Giardia* as being sluggish and having rough hair and enlarged abdomens, but lacking diarrhea. At autopsy he found that the small bowel had pale, translucent lesions, yellow or white watery fluid and large numbers of *Giardia* trophozoites. In some mice, he noted the presence of a pale liver and edematous pancreas.

Csiza and Abelseth[63] encountered an episode of protozoan enteritis among mice in a closed colony. The only protozoans found in the mice were *Giardia* and *Hexamita,* and the signs of the disease included diarrhea (mucoid and occasionally blood-tinged) with fetid odor, low morbidity rate, protracted course, and sporadic mortality. The disease appeared to be self-limiting in these animals. Csiza and Abelseth[63] attributed the outbreak to a change in the diet of the mice which triggered an imbalance in their gut flora. They believe that this alteration allowed massive proliferation of the protozoans normally present only in small numbers in the intestines of these mice.

In a paper by Roberts-Thomson et al.,[64] the mouse-*Giardia muris* system was proposed as a model with which to study human giardiasis. These investigators used outbred Swiss albino mice, apparently free of *Giardia* infection, and infected them with *G. muris* cysts. The number of trophozoites and cysts in the infected animals reached a peak within 5 to 14 days after cyst inoculation. Spontaneous clearing of the infection was observed in most of the animals within 21 to 28 days. These authors observed that the attainment of the maximum parasite burden in a mouse was independent of the number of cysts inoculated, but that the time required to attain the maximum parasite burden was dependent on the size of the inoculum. Such is likely to be the case in most, if not all, of the vertebrates that harbor *Giardia.* Stevens and Roberts-Thomson[65] noted that the mice in their model studies exhibited impaired weight gain, decreased villus to crypt ratios, and increased numbers of inflammatory cells in the lamina propria.

The ability or inability of an animal to clear *Giardia* infection spontaneously has been associated with strain differences among mice.[66-67] It was found that mice of strain C3H/He produced cysts at a relatively constant rate during the 10-week study while those of strains CBA/H, SJL, A/J, BALB/c, and DBA/2 showed a steady decline in cyst production after reaching an initial peak. Except for the C3H/He mice, all of the other strains showed greater resistance to reinfection with *G. muris.*

Studies using athymic (nude) mice,[67,68] have demonstrated the inability of immunosuppressed mice to resolve a *Giardia* infection spontaneously or to resist reinfection. Nude mice whose lymphoid systems were reconstituted with lymphoid cells from syngeneic, thymus-intact mice showed a progressive reduction in cyst numbers.[67] If the thymus-intact mice used had been previously exposed to *Giardia,* then clearing of the infection was accelerated.

Stevens and Frank[51] suggested the possibility that a humoral as well as a cellular immune response to *Giardia* infections occurs in mice. Using the mouse model of Roberts-Thomson et al.,[64] these workers attempted to show that female mice transfer immunity to their offspring. The immunity appeared to be conferred to the suckling mice via mother's milk rather than transplacentally. They did not rule out the possibility that both cellular and humoral (as secretory IgA) immunity were involved. Parenthetically, pregnant mice that had seemingly cleared their *Giardia* infection began producing cysts again just prior to delivery. The cyst production decreased after the sucklings were weaned. It was suggested that this could represent a migration of *Giardia*-sensitized lymphoid cells away from the small intestine and into mammary sites during lactation.[51] Another possibility, not discussed by these authors, could be that a relationship exists between hormonal changes in pregnant mice, and *Giardia* trophozoite proliferation and cyst production. Such a mechanism could serve to ensure perpetuation of the *Giardia* from one host generation to another.

Many reports, all supported by light micrographs, exist in the literature which suggest that *Giardia* may penetrate mucosal cells of the intestine as well as extraintestinal tissues of rodents.[59,69-74] Two groups of these workers[73,74] have studied mice concomitantly infected with *Giardia* and *Plasmodium*. They disagreed as to whether concomitant infection with *Plasmodium* increased the likelihood of tissue penetration by *Giardia*, but they agreed that tissue penetration by *Giardia* occurred. Questions such as (1) whether tissue invasion by *Giardia* was found only in compromised hosts, or (2) whether invasion was initiated by the *Giardia* alone, the *Giardia* and a synergist, or by another pathogen alone await further investigation. The interpretation of future investigations of cellular penetration by *Giardia* would be benefited by transmission electron micrographs.

Brightman and Slonka[75] described five cases of clinical giardiasis in domestic cats. They noted signs which included loss of weight, soft, mucoid stools, and the presence of split and unsplit fats in the feces.

Bemrick[76] and Johnson[77] suggested that dogs less than 1 year old are more likely to have symptomatic giardiasis than older dogs. Canine symptoms may include diarrhea with mucus and fats, anorexia, and listlessness. Complications from growth retardation to death have been reported in puppies with severe giardiasis.[78]

The clinical picture of symptomatic giardiasis in apes at a Kansas City, Mo. zoo[79] was quite similar to that seen in their human attendants who also contracted the disease. The signs observed were loose stools, diarrhea, and vomiting; no fatalities were reported. Presently, it is unknown if giardiasis in apes is self-limiting since in this case at least some chemotherapy was administered to the animals. Chemotherapy for the apes was suspended prior to completion of the course because administration of the drug proved to be very difficult. Despite the early cessation of treatment, no recurrence of symptoms was observed.

Disease in Man

Symptomatic giardiasis, although occurring less frequently than asymptomatic infections,[80] is commonly encountered and is often associated with epidemics.[38-44]

A multiplicity of signs and symptoms have been associated with giardiasis in humans, and a recent review discusses them at some length.[8] Among the more common signs and symptoms are epigastric pain and distress, abdominal pain, cramps, weight loss, diarrhea with foul-smelling flatus, loose stools, and steatorrhea.

In addition to the typical symptoms often associated with *Giardia* infection, other complications have been cited. Carroll et al.[81] linked a case of uveitis in a 9-year-old female to her *Giardia* infection. Although no direct connection between the giardiasis and the uveitis was demonstrated, the elimination of *Giardia* cysts from her feces and a slow, steady improvement in her uveitis followed antigiardial therapy.

Giardiasis has also been associated with hypersensitivities. Harris and Mitchell[82] described urticaria in a 16-year-old male with symptomatic *Giardia* infection. Both the urticaria and the giardiasis disappeared after quinacrine therapy.

Halstead and Sadun[83] noted an intolerance to mammalian meat in a 29-year-old male physician with giardiasis. These investigators kept a record of the patient's diet and the symptoms that he experienced during the course of his infection. They observed moderate to severe intestinal symptoms in the patient only when the meals included mammalian meat. Shrimp, swordfish, chicken, and vegetables did not precipitate a reaction. Treatment of the giardiasis relieved the hypersensitivity to the mammalian meat.

Goobar,[84] upon examining 66 children younger than 16, found inflammation of the synovial membranes of major joints in 42 of them and *Giardia* cysts in the feces of 62. Intestinal symptoms attributed to the *Giardia* were also observed. After quinacrine or metronidazole therapy, the intestinal and synovial symptoms abated.

Celiac-like syndrome, failure to thrive, and malabsorption have been attributed to more severe *Giardia* infections.[85-91] On the other hand, Carswell et al.[92] were unable to associate these severe complications with giardiasis. Rather, they found that the incidence of *Giardia* infection in children with and without celiac syndrome was essentially the same. Further, after comparing jejunal biopsies from 57 celiac patients with and without *Giardia* infection, they found that the patients with giardiasis had less severe histological changes than those without the disease. In a more recent study by Duncombe et al.,[93] a positive correlation was found between the severity of the villus atrophy and the severity of the diarrhea in patients harboring *Giardia.* They hypothesized that an immune response by the host rather than a direct toxic effect by the parasite could account for the villus atrophy.

Only two deaths have been attributed to giardiasis in humans. One of these was in Germany[94] and the other in Ireland.[95] Although *Giardia* was present in both patients, no evidence was presented that conclusively identified the lethal agents.

As discussed previously in the animal disease section, the incubation period before the onset of disease varies greatly from one individual to another. Generally, the incubation period is directly related to the number of viable cysts ingested, but may also depend on the immunologic and physiologic status of the host.

Invasion of cells and tissues by *Giardia* trophozoites has been described in humans[89,91,96,97] as well as in lower animals. However, unike the reports in lower animals, at least one of those from humans has included transmission electron micrographs[89] in addition to light micrographs.[91,96,97] The results obtained using transmission electron microscopy appear more convincing than those obtained from light microscopy alone.

Despite the numerous reports of histopathology and tissue invasion described in some cases of giardiasis, the existence of a well-defined immune response to this flagellate remains unproven. The presence of such a response can only be inferred. For example, individuals with gamma-globulin deficiencies, either partial or complete, are likely to exhibit more severe symptoms[98-101] than those who have normal gamma-globulin levels.

A number of hypotheses for the role of immunoglobulins have been proposed. In the jejunal lamina, for instance, the early immune response may be immunoglobulin IgM followed by IgA and IgG.[102] Additionally, Zinneman and Kaplan[103] compared serum IgA levels to those found in duodenal aspirates of ten patients with symptomatic giardiasis and ten control patients and found lowered IgA levels in patients with *Giardia.* However, McClelland et al.[105] maintained that the method Zinneman and Kaplan[103] used to collect the duodenal aspirates might have allowed for the dilution of the IgA in their samples.

The serum IgE level does not appear to be affected by the presence of *Giardia.*[106,107]

Numerous attempts have been made to demonstrate an immune response to *Giardia* infection in humans using serologic and skin testing techniques. Success in demonstrating serum antibodies to *Giardia* cysts or trophozoites has been reported using immunofluorescence,[108,109] immunodiffusion,[110] complement fixation,[111] and intradermal skin tests.[112] Without exception, these investigators relied on trophozoites from duodenal contents or cysts from human feces as a source of antigen for their tests. Thus, nonspecific antigens, which were undoubtedly present in these crude antigen preparations, make the results of the tests questionable. Clearly, these experiments would have benefited from a consistent supply of antigen free from contamination. Such a source of trophozoite antigen is now available using axenically cultured trophozoites,[113,114] but a source of pure cyst antigen is still lacking.

The role of immunity in *Giardia* infections could be more clearly elucidated by the development of an appropriate animal model for the disease. While the *Giardia muris* mouse model of Roberts-Thomson et al.[64] has yielded promising results, the inability to cultivate *G. muris* in vitro is a serious stumbling block. Thus separation of the *G. muris* trophozoites from other murine gut contents remains the only means by which ample quantities of antigen may be collected.[115] Another concern might be the fact that *G. muris* is morphologically and probably physiologically distinct from *Giardia duodenalis* and the immune response(s) elicited against the former may differ from the response(s) elicited against the latter.

General Mode of Transmission

The life cycle of *Giardia*, as that of many intestinal protozoans, is simple and direct (Figure 1) and includes a trophozoite and cyst form (see Section on Etiologic Agent). The chemical nature of the cyst wall, the stimulus for its production and the mechanism by which it is produced remain a mystery. However, the importance of the cyst to *Giardia* survival outside the host and transmission to another host is clear. Survival of the *Giardia* in the external environment is due to the resistant nature of their cysts,[116,117] and infection of a suitable host occurs upon ingestion of viable cysts.

Transmission of the *Giardia* cyst from one host to another is usually accomplished by the fecal-oral route. In humans, fingers and food contaminated with feces seem to be a common means of infection. Evidence is increasing that drinking water may also be a common mode of infection. Numerous outbreaks of giardiasis associated with drinking water have been reported in recent years (see the following Section).

Similar modes of infection must also be considered likely in animals. Additionally, the intimate association of young animals with parents and the increased possibility that the lactating mother is excreting cysts[51] could improve the chance of the offspring being infected via a direct fecal-oral route.

Venereal transmission of *Giardia* as a possible mode of infection has gained recognition in recent years. Numerous case histories point to oral-anal sexual activity as the route of infection, especially among male homosexuals (see the following Section).

Epidemiology

The circumstances in which *Giardia* organisms are spread are similar to those of a number of other organisms which are excreted in the feces of one vertebrate host and ingested by another host. The traditional concept of giardiasis in humans thus is that of a disease which is particularly prevalent where standards of sanitation are in need of improvement. Although infection with this organism is world-wide, its incidence is usually greater in developing countries,[35] in the tropics,[35] and in day-care facilities.[36,118,120] The disease occurs in persons of all ages, with greatest incidence in infants and children; this may be because those in this age group are least likely to (1) have acquired an active immune response, and (2) exercise adequate hygienic care. The transfer of *Giardia* from host to host in warmer climates must be relatively direct since it is known that temperature affects *Giardia* cyst survival: at 21°C, *Giardia* cysts survived 5 to 24 days, while at 37°C cysts were never observed to survive more than 4 days.[117]

In recent years it has become evident that giardiasis can be spread in epidemic form in humans in temperate and cold climates and that the vehicle of spread is drinking water. The observation that some of the suspect water was more likely to have been polluted by animal than human excreta raised the possibility, not widely considered before that time, that humans might be subject to infection by *Giardia* not only from other humans but from other vertebrates as well. The observation was strengthened when evidence was presented that *Giardia* from one vertebrate species would infect another species and that human to animal transmission, and animal to human transmission of these infections was possible.[7,8,121] The finding that some *Giardia* cysts would survive in cold (8°C) water for upwards of 70 days increases the chances that cold drinking water, once contaminated with cysts, can serve as a successful vehicle for transmitting this disease to a new host. Although the suspect animal sources of epidemic waterborne giardiasis include any vertebrate species which harbors *Giardia* of the appropriate type and whose feces reach drinking water, animals which spend at least part of their time in water are considered prime candidates. *Giardia*-infected beaver and muskrat in the affected watersheds are deemed likely sources of human disease.[43]

Waterborne giardiasis has been reported in North America from New York State,[39] New Hampshire,[40] Pennsylvania,[44] Colorado,[44] Utah,[41] Oregon,[44] and Washington State.[43,122] Other outbreaks have been documented in Leningrad, U.S.S.R.,[42,123] the Mediterranean,[124] and the island of Madeira.[38]

In recent years, a number of reports have appeared which suggest that giardiasis may be spread from person to person as a result of sexual activity particularly among homosexuals.[121]

Animal to animal spread of this infection is presumably through ingestion of fecal material or by ingestion of water contaminated by other animals. The fact that it is the young of the species, whether human or other vertebrate, that is more likely to have symptomatic giardiasis, suggests that the infection is often acquired early in life and at a time when the host is unlikely to have active immunity against the causative organisms.

Diagnosis

The usual initial procedure employed to diagnose giardiasis is the demonstration of the causative organisms, either in the cyst or the trophozoite form, in the host's excreta.[125,126] Cysts are more likely to be found in a formed stool; trophozoites, in a diarrheic one. Trophozoites with their typical "falling leaf" motility are more likely to be seen if the specimen is fresh (not more than a few hours old). Since cyst excretion is not continuous but periodic, and since some infected hosts never excrete large numbers of cysts,[35] repeated stool examinations may be necessary to confirm diagnosis. The examination of three fecal samples obtained at 48 hr intervals will successfully yield organisms in 90% or more cases of giardiasis.[127,128] In addition to examination of fresh, unconcentrated material, concentration of fecal specimens may be necessary to detect organisms in light infections.

In humans whose undiagnosed disease is suggestive of giardiasis, but whose stools are consistently negative for the causative organisms, diagnosis may require obtaining and identifying motile trophozoites in specimens from the upper small intestine. Duodenal intubation or biopsy may be used for this purpose.[126,128] Because of the difficulty in using these procedures, particularly in the young, another diagnostic device, called the Enterotest, may be used.[128,129] This consists of a nylon thread about a meter long attached to a weight and embedded in a gelatin capsule. Holding the free end of the string, the patient swallows the capsule and as the gelatin dissolves the string unwinds. After an hour or more the thread is fully extended and part of it is in the jejunum. Trophozoites, if present, attach to the thread just as they attach to intestinal epithelium. The thread is gently retrieved and some of the fluid attached to it is transferred to a microscope slide and examined. In a recent study it was reported that the rate of positive diagnoses using the Enterotest device was the same as that when duodenal intubation was employed.[130] The use of purgatives has been found not to increase the rate of parasite excretion.[35]

Although no serologic method for diagnosing giardiasis is presently available, experimental efforts directed at perfecting such a test are under way. Visvesvara and Healy[131] reported studying the use of an indirect immunofluorescent test for diagnosing giardiasis. As antigen, axenically grown *Giardia* trophozoites originally isolated from a human were used. The anti-*Giardia* antibody content in 108 sera from patients with symptomatic and asymptomatic giardiasis and of 53 normal sera was determined. They reported positive, reproducible titers in two thirds of the patients; none of the 53 control sera yielded a response considered positive. They believe that lack of sensitivity is a major drawback of the indirect immunofluorescent test; although no false positives were detected, the test failed to demonstrate a number of known cases of giardiasis. The explanation of failure to demonstrate antibodies in these patients, as in some cases of amebiasis, may stem from the fact that in both instances, infection may occur with little if any invasion and subsequent stimulation of the antibody mechanism.

In small animals the repeated examination of stool specimens is presently the only practical method of diagnosing giardiasis; in larger animals, intubation or duodenal biopsies may be attempted.

Prevention and Control

Prevention of giardiasis in human populations is difficult at best. In areas of the world where sanitation and personal hygiene are poor, major improvements in water treatment, sewage disposal, and personal habits would be necessary. Since the prevalence of giardiasis is highest among infants and young children,[132] preventing spread of this disease by correcting poor personal hygiene may be difficult.

At present, there are no vaccines or oral medications that can be used as prophylaxis against *Giardia* infection. However, the Centers for Disease Control has published measures designed for travelers that can lower the risk of acquiring giardiasis as well as other gastrointestinal diseases.[133] Included among these are cooking food and peeling raw fruits and vegetables before they are eaten.

Boiling water kills *Giardia* cysts immediately,[117] but when this is impractical or impossible, some chemical disinfection methods are available.[116] Disinfectants containing chlorine (Halazone®; Bleach) and iodine (Globaline; Emergency Drinking Water Germicidal Tablets, (Coghlan, Ltd.); tincture of iodine; saturated iodine solutions) were tested in the laboratory under conditions approximating those which might be encountered in practice.[116] Water was treated with each disinfectant as specified by the label directions or the article describing the method. Halazone® and Emergency Drinking Water Germicidal Tablets were effective under all of the conditions tested while the others had some deficiencies. The reader should be cautioned that some halogen-containing disinfectants have a limited shelf life, especially after the container is opened. Thus only fresh disinfecting agents should be used. Furthermore, because *Giardia* cysts survive longer in cold than in warm water, and because more halogen is required to kill cysts in cold than in warm water,[116] special care must be taken to follow label directions regarding water temperature when disinfecting drinking water in climates where the water temperature may be below 10°C.

Freezing water has been shown to destroy most *Giardia* cysts;[117] however, some cysts survived for several days at −13°C. These findings suggest that ice may serve as a source of infection, and that water used to make ice for cooling drinks should be treated before it is frozen.

In the above experiments, the effect of boiling, freezing, or chemically treating water containing *Giardia* cysts was assessed by using the inability of *Giardia* to excyst in vitro as the criterion of cyst destruction. There is no evidence that proves conclusively that cysts which are incapable of in vitro excystation are also incapable of infecting an animal.

Domestic animals such as dogs and cats harbor *Giardia* of the *duodenalis* type,[20,22] and may have symptomatic disease.[75-78] Since humans, especially children, often have close personal contact with these domestic animals, it seems logical that treatment of pets infected with *Giardia* would help prevent animal to human transmission of the organism. Successful treatment of various animals has been reported using metronidazole,[57,77,79] and quinacrine hydrochloride.[75] According to Johnson,[77] metronidazole is the drug of choice for treating canine giardiasis. Treatment of livestock should be on a herd basis.

The drug of choice for treating human giardiasis is quinacrine hydrochloride;[134] an alternative is metronidazole.[134] The latter is contraindicated for treating pregnant women; it has been shown to be carcinogenic in rodents and mutagenic in bacteria.[134] Furazolidone has been recommended for treating small children because it is available in a suspension; its cure rate (80%), however, is not as high as that of quinacrine.[126]

REFERENCES

1. **Benenson, A. S.,** *Control of Communicable Diseases in Man,* The American Public Health Association, Washington, D.C., 1975, 129.
2. **Babb, R., Peck, O., and Vescia, F.,** Giardiasis: a cause of traveler's diarrhea, *JAMA,* 217, 1359, 1971.
3. **Merson, M. H., Morris, G. K., Sack, D. A., Wells, J. G., Feeley, J. C., Sack, R. B., Creech, W. B., Kapikian, A. Z., and Gangarosa, E. J.,** Traveler's diarrhea in Mexico, *N. Engl. J. Med.,* 294, 1299, 1976.
4. **Dobell, C.,** Vilem Lambl (1824—1895), a portrait and a biographical note, *Parasitology,* 32, 122, 1940.
5. **Filice, F.,** Studies on the cytology and life history of a *Giardia* from the laboratory rat, *Univ. Calif. Publ. Zool.,* 57, 53, 1952.
6. **Grant, D. and Woo, P. T.,** Comparative studies of *Giardia* spp. in small mammals in Southern Ontario. II. Host specificity and infectivity of stored cysts, *Can. J. Zool.,* 56, 1360, 1978.
7. **Davies, R. B. and Hibler, C. F.,** Animal reservoirs and cross-species transmission of *Giardia,* in EPA Symp. Waterborne Giardiasis, EPA Publ. 600/9-79-001, Jakubowski, W. and Hoff, J. C., Eds., Environmental Protection Agency, Cincinnati, 1978.
8. **Meyer, E. A. and Radulescu, S.,** *Giardia* and Giardiasis, in *Advances in Parasitology,* Academic Press, London, 17, 1979, 1.
9. **Ansari, M.,** Contribution a l'etude du genre *Giardia,* Kuntsler, 1882, (Mastigophora, Octomitidae), *Ann. Parasitol. Hum. Comp.,* 27, 421, 1952.
10. **Kulda, J. and Nohynkova, E.,** Flagellates of the human intestine and of intestines of other species, in *Protozoa of Veterinary and Medical Interest,* Vol. 2, Kreier, J. P., Ed., Academic Press, New York, 1978, 69.
11. **Tsuchiya, H.,** A comparative study of two diverse strains of *Giardia lamblia,* Stiles, 1915, *Am. J. Hyg.,* 12, 467, 1930.
12. **Tsuchiya H.,** Changes in morphology of *Giardia canis* as affected by diet, *Proc. Soc. Exp. Biol. N.Y.,* 28, 708, 1931.

13. **Grant, D. R. and Woo, P. T.,** Comparative study of *Giardia* spp. in small mammals in southern Ontario. I. Prevalence and identity of the parasite with a taxonomic discussion of the genus, *Can. J. Zool.,* 56, 1348, 1978.

14. **Lambl, W.,** Mikroskopische Untersuchungen der Darm-Excrete, *Vierteljahresschr. Prakt. Hei. Praug.,* 61, 1, 1859.

15. **Blanchard, R.,** Remarques sur le *Megastome intestinal, Bull. Soc. Zool. Fr.,* 30, 18, 1888.

16. **Abraham, R.,** On two new species of *Giardia* parasitic in Indian mammals, *Parasitology,* 52, 159, 1962.

17. **Fantham, H. B.,** Some parasitic protozoa found in South Africa, *S. Afr. J. Sci.,* 18, 164, 1921.

18. **Nieschultz, O.,** Uber den Bau von *Giardia caprae* miki, *Arch. Protistenkd.,* 49, 278, 1924.

19. **Hegner, R. W. and Schumaker, E.,** Some intestinal amoebac and flagellates from the chimpanzee, three-toed sloth, sheep and guinea-pig, *J. Parasitol.,* 15, 31, 1928.

20. **Hegner, R. W.,** A comparative study of the Giardias living in man, rabbit and dog, *Am. J. Hyg.,* 2, 435, 1922.

21. **MacKinnon, D. and Debb, M.,** Report on intestinal protozoa of some mammals in the zoological gardens at Regents Park, *Proc. Zool. Soc. Lond.,* 108, 323, 1938.

22. **Deschiens, R.,** *Giardia cati* (n. sp.) du Chat domestique, *C. R. Soc. Biol. Paris,* 92, 1271, 1925.

23. **Hegner, R. W.,** *Giardia felis* n. sp. from the domestic cat and giardias from birds, *Am. J. Hyg.,* 5, 258, 1925.

24. **Chu, H.,** *Giardia hegneri* n. sp. from a Philippine civet cat, *J. Parasitol.,* 16, 231, 1929.

25. **Davaine, C.,** Monadiens, in *Dictionnaire Encyclopedique des Sciences Medicales,* Asselin, P. and Masson, G., Place de L'Ecole-de-Medecine, Paris, 1875.

26. **Hegner, R. W.,** *Giardia beckeri* n. sp. from the ground squirrel and *Endamoeba dipodomysi* n. sp. from the kangaroo rat, *J. Parasitol.,* 12, 203, 1926.

27. **Hegner, R. W.,** Giardias from wild rats and mice and *Giardia caviae* sp. n. from the guinea pig, *Am. J. Hyg.,* 3, 345, 1923.

28. **Kofoid, C. and Christiansen, E.,** On *Giardia microti* sp. nov., from the meadow mouse, *Univ. Calif. Publ. Zool.,* 16, 23, 1915.

29. **Travis, B.,** Description of five new species of flagellate protozoa of the genus *Giardia, J. Parasitol.,* 25, 11, 1939.

30. **Carini, A.,** Sobre uma *Giardia* parasita do intestino da Irara (*Tyra baibara*), *Arq. Biol. Sao Paulo,* 23, 1, 1939.

31. **Splendore, A.,** Sui parassiti della avicole, *Ann. D'Igiene,* 30, 561, 1920.

32. **Lavier, G.,** Deux especes de *Giardia* du rat d'egout parisien (*Epimys norvegicus*), *Ann. Parasitol. Hum. Comp.,* 2, 161, 1924.

33. **Lavier, G.,** Sur deux especes nouvelles du genre *Giardia: G. viscaciae* de la viscache (*Viscacia viscacia*) et *G. varani* (*Varanus niloticus*), *Ann. Parasitol. Hum. Comp.,* 1, 147, 1923.

34. **Kotlán, A.,** Giardien (Lamblien) in Vögeln, *Zentralbl. Bakteriol. Parasitenkd. u. Infektionskr. Orig. Hyg. Abt. Rlhea,* 88, 54, 1922.

35. **Danciger, M. and Lopez, M.,** Numbers of *Giardia* in the feces of infected children, *Am. J. Trop. Med. Hyg.,* 24, 237, 1975.

36. **Court, J. and Stanton, C.,** The incidence of *Giardia lamblia* infestation of children in Victoria, *Med. J. Aust.,* 2, 438, 1959.

37. **Babbott, F. L., Frye, W. W., and Gordon, J. E.,** Intestinal parasites of man in arctic Greenland, *Am. J. Trop. Med. Hyg.,* 10, 185, 1961.

38. **Lopez, C. E., Juranek, D. D., Sinclair, S. F., and Schultz, M. G.,** Giardiasis in American travelers to Madeira Island, Portugal, *Am. J. Trop. Med. Hyg.,* 27, 1128, 1978.

39. **Shaw, P. K., Brodsky, R. E., Lyman, D. O., Wood, B. T., Hibler, C. P., Healy, G. R., MacLeod, K. I. E., Stahy, W., and Schultz, M. G.,** A communitywide-outbreak of giardiasis with evidence of transmission by municipal water supply, *Ann. Intern. Med.,* 87, 426, 1977.

40. **Lippy, E. C.,** Tracing a giardiasis outbreak at Berlin, New Hampshire, *J. Am. Water Works Assoc.,* 70, 512, 1978.

41. **Barbour, A. G., Nichols, C. F., and Fukushima, T.,** An outbreak of giardiasis in a group of campers, *Am. J. Trop. Med. Hyg.,* 25, 384, 1976.

42. **Brodsky, R. E., Spencer, H. C., and Schultz, M. G.,** Giardiasis in American travelers to the Soviet Union, *J. Infect. Dis.,* 130, 319, 1974.

43. **Dykes, A. C., Juranek, D., Lorenz, R., Sinclair, S., Jakubowski, W., and Davies, R.,** Municipal waterborne giardiasis: an epidemiologic investigation, *Ann. Intern. Med.,* 92, 165, 1980.

44. **Waterborne Giardiasis — California, Colorado, Oregon, Pennsylvania,** *Morbid. Mortal. Weekly Rep.,* 29, 121, 1980.

45. **Petersen, H.,** Giardiasis (Lambliasis), *Scand. J. Gastroenterol.,* 7 (Suppl. 14), 1, 1972.

46. **Ansari, M.,** An epitome on the present state of our knowledge of the parasitic duodenal flagellate of man — *Giardia intestinalis* (Lambl 1859), *Pakistan J. Health,* 4, 131, 1954.

47. Public Health Service, Intestinal Parasite Surveillance (Annual Summary, 1978), HEW Publ. No. (CDC) 79-8352, U.S. Department of Health, Education and Welfare, Washington, D.C., 1979, 1.

48. Communicable Disease Weekly Report, Public Health Service, London, 1977.

49. **Shelton, G. C.,** Giardiasis in the chinchilla. I. Observations on morphology, location in the intestinal tract and host specificity, *Am. J. Vet. Res.,* 15, 71, 1954.

50. **Haiba, M. H.,** Further study of the susceptibility of murines to human giardiasis, *Z. Parasitenkd.,* 17, 339, 1956.

51. **Stevens, D. P. and Frank, D. M.,** Local immunity in murine giardiasis: is milk protective at the expense of maternal gut?, *Trans. Assoc. Am. Phys.,* 91, 268, 1978.

52. **Rendtorff, R. C.,** The experimental transmission of human intestinal protozoan parasites. II. *Giardia lamblia* cysts given in capsules, *Am. J. Hyg.,* 59, 209, 1954.

53. **Rendtorff, R. C. and Holt, C. J.,** The experimental transmission of human intestinal protozoan parasites. IV. Attempts to transmit *Endamoeba coli* and *Giardia lamblia* cysts by water, *Am. J. Hyg.,* 60, 327, 1954.

54. **Burrows, R. B. and Hunt, G. R.,** Intestinal protozoan infections in cats, *J. Am. Vet. Med. Assoc.,* 157, 2065, 1970.

55. **Thomas, R. F.,** Incidence of intestinal parasites in German Shepherd dogs, *J. Am. Vet. Med. Assoc.,* 136, 25, 1960.

56. **Burrows, R. B. and Lillis, W. G.,** Intestinal protozoan infections in dogs, *J. Am. Vet. Med. Assoc.,* 150, 880, 1967.

57. **Barlough, J. E.,** Canine giardiasis: a review, *J. Small Anim. Pract.,* 20, 613, 1979.

58. **Panigrahy, B., Grimes, J. E., Rideout, M. I., Simpson, R. B., and Grumbles, L. C.,** Zoonotic diseases in psittacine birds: apparent increased occurrence of chlamydiosis (psittacosis), salmonellosis and giardiasis, *J. Am. Vet. Med. Assoc.,* 175, 359, 1979.

59. **Sachs, R.,** *Giardia* in the blood of chinchilla, *J. S. Afr. Vet. Med. Assoc.,* 34, 445, 1963.

60. **Schneider, von C. C.,** Infektionsversuche mit *Lamblia muris.* II. Der Einfluss der Ernahrung und anderer Faktoren auf den Infektionsverlauf, *Z. Tropenmed. Parasitol.,* 12, 368, 1961.

61. **Kofoid, C. A. and Christiansen, E. H.,** On the life-history of *Giardia, Proc. Nat. Acad. Sci.,* 1, 547, 1915.

62. **Sebesteny, A.,** Pathogenicity of intestinal flagellates in mice, *Lab. Anim.,* 3, 71, 1969.

63. **Csiza, C. K. and Abelseth, M. K.,** An epizootic of protozoan enteritis in a closed mouse colony, *Lab. Anim. Sci.,* 23, 858, 1973.

64. **Roberts-Thomson, I. C., Stevens, D. P., Mahmoud, A. F., and Warren, K. F.,** Giardiasis in the mouse: an animal model, *Gastroenterol.,* 71, 57, 1976.

65. **Stevens, D. P. and Roberts-Thomson, I. C.,** Animal model of human disease: Giardiasis, *Am. J. Pathol.,* 90, 529, 1978.

66. **Roberts-Thomson, I. C. and Mitchell, G. F.,** Giardiasis in mice. I. Prolonged infections in certain mouse strains and hypothymic (nude) mice, *Gastroenterology,* 75, 42, 1978.

67. **Roberts-Thomson, I. C., Stevens, D. P., Mahmoud, A. A., and Warren, K. S.,** Acquired resistance to infection in an animal model of giardiasis, *J. Immunol.,* 117, 2036, 1976.

68. **Boorman, G. A., Lina, P. H. C., Zurcher, C., and Nieuwerkerk, H. T.,** *Hexamita* and *Giardia* as a cause of mortality in congenitally thymus-less (nude) mice, *Clin. Exp. Immunol.,* 15, 623, 1973.

69. **Manson-Bahr, P. H.,** *Manson's Tropical Diseases. A Manual of the Diseases of Warm Climates,* 9th ed., Cassell, London, 1929, 437.

70. **Herman, C. M.,** *Giardia* in the blood of a kangaroo rat, *J. Parasitol.,* 29, 423, 1943.

71. **Tumka, A. F.,** Spread of parasitic flagellates in the intestines of mice irradiated by X-rays, *Parazitologiia,* 6, 222, 1972.

72. **Lupascu, G., Radulescu, S., and Cernat, M. J.,** The presence of *Lamblia muris* in the tissue and organs of mice spontaneously infected, *J. Parasitol.,* 56, 444, 1970.

73. **Radulescu, S., Lupascu, G., and Ciplea, A.,** Presence of the flagellate *Giardia muris* in tissues and organs of spontaneously infected mice, *Arch. Roum. Pathol. Exp. Microbiol.,* 30, 405, 1971.

74. **Akimova, R. F. and Solov'ev, M.,** Problems of finding *Lamblia* in tissues of small intestine and other organs of rodents, *Med. Parazitol. Parazit. Bol.,* 52, 585, 1973.

75. **Brightman, A. H. and Slonka, G. F.,** A review of five clinical cases of giardiasis in cats, *J. Am. Anim. Hosp. Assoc.,* 12, 492, 1976.

76. **Bemrick, W. S.,** A note on the incidence of three species of *Giardia* in Minnesota, *J. Parasitol.,* 47, 87, 1961.

77. **Johnson, G.,** Giardiasis, in *Current Veterinary Therapy,* Vol. 6, Kirk, R., Ed., W. B. Saunders, Philadelphia, 1977.

78. **Craige, J.,** Differential diagnosis and specific therapy of dysenteries in dogs, *J. Am. Vet. Med. Assoc.,* 113, 343, 1948.

79. Public Health Service, Giardiasis in Apes and Zoo Attendants, Kansas City, Missouri, (CDC) Vet. Public Health Notes, U.S. Department of Health, Education and Welfare, Washington, D.C., January 1979, 7.

80. Jokipii, L., Occurrence of *Giardia lamblia* in adult patients with abdominal symptoms and in symptomless young adults, *Ann. Clin. Res.,* 3, 286, 1971.

81. Carroll, M., Anast, B. P., and Birch, C., Giardiasis and uveitis, *Arch. Ophthalmol.,* 65, 775, 1961.

82. Harris, R. and Mitchell, J., Chronic urticaria due to *Giardia lamblia, Arch. Dermatol. Syphilol.,* 59, 587, 1949.

83. Halstead, S. and Sadun, E., Alimentary hypersensitivity induced by *Giardia lamblia, Ann. Intern. Med.,* 62, 564, 1965.

84. Goobar, J., Joint symptoms in giardiasis, *Lancet,* 1, 1010, 1977.

85. Veghelyi, P., Coeliac disease imitated by giardiasis, *Am. J. Dis. Child.,* 57, 894, 1939.

86. Cortner, J. A., Giardiasis, a cause of coeliac syndrome, *Am. J. Dis. Child.,* 98, 311, 1959.

87. Court, J. M. and Anderson , C. M., The pathogenesis of *Giardia lamblia* in children, *Med. J. Aust.,* 2, 436, 1959.

88. Hoskins, L., Winawer, S., Broitman, S., Gottlieb, L., and Zamcheck, N., Clinical giardiasis and intestinal malabsorption, *Gastroenterology,* 53, 265, 1967.

89. Morecki, R. and Parker, J., Ultrastructural studies of the human *Giardia lamblia* and subjacent jejunal mucosa in a subject with steatorrhea, *Gastroenterology,* 52, 151, 1967.

90. Barbieri, D., deBrito, T., Hoshino, S., Nascimento, O., Campos, J., Quartentii, G., and Marcondes, E., Giardiasis in childhood: absorption tests and biochemistry, light and electron microscopy of jejunal mucosa, *Arch. Dis. Child.,* 45, 466, 1970.

91. Brandborg, L. L., Structure and function of the small intestine in some parasite diseases, *Am. J. Clin. Nutr.,* 24, 124, 1971.

92. Carswell, F., Gibson, A., and McAllister, T., Giardiasis and coeliac disease, *Arch. Dis. Child.,* 48, 414, 1973.

93. Duncombe, V. M., Bolin, T. D., Davis, A. E., Cummins, A. G., and Crouch, R. L., Histopathology in giardiasis: a correlation with diarrhoea, *Aust. N. Z. J. Med.,* 8, 392, 1978.

94. Friederici, L., Lamblien-cholecystitis mit septischem charakter, *Arztl. Wochenschr.,* 3, 89, 1948.

95. McGrath, J., O'Farrell, P., and Boland, S., Giardial steatorrhea — a fatal case with organic lesions, *Ir. J. Med. Sci.,* 6, 802, 1940.

96. Yardley, J., Takano, J., and Hendrix, T., Epithelial and other mucosal lesions of the jejunum in giardiasis. Jejunal biopsy studies, *Bull. Johns Hopkins Hosp.,* 115, 389, 1964.

97. Saha, T. K. and Ghosh, T. P., Invasion of small intestinal mucosa by *Giardia lamblia* in man, *Gastroenterology,* 72, 402, 1977.

98. Parkin, D., McClelland, D., Percy-Robb, I., O'Moore, R., and Shearman, D., Intestinal immunoglobulin levels and bacterial flora in hypogammaglobulinemic adults in relation to intestinal absorptive function, *Gut,* 11, 1064, 1970.

99. Brown, W., Butterfield, D., Savage, D., and Tada, T., Clinical, microbiological, and immunological studies in patients with immunoglobulin deficiencies and gastrointestinal disorders, *Gut,* 13, 441, 1972.

100. Ament, M., Immunodeficiency syndromes and gastrointestinal disease, *Pediatr. Clin. N. Am.,* 22, 807, 1975.

101. Hermans, P., Diaz-Buxo, J., and Stobo, J., Idiopathic late-onset immunoglobulin deficiency. Clinical observations in 50 patients, *Am. J. Med.,* 61, 221, 1976.

102. Thompson, A., Rowland, R., Hecker, R., Gibson, G., and Reid, D., Immunoglobulin-bearing cells in giardiasis, *J. Clin. Pathol.,* 30, 292, 1977.

103. Zinneman, H. and Kaplan, A., The association of giardiasis with reduced intestinal secretory immunoglobulin A, *Am. J. Dig. Dis.,* 17, 793, 1972.

104. Popovic, O., Pendic, B., Paljm, A., Andrejevic, M., and Trpkovic, D., Giardiasis, local immune defense and responses, *Eur. J. Clin. Invest.,* 4, 380, 1974.

105. McClelland, D., Warwick, R., and Shearman, D., IgA concentration, *Am. J. Dig. Dis.,* 18, 347, 1973.

106. McLaughlan, P., Stanworth, D., Webster, A., and Asherson, G., Serum IgE in immune deficiency disorders, *Clin. Exp. Immunol.,* 16, 375, 1974.

107. Geller, M., Geller, M., Flaherty, K., Black, P., and Madruga, M., Serum IgE levels in giardiasis, *Clin. Allergy,* 8, 69, 1978.

108. Ridley, M. and Ridley, D., Serum antibodies and jejunal histology in giardiasis associated with malabsorption, *J. Clin. Pathol.,* 29, 30, 1976.

109. Radulescu, S., Iancu, L., Simionescu, O., and Meyer, E. A., Serum antibodies in giardiasis, *J. Clin. Pathol.,* 29, 963, 1976.

110. Vinayak, V., Jain, P., and Naik, S., Demonstration of antibodies in giardiasis using immunodiffusion technique with *Giardia* cysts as antigen, *Ann. Trop. Med. Parasitol.,* 72, 581, 1978.

111. **Halita, M. and Isaicu, L.**, Reacti de fixare a complementului in lambliaza intestinala, *Ardeal. Med.*, 6, 154, 1946.
112. **Vinnikov, M.**, Lamblioza, *Sov. Med.*, 12, 18, 1949.
113. **Meyer, E. A.**, Isolation and axenic cultivation of *Giardia* trophozoites from the rabbit, chinchilla and cat, *Exp. Parasitol.*, 27, 179, 1970.
114. **Meyer, E. A.**, *Giardia lamblia:* isolation and axenic cultivation, *Exp. Parasitol.*, 39, 101, 1976.
115. **Andrews, J., Ellner, J., and Stevens, D.**, Purification of *Giardia muris* trophozoites by using nylon fiber columns, *Am. J. Trop. Med. Hyg.*, 29, 12, 1980.
116. **Jarroll, E. L., Bingham, A. K., and Meyer, E. A.**, *Giardia* cyst destruction: effectiveness of six small-quantity water disinfection methods, *Am. J. Trop. Med. Hyg.*, 29, 8, 1980.
117. **Bingham, A. K., Jarroll, E. L., Meyer, E. A., and Radulescu, S.**, *Giardia* sp.: physical factors of excystation *in vitro* and excystation vs. eosin exclusion as determinants of viability, *Exp. Parasitol.*, 47, 284, 1979.
118. **Dancescu, P. and Tintareanu, J.**, Investigations concerning the spread of giardiasis in a children's community, *Microbiol. Parazitol. Epidemiol.*, 9, 343, 1964.
119. **Black, R. E., Dykes, A. C., Sinclair, S. F., and Wells, J. G.**, Giardiasis in day-care centers: evidence of person to person transmission, *Pediatrics*, 60, 486, 1977.
120. **Keystone, J. S., Krajden, S., and Warren, M. R.**, Person to person transmission of *Giardia lamblia* in day-care nurseries, *Can. Med. Assoc. J.*, 119, 241, 1978.
121. **Meyer, E. A. and Jarroll, E. L.**, Giardiasis, *Am. J. Epidemiol.*, 111, 1, 1980.
122. **Kirner, J. C., Littler, J. D., and Angelo, L. A.**, A waterborne outbreak of giardiasis in Camas, Wash., *J. Am. Water Works Assoc.*, 70, 35, 1978.
123. **Fiumara, N.**, Giardiasis in travelers to the Soviet Union, *N. Engl. J. Med.*, 288, 1410, 1973.
124. **Thompson, R., Karandikan, D., and Leek, J.**, Giardiasis, an unusual cause of epidemic diarrhoea, *Lancet*, 1, 615, 1974.
125. **Burke, J. A.**, The clinical and laboratory diagnosis of giardiasis, in *CRC Critical Reviews in Clinical Laboratory Sciences*, Vol. 7, 1977, 373.
126. **Wolfe, M. S.**, Giardiasis, *Pediatr. Clin. North Am.*, 26, 295, 1979.
127. **Faust, E. C., Russell, P. F., and Jung, R. C.**, *Craig and Faust's Clinical Parasitology*, 8th ed., Lea & Febiger, Philadelphia, 1970.
128. Council for the American Society of Parasitologists, Procedure suggested for use in examination of clinical specimens for parasitic infections, *J. Parasitol.*, 63, 959, 1977.
129. **Beal, C. B., Viens, P., Grant, R. C. L., and Hughes, J. M.**, A new technique for sampling duodenal contents., *Am. J. Trop. Med. Hyg.*, 19, 349, 1970.
130. **Rosenthal, P. and Liebman, W. M.**, Comparative study of stool examinations, duodenal aspiration, and pediatric Enterotest for giardiasis in children, *J. Pediatr.*, 96, 278, 1980.
131. **Visvesvara, G. S. and Healy, G. R.**, The possible use of an indirect immunofluorescent test using axenically grown *Giardia lamblia* antigens in diagnosing giardiasis, in Waterborne Transmission of Giardiasis, EPA 600/9-79-001, Jakubowski, W., and Hoff, J. C., Eds., Environmental Protection Agency, Cincinnati, 1979, 53.
132. **Meuwissen, J. H. E., Tongeren, J. H. M., and Werkman, H. P. T.**, Giardiasis, *Lancet*, 32, July 2, 1977.
133. Center for Disease Control, Health Information for International Travel, HEW Publ. No. (CDC) 79-8280, Atlanta, Ga., U.S. Department of Health, Education and Welfare, Washington, D.C., 1979.
134. Drugs for Parasitic Infections, *The Medical Letter on Drugs and Therapeutics*, 21(26), 106, 1979.
135. **Box, E. D.**, Observations on Giardia of budgerigars, *J. Protozool.*, 28, 491, 1981.

LEISHMANIASIS

Ralph Lainson

INTRODUCTION

Disease
Visceral, cutaneous and mucocutaneous leishmaniasis.

Etiologic Agent
Various species and subspecies of the genus *Leishmania* Ross 1903 (Phylum Sarco-mastigophora: Order Kinetoplastida: Family Trypanosomatidae).

The genus *Leishmania* may be defined as a unicellular parasite, closely related to the trypanosomes and loosely included with these organisms in the "hemoflagellates". It is a digenetic parasite: that is to say, its life cycle is completed in two different hosts, in this case a vertebrate and an insect. As far as is known, this life cycle consists only of asexual division, in both hosts.

The vertebrate hosts of *Leishmania* include a wide variety of mammals, and some reptiles: among the mammals, infections are particularly common in rodents and canids, but important hosts are also known in edentates, marsupials, procyonids and primates (including man). No infections have yet been recorded in birds or amphibians, but this may simply be because such animals are seldom examined for this parasite. Within the vertebrate, *Leishmania* is in the amastigote form (Figures 1 and 2), as obligate, intracellular inhabitants of the macrophage cells, either in the skin, the viscera, or both.*

The insect hosts appear to be strictly limited to phlebotomine sandflies (Order Diptera: Family Psychodidae: Sub-Family Phlebotominae) in which a definite cycle of development takes place in the alimentary tract, and at times attached to the gut wall. Here the parasite assumes the flagellate or promastigote form (Figure 3) and, in the life cycle of most leishmanias, the flagellates migrate to the biting mouthparts; in such cases transmission to another vertebrate takes place following the bite of the infected sandfly. Some lizard leishmanias, however, migrate to a posterior position in the intestine of the sandfly, when transmission is most probably achieved after the insect is eaten by another lizard. Once within the vertebrate host, the promastigote rounds up and once more assumes the amastigote form within the macrophages; the cycle is now complete.

Species and subspecies of *Leishmania* have a remarkably wide distribution in most tropical and sub-tropical countries, extending through most of Central and South America, Central and South-East Asia, India, China, the Mediterranean Basin and Africa. Interestingly, *Leishmania* was thought to be absent from North America, north of Mexico, until very recently; three cases of human cutaneous leishmaniasis, probably due to *Leishmania mexicana mexicana* have now been reported from Texas, however,[155,161] and canine visceral leishmaniasis was recorded among foxhounds from a kennel in Oklahoma.[13] The exact origin of the human infections remains questionable, as all patients had made sporadic visits to Mexico. The canine disease was shown to be due to a parasite biochemically indistinguishable from *Leishmania donovani infantum,* the causative agent of human and canine visceral leishmaniasis in many parts of the Old World. It is possible that it was imported into the U.S.A. in a dog from Europe, and transmitted to other dogs by a local sandfly.

---

*   In reptiles the parasites may sometimes exist in both the amastigote and promastigote form.

There are no records of *Leishmania* in the Australian Region, although phlebotomine sandflies do occur in certain parts of Australia (one species of *Phlebotomus* and two species of *Sergentomyia*). A single case of mucocutaneous leishmaniasis in Japan remains of doubtful origin.

From the standpoint of human suffering and economics, leishmaniasis is probably second in importance only to malaria among the protozoal diseases — with the important difference that both treatment and control are much more difficult. From antiquity, visceral leishmaniasis ("kala azar") has exacted a heavy toll of human life, particularly in Asia, while American cutaneous and mucocutaneous leishmaniasis have debilitated and mutilated man for centuries.

Historical Background

There seems little doubt that both cutaneous and visceral leishmaniasis are ancient afflictions of man. Descriptions of the cutaneous disease can be traced back to at least the first century A.D., in Central Asia, where it was referred to as "Balkh Sore" (from the name of a town in north Afghanistan, near the Russian border), and to early travelers' accounts of "Aleppo Boil" in Syria, and "Baghdad Boil" in Iraq. In the Americas, Peruvian and Ecuadorean pottery from the era 400 to 900 A.D. depicts human faces with mutilations very similar to those caused by cutaneous and mucocutaneous leishmaniasis today; and Spanish historians at the time of the Conquest noted severely mutilating sores on the faces of the Peruvian Indians.

The major signs or symptoms of visceral leishmaniasis, such as fever, and marked enlargement of spleen and liver, are characteristic of a number of other tropical diseases and it is consequently difficult to trace early, clear-cut references to visceral leishmaniasis in ancient writings of either the Old or the New World. Its recognition as a clinical entity before the discovery of the causative agent, in the Old World, was doubtless due to the relatively high standard of medical service available during the period of colonialism in the Far East, and "kala azar" was well known to military clinicians in India as early as the 1880s. In the Mediterranean region, at the same period, the condition was referred to as "infectious splenic anemia" or "infantile splenic anemia".

The fact that visceral leishmaniasis appears not to have been recognized as a distinct disease state in Latin America until the time of the first parasitologically proven case, in Paraguay, in 1913, had led to the suggestion that it was imported into the New World in recent times. Some support for this hypothesis does come from close similarities in the clinical and epidemiological features of Mediterranean and American visceral leishmaniasis, and the undoubtedly close biochemical relationship of the causative agents.

Although it has long been textbook practice to discuss visceral and cutaneous leishmaniasis separately, as two distinctly different diseases, this division is misleading and by no means sharply defined. The old custom of treating the parasites of the eastern and western hemispheres as two separate groups is equally artificial, and has hampered our progress in formulating a basic, global classification of the leishmanias. As far as possible, therefore, major advances in the history of leishmaniasis are presented here in chronological order, although it has been necessary to abandon this idealistic approach at times, particularly when lengthy sequences of events concerning different parasites have paralleled one another in time, in different geographic regions.

It was natural that past studies on the leishmanias in their vertebrate and invertebrate hosts should go hand-in-hand, but it is clearly more convenient and less confusing to review them separately. Finally, the immense bibliography on *Leishmania* and leishmaniasis makes it impracticable to cite all references to the historical events mentioned, without seriously impairing the continuity of text. Almost all such references may be traced, however, in the more extensive review papers listed in the Recommended Reading given at the end of this chapter.

Leishmania in the Vertebrate Host

Cunningham[42] was apparently the first to see the parasite, during his examination of sections of "Delhi Boil" in India, in 1885; his first impression, however, was that the organism was a member of the Mycetozoa, or "slime fungi". Credit must go to the Russian army doctor, Borovsky,[21] in 1898, for the first suggestion that the causative agent of cutaneous leishmaniasis ("Sart Sore") in Turkestan was in fact a protozoon. He refrained, however, from giving it a name.

Leishman[106] discovered the organism associated with visceral leishmaniasis of man in 1900, in cases of "kala azar" in India, and astutely recognized it as related to the trypanosomes; in the same year Donovan published his own observations on the same parasite. Visceral leishmaniasis had also been recognized in China, in 1900, but the diagnosis was not confirmed until 1904, by Marchand and Ledingham.[39] Temporary confusion reigned in the taxonomy of the causative organism when Laveran and Mesnil named it *Piroplasma donovani*, but Ross[141] correctly and justly amended the name to *Leishmania donovani* in 1903.

In the meantime, the causative agent of the cutaneous disease encountered by Cunningham and Borovsky remained unnamed, although it was soon appreciated that it was responsible for dermal lesions known under a bewildering array of local names in many parts of Asia, the Middle East, and the Mediterranean Basin.

Wright, in 1903,[185] gave the name of *Helcosoma tropicum* to the organism he described from a case of "oriental sore" on the cheek of an Armenian child who had been brought to Boston; he was under the impression that the parasite was a microsporidian. The German parasitologist Lühe[109] followed a general concensus of opinion that there were close similarities between the parasites of cutaneous and visceral leishmaniasis and, in 1906, amended the name to *Leishmania tropica*. He still clung to the French workers' view that the organism was a piroplasm, however, although any doubt as to the parasite's true affinities had already been removed in 1904, when Rogers demonstrated the flagellate stage of *L. donovani* in in vitro culture; these "leptomonad" forms were later obtained by Nicolle, when he cultured *L. tropica* in blood-agar medium (NNN) in 1908.

The known geographic distribution of leishmaniasis took a dramatic jump from the Far East to the Mediterranean, when Cathoire and Laveran[29] described a fatal case of the visceral disease in a 7-month-old child from Tunisia and over the following years foci of "infantile kala azar" were found to extend throughout the whole of the Mediterranean littoral, including the south of France.

By 1909 visceral leishmaniasis, confirmed parasitologically, had been reported from India, China, Russia, Italy, Tunisia, Egypt, and the Sudan, while the leishmanial origin of cutaneous lesions had been established in India, Russia, Persia, Egypt, Italy, and Tunisia. Inevitably, there was much discussion, and dissension, over the early taxonomy of parasites associated with leishmaniasis over such a wide geographic area. In 1908, Nicolle considered that the clinical and epidemiological features of Indian and Mediterranean visceral leishmaniasis were sufficiently different to warrant a separate name for the parasite causing the latter disease, and called it *Leishmania infantum* because of its virtual restriction to children. He proposed that the organism responsible for cutaneous leishmaniasis should be named *Leishmania wrighti*, overlooking the fact that *L. tropica* already had priority.

In the meantime, studies on monogenetic flagellates (*Leptomonas* and *Herpetomonas*), in a variety of insects, had led some workers to overstress the undoubtedly close relationship of these parasites to *Leishmania*. Some actually suggested that the

name *Leishmania* must be dropped, and that the correct name for the parasite of Indian "kala azar" was *Leptomonas donovani*. Patton,[130] for example, used the names
Herpetomonas donovani, H. infantum and *H. tropica*, and the term "herpetomon-
iases" for the diseases they caused in man. A number of notable figures in the history
of leishmaniasis[159] for some time used the generic name of *Herpetomonas*, but Wenyon
(see Recommended Reading) was never in agreement. He pointed out that *Leishmania*
parasitized vertebrates, whereas *Herpetomonas* and *Leptomonas* were purely insect
flagellates, which had never, to his satisfaction, been shown capable of infecting vertebrate hosts.

It came as no great surprise when leishmaniasis was eventually shown also to exist
on the American continent; for as long ago as 1898 a certain Dr. L. Villar in Peru had
written that "uta", "was very like the Aleppo button". The first records of South
American cutaneous leishmaniasis, however, were made independently by Lindenberg,[108] and Carini and Paranhos,[27] in South Brazil in 1909. From the first uncomplicated skin lesions examined, it was understandable that these authors considered the
infections to be due to *L. tropica*, but in 1911 the Brazilian parasitologist Vianna[176]
felt that there were morphological differences which warranted the new name of *L.
braziliensis** for the parasite in Brazil. However slender these reasons may have
seemed, the finding of similar organisms in the nasopharyngeal lesions of cases of
mucocutaneous leishmaniasis 2 years later, by Splendore[166] justified Vianna's decision,
for such a clinical picture is not characteristic of infection with *L. tropica*.

In 1910, a Dr. A. L. Barton of Lima claimed to have seen amastigotes in smears
made from a skin lesion of a patient suffering from "uta", a cutaneous disease long
known to be common in the Peruvian Andes; he regarded the parasite as *L. tropica*,
however, and did not bother to publish his observation.[174] Velez,[175] on the other hand,
was clearly much influenced by Vianna's recent creation of the name *L. braziliensis*,
and called the Peruvian parasite *Leishmania peruviana*. Some authorities still clung to
the view that "uta" was due to *L. tropica* which had been imported into Peru by the
conquistadores, in post-Columbian times. This fanciful view persisted until quite recently, but had to be abandoned when it was shown that the developmental pattern of
L. peruviana in the sandfly was quite different from that of *L. tropica*, and more
closely resembled the development of *L. braziliensis*.[98]

The first record of undoubtedly autochthonous visceral leishmaniasis of man in the
New World was made by Migone, in Paraguay in 1913; the patient had spent some
time in the state of Mato Grosso, Brazil, however, where he had almost certainly acquired the infection. Since that time the disease has been recorded in 13 other states
of Brazil, as well as in Argentina, Venezuela, Bolivia, Colombia, Paraguay, Guatemala, El Salvador, Mexico, Surinam, Ecuador, Honduras, and even the tiny West
Indian island of Guadaloupe. Although the Brazilians, Cunha and Chagas,[41] later gave
the name of *Leishmania chagasi* for the parasite causing visceral leishmaniasis in Brazil, in 1937, some authorities have preferred to regard the disease as an importation
from the Old World, and consider that the causative agent is therefore synonomous
with *L. infantum*. In the grouping of the leishmanias given in the following pages, I
have followed previous authors' use of the subspecific names *L. donovani donovani,
L. donovani infantum,* and *L. donovani chagasi*.

In 1908, Nicolle and Comte[127] recorded the important discovery of a natural infection with *L. donovani infantum* in a dog, supporting the growing suspicion that at
least some forms of human leishmaniasis had their origin in animal reservoirs. By
1912, canine visceral leishmaniasis was known in all those Mediterranean countries
where the human disease occurred, and was subsequently reported in other endemic

*   This was Vianna's original spelling, not *brasiliensis* as is frequently written.

areas in Europe (Rumania), Russia, China, Africa, and Latin America (Brazil, Argentina, and Venezuela). Strangely, no similar canine reservoir could be found for *L. donovani donovani* in India, altbough Patton,[131] in 1913, examined the spleens of 1438 dogs in Madras. It was concluded that Indian "kala azar" was transmitted directly from man to man, and till this day no firm evidence of a domestic or wild animal reservoir has been found.

In the meantime the source of cutaneous leishmaniasis due to *L. tropica* remained obscure. Neligan[123] discovered skin lesions containing amastigotes in dogs of Teheran, Iran, as early as 1913; the causative organism was not identified, however, and could well have been *L. donovani infantum* — which we now know to commonly produce skin lesions during the evolution of visceral leishmaniasis of the dog — or another parasite, *Leishmania major,* discussed in later pages.

As the enormous geographical range of *Leishmania* became apparent, more attention was devoted to the epidemiological features peculiar to the different foci throughout the world, and to differences in the organisms responsible.

It became clear to early workers in leishmaniasis that there were two nosological forms of the cutaneous disease variously distributed in the major endemic areas of the Mediterranean basin, Central Asia, and the Indian continent; Russian clinicians referred to them as "dry, urban" and "wet, rural" forms, although these descriptions did not find wide use in other countries. (It is historically interesting to note, however,[138] that in 1756 an English physician in Aleppo, Syria gave a very good description of what was clearly cutaneous leishmaniasis, and wrote of "male" nonulcerative sores, and "female" moist or ulcerative sores). The "wet, rural" disease was found to be associated with the edges of arid or semiarid regions, with particularly conspicuous foci around the oases of the Syrian, Kara-kum, and Kyzylkum deserts. In contrast, foci of "dry, urban" cutaneous leishmaniasis (classical "oriental sore") were in the vicinity of townships and ancient settlements — hence such local names as "Ashkabad Sore", Aleppo Button", Baghdad Boil", etc.

In 1914, the Russian workers Yakimoff and Schokhor[186] used the subspecific names of *Leishmania tropica major* and *Leishmania tropica minor* to distinguish the causative agents of "wet, rural" and "dry, urban" cutaneous leishmaniasis in southern Russia; this distinction was largely based on a difference in the size of the amastigotes of the two parasites — a taxonomic feature curiously ignored until very recently.[152] Modern specialists now refer to them simply as *Leishmania major* and *Leishmania tropica.* Finally, Latyšev and Krjukova,[105] working in desert regions of Turkmenia, S. S. R., reported that up to 25% of the burrowing rodents *Rhombomys opimus* (the great gerbil) harbored *L. major* in their skin, and acted as a vast reservoir of infection for man. Infections were less frequently found in other rodent species and in a few nonrodents, although these would appear to play a less important role as reservoirs.

In contrast, the Russian workers were unable to find a wild animal reservoir for the "dry, urban" disease, caused by *L. tropica,* which appeared to be restricted to man and, more rarely, dogs.

These observations were to have a profound influence on subsequent epidemiological studies on the leishmaniases the world over. Thus, foci of zoonotic "wet, rural" cutaneous leishmaniasis have been shown to exist in most of the desert or semi-desert regions, extending in a broad band from N.W. China, N.W. India and Pakistan, Turkmenia, Usbekistan, S. Tadjikistan and Kazakhstan S.S.R., through Southeast Asia, and into North, East and Central Africa. Wild rodents incriminated as reservoir-hosts include *Rhombomys, Meriones, Psammomys, Arvicanthis, Mastomys, Tatera* and *Xerus.*

Early studies in the Mediterranean littoral zone, including Morocco, Tunisia, and Algeria in North Africa, suggested the presence of both "wet, rural" *(L. major)* and "dry, urban" *(L. tropica tropica)* forms of cutaneous leishmaniasis. Modern methods for the identification of *Leishmania* species and subspecies, however, are beginning to cast doubt on the existence of the latter parasite in Europe and Africa. In Europe, for example, some cutaneous lesions of man have been shown to be due to an unusual (?) clinical manifestation of infection with *L. d. infantum*,[143] and isolates from skin lesions in most parts of Africa are either indistinguishable from *L. major,* or very closely related.[33] It may well be, therefore, that the true "home" of *L. t. tropica* does not extend beyond the Indian continent, and Central and South East Asia.

In addition to the Mediterranean countries of North Africa, visceral leishmaniasis was early on shown to be widespread on the rest of the African continent. Neave[122] registered the existence of the disease in Anglo-Egyptian Sudan in 1904, where it has long been notorious for its explosive and lethal nature, and its poor response to anti-leishmanial drugs. In 1919, Castellani and Chalmers[28] differentiated the causative parasite as *L. donovani* var *archibaldi.* What was probably a cutaneous form of the disease had already been attributed to *"L. nilotica"* by Brumpt,[26] in 1913; there is no means of confirming that the condition was caused by the same parasite, however, and if a subspecific name is to be used for the organism of Sudanese visceral leishmaniasis, it should be *L. d. archibaldi,* as already indicated by Lysenko[110] and Bray.[23]

In spite of exhaustive epidemiological studies in the Sudan, the incrimination of reservoir-hosts of *L. d. archibaldi* s.l. was not achieved until 1962, when Hoogstraal and colleagues[77] found visceral infections in rodents *(Arvicanthis niloticus, Acomys albigens* and *Rattus rattus)* and carnivores *(Genetta genetta* and *Felis serval).* Sporadic case reports of human visceral leishmaniasis in Western Ethiopia, Chad, Central African Republic and Niger, may possibly represent part of the same focus.

Visceral leishmaniasis remained sporadic in Kenya until the second World War, when troop movements were probably responsible for a sharp rise in the incidence of infection, with 136 cases between 1941 and 1943. The most serious epidemic, however, was in 1952—1953, when over 2,000 cases were registered. Although sporadic visceral infections have been recorded in dogs, these are possibly of little significance in the epidemiology of the disease, and the fact that troops commonly acquired infection when penetrating virtually uninhabited areas, strongly indicates a wild animal reservoir. Isolates of a *Leishmania* from the spleens of the rodents *Tatera rutilis, T. robustis, T. nigricauda* and *Xerus* sp., by Heisch et al.,[68,69] have since been shown to be parasites of the *L. major* complex. Visceral leishmaniasis in South Ethiopia and Somalia is probably part of the Kenyan focus.

Sporadic cases of visceral leishmaniasis have been recorded in other countries of Central and West Africa, including Mali, Upper Volta, Zaire, Uganda, Nigeria, Congo, Gabon, Ivory Coast, Niger, Zambia and Malawi. Their relationship to the principal Sudanese and Kenyan foci remains obscure, and virtually nothing is known of their epidemiology except the registration of isolated cases of canine visceral leishmaniasis in Congo, Niger and Somalia. Infected dogs have been frequently found in Senegal, but till now the human disease is unknown.

In Ethiopia, cutaneous and visceral leishmaniasis had long been known to exist, but there remained little epidemiological data concerning these diseases until the studies of Bray and co-workers.[25] They considered the causative agent of cutaneous and diffuse cutaneous leishmaniasis (DCL) in the Ethiopian and Kenyan Highlands to differ from *L. tropica,* and gave it the name of *L. aethiopica.* They also suggested that *L. tropica major* should be raised to specific rank, as *L. major,* while *L. tropica minor* should be referred to simply as *L. tropica.* The same workers[17] showed the hyraxes *Procavia habessinica* and *Heterohyrax brucei* to be the reservoir hosts of *L. aethiopica,* and to harbor parasites in their skin.

The clear-cut morphological, biochemical and immunological differences between

L. major and *L. tropica* clearly warrant the use of these specific names, but the differences between *L. tropica* and *L. aethiopica* are much less striking on all counts. In this chapter it is proposed to use the names *L. major, L. tropica tropica* and *L. tropica aethiopica*. There is increasing evidence of a multiplicity of parasites causing Old World cutaneous leishmaniasis, and at least some of these may be grouped as subspecies within the *L. major* and *L. tropica* complexes.

South Africa seemed to be completely free of any form of leishmaniasis until as recently as 1970, when Grové[65] reported four cases of the cutaneous disease in S.W. Africa. Grové and Ledger[66] isolated a *Leishmania* from the skin of some specimens of the hyrax, *Procavia capensis*, and from the sandfly, *Phlebotomus rossi*, in the same area. Surprisingly, enzyme electrophoretic studies suggested that the parasite from the hyrax was not the same as that isolated from man,[33] although Grové had found evidence to suggest that there was an association of human infection with an increase in the hyrax population. Biochemically, the parasite(s) appears most closely related to *L. tropica* and possibly represents a further subspecies of this leishmania.

In the Americas, studies on the leishmaniases were long limited to case reports of cutaneous and mucocutaneous leishmaniasis, by clinicians largely obsessed with differing clinical aspects of the disease. It seemed that cutaneous leishmaniasis extended from Mexico in the north, to Argentina in the south, and that the disease was most prevalent in the forested areas, suggesting the existence of a wild animal reservoir.

The importance of visceral leishmaniasis in the Americas did not really become apparent until 1934, when Penna,[132] in Brazil, used the viscerotome to examine liver samples from fatal cases of undiagnosed fever. He rapidly uncovered 41 deaths from visceral leishmaniasis and pinpointed the major endemic areas in the drier, poorly forested areas of the country, in particular the State of Ceará. Chagas and colleagues[32] studied an area of low endemicity in the State of Pará, Brazil, and found a small number of dogs with visceral infections to be infected.

Herrer[70,71] studied cutaneous leishmaniasis, or "uta", in Peru, due to the parasite referred to as *L. peruviana*. The endemic areas were restricted to regions between 900—3000 m above sea level, in non-forested areas on the Peruvian Andes. Cases occurred in up to 94% of the schoolchildren, but infection was usually mild, self-healing, and it imparted a firm immunity to re-infection; there was no tendency for the disease to progress to mucocutaneous leishmaniasis. Dogs commonly showed amastigotes in discrete lesions of the nose and ears, with parasites sometimes present in apparently normal skin. No wild animals were found infected, but examination of these was largely restricted to a search for skin lesions.

In Brazil, in 1948, Muniz and Medina[119] discovered the enigmatic *Leishmania enriettii*, forming tumor-like lesions in the skin of laboratory guinea pigs in Paraná State. Although the parasite does not appear to infect man, and nothing is known of its natural hosts, the discovery of *L. enriettii* provided an excellent laboratory model for immunological studies: it also increased our awareness of a multiplicity of different parasites within the genus *Leishmania,* and the need for a fresh look at the nature of those already known to infect man. In spite of misgivings on the part of many notable parasitologists, specific or subspecific distinction began to be made between a number of leishmanias hidden under a common specific name, in the same manner in which the Russian workers had sub-divided *L. tropica*.

There had long been known a form of cutaneous leishmaniasis in the Yucatan Peninsula, Belize and Guatemala, in which the parasite showed a strange predilection for development in the tissues of the external ear. The disease, "chiclero's ulcer" or "Bay Sore", is mostly contracted by forest workers, in particular those collecting chewing-gum latex from the sapodilla trees *(Achras sapota)*, deep in the forest. From studies on the disease in man, Biagi[19] concluded that the etiologic agent differed from *L.*

braziliensis described by Vianna in Brazil, and in 1953 he proposed that it should be called *Leishmania tropica mexicana*. The same trinomial taxonomy was àdopted by Floch,[54] in 1954, who proposed the name of *L. tropica guyanensis* for the parasite causing "pian-bois", a form of cutaneous leishmaniasis in the Guyanas of South America. Unfortunately, as subsequent studies were to show, he made the mistake of lumping *L. peruviana* or Peruvian "uta", and *L. braziliensis* of Brazilian cutaneous and mucocutaneous leishmaniasis, under the common name of *L. tropica braziliensis*.

In Brazil, interest in leishmaniasis had slowly waned until 1953, when an explosive outbreak of the visceral disease accounted for the death of a hundred or more persons in the small town of Sobral in the State of Ceará, and startled the health authorities into a fervor of epidemiological enquiries. Deane and Deane,[43,44] to whom we owe much of our present knowledge on American visceral leishmaniasis, confirmed the important role of the dog as the major, domestic reservoir of infection for man, and also demonstrated natural infections in wild foxes *(Lycalopex vetulus)*. Infected wild canids have also been found in the Old World: foxes, wolves and jackals in Russia, and foxes in France and Italy. Subsequent case reports of visceral leishmaniasis in Latin America added little new epidemiological data, except to extend the geographical range throughout most of Central and South America.

In studies on the epidemiology of cutaneous leishmaniasis in Panama, workers at the Gorgas Memorial Laboratories cultured heart-blood from a large number of wild animals in attempts to find a silvatic reservoir of the disease. A *Leishmania* was isolated from some "spiny-rats", *Hoplomys gymnurus* and *Proechimys semispinosus*,[14,15] and both hamsters and a volunteer were infected by the intradermal inoculation of flagellates from the blood-agar cultures. In 1960, Forattini[56] worked on similar lines in Brazil, and found three wild animals infected with *Leishmania*; amastigotes were seen in skin lesions of an agouti *(Dasyprocta azarae)* and a "rat" *(Kannabateomys amblyonyx)*, and promastigotes were isolated following the culture of heart-blood from a "paca" *(Agouti paca)*. Although the precise identity of these leishmanias from Panamanian and Brazilian animals was not determined, their discovery did represent the first concrete evidence of the long suspected zoonotic nature of American cutaneous leishmaniasis, and provided a much needed stimulus for others in the field.

In Venezuela, in 1959, Medina and Romero[114] described a strange form of cutaneous leishmaniasis of man, characterized by large histiocytoma-like nodules scattered over the body, and containing enormous numbers of large amastigotes. The disease would not respond to treatment with drugs active against other forms of leishmaniasis, and the patients always showed a negative response to intradermal "leishmanin" tests. Largely based on these criteria, the causative organism received the new name of *Leishmania braziliensis pifanoi,* although we now know that this form of leishmaniasis in the Americas (DCL) is the relatively rare coincidence of immunologically incompetent persons infected with sub-species of *L. mexicana*. At least one member of the *L. tropica* complex is capable of producing the same clinical picture in man (see *L. mexicana pifanoi, L. m. mexicana, L. m. amazonensis* and *L. tropica aethiopica*, on later pages).

The Brazilian parasitologist Pessoa[133] agreed with Floch's[54,55] trinomial subdivision of New World leishmanias, but in 1961 he listed them as *L. braziliensis braziliensis, L. b. guyanensis, L. b. peruviana, L. b. pifanoi* and *L. b. mexicana*. Garnham,[62] however, preferred to give specific rank to the latter parasite and simply called it *L. mexicana*.

Pessoa's classification might well have remained unchanged to this day, were it not for a remarkable sequence of events which led to the uncovering of a hitherto unsuspected complex of subspecies of *L. mexicana* throughout the forests of Central and South America, and unquestionably confirmed the specific status of this parasite.

Lainson and Strangways-Dixon[96] found the reservoirs of *L. mexicana* in Belize (British Honduras), when they showed three different rodents to harbor the parasite in the skin — *Ototylomys phyllotis, Heteromys desmarestianus* and *Nyctomys sumichrasti.* The infections were characterized by inconspicuous lesions on the tail, containing abundant amastigotes; the parasite has been shown to be identical to that causing "chiclero's ulcer" of man, by the inoculation of volunteers and by comparative biological and biochemical studies.

During a visit to the Instituto Evandro Chagas in Belém, Pará, Brazil, in 1963, the present author was shown a capture-release program for forest mammals carried out by the virologist, Dr. Otis Causey. The findings in Belize were discussed, and Causey was impressed by the similarities of the tail-lesions due to *L. mexicana* and lesions he had noted in some specimens of a local, Brazilian rodent, *Oryzomys capito.* His promise to examine such animals at the next opportunity was well kept, and within two weeks he presented the author with stained smears which were teeming with amastigotes.

At first it was thought that Causey had uncovered an enormous reservoir of *L. braziliensis,* but after lengthy study the parasite was shown to be closely related to *L. mexicana* and, in 1972, Lainson & Shaw[88] named the organism *L. mexicana amazonensis.* The parasite of "chiclero's ulcer" thus became *L. mexicana mexicana;* while *L. b. pifanoi,* for reason of its obvious affinities to the *mexicana* complex, was re-named *L. mexicana pifanoi. L. m. amazonensis* has a remarkably wide range of hosts among silvatic mammals; thirteen different species have been incriminated in the forests near Belém, including rodents, marsupials and foxes. The infection rate in the major rodent reservoir-host, *Proechimys guyannensis,* may sometimes be as high as 25%.

A further subspecies of *L. mexicana* was discovered in a number of rodents and an opossum in Panama, by Herrer and colleagues[73] (see *L. m. aristedesi,* later in this chapter), and biochemical evidence[33] has indicated the existence of yet others (unnamed) in the States of Mato Grosso and Minas Gerais in Brazil. Others are likely to be discovered, and the range of *L. mexicana* will probably be shown to extend through all the forested areas of Central and South America. An undoubted subspecies of *L. mexicana* was, for example, discovered in rodents and marsupials of Trinidad, by Tikasingh[173] in 1969. He regarded it as *L. m. amazonensis,* but as Trinidad is over 2000 km from the type locality of this parasite, he may well have been dealing with a different subspecies.

Continuing their studies in Panama, Herrer et al.[74] made several isolations of *Leishmania* from a number of different silvatic mammals, including monkeys and procyonids. These animals were considered to be of minor importance in the epidemiology of Panamanian cutaneous leishmaniasis, however, and it was finally concluded that the major reservoir host was the sloth *Chloepus hoffmanni,* in which a very high infection rate was recorded. Infections were always inapparent, with amastigotes scattered through the skin and sometimes the viscera. Throughout their extensive publications in Panama, workers have always guardedly referred to the parasite simply as *L. braziliensis.* Lainson and Shaw[88] gave it the name *L. braziliensis panamensis,* however, and enzyme electrophoresis has confirmed the validity of this separation from the other subspecies of *L. braziliensis.* At the same time the latter authors divided the leishmanias of the New World into two major groups: the *Leishmania mexicana* complex, containing four subspecies of this parasite and *L. enriettii;* and the *L. braziliensis* complex containing three subspecies of that organism, *L. peruviana,* and a strange parasite of tree-porcupines, *L. hertigi,* described by Herrer in Panama in 1971.[72] This broad grouping was based on all criteria available at that time, including behavior in sandfly vectors, in vitro culture and experimental vertebrate hosts (hamster), immunology and biochemistry.

Two characteristics noted for the Brazilian isolates of *L. b. braziliensis* s. l. by Lainson and Shaw[88] were the very poor growth of the parasite in the skin of the hamster and the great difficulty in maintaining it in a wide variety of blood-agar media; variations in in vivo and in vitro growth were found with parasites isolated in a number of different regions — doubtless an indication of the existence of a variety of leishmanias within the *braziliensis* complex. The poor growth in both hamster and culture has seriously hampered efforts to indicate the reservoir hosts of *L. b. braziliensis.* Thus, in epidemiological studies in Mato Grosso, Brazil, Lainson and Shaw[87] confirmed that human cutaneous and mucocutaneous leishmaniasis in the area of study was due to *L. b. braziliensis* s.l. However, although a high rate of infection with *L. m. amazonensis* in wild rodents and marsupials was readily demonstrated due to the luxurious growth of this parasite in both the hamster and blood-agar media, only one isolate was made of *L. b. braziliensis* from the skin of one of these animals *(Oryzomys concolor).* This was possibly explained by the fact that even when amastigotes were microscopically detected in smears from the skin lesions of patients, their intradermal inoculation into hamsters frequently failed to produce detectable infections. Other isolations of parasites considered as *L. b. braziliensis* s.l. were made by Forattini[57,59] from the tail skin of the rodents *Akodon arviculoides, Oryzomys nigripes* and *O. capito,* and by Lainson and Shaw[89] from the viscera of another rodent, *Proechimys guyannensis,* in the State of Pará.

Herrer[72] described a new leishmania, *L. hertigi,* from the skin and viscera of tree-porcupines in Panama. Infections were always inapparent, long-lasting, and with amastigotes scattered throughout the skin, in the absence of any host-cell reaction. Deane et al.[47] found extremely large amastigotes in liver smears of another species of porcupine, *Coendou* sp., from the State of Piauí, Brazil. On size alone, the organism was clearly different from *L. hertigi* of Panamanian porcupines, but no isolations were made and the authors were only able to conclude that the parasite was a *"Leishmania* proper to the porcupines". Lainson and Shaw rediscovered this leishmania in *Coendou prehensilis* and an unnamed *Coendou* sp., in Pará State, Brazil,[90] and gave it the name of *L. hertigi deanei* ; the type species described by Herrer in Panama thus became *L. hertigi hertigi. L. h. deanei* has the largest amastigotes of any known *Leishmania* species, averaging $6.1 \times 3.7 \mu m$.

In Costa Rica, Zelodón et al.,[189] recorded *Leishmania* infection in a number of sloths, *Choloepus griseus* and *C. hoffmanni* ; the parasites were regarded as *"L. braziliensis"* and it is likely that at least some isolations were of *L. b. panamensis,* as found by Herrer and colleagues in neighboring Panamanian sloths. In 1979, however, Zelodón et al.[188] made further isolations of promatigotes in cultures of blood, skin, and viscera from the same species of sloths, which were clearly mixtures of *Endotrypanum* and *Leishmania.* One isolation from *C. griseus* was considered to be only *Leishmania,* and inoculation of culture forms into the skin of hamsters gave rise to inapparent infections, with the presence of parasites referred to as "sphaeromastigotes". The organism produced amastigotes in tissue-cultures of hamster cells, and was given the name of *Leishmania herreri.* Apparently the biochemistry (DNA buoyant densities and enzyme profiles) was totally different from any other known *Leishmania,* but no details were given regarding this data.

Another new *Leishmania, L. garnhami,* was described by Scorza et al.,[144] from patients suffering from cutaneous leishmaniasis in forested areas in the Venezuelan Andes; a single opossum, *Didelphis marsupialis,* was found infected. From the parasite's behavior in hamsters and NNN culture, and its enzyme profiles, however,[97a] it is so close to *L. m. amazonensis* that it would be wisest to refer to it as *L. m. garnhami* for the time being. The organism is said to frequently contain a refractile granule, visible by ordinary light microscopy, but this does not seem to be a constant feature usable as a diagnostic feature.

Lainson et al.,[104] found a high percentage of armadillos (*Dasypus novemcinctus*) from Pará State, Brazil, to be infected with a hitherto unnamed *Leishmania* with amastigotes of extremely small size. The parasites were localized in the viscera and were sometimes demonstrable in the peripheral blood; the relationship of the organism to human leishmaniasis remains obscure, although it is clearly most closely related to parasites of the *L. braziliensis* complex on its enzyme profiles.

The same workers examined large numbers of wild mammals from a highly endemic area of "pian-bois", due to *L. b. guyanensis*, in north Pará. Infections with this parasite were found in a small percentage of rodents and opossums, and one of two anteaters, *Tamandua tetradactyla*.[103] Subsequent examination of further specimens of edentates from the same general area revealed an infection rate of 46.0% in the two-toed sloth, *Coloepus didactylus* (27/59) and 22.2% in *T. tetradactyla* (6/27).[99] The parasite was almost always isolated from the liver and spleen, rarely from the skin. Gentile et al.,[63] found 46.7% (7/15) of *C. didactylus* to be infected in French Guyana, and it is likely that both edentates are the major reservoir of *L. b. guyanensis* throughout its geographical range in the northern Amazon Basin.

Very recent studies on the epidemiology of the leishmaniases in the Old World have largely concerned the incrimination of reservoir hosts and the identification of isolates of *Leishmania* from man and animals by enzyme electrophoresis, serology and other methods.

Mutinga[120] demonstrated natural infections with *L. tropica aethiopica* in the skin of the hyraxes *Dendrohyrax arboreus* and *Procavia johnstoni*, and the "giant-rat" *Cricetomys*, trapped on Mount Elgon, Kenya, thus confirming previous authors' views[17] that the epidemiology of cutaneous leishmaniasis in the Kenyan highlands was an extension of that in the highlands of Ethiopia.

Natural visceral infections with *L. d. infantum* in domestic rats have excited considerable interest: in Yugoslavia, Petrović et al.,[135] found *Rattus rattus* and *Rattus norvegicus* infected, and Bettini et al.,[18] have confirmed the existence of natural infections in *R. rattus* in Italy. Whether or not these non-canine hosts have any real epidemiological significance is debatable, and they may simply represent circumstantial "victims", like man.

Chance et al.,[36] studied 68 stocks of *Leishmania* from Ethiopia; they found them to fall into three main groups, identified as *L. donovani* s.l., *L. major* and *L. aethiopica*. Three other groups occurred, however, which differed from these parasites.

From their own and other authors' observations on the development of different leishmanias in sandfly vectors, Lainson and Shaw[92] placed more stress on this feature in a revision of their previous (1972) classification[88] of the genus *Leishmania*. Among their modifications were the removal of *L. hertigi* from the *L. braziliensis* complex, and the inclusion of a number of newly discovered leishmanias.

Leishmania in the Insect Vector

Rogers' observation in 1904,[140] on the development of *L. d. donovani* into "leptomonad" forms (promastigotes) in in vitro culture, in a blood-agar medium, suggested an arthropod vector for the leishmanias, for similar organisms (e.g. *Leptomonas*) were already known to be natural, monogenetic parasites of insects. The subsequent search for the vector of "kala azar" and "oriental sore" thus encompassed a wide range of suspects, including bed-bugs, fleas, house-flies, mosquitoes, hippoboscids and even blood-sucking helminths such as ancylostomes.

These epidemiological "red herrings" were to delay progress in the elucidation of the transmission of *Leishmania* for many years, although the coincidental distribution of phlebotomine sandflies and leishmaniasis had attracted the attention of Pressat[137] and Sergent et al.,[145] in foci of "oriental sore" in the Mediterranean Region. In 1911,

Wenyon[182] provided the first real evidence of the role of these insects as vectors, when he found 6% of wild-caught *Phlebotomus papatasi* and/or *P. sergenti*, from Aleppo, to harbor intestinal flagellates; they were indistinguishable from the developmental forms that Rogers and Nicolle obtained in their in vitro cultures. In India, Mackie[111] dissected sandflies he had caught on sticky fly-papers hung in houses or hospital wards housing patients with "kala azar", and reported the presence of "herpetomonads". As no infections with monogenetic flagellates are yet known in members of the Psychodidae, it is highly likely that Mackie, too, was dealing with *Leishmania*.

Sergent et al.,[146] again drew attention to the possible role of sandflies (*P. papatasi*) in the transmission of "oriental sore", when they discussed the disease in Biskra. They finally obtained a number of female *P. papatasi* from that area, crushed them in saline, and inoculated the material intradermally into volunteers: typical "oriental sores" developed at the inoculation sites, and were shown to contain amastigotes.

Meanwhile Sinton,[162] in 1922, had drawn attention to the strictly coincidental distribution of "kala azar" and sandflies in India, and suggested these insects to be the most likely vectors. A "Kala Azar Commission" was set up in 1924, under the Directorship of Christophers, and they soon succeeded in rearing the most likely sandfly suspect, *Phlebotomus argentipes*, in the laboratory. When these were fed on patients with "kala azar" a prolific development of flagellates took place in the gut of the insect, and Christophers et al.[38] concluded that *P. argentipes* was the major suspect as the vector of *L. d. donovani* because it was the only arthropod in which the parasite developed with ease.

At the same time, Adler and Theodor[4] studied the transmission of "oriental sore" in Palestine. They found a specimen of the sandfly *P. papatasi* heavily infected with flagellates, which were seen to be attached to the esophageal valve. A volunteer was inoculated with the parasites by scarification of the arm, and one month later a small papule containing amastigotes appeared at the point of entry.

Evidence that sandflies were the vectors of *Leishmania* mounted quickly. Shortt, who had assumed Directorship of the Indian Kala Azar Commission in 1925, wrote of their progress in 1926 as "...all that is required, short of the final proof of a transmission experiment, to demonstrate that kala azar is transmitted by the bite of the sandfly".[159] Infections had been obtained in *P. argentipes*, with active flagellates reaching almost to the biting mouthparts; a naturally infected specimen of this insect was found in a house with a case of "kala azar", and the flagellates were associated with the remains of a bloodmeal; finally, it was established that in endemic areas, every house was infested with *P. argentipes*. In China, other investigators had succeeded in obtaining heavy infections in the sandfly *P. chinensis*, fed on patients with visceral leishmaniasis.

Adler and Theodor[5] made it quite clear that in their opinion they had provided sufficient proof of the role of sandflies as major vectors of *Leishmania*, by their scarification transmission from a naturally infected fly. Wenyon[183a] criticized this view, however, and emphasized the need to demonstrate transmission by the natural bite of the insect. Adler and Theodor's reply to this was an ingenious experiment,[7] by which they did in fact demonstrate the capability of the sandfly to transmit *Leishmania* by bite, although it was not from man to man. *P. papatasi* were fed through a rabbit-skin membrane on a culture of *L. t. tropica* and, eight days later, through another membrane on sterile inactivated rabbit serum. Some of this serum was then sown into the customary blood-agar medium used for cultivating *Leishmania* and flagellates were demonstrable six days later. The same authors[8] quite possibly did actually transmit *Leishmania* to man by the bite of a sandfly, one year later (1929). They fed experimentally infected *Phlebotomus sergenti* on a number of volunteers and obtained a positive lesion on the arm of one man. Unfortunately the incubation period was so long that he had since visited endemic areas of "oriental sore", and could possibly have acquired the infection there.

With indefatigable patience, Shortt et al.,[160] continued their transmission experiments in India, having fed a total of nearly 80,000 sandflies on infected persons and many hundreds of these on volunteers, without any evidence of transmission. In his summary of the work, he bitterly concluded that either some essential factor was missing in the experiments, or that all this vast amount of work over the past 5 years had been on an insect which was not an essential link in the chain of infection. In 1931, however, Shortt's patience was finally rewarded, and a brief note appeared in *Nature* on the 28th of February,[158] stating that a general infection had resulted in a hamster on which infected *P. argentipes* had been fed over a period of 12 months. The infection was only discovered 17 months after the commencement of the experiment.

Although three more transmissions of *L. d. donovani* to hamsters by the bite of *P. argentipes* were reported by Napier et al.,[121] and Smith et al.,[163] the results were disappointing, and extremely puzzling in view of the now overwhelming evidence suggesting sandflies to be the natural and efficient vectors of *Leishmania*. In 1940, however, Smith et al.,[164] made a vitally important observation. They noted that sandflies survived better if given moistened raisins to feed on after the first, infective bloodmeal, rather than more blood. Furthermore, the flagellate infections in such flies were very much heavier. In subsequent experiments[165] they were now able to make repeated transmissions of *L. d. donovani* to hamsters and mice, with relative ease. The final piece of the jigsaw puzzle had been found, and the complicated picture of the life-history of *Leishmania* completed.

In North Africa, *P. papatasi* was long suspected as a vector of "oriental sore" on the grounds of coincidental distribution, and Parrott and Donatien[129] had experimentally infected this fly on infected mice, and found a natural infection in a wild-caught fly. Furthermore, Adler and Theodor[6] (1926) had been able to show that parasites isolated from a naturally infected *P. papatasi* and "oriental sore" of man were serologically identical. Finally, Adler and Ber[3] succeeded in transmitting the parasite by the bite of *P. papatasi* that had been fed through a membrane on flagellates in a mixture of 3 parts 2.7% saline and 1 part inactivated, defibrinated rabbit blood. Their transmissions were made with astonishing ease, producing a total of 28 lesions in 5 out of 8 volunteers. This unprecedented transmission rate was attributed to the addition of the saline to the suspension of flagellates.

The coincidental limitation of visceral leishmaniasis and the sandfly *P. chinensis* to that part of China north of the Yangtze River, clearly indicated this insect as the vector of the disease. The first serious attempts to incriminate this sandfly began in 1926, when Young and Hertig[187] experimentally infected local sandflies, including *P. chinensis*, *P. sergenti* and *P. perturbans*. They noted good infections in the first species, but the parasites tended to die out in the latter two; their attempts to transmit the infection to hamsters by the bite of the infected sandflies failed. Sun et al.,[171] and Sun and Wu[170] made similar studies, and also demonstrated promastigotes in 7 out of 21 *P. chinensis* caught in houses with cases of visceral leishmaniasis. Successful transmission to hamsters by the bite of *P. chinensis* was finally recorded by Feng and Chung.[52]

Mention is made of the experimental transmission of *L. major* to gerbils by the bite of *P. papatasi* and *P. mongolensis* by the Russian worker, Strelkova, in 1975.[169]

Overwhelming epidemiological evidence of the role of *P. ariasi* as the vector of *L. d. infantum* in the Cévennes, southern France, had slowly been accumulated by Rioux and colleagues,[139] but it was not until 1979 that these workers finally transmitted the parasite to a dog by the bite of an experimentally infected sandfly.

The series of investigations mentioned above may be regarded as the ideal, in attempts to incriminate a given sandfly vector. Unhappily, experimental transmission by the bite of sandflies is rarely attempted; nevertheless, coincidental distribution of leishmaniasis and a sandfly species, the finding of significant numbers of that species with natural infections (particularly in the foregut), and the ability to infect that insect readily in the laboratory, are all important criteria. They are all we have regarding some sandflies, which are nevertheless frequently referred to as "proven" vectors, e.g., *P. sergenti (L. t. tropica); P. perniciosus,* and *P. major (L. d. infantum); P. orientalis (L. d. archibaldi),* and others. Proven or highly suspect vectors are given in the sections dealing with the different *Leishmania* species and subspecies, on subsequent pages.

The incrimination of sandfly vectors associated with leishmaniasis in the New World has been complicated by the extremely wide variety of sandfly species, the failure to appreciate the existence of a multiplicity of leishmanial parasites on the part of many Latin American investigators, and the arduous task of working in dense tropical rain-forest.

The peri-domestic nature of American visceral leishmaniasis due to *L. d. chagasi,* however, led to a fairly rapid incrimination of the sandfly *Lutzomyia longipalpis,* the distribution of which was generally found to coincide with the disease throughout all of Latin America; another peri-domestic species, *Lu. intermedia,** was less strongly suspected.

Chagas, in 1936,[31] reported the presence of *Lu. longipalpis* in the house of the first living case of visceral leishmaniasis to be studied in South America, in Sergipe, Brazil. This prompted others (Ferreira et al., 1938;[53] Paraense and Chagas, 1940[128]) to feed this insect on infected dogs; promastigotes developed in the gut of these sandflies and their inoculation into hamsters gave rise to visceral leishmaniasis. Unfortunately, interest in visceral leishmaniasis seemed to die with Evandro Chagas in 1940, and it was not until 1954 that Deane and Deane,[45] investigating the serious outbreaks of the disease at the State of Ceará, first found wild-caught *Lu. longipalpis* heavily infected with promastigotes. They fed others on a naturally infected fox, and noted highly active flagellates in the biting mouthparts of these flies 8 days later.

The promastigotes seen by the Deanes in the wild-caught sandflies were not proven to be those of *L. d. chagasi,* but the epidemiological evidence presented was so strong that there remained little doubt as to the importance of this sandfly as the major vector. It was not until 1977, however, that the chain of evidence against *Lu. longipalpis* was finally completed, when Lainson and colleagues[101] achieved five separate transmissions of *L. d. chagasi,* in hamsters, by the bites of infected, laboratory-bred insects.

Although a wide range of silvatic sandfly species had previously been experimentally infected with parasites causing New World cutaneous leishmaniasis, the first experimental transmission was not achieved until 1962, by Strangways-Dixon and Lainson.[167,168] These authors infected nine different species of sandflies on hamsters with skin lesions due to *L. m. mexicana,* and subsequently transmitted the parasite to a volunteer by the bite of one of them, *Psychodopygus pessoanus.* In the same year, Coelho and Falcão[40] transmitted *L. m. mexicana* to hamsters using *Lu. longipalpis* and *Lu. renei.* Both groups of workers did little more than show that neotropical sandflies (as expected) were the most likely vectors of the various forms of leishmaniasis in the Americas, and more precise details as to the actual species involved had to await epidemiological studies in the different endemic areas.[84,92]

Although natural flagellate infections were recorded in numerous neotropical sandfly species, on no occasion had they been proven to be *Leishmania* until the extensive studies carried out at the Gorgas Memorial Laboratories, in Panama, by Hertig, Fairchild, Johnson and McConnell. After many years of patient work they found natural promastigote infections in more than 400 man-biting Panamanian sandflies and

---

*   The abbreviation *Lu.* for *Lutzomyia* is used to avoid confusion with *L.* for *Leishmania.*

had incriminated 3 species, *Lu. trapidoi*, *Lu. ylephiletor* and *Lu. gomezi*, as vectors of Panamanian cutaneous leishmaniasis.[78] *Psychodopygus panamensis* was also found infected by Christensen and colleagues.[37] It is not certain exactly what proportion of the promastigote infections seen were *Leishmania*, and McConnell[113] concluded that a great many certainly were not developmental stages of this parasite. Quite probably many infections were due to *Endotrypanum*, a blood parasite of sloths which also develops as promastigotes in sandflies; again, a high proportion may have been infections with *Leishmania* species unconnected with the human disease, such as *L. hertigi* of porcupines. What did clearly emerge from this rather complicated situation, however, was the fact that *Lu. trapidoi* undoubtedly did frequently harbor promastigotes of *L. b. panamensis*, as shown by the inoculation of volunteers, and that this sandfly was largely arboreal. The latter observation was to lead to the eventual incrimination of sloths as the major reservoir host of *L. b. panamensis*.

In his search for the vector of *L. m. mexicana* in the forests of Belize in Central America, Disney[50] designed a trap to catch sandflies attracted to the rodent reservoirs. He found that one particular fly, *Lu. olmeca olmeca* was highly attracted to the rodents and, in October 1965, found this sandfly naturally infected with *L. m. mexicana*.[51] In December of the same year, in neighboring Yucatan Peninsula, Biagi et al.,[20] confirmed the importance of *Lu. o. olmeca* as a vector, and transmitted the parasite to a volunteer by the bite of a naturally infected fly.

In Surinam, Wijers and Linger[184] dissected large numbers of anthropophilic sandflies, caught off human bait in areas endemic for "pian-bois" due to *L. b. guyanensis*. The most common man-biting species was recorded as *Ps. squamiventris,** but on no occasion was this insect found infected. Dissections of another fly, described as *"Lu. anduzei"*, and found resting on tree-trunks, however, revealed numerous infections with promastigotes; unfortunately, attempts to infect a hamster with the parasite failed and the role of this sandfly as a vector remained speculative.

Lainson et al.[100] studied the epidemiology of "pian-bois" in the region of Monte Dourado, north Pará State, Brazil; they found a 7% infection rate in *"Lu. anduzei"*, mostly taken from large tree trunks. This time the parasite was isolated on all occasions after the intradermal inoculations of the flagellates into hamsters, and it was shown to be identical, biologically and biochemically, with that causing the disease in man. Interestingly, the vector showed differences from the type material of *Lu. anduzei* Rozeboom, and has now been given the new name of *Lutzomyia umbratilis* Ward and Fraiha.[181] *Lu. umbratilis* was subsequently incriminated as the vector of *L. b. guyanensis* in the neighboring state of Amazonas, Brazil, by Arias and Freitas in 1977.[16] Finally, Lainson et al.,[104] disclosed heavy infections in seven specimens of another tree trunk inhabiting sandfly, *Lu. whitmani*. Unlike *Lu. umbratilis*, this insect has not been found to be particularly anthropophilic in the area, and it was suggested that its importance is probably limited to secondary transmission among the wild animal reservoirs.

Using Disney traps in the Amazonian forests of Brazil, in 1968, Lainson and Shaw,[86] showed the vector of *L. m. amazonensis* to be the sandfly *Lu. flaviscutellata*, which is highly attracted to the principal reservoir host, the rodent *Proechimys guyannensis*. During this and later work, 45 infections were found among 7,498 *Lu. flaviscutellata* dissected (0.6%), and the inoculation of the flagellates intradermally into hamsters, in 18 instances, isolated *L. m. amazonensis* on 15 occasions. This, the failure to find the parasite in any other species of sandfly dissected in the same forest region, and the subsequent experimental transmission of the parasite from hamster to hamster on four

---

*   The abbreviation *Ps.* for *Psychodopygus* is used to avoid confusion with that of *P.* for *Phlebotomus*.

occasions, using laboratory-bred *Lu. flaviscutellata*, left the authors with no doubt as to the importance of this fly as the principal and probably only vector of *L. m. amazonensis* in the Amazon Region.[92]

Sandfly vectors of *L. b. braziliensis* have proved more difficult to pinpoint, due to the poor growth of this parasite in laboratory animals and blood-agar media, and problems in the raising of workable colonies of suspected vectors for transmission experiments. Working in São Paulo State, Brazil, Forattini et al.,[58] did succeed in infecting hamsters with promastigotes found in two naturally infected sandflies, *Lu. intermedia* and *Lu. pessoai*, however, and considered the parasite as *L. b. braziliensis*. *Lu. intermedia* is found in low, secondary forest and is known to also invade houses. The other sandfly, *Lu. pessoai* is essentially silvatic, but has been recorded in houses which were up to 300 m away from the forest edge. These observations have led to the suggestion that cutaneous leishmaniasis in the south of Brazil may have a peridomestic transmission; the original source of infection doubtless still lies in the nearby wooded areas, however.

Lainson et al.,[102] worked in the Serra dos Carajás, Pará State, north Brazil, where cutaneous and mucocutaneous leishmaniasis were serious public health problems, and they concluded that *Psychodopygus wellcomei* was a major vector to man. Promastigotes from this fly grew very poorly in hamster skin and blood-agar cultures, but served to show that the parasite was the same as that infecting man in the same area. *Ps. wellcomei* was considered to be of particular importance because of the avidity with which it attacks man both during the night *and* the day.

As in the Old World, there have been numerous reports of unidentified flagellates in wild-caught neotropical sandflies, and these have sometimes led to unfounded conclusions regarding the importance of certain sandfly species in a given region. In other instances claims have been made to have produced cutaneous leishmaniasis in volunteers after feeding wild-caught sandflies on them. In most cases, however, the possibility has not been excluded that resulting lesions could have originated from unnoticed bites of free-flying sandflies before, during, or after the experiment. While all these observations are clearly of importance as indications for further studies, they cannot be taken to indicate the definite incrimination of any particular sandfly species as an important vector. In subsequent pages they are referred to as probable or possible vectors.

Morphology and Transmission

Apart from some very marked differences in size, and disposition of the nucleus and kinetoplast, all the known leishmanias do share a basic morphology in both the amastigote (Leishman-Donovan body), found in the vertebrate host, and the promastigote (leptomonad) in the insect vector. It is appropriate, therefore, to give a general account of these forms here, which will serve for each of the species or subspecies discussed later.

The Amastigote (Figure 1)

In smears stained with the Romanovsky stains, the organism appears as a rounded or oval body which measures ~ 1.5 × 2.5 to 3.0 × 6.5 μm, depending on the species or subspecies.[84,152] The cytoplasm stains a pale blue and may contain a variable number of vacuoles; the single, round to oval nucleus and the rod-shaped kinetoplast both stain a deep reddish-purple. There is no *free* flagellum.

Electron micrographs reveal several other details which are not apparent by ordinary light-microscopy (Figure 2). The parasite is bounded by a two-layered membrane or periplast, beneath which there is a layer of peripheral fibrils. The nucleus measures about 1.0 × 1.5 μm, having a double wall with a number of conspicuous pores; it

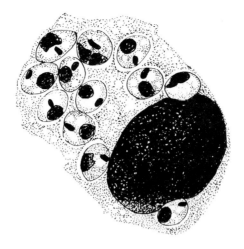

FIGURE 1. Amastigotes of *Leishmania* in a macrophage. Impression film of hamster spleen.

contains a well-defined nucleolus and peripherally disposed chromatin masses. Near the nucleus, the kinetoplast is seen to be an expansion of the mitochondrial apparatus, which is highly branched. This expansion contains a distinct fibrillar DNA band and conspicuous cristae. A little above the kinetoplast there is a flask-shaped invagination of the surface membrane which forms a small vacuole, the "flagellar pocket". In this lies the short, rudimentary flagellum, which does not protrude above the surface of the amastigote; the flagellum arises from the "basal body", within the cytoplasm and close to the nucleus, and shows the familiar collection of nine pairs of peripherally disposed micro-tubules and a single central pair, all of which run the length of the flagellum. There is a well developed Golgi apparatus.

Within the reticulo-endothelial cells, the amastigotes undergo binary fission, often packing the cells with parasites. Spread of infection in the host results when infected macrophages divide and share their parasites between daughter cells, or after the rupture of heavily parasitized cells and ingestion of the liberated amastigotes by other macrophages. It is a paradoxical fact, then, that the parasite lives in the very cells which should be protecting the host against their invasion. The mechanism of nutrition is poorly known. One school of thought suggests that food particles are actually taken into the flagellar pocket and digested within that organelle.

The Promastigote (Figure 3)

Phlebotomine sandflies are "pool-feeders", the biting mouthparts cutting the tissues of the host's skin to form a tiny pool of blood, which is sucked up the proboscis and into the midgut (stomach) by a muscular pharynx. If the vertebrate host is infected with *Leishmania*, free and/or intracellular amastigotes may be taken up with the bloodmeal, originating either directly from the peripheral blood (e.g., *L. d. donovani*, in man) or from parasites released from the traumatized skin (e.g., *L. d. infantum* and *L. d. chagasi* in dogs).

During the first 72 hours, and before the fly defecates, the amastigotes elongate and the rudimentary flagellum grows out into a long, whip-like structure extruding from the flagellar pocket. There may be a prior division as amastigotes before this elongation takes place.

The resulting promastigotes (Figure 3) may be seen swimming within the bloodmeal from 24 to 48 hours after the insect has fed, both blood and parasites being confined to the posterior part of the midgut, within a diffuse peritrophic membrane which is

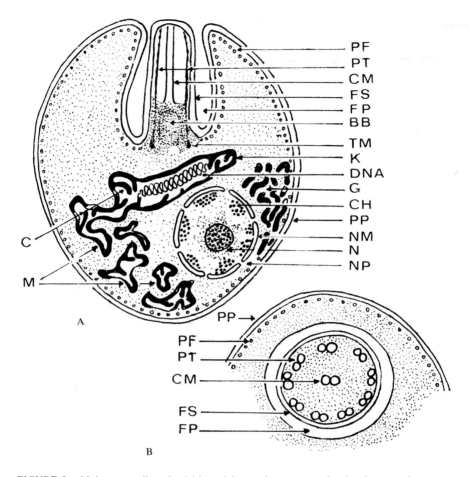

FIGURE 2.   Major organelles of a leishmanial amastigote as seen by the electron-microscope (schematic). (A) Longitudinal section: PF, peripheral fibrils; PT, peripheral microtubules of flagellum (nine pairs); CM, central, paired microtubules of flagellum; FS, flagellar sheath; FP, flagellar pocket; BB, basal body; TM, basal, triple microtubules; K, kinetoplast; DNA, fibrillar DNA band; G, Golgi apparatus; CH, peripherally disposed chromatin masses of nucleus; PP, periplast; NM, nuclear membrane; N, nucleolus; NP, nuclear pore; M, mitochondrion, cut in various planes; C, cristae of mitochondrion. (B) Transverse section through flagellum and flagellar pocket, showing the peripheral and central microtubules and peripheral fibrils.

secreted by the epithelial cells of this part of the intestine. At this stage, the flagellates are highly motile and undergo profuse multiplication by longitudinal binary fission.

Measurements of the promastigotes are highly variable, depending on whether or not the parasite is in the process of division or recently divided. There is no doubt, too, that the overall size of some parasites (e.g., subspecies of *L. mexicana)* is much larger than that of others (e.g., subspecies of *L. braziliensis).* In general, however, the body measures from about 10.0 — 20.0 × 1.5 — 3.0 μm, with the flagellum often longer than the body. The nucleus, spherical to oval in shape, is placed centrally in the cell, or slightly more anterior in position. The kinetoplast, flagellar pocket and flagellum are all situated at the anterior end. Apart from the free flagellum, the electron microscopic appearance of the promastigote is essentially a highly elongated version of the amastigote, although some ultrastructures, such as vesicles and lysosomes, are more highly developed.

Subsequent development of the infection in the sandfly host varies somewhat in the different leishmanias, principally in the time required for the production of the infec-

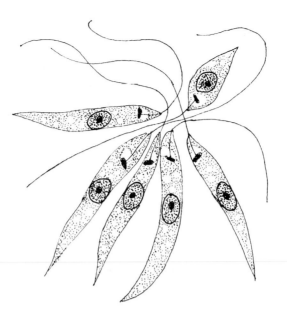

FIGURE 3.   Promastigotes of *Leishmania*. From in vitro culture.

tive promastigotes invading the biting mouthparts, and in the position of attachment sites of the parasites throughout the intestine.[80,92] In the development of *L. mexicana* subspecies, the long slender promastigotes continue to divide during the second and third days after the infective bloodmeal. With rupture of the peritrophic membrane and the passage of the digested blood to the hindgut, however, the flagellates become attached to the midgut by inserting the flagellum deep between the micro-villi lining the gut wall. Migration of other promastigotes takes place to the anterior part of the midgut and, in the cardia, they lose their long, slender form and transform into shorter, fatter bodies which become tightly packed against each other and the micro-villi of the gut wall; they do not attach, however, but slowly migrate forward to the esophageal valve. This, being ectodermal in origin, is lined with cuticle, to which the parasites now anchor themselves firmly by the tip of the flagellum, which becomes expanded into a foot-like hemidesmosome. A further transformation takes place when parasites migrate further forward, to the pharynx; where they can be seen in dissected sandflies as small, elongated, free promastigotes which move with extreme rapidity. Finally, from 4 to 5 days after the infective bloodmeal, small numbers of these forms may be found swimming up and down in the lumen of the proboscis; these infective forms may be injected into the next vertebrate host during subsequent bloodmeals.

Subspecies of *L. braziliensis* undergo an additional phase of development as small, rounded or pear-shaped flagellates (paramastigotes, spheromastigotes and promastigotes) firmly attached to the hindgut wall (Figure 4) by flagellar hemidesmosomes. The significance of this hindgut development is as yet unknown, but it is apparently an integral part of the life-cycle of leishmanias of the *braziliensis* complex in their sandfly vectors; it takes place even when sandflies are experimentally infected by feeding them directly with fully developed promastigotes, from in vitro cultures, through membranes. A similar hindgut development is shown by lizard leishmanias in their sandfly vectors, suggesting that parasites of the *braziliensis* complex have retained some primitive characteristics which have been lost by all other known leishmanias of mammals. The different development of species and subspecies of *Leishmania* in the sandfly is an important characteristic now used in the classification of these organisms.

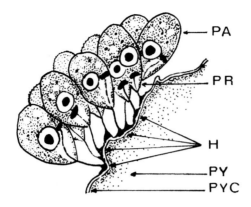

FIGURE 4.   Cluster of paramastigotes and promastigotes of *Leishmania braziliensis* attached to the hindgut (pylorus) wall of the sandfly vector. PA, paramastigote; PR, dividing promastigote; H, hemidesmosomes of flagella (expanded tips) attaching flagellates to cuticular surface of gut; PY, pylorus; PYC, chitinous cuticle of pylorus.

Diagnosis

As in all parasitic infections, the microscopic detection of the organism is the unequivocal method of diagnosis, and should be given priority over all other techniques. For greater details on techniques in this sub-head, see Lainson,[84] Lainson and Shaw.[93]

Parasitological Diagnosis

When infection of man or other animals is accompanied by visible skin lesions, amastigotes may be detected by the direct microscopic examination of stained smears prepared from tissue removed from the edge of ulcers or incised nodules. Well stained smears are of the utmost importance, and great care should be taken to avoid the central, necrotic area of ulcers, when secondary fungal and bacterial contaminants may cause considerable confusion in diagnosis, or ruin any attempts at sterile, in vitro culture. If dermal lesions do have a heavy bacterial contamination, it is advisable to first treat the patient with a course of a suitable antibiotic, and to postpone any examination for *Leishmania* until such treatment has been completed.

Direct examination of smears for amastigotes may be all that is required in about 50% of active lesions of man or other animals. Parasites may be extremely scanty, however, and a considerable degree of practice and patience is needed to find them. Finally, stained smears from highly suspect cases may appear completely devoid of parasites, and this is particularly the case in skin and naso-pharyngeal lesions due to *L. b. braziliensis*. Diagnosis must now depend on isolation of the parasite in in vitro culture of tissue in a suitable medium (usually a variety of rabbit-blood-agar mixtures), or the intradermal inoculation of such material into susceptible laboratory animals, in particular the hamster; wherever possible, both methods should be used. The author has found punch-biopsies of tissue from the borders of skin lesions to be much more effective than the method of aspirating material with a syringe. Two or three small biopsies are made to give sufficient tissue for culture, hamster inoculation, smears and histology. Histological sections have limited use in the diagnosis of cutaneous leishmaniasis, especially when parasites are very scanty, and the time devoted to their preparation would be better spent in the examination of a few well-prepared Giemsa-stained smears. In cases of advanced naso-pharyngeal lesions the hazard of contamination following in vitro culture of biopsied material is particularly high, and the examination of smears and inoculation of hamsters remain the most reliable diagnostic methods.

Blood-agar cultures should be examined at intervals of 7 to 10 days, when any isolated *Leishmania* will be found growing in the promastigote form, similar to that seen in the infected sandfly. The tubes should not be discarded as negative until at least one month after inoculation of the suspect material. It should be remembered that certain leishmanias grow poorly in a wide variety of blood-agar media; this is particularly the case for some subspecies of *L. braziliensis* and certain stocks of *L. donovani* subspecies.

Theoretically, the in vitro culture method is the most rapid and sensitive means of diagnosis, with results generally available in from 1 to 3 weeks. In practice, however, bacterial and fungal contamination may make diagnosis impossible. The former can to a great extent be controlled by the incorporation of a broad-spectrum antibiotic in the fluid phase of the medium (gentamycin, 250 μg mℓ^{-1} is particularly useful), or by prior incubation of tissue in saline containing much higher concentration (approximately 24 hr at 4°C). Fungal contaminants are more difficult to eradicate, as most fungicides are also lethal to leishmanial promastigotes. Kimber et al.,[82] however, claim that the incorporation of 500 μg mℓ^{-1} of 5-fluorocytosine in certain culture media eliminated problems of fungal contaminants without affecting the growth of leishmanial promastigotes.

The development of visible skin lesions in hamsters inoculated with triturated material from suspected leishmaniotic lesions is very variable, depending greatly on the *Leishmania* involved and the number of parasites that have been inoculated. Nodules, with very abundant amastigotes, may appear in only a few weeks in animals that have been inoculated with certain subspecies of *L. mexicana*. On the other hand, other parasites such as some members of the *L. braziliensis* complex, may only produce visible skin alterations after 6 to 12 months.

In cases of suspected visceral leishmaniasis, material is usually obtained by the aspiration of bone-marrow, following sternal puncture, or by spleen-puncture. Amastigotes are usually far more abundant in the spleen than they are in the bone-marrow; the undoubted medical risks entailed in spleen-puncture should always be considered however, especially when there is extreme splenomegaly. Direct examination of stained smears is usually sufficient for diagnosis, but in vitro culture and hamster inoculation should also be practiced wherever possible. Hamsters are usually inoculated by the intraperitoneal route, and a few months are generally needed before parasites become abundant in the viscera.

In the examination of wild animals for either cutaneous or visceral leishmaniasis, it should be remembered that infections in the natural hosts are likely to be of the inapparent type, with parasites scattered throughout apparently normal skin or viscera. In epidemiological studies on the importance of certain animals as reservoirs of *Leishmania* it is necessary, therefore, to examine skin-snips from different parts of the body, such as the ears, nose, feet and tail. The skin tissue is triturated in sterile saline solution with antibiotics, as indicated above, inoculated intradermally into hamsters, and cultured in blood-agar medium. Portions of liver and spleen should be treated similarly, for so-called "cutaneous" parasites such as *L. major* and *L. braziliensis* may also be isolated from the viscera of wild animals.

Isolation and subsequent identification of *Leishmania*, from man and other animals, has assumed considerable importance in recent years with our increasing awareness of a multiplicity of leishmanial parasites causing the human disease, in particular in neotropical regions. It is no longer sufficient to simply say that a patient has "cutaneous leishmaniasis", for prognosis greatly depends on which species or subspecies of *Leishmania* is involved. Thus, infection with *L. b. guyanensis* ("pian-bois") is rarely, if ever, associated with subsequent metastasis to the naso-pharyngeal tissues, whereas mucocutaneous leishmaniasis is a common sequel to infection with *L. b. braziliensis* ("espundia"), sometimes 20 or more years after the initial skin lesion has healed.

Again, although skin lesions due to *L. m. amazonensis,* in Brazil, are relatively mild compared with those of *L. b. braziliensis,* and unassociated with spread to the naso-pharynx, there is the unpleasant fact that up to 40% of the recorded cases have developed into incurable and highly mutilating diffuse cutaneous leishmaniasis (DCL).

Clearly, it is beyond the scope of most clinicians to bring diagnosis down to the specific or subspecific nature of the *Leishmania* concerned, particularly when dealing with American cutaneous leishmaniasis; however, attempts should be made to have the organism isolated and passed on to experts for more accurate identification.

Skin tests

The intradermal injection of suspensions of dead promastigotes, or extracts of the disrupted flagellates, usually provokes a typical delayed hypersensitivity reaction in patients recovered from, or with, cutaneous leishmaniasis.

Erythema and induration develop at the site of inoculation after 24 to 48 hr, the test routinely being read at 48 and 72 hr. More sophisticated "exo-antigens" are prepared by growing the promastigotes in dialysis-sacs suspended in the liquid phase of a suitable medium; in this case the antigen consists of the metabolic by-products of the flagellates, in the absence of any organisms. Such exo-antigens are particularly useful because they produce an "immediate" skin reaction, in the form of a pronounced erythema, which can be read within about 15 min; they also produce the characteristic, delayed induration at 24 to 72 hours.[150,151]

The leishmanin test is group specific, in that antigen from one *Leishmania* species or subspecies will reveal the development of delayed hypersensitivity to the same or *other* leishmanias. Its major use is in large scale epidemiological surveys, but it is a useful confirmatory tool to back up parasitological diagnosis. Recovered patients usually show positive reactions for many years after cure.

Weak or negative responses are, however, common in cases of infection with *L. b. braziliensis,* and a negative response is the rule in cases of DCL. In visceral leishmaniasis there is a positive reaction only following cure. Finally, it should be remembered that a positive leishmanin test is no indication of *protective* immunity in cutaneous leishmaniasis.

In general, leishmanin skin tests have proved of limited value in the detection of *Leishmania* infections in animals other than man.

Serodiagnosis

In visceral leishmaniasis, the excessive rise in serum globulins has formed the basis of the "formol-gel" or similar tests.[93] They are not serological tests in the strict sense of the word, since the globulins are non-specific and are not anti-leishmanial antibody. In Indian kala azar, at least, the formol-gel test is still of value in the field.

Almost all known serological tests have been applied to leishmaniasis, with somewhat inconsistent results — possibly due to lack of standardization of methods and interpretation of the results. Of these, circulating antibodies seem best detected by the indirect fluorescent antibody test (IFAT), using amastigotes or promastigotes as antigen. Shaw and Lainson[154] have reviewed the literature on this test in various forms of leishmaniasis, and demonstrated leishmanial IgA antibody in the sera of patients with the cutaneous and mucocutaneous disease, in Brazil. There were significantly more positive reactions with IgA conjugate in cases of mucocutaneous leishmaniasis than in those with other forms, and no association was noted between IgA and IgG titers. It would seem that IgA antibodies may be useful diagnostically, especially in that phase of the disease, due to *L. b. braziliensis* s.l., when lesions are predominantly in the mucosae.

Antibodies against *Leishmania* usually disappear after cure, and persistence after treatment is taken to indicate treatment failure and the survival of parasites in an occult infection. As is the case with positive skin-tests, circulating antibodies detected by the IFAT are probably unconnected with protection, since protective immunity in leishmaniasis seems largely related to cell-mediated rather than humoral responses.

The Infection in Wild and Domestic Animals

Two common misconceptions have developed regarding *Leishmania:* firstly that infection is always associated with disease and, secondly, that there is a sharp division between "visceral" and "cutaneous" leishmaniasis. Both are largely due to past emphasis on the human disease, although the virulence of certain parasites such as *L. d. infantum* and *L. d. chagasi* in the dog and the fox have doubtless contributed to our misunderstanding.

It is not appropriate, here, to discuss theories on the evolution of the leishmanias, but there is much evidence to suggest that they represent a very ancient group of parasites. As is normally the case with long-established parasitic associations, a well-balanced host-parasite relationship is the general rule and infection is inapparent, with little or no pathological effect. Accumulated evidence, particularly in regard to the neotropical leishmanias, has in fact shown that infection in the *natural* hosts is almost always benign and inapparent. The parasites are scattered, in small numbers, throughout the dermis or the viscera, where they produce little or no host-cell reaction. Such disseminated skin infection provides a ready source of parasites for the sandfly vectors, while visceral involvement will provide additional leishmaniae, as they gain entrance to the peripheral blood.

Infection in the natural hosts is, therefore, usually detected only by the culture of portions of skin or viscera in blood-agar medium, or by the inoculation of highly susceptible laboratory animals such as the hamster. Almost nothing is known of the normal course of infection of the different leishmanias in their wild mammalian hosts.

Visible dermal lesions are sometimes seen, however, in wild animals which normally show no signs of infection. Among rodents and marsupials the tail is the most frequent site of such lesions, less frequently the ears and the feet. They may appear as quite severe, destructive ulcers, but are more usually in the form of inconspicuous nodules or flat, depigmented and depilated areas of unbroken skin. Why a minority of animals should show destructive skin lesions is not known; possibly they mark the site of mechanical trauma which has resulted in the local formation of unusually favorable conditions for multiplication of the parasites. Factors such as stress, and the age at which individual animals become infected, have also to be considered.

When their preferred blood-source is scarce, many sandfly species will feed on unusual hosts, including man, and inoculated *Leishmania* species may find themselves in unaccustomed surroundings. Very often they will be rapidly destroyed, but on other occasions they may multiply and evoke a violent host reaction which will be manifested by a variety of skin lesions, or severe pathological changes in the internal organs. Such accidental hosts play a minor role in the maintenance of the parasite in nature, for leishmaniae localized in discrete ulcers (e.g. in man) are not so readily available to the sandfly vector as are those scattered throughout healthy skin. Sick animals, such as dogs and foxes infected with *L. d. infantum* or *L. d. chagasi* will die from the disease, or fall more ready prey to predators; they will thus be removed as effective long-term reservoirs of infection. Their importance as a temporary source of infection for man nevertheless remains high.

L. d. infantum and *L. d. chagasi* produce a fatal disease in dogs and the fox *Lycalopex retulus.* In the final phase there is extreme wasting; weakness of the legs, with pronounced edema of the feet and exaggerated elongation of the claws; ulcerative and nodular lesions of the skin, with frequent depigmentation and depilation; various eye conditions such as conjunctivitis, blepharitis and keratitis, leading to blindness; and diarrhea. Death may occur after only a few months of infection, although acutely infected animals may survive as long as two years.

Such a poor host-parasite relationship in the canine infection does not suggest either the dog or the fox, L. retulus, to be primary hosts of *L. d. infantum* or *L. d. chagasi*, however great their importance as reservoirs of infection for man. The parasites possibly originate from a hitherto undetected source in some wild animal(s). Pathology of the skin lesions and acute visceral leishmaniasis in wild and domestic animals is similar to that described below, in man.

It has long been customary to distinguish between "visceral" and "dermal" leishmaniasis, but this division is by no means always maintained.[92] Thus, the parasites responsible for East African and Sudanese "visceral" leishmaniasis may produce primary cutaneous lesions, several months before the onset of a visceral disease, and in some cases the infection does not proceed past the cutaneous stage. *L. d. donovani*, the causative agent of Indian "kala azar", occasionally shows a striking invasion of the skin in the form of the disease referred to as "post kala azar dermal leishmanoid". Again, in dogs infected with *L. d. infantum* or *L. d. chagasi* there are abundant parasites in the skin, which makes these animals particularly important domestic reservoirs of infection for man. At least *L. major* and subspecies of *L. braziliensis* are commonly found in the viscera of both natural and experimental hosts, although most textbooks regard them as essentially "cutaneous" leishmanias, based on the infection seen in man. Very recently, isolates of *Leishmania* from cases of visceral leishmaniasis of man in India and Israel have been identified as *L. t. tropica*,[33] while others from cutaneous lesions of patients in Europe have been found to be *L. d. infantum*.[143] Isolates of *L. b. guyanensis* from sloths and anteaters[99] have been almost exclusively from the viscera. The disease in man, however, is known only in the form of skin lesions; whether or not the organism is also present in the viscera of the infected person is not known, but it is of interest that hamsters with cutaneous lesions due to intradermally inoculated promastigotes of *L. b. guyanensis,* also develop visceral infections.

It is beyond the scope of this review to further discuss the behavioristic differences of the various leishmanias in laboratory animals. They may sometimes be sufficiently striking, however, to enable the differentiation of certain species of *Leishmania* in a *given geographic area.* Thus, most subspecies of *L. mexicana* produce large tumor-like lesions containing extremely large numbers of amastigotes, but evoke very little host-cell response. On the other hand, subspecies of *L. braziliensis* grow much less luxuriantly in hamster skin, in which they tend to produce smaller, fleshy nodules containing fewer parasites, associated with a great deal of host-cell reaction. (For further details under this sub-head, see Reference 84.)

The Infection in Man
Signs and Symptomology of Visceral Leishmaniasis

The incubation period is extremely variable, with periods as little as 2 weeks and as long as 9 years having been estimated between the most likely date of infection and the onset of symptoms; in most cases, however, the period of incubation lies between 6 weeks to 6 months.

Early on, symptoms are restricted to a mild, irregular fever, which is later of daily occurrence and frequently accompanied by sweats and chills. This initial symptomology may be more dramatic with non-indigenous patients, who may develop very high fever and severe chills from the onset. Associated symptoms include cough, diarrhea, dizziness, vomiting, bleeding gums, pains in the limbs and weight loss.

As the disease progresses, fever becomes an almost constant feature. Physically, the patient now begins to manifest lymphadenopathy and the onset of splenomegaly. The extent of the latter is variable, and at times at variance with the duration of infection. Enlargement of the liver is usual, although less striking than that of the spleen; hypertrophy of both organs is associated more with a feeling of discomfort rather than pain. Lymphadenopathy is a conspicuous feature, but more so in infections with *L. d. infantum* and the Kenyan and Sudanese parasites than in that due to *L. donovani*.

Skin changes are commonly associated with visceral leishmaniasis. The local Hindu name of "kala azar" in fact stems from the strange, earthy-grey hue of the skin in patients with the Indian form of the disease (i.e. "black sickness"); it is particularly noticeable on the legs and feet, and is most conspicuous in light-skinned races. In Kenyan, Sudanese and Mediterranean visceral leishmaniasis there may be nodular or even ulcerative skin lesions.

Without treatment, visceral leishmaniasis of man usually has a fatal outcome* and, after a period varying from a few months to several years, the patient becomes emaciated and exhausted. Anemia is very pronounced and there is serious imbalance in the serum globulins. Increase of the IgG fraction of gamma globulin results in an increase of total serum proteins to over 10 g/100 mℓ, in some instances; and this shows up markedly in immunoelectrophoretic studies. IgM may show some increase, but reverts to normal after treatment; serum albumin levels are low in advanced visceral leishmaniasis.

Most striking of the blood changes is the leukopenia, with a drop to approximately 2,000 cells per cubic millimeter in up to 75% of cases; peripheral blood eosinophils and neutrophils become non-existent, with corresponding relative monocytosis and lymphocytosis. Anemia is particularly severe late in the infection, and principally due to the shortened life-span of the erythrocytes. Thrombocytopenia tends to increase progressively with duration of the infection, accompanied by prolongation of the time in clotting tests.

Pathology of Visceral Leishmaniasis

The overall, characteristic pathology of this disease is parasitic blockage and destruction of the reticulo-endothelial system, with the most severe effects reflected in such organs as the spleen, liver, bone marrow, lymph glands and intestines.

The spleen becomes grossly enlarged, due to congestion and excessive reticulo-endothelial proliferation, with cells packed with parasites. The capsule is smooth and considerably thickened, and the pulp greatly increased in amount and friability; there are usually frequent infarcts.

The liver is usually enlarged and often with a mottled, brownish appearance. Pressure atrophy of the parenchyma cells may occur, with fibrosis and cirrhosis in untreated cases of long duration. Parasites are abundant in the Küpffer cells.

The bone marrow assumes a reddish color and usually contains abundant intra-cellular amastigotes. Initially there is normal erythropoiesis and granulopoiesis, but these become depressed, and destruction of the bone-marrow may become so extensive that little blood-forming tissue is left.

The kidney and lungs are not usually extensively parasitized, but there may be cloudy swelling of the tubule cells and amyloidosis. Secondary bacterial infections of the lungs may occur, due to the overriding leukopenia.

In the intestines there is often excessive reticulo-endothelial cell proliferation, especially in the jejunum and duodenum. The villi may become packed with infected cells.

Lymph glands are enlarged, especially those of the mesenteries; there is hypertrophy of the retro-pharyngeal lymph tissues, and amastigotes of *Leishmania* can often be demonstrated in pharyngeal and nasal secretions.

---

* Evidence in recent years, however, suggests that both *L. d. donovani* and *L. d. infantum* may produce inapparent, chronic infection in some individuals.

Parasites may sometimes be detected in apparently normal skin, but are more usually associated with the nodular lesions seen in cases of "post kala azar dermal leishmanoid".

Symptomology of Cutaneous Leishmaniasis

In oriental sore, due to parasites of the *L. tropica* complex, the incubation period varies from about 14 days to a month after the bite of the infected sandfly. The lesion appears, at the site of the bite, as a tiny papule about 1 to 3 mm in diameter and is usually overlooked as "an insect-bite"; it may itch, but is certainly not painful.

In infection with *L. t. tropica* ("dry", urban cutaneous leishmaniasis), the skin above the papule commences to flake away after a further week or two; a moist crust is formed which, when it falls or is scratched off, reveals a small, shallow ulcer. Over a period of some months the ulcer slowly extends, by erosion of its edges. Subsidiary or satellite lesions sometimes appear around the primary sore. Secondary infection with bacteria is a common complication, with discharge of pus, and this can cause clinical confusion with other skin conditions such as "tropical ulcer".

The final size of the lesions, prior to healing, is variable and very much depends on the degree of secondary infection; in general they may be from 1 to 3 in. in diameter. Multiple lesions are sometimes seen; when in small numbers, and on exposed parts, they are probably the result of separate bites from the infected sandfly or sandflies, but very large numbers of lesions are probably due to blood or lymph-borne metastases.

Development of spontaneous healing is relatively slow; seldom less than a year, and sometimes as long as two or more years. Considerable deformative scarring may occur, especially disfiguring when on the face.

An aberrant form of chronic oriental-sore, "leishmaniasis recidiva" (LR), is probably due to immune deficiencies (allergic state) in which cell-mediated reactions are over-developed; the patient develops multiple and long-lasting lesions which are chronically and histologically comparable with tuberculosis of the skin. The lesions appear during or after the healing of the initial ulcer, and the course of the disease is very slow and long. The condition has been recorded mostly in children, and the most seriously affected parts of the body appear to be those most exposed to the sun.

The development of infection with *L. major* ("wet" rural cutaneous leishmaniasis), is more rapid. The initial papule often simulates a boil, is often of large size (5 to 10 mm), and produces a rapidly growing, uneven ulcer which quickly heals in only 3 to 6 months. This zoonotic form of "oriental sore" is characterized, too, by the occurrence of lymphangitis, lymphadenitis, and the common production of secondary satellite papules.

In the Ethiopian highlands *L. t. aethiopica* is associated with both typical "oriental-sore", which heals spontaneously and is not particularly disfiguring, and diffuse cutaneous leishmaniasis which is highly disfiguring and till now incurable. The latter condition (DCL) is generally considered related to immunological incompetence of the patient, and it takes the form of large disseminated nodules which are extremely rich in parasites.

The incubation period and initial development of the various forms of American cutaneous leishmaniasis, due to subspecies of *L. mexicana* and *L. braziliensis*, is similar to that already described for *L. t. tropica*. A multitude of clinical manifestations have been recorded for infections which are in many cases due to the same organism, and which probably reflect different individual responses, depending on the patient's immunological idiosyncrasies more than anything else.

In infection with *L. m. mexicana* ("chiclero's ulcer"), the disease may follow a course similar to that of "oriental sore", with eventual spontaneous healing after periods of up to a year or more. Lainson and Strangways-Dixon[95] noted a tendency of many body lesions to apparently cure spontaneously within only a few weeks of their appearance, and when they had reached only a few mm in diameter. This fact suggests that chronic, inapparent skin infection may exist in some persons, and would help to explain why many individuals deny having acquired the infection, although showing a strongly positive delayed hypersensitivity (skin test) reaction.

For reasons not fully understood, however, 40.0% of "chiclero's ulcers" are on the external ear. Here, the infection is extremely long-lasting (up to 30 years has been recorded), and very frequently results in complete destruction of the pinna. As in oriental sore, recovery from *L. m. mexicana* imparts strong immunity to reinfection with the same parasite.

The clinical course of "uta", due to *L. b. peruviana,* is so similar to that of *L. t. tropica,* that many authorities considered that the disease was in fact caused by the latter parasite, which was presumed to have been introduced into Peru by the Spanish "conquistadores". As already discussed, however, the similarities are purely coincidental, and there is no longer any doubt regarding the taxonomic position of the causative agent of "uta", within the *L. braziliensis* complex.

In infections with *L. b. guyanensis* ("pian-bois"), development of the initial lesion follows the usual pattern, the incubation period having been accurately shown to be about 14 days following the bite of the infected sandfly. Multiple lesions are commonly seen, with some patients showing up to 50 or more lesions spread all over the body. There is no doubt that such a condition may be the result of an extremely high rate of infection in the sandfly vector of a given region, and an unnaturally close contact with these insects. Thus, men collecting the vector, *Lu. umbratilis,* from tree trunks have often developed a great many lesions simultaneously, on their arms.[104] At times, however, multiplicity of lesions is clearly due to metastatic spread, and developing nodules may be traced along the course of the lymphatics. Spontaneous cure probably does take place, but it would appear to be a slow process, and leaves considerable scarring. There is no conclusive evidence that subsequent naso-pharyngeal involvement occurs, and cases of mucocutaneous leishmaniasis in the same geographical area are considered to be due to overlapping *L. b. braziliensis* s.1.

Panamanian cutaneous leishmaniasis, due to *L. b. panamensis,* is similar to "pian-bois", although multiple lesions appear to occur less frequently. Literature refers to occasional cases of mucocutaneous leishmaniasis in Panama but, once again, there is evidence that these are due to another parasite.[178]

By far the most mutilating form of cutaneous leishmaniasis (apart from the rather exceptional DCL cases caused by subspecies of *L. mexicana*) is that due to *L. b. braziliensis* s.1. Initially, the skin lesion follows the same developmental pattern as that described for *L. t. tropica,* the incubation period being about 14 days. Multiple lesions are relatively rare, and are most likely due to the separate bites of infected sandflies. Evolution of the ulcer is slow and often over many years, producing extensive lesions which may become several inches across. Shortly after ulceration of the initial skin lesion, the parasites may migrate to and invade the tissues of the naso-pharynx or palate, where they may sometimes be detected in biopsied material as little as 4 — 6 weeks after the primary lesion has become apparent. Here the parasites may remain, seemingly dormant, for many years after the skin lesion has spontaneously healed, or sometimes when it has apparently been resolved by drug treatment.

Some time later, varying from a few months to as long as 20 years or more, lesions may appear in the naso-pharyngeal mucosae. There now ensues a slow but relentless erosion of these tissues, leading to destruction of the septum of the nose and frequent spread of infection to surrounding areas, such as the lips. Disfiguration is often extreme, and there is usually serious impairment of speech, respiration and the process of eating; in advanced cases, secondary bacterial infection may lead to death from pneumonia.

Pathology of Cutaneous Leishmaniasis

"Oriental-sore" is characterized by an initial, massive invasion of monocytes and histiocytes which ingest amastigotes and thus contribute to the continuing multiplication of the parasite. The lesion is then walled off, or infiltrated, by the invasion of lymphocytes, plasma cells, and macrophages, which usually results in a diminution of parasites. This protective mechanism is of only partial success, however, for the lesion persists, albeit with reduced numbers of parasites, often for many years. The overlying dermis now ulcerates and the epidermis shows variable degrees of acanthosis, intraepidermal necrosis, pseudoepitheliomatous hyperplasia, and hyperkeratosis.

After a very variable time, the process of healing is initiated, accompanied by the usual fibrosis and formation of scar tissue. Recovery from infection, in general, imparts a long-term immunity to reinfection with the homologous parasite.

If the patient fails to develop cell-mediated immunity, there is no parasite check and the result is diffuse cutaneous leishmaniasis, till now incurable. The skin nodules in this condition are composed largely of masses of macrophages, packed with parasites, in the absence of any notable host-cell reaction.

At the opposite pole of the spectrum, the patient with "oriental-sore" may show a failure to heal due to an allergic state (leishmaniasis recidiva); antibody production is marked and cell-mediated reaction overdeveloped, but destruction of parasites is nevertheless suppressed. The condition thus arises of long-lasting lesions of the skin which contain very scanty parasites.

The sequence of events is similar in the various forms of American cutaneous leishmaniasis. The extremely chronic and destructive nasopharyngeal lesions due to *L. b. braziliensis* are regarded as another expression of allergic state, similar to that of LR in infection with *L. t. tropica*. Diffuse cutaneous leishmaniasis in the Americas seems limited to infections with subspecies of *L. mexicana*.

Classification of the Leishmanias

The systematic position of the genus *Leishmania* is as given by Levine et al.[107] The grouping of species and subspecies broadly follows that of Lainson and Shaw,[92] with some modifications (see Figure 5).

Kingdom Protista Haeckel, 1866
Sub-Kingdom Protozoa Goldfuss, 1817
Phylum Sarcomastigophora Honigberg and Balamuth, 1963
Sub-phylum Mastigophora Diesing, 1866
Class Zoomastigophorea Calkins, 1909
Order Kinetoplastida Honigberg, 1963, emend. Vickerman, 1976
Sub-Order Trypanosomatina Kent, 1880
Family Trypanosomatidae Doflein, 1901, emend. Grobben, 1905
Genus *Leishmania* Ross, 1903

Section Hypopylaria (from Gk. hypo = under; Gk. pyl = gate)

These are primitive leishmanias. In the sandfly the flagellates move to a posterior station in the intestine, in the pylorus, ileum and rectum. The only known hosts are some lizards of the Eastern Hemisphere, in which the parasites apparently can occur in both the promastigote *and* amastigote forms. As infection is limited to the hindgut of the insect, transmission presumably takes place when the lizard eats infected sandflies.

1.   *L. agamae* David, 1929
2.   *L. ceramodactyli* Adler and Theodor, 1929

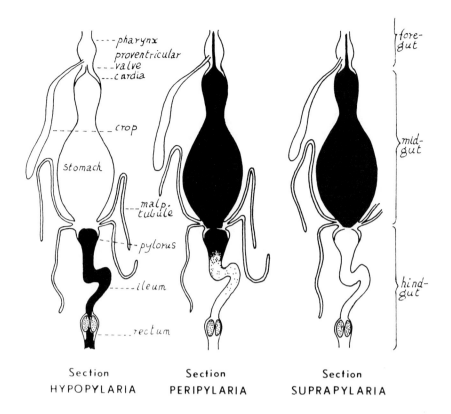

Section
HYPOPYLARIA

Section
PERIPYLARIA

Section
SUPRAPYLARIA

FIGURE 5.   Classification of the leishmaniae, based on their behavior in the sandfly vectors. Section HYPOPYLARIA: flagellates restricted to the hindgut, and transmission presumed to be after the ingestion of the infected insect. In lizards of the Old World. Section PERIPYLARIA: hindgut development retained, but parasites also migrating to the midgut and foregut and transmission now by the bite of the sandfly. In some lizards of the Old World, and represented by the *L. braziliensis* complex among the neotropical mammals. Section SUPRAPYLARIA: hindgut development completely lost, and parasites restricted to the midgut and the foregut, with transmission by bite. In mammals of both the Old and the New Worlds. Distribution of the parasites is shown in black. (After Lainson, R. and Shaw, J. J., *Biology of the Kinetoplastida,* Vol. 2, Lumsden, W. H. R. and Evans, D. A., Eds., Academic Press, London, 1979, 1. With permission.)

Section Peripylaria (from Gk. peri = on all sides; Gk. pyl = gate)

These are leishmanias which have retained the development of rounded paramastigotes and promastigotes attached to the wall of the sandfly hindgut, but which also undergo an anterior migration of the flagellates to the midgut and the foregut. This section includes some parasites of Old World lizards (and snakes?), but is mainly notable for inclusion of members of the *L. braziliensis* complex, which are important parasites of mammals, including man, in neotropical regions.

There is little information on the form adopted by those parasites infecting reptiles, but both promastigotes and amastigotes possibly occur, in the blood and/or viscera.

In mammals the peripylarian leishmanias occur only in the amastigote form, as far as is known, in macrophages of the skin and viscera. With development of the flagellates in the foregut of the sandfly, and subsequent invasion of the biting mouthparts, transmission is now *inoculative,* following the bite of the infected insect.

1.   In Old World lizards
    a.   *L. adleri* Heisch, 1958
    b.   *L. tarentolae* Wenyon, 1921

2.   In New World mammals
    a.   *L. braziliensis braziliensis* Vianna, 1911
    b.   *L. b. guyanensis* Floch, 1954
    c.   *L. b. panamensis* Lainson and Shaw, 1972
    d.   *L. b. peruviana* Velez, 1913

Section Suprapylaria (from Lat. supra = above; Gk. *pyl =* gate)
   These leishmanias have lost the primitive attached forms in the hindgut of the sandfly host, and development is now restricted to the midgut and the foregut; transmission is inoculative, by bite of the infected insect.
   Vertebrate hosts are limited to wild and domestic mammals, including man, in which the parasites are found only in the amastigote form, in macrophages of the skin, viscera, and blood.
   The Section Suprapylaria contains parasites of the *L. mexicana* and *L. hertigi* complexes (New World), the *L. tropica* and *L. major* complexes (Old World), and the *L. donovani* complex (Old and New Worlds).
   Subspecies of *L. mexicana* are well adapted parasites of rodents and marsupials of the Americas; *L. hertigi hertigi* and *L. hertigi deanei* appear to be restricted to neotropical tree-porcupines, and are so far unknown in man. Hyraxes (primitive ungulates) are the principal natural hosts of *L. tropica aethiopica* and an unnamed subspecies of *L. tropica* in South Africa, but a feral reservoir has yet to be found for *L. tropica tropica*. Like *L. mexicana, L. major* has a wide geographical distribution in a variety of wild rodents.
   In man, *L. mexicana, L. tropica* and *L. major* generally produce a variety of relatively mild and easily treated skin lesions. *L. tropica tropica* may, however, produce a condition known as "leishmaniasis recidiva", with long-lasting multiple lesions, and on rare occasions has given rise to visceral leishmaniasis in juveniles. *L. tropica aethiopica* infection may sometimes lead to involvement of the naso-pharyngeal mucosae (mucocutaneous leishmaniasis) or, in immunologically incompetent patients, incurable diffuse cutaneous leishmaniasis (DCL). At least three subspecies of *L. mexicana* may also produce DCL.
   Representatives of the *L. donovani* complex are closely related leishmanias which are particularly common in members of the Canidae (with the apparent exception of *L. donovani donovani*). Usually they are associated with visceral leishmaniasis, but *L. d. infantum* is also known to produce skin lesions which may easily be confused with those of *L. tropica* or *L. major*.

1.   The *L. mexicana* complex
    a.   *L. mexicana mexicana* Biagi, 1953
    b.   *L. m. amazonensis* Lainson and Shaw, 1972
    c.   *L. m. pifanoi* Medina and Romero, 1959
    d.   *L. m. aristedesi* Lainson and Shaw, 1979
    e.   *L. m. garnhami* Scorza et al., 1979
    f.   *L. m. enriettii* Muniz and Medina, 1948
    g.   *L. m.* subsp. (Mato Grosso State, Brazil)
    h.   *L. m.* subsp. (Minas Gerais State, Brazil)

2.   The *L. hertigi* complex (New World)
    a.   *L. hertigi hertigi* Herrer, 1971
    b.   *L. h. deanei* Lainson and Shaw, 1977

3.   The *L. tropica* complex (Old World)
    a.   *L. tropica tropica* (Wright, 1903)

   b. *L. t. aethiopica* Bray, Ashford and Bray, 1973
   c. *L. t.* subsp. (Namibia, S. Africa)
   d. *L. t.* subsp. (Ethiopia)

4. The *L. major* complex (Old World)
   a. *L. major* Yakimoff and Schokhor, 1914
   b. *L. m.* subsp.? (N.W. India)
   c. *L. gerbilli* Wang, Qu and Guan, 1964

5. The *L. donovani* complex (Old World)
   a. *L. donovani donovani* (Laveran and Mesnil, 1903)
   b. *L. d. infantum* Nicolle, 1909
   c. *L. d. archibaldi* Castellani and Chalmers, 1919
   d. *L. d.* subsp.? (Kenya)

6. The *L. donovani* complex (New World)
   a. *L. donovani chagasi* Cunha and Chagas, 1937

Leishmanias of Uncertain Taxonomic Position
1. In lizards of the Old World
   a. *L. gymnodactyli* Khodukin and Sofiev, 1947
   b. *L. hemidactyli* Mackie, Gupta and Swaminath, 1923
   c. *L. hoogstraali* McMillan, 1965
   d. *L. smeevi* Andrushko and Markov, 1955
2. In mammals of the New World
   a. *L. herreri* Zelódon, Ponce and Murillo, 1979

It is not proposed to deal with lizard leishmanias in the following, more detailed accounts of the above listed parasites. It may be mentioned, however, that *L. adleri* has been shown experimentally to produce fleeting skin infections in man. While the parasite is apparently of no importance as a pathogen in man, it may well be that natural, transient infections with *L. adleri* might provoke a positive leishmanin skin-test, and even influence the course of subsequent infection with *L. donovani* in Kenya. In that country, *L. adleri* is commonly found in the lizard *Latastia longicaudata,* and the parasite is apparently transmitted by the sandfly *Sergentomyia clydei*. This sandfly is also known to bite man in the Sudan.

There is no available information on the behavior of the leishmania described by Zelódon et al., in sandflies. In addition to sloths, they also claim to have isolated it from naturally infected sandflies, *Lu. ylephiletor, Lu. shannoni* and *Lu. trapidoi*. It was considered in most cases, however, that the infections were mixed with *Endotrypanum* and/or *"L. braziliensis" (L. b. panamensis?),* so the site of development of *L. herreri* in the sandfly gut was presumably impossible to ascertain. The fact that the parasite produced "sphaeromastigotes" in hamster skin is strange, and not characteristic of the genus *Leishmania*. Dr. M. L. Chance is acknowledged as having indicated *L. herreri* to have biochemical characteristics (not stated) which are "different from other known hemoflagellates". Presumably this includes the genera *Leishmania Trypanosoma* and *Endotrypanum;* it may be, therefore, that *"L. herreri"* is not in fact a *Leishmania*. It is provisionally included in the present classification, pending further observations on this interesting parasite.

Biochemical Identification of the Leishmanias

Early studies used comparative buoyant densities of nuclear and kinetoplastic

DNA.[33,35] The method proved of particular value in studies on the relationship of members of the Kinetoplastida at generic and specific levels, but of limited sensitivity at lower taxa. For example, there is clear separation of *L. mexicana*, *L. braziliensis*, *L. donovani* and *L. hertigi*, but failure to separate *L. t. tropica* and *L. t. aethiopica*, or *L. b. braziliensis* and *L. b. guyanensis*. Limitations have been particularly notable with leishmanias of the Old World "... because the results are tightly clustered about similar values..."[33] An added disadvantage to the DNA buoyant density method is the bulky and costly apparatus needed, virtually limiting its use to a handful of "typing centers" throughout the world.

Characterization of kinetoplastids by enzyme electrophoresis has been brought to a high level of efficiency.[33,64,117] Early results were somewhat disappointing, principally due to the small number of enzymes used. Thus, in spite of strong biological, clinical, and epidemiological evidence for the separation of the New World leishmanias *L. b. braziliensis* and *L. b. guyanensis,* early attempts to separate them on four enzyme profiles failed;[33] they could be separated, however, when the battery of enzymes was substantially enlarged.[116]

Another biochemical technique more recently applied to the leishmanias is the comparison of restriction endonuclease "fingerprints" of the minicircle component of kinetoplast DNA. Although considered a more powerful tool than enzyme electrophoresis,[112,118] it is possible that the rapid rate of evolution of kinetoplastic DNA minicircles may render the technique unsuitable for identification of kinetoplastid parasites.[67]

Radiorespirometry (as used so successfully in bacteriology) has been applied to the leishmanias[48] but is still very much under trial. There is the problem that this, and other increasingly sophisticated methods may indicate differences so fine as to render their significance difficult to evaluate in terms of classification. With the application of each new technical aid, there develops a tendency to regard it as some sort of "instant taxonomy kit", with which to bypass a tiresome process of basic parasitological investigation; even striking morphological differences may become overlooked or ignored. The various techniques are, without doubt, valuable tools with which to *identify* organisms but they are not, per se, the key to their *taxonomy*. For this we must still rely on a critical assessment of *all* available characters, including morphology, life cycle features, immunology, serology, etc., with which our new biochemical data should be incorporated.

Immunological Identification of the Leishmanias

An agglutination test has for a long time been used to differentiate leishmanias, usually at specific level, sometimes to subspecies. Known as the "Noguchi-Adler test" or the "Adler test", the technique makes use of the fact that when *Leishmania* is grown in a culture medium containing homologous antiserum, the flagellates form immobile masses resembling syncytia. As seen by the electron-microscope, the rounded promastigotes are actually individual bodies which are separated by a precipitate which is believed to be produced by the flagellar pocket; it is notable that this structure becomes greatly enlarged. By using tubes of media with varying dilutions of the homologous antiserum, a titer can be obtained by determining the lowest dilution at which no agglutination occurs, or when free, motile promastigotes begin to appear. The Noguchi-Adler test separates *L. major, L. t. tropica, L. mexicana, L. braziliensis, L. d. donovani* and *L. d. infantum,* and indicated the common identity of *L. d. archibaldi* s.l. from wild mammals, sandflies, and man in the Sudan.[1,2,10]

Using monoclonal antibodies in radioimmune assay, Pratt and David[136] were able to differentiate between *L. mexicana* and some subspecies of *L. braziliensis,* and the method would appear to hold great promise for the future. Lainson and Shaw[93a] have used antisera prepared in rabbits in immunofluorescence tests to distinguish *L. m. amazonensis* from a number of suprapylarian and peripylarian parasites.

Promastigotes of *Leishmania* at log-phase of growth release a substance(s) referred to as "excretory factor" (EF) into the culture fluid. It is thought to be a polysaccharide, and as different leishmanias produce various "types" of EF, this exoantigen can be used as a taxonomic marker.[143] Comparison of the various EFs is made by gel-immunodiffusion, using homologous and heterologous anti-promastigote sera obtained by inoculating rabbits. The EF technique probably measures the same antigens as the Noguchi-Adler test.

The complement-fixation test and the indirect immunofluorescent antibody test have till recently been found to be of limited use in differentiating the leishmanias, due to an overall cross-reaction between the different organisms. Recent modifications of the latter test, however, have reawakened interest in its use to identify leishmanias even to subspecific level.[93a]

Passive hemagglutination tests, using soluble antigen adsorbed onto the surface of tanned red blood cells, has been found of limited use in separating some leishmanias of the Old World, but the technique does not appear to differentiate parasites of the Americas.[24]

Providing infection is allowed to continue for sufficient time, a given *Leishmania* will usually produce a firm immunity to reinfection in the recovered patient or experimental animal with the same parasite; this immunity may persist for many years. There is, however, a striking lack of cross immunity between the different leishmanias. Sometimes this may be of a partial nature; thus, a volunteer recovered from an infection with *L. m. mexicana* was firmly resistant to reinfection with this parasite but susceptible to infection with *L. b. panamensis*,[85] and *L. b. braziliensis*.[93a] On the other hand, another volunteer who had recovered from infection with *L. b. panamensis* was protected against reinfection with this parasite *and* challenge with *L. m. mexicana,* but susceptible to *L. b. braziliensis*.[85,93a] Even bearing in mind the existence of some experimental variables (e.g., length of primary infection, virulence and number of challenging organisms, etc.), such experimental data are nevertheless strong supportive evidence for differentiating many leishmanias. Additional criteria are to be found in the behavior of parasites in vitro culture and experimental animal models, vector-specificity and morphology.

Section Peripylaria
The L. braziliensis Complex

This is a specific name which clearly embodies a number of different subspecies, some of which have yet to be defined. It is applied to those neotropical Peripylaria having nuclear and kinetoplastic DNA buoyant densities of 1.716-7 and 1.691-4, respectively, and having small amastigotes (approximating 2.4×1.8 μm) and small promastigotes. Growth in blood-agar media is very variable, depending on the subspecies, but these parasites are undoubtedly much more fastidious than those of the *L. mexicana* complex; nutrient-agars are recommended. Growth in hamster skin is very different from that of most parasites of the *L. mexicana* complex, from which *L. braziliensis* has most frequently to be differentiated. Some members, such as the unnamed parasite of the nine-banded armadillo,[104] may produce no visible lesion after intradermal inoculation in hamsters, and the parasite can only be detected by in vitro culture from the inoculation site. Others, loosely referred to as *L. b. braziliensis,* only give rise to a visible lesion, usually nodular, after an incubation period of many months — even as long as 9 to 12 months. The lesion remains small for the hamster's lifespan, and it is typically vascular and (compared with lesions due to *L. mexicana*) with marked host-cell reaction in the presence of relatively scanty amastigotes.

Although the primary skin lesion of *L. b. guyanensis* may appear within only a few weeks of inoculation into hamster skin, its growth, like that of *L. b. braziliensis*, soon becomes checked, and it remains discrete for the hamster's lifespan. Metastases may take place to the animal's extremities but they, too, share the same characteristics as the primary lesion. Parasites may become quite abundant in the viscera of hamsters infected with *L. b. guyanensis*.

There is a lack of cross immunity between the known subspecies of *L. braziliensis*.

Leishmania braziliensis braziliensis

It is a sad fact that as Vianna's parasite is no longer available for re-study, present-day workers on American leishmaniasis are in the difficult position of attempting to define new isolations of *L. b. braziliensis* s.l. in the absence of an adequate description of the type material (by modern standards). Taxonomic priority for this subspecies should, of course, go to a parasite from the general area of São João de Além Paraiba, Minas Gerais State, Brazil, where Vianna first described the organism from a case of disseminated cutaneous leishmaniasis, in 1911. The chances of obtaining material from the same area may prove difficult, however, in view of the drastic ecological upheavals (deforestation) that have taken place during the past decades.

Largely as a result of early failure to appreciate the multiplicity of leishmanias in the new World, the name *L. b. braziliensis* has been loosely used for parasites associated with leishmanial skin lesions of man in general, throughout Latin America, and in particular (why?) with that (or those?) producing mucocutaneous leishmaniasis after metastasis to the nasopharyngeal tissues; this was not the clinical picture, however, in the case of Vianna's patient. Lainson and Shaw[92] have suggested that "all it is possible to do at this stage is to regard those parasites referred to as *L. b. braziliensis* as being the same, until comparative studies prove otherwise".

The disease in man — Cutaneous and mucocutaneous leishmaniasis: "úlcera de Baurú", "ferida brava", "ferida sêca", "bouba", "buba", "nariz de anta" ("tapir nose"), "espundia".

Recorded mammalian hosts — Man (accidental "victim" host): wild animal hosts uncertain, possibly some of those listed under "unidentified parasites" of the *L. braziliensis* complex, below.

Recorded sandfly hosts — In South Brazil, *Lutzomyia intermedia* and *Lu. pessoai*. Promastigotes in *Lu. migonei* and *Lu. whitmani* from the same general region were not proven to be *Leishmania*. In North Brazil, *Psychodopygus wellcomei*.

Known geographic distribution — S.E. Brazil (Minas Gerais State). Distribution ill-defined due to lack of information on the true identity of the parasite.

Differential characters — Separated from *L. b. guyanensis* biochemically on enzyme profiles of aspartate aminotransferase E.C.2.6.1.1. (ASAT); analine aminotransferase E.C.2.6.1.2. (ALAT); phosphoglucomutase E.C.2.7.5.1. (PGM) and mannosephosphate isomerase E.C.5.3.1.8. (MPI).[116] Distinguished from *L. b. panamensis* on nuclear and kinetoplastic DNA buoyant densities of 1.716 g/ml and 1.691 g/ml, and 1.717 g/ml and 1.694 g/ml, respectively; also by enzyme profiles for 6-phosphogluconate dehydrogenase (6PGDH).[33a,34] Recovery from *L. b. braziliensis* infection confers no immunity against *L. b. guyanensis* in the monkey *Cebus apella*. Differences between *L. b. braziliensis* and *L. b. panamensis* are further indicated by lack of cross immunity between the two parasites, in man.[93a]

L. b. braziliensis grows very poorly and is difficult to maintain in most blood-agar media, whereas both *L. b. guyanensis* and *L. b. panamensis* grow relatively well in certain nutrient blood-agar media. Growth of *L. b. braziliensis* in hamster skin is poor; the lesion may become apparent only after some 6—12 months incubation, and it usually contains scanty parasites. On the other hand, both *L. b. guyanensis* and *L. b.*

panamensis grow relatively well in hamster skin, with a visible lesion often appearing within a few weeks after inoculation of the infective material; it usually contains abundant amastigotes.

Leishmania braziliensis guyanensis

The disease in man — Cutaneous leishmaniasis, often with multiple lesions. No evidence of the mucocutaneous disease. "Pian-bois", "bosch-yaws", "forest-yaws".

Recorded mammalian hosts — The sloth, *Choloepus didactylus,* and the lesser anteater, *Tamandua tetradactyla,* are the primary hosts. Secondary hosts occur in marsupials *(Didelphis marsupialis)* and rodents *(Proechimys guyannensis).* Primates: man (accidental host).

Recorded sandfly hosts — *Lutzomyia umbratilis* is the major vector, with *Lu. whitmani* and *Lu. anduzei* acting as secondary vectors among the wild animal hosts.

Known geographical distribution — The Amazon Basin, *north* of the river Amazonas, i.e., Guyana, Surinam, French Guyana and, in Brazil, Federal Territory of Amapá, north Pará and Amazonas States, possibly extending into Roraima.

Differential characters — See under *L. b. braziliensis. L. b. guyanensis* is differentiated from *L. b. panamensis* on nuclear and kinetoplastic DNA buoyant densities of 1.716 g/mℓ and 1.692 g/mℓ, and 1.717 g/mℓ and 1.694 g/mℓ, respectively, and enzyme mobilities for 6PGDH.[33a,34] *L. b. guyanensis* infections are treated with considerable difficulty with the antimonials "Glucantime" and "Pentostam", whereas *L. b. panamensis* is readily eliminated by these drugs.

Leishmania braziliensis panamensis

The disease in man — Panamanian cutaneous leishmaniasis, usually with single or a limited number of lesions. No evidence of mucocutaneous disease; cases of this disease in Panama are thought to be due to another parasite.[178]

Recorded mammalian hosts — Edentates: the sloths *Choloepus hoffmanni* (primary host) and *Bradypus infuscatus* (secondary host). Procyonids: *Bassaricyon gabbii, Nasua nasua* and *Potos flavus* (secondary hosts). Primates: the monkeys *Aotus trivergatus* and *Saguinus geoffroyi* (secondary hosts), and man (accidental host). Carnivores: the domestic dog (accidental host).

Recorded sandfly hosts — *Lutzomyia trapidoi* is the major vector, with *Lu. ylephiletor, Lu. gomezi* and *Psychodopygus panamensis* considered as secondary vectors.

Known geographical distribution — Panama and Costa Rica.

Differential characters — See under *L. b. braziliensis* and *L. b. guyanensis.* The parasite is clearly closest to *L. b. guyanensis.*[116]

Leishmania braziliensis peruviana

The disease in man — Cutaneous leishmaniasis, very similar to "oriental-sore" caused by *L. tropica tropica.* Not associated with the mucocutaneous disease. "Uta", "tiacc-araña", "llaga".

Recorded mammalian hosts — The domestic dog, *Canis familiaris,* is the only known host, other than man, till now. Whether or not the dog is a primary, secondary or accidental host, is difficult to say. Wild animals have not been adequately examined in the endemic areas of "uta" to date, and the infection in the dog seems localized in small skin lesions, which do not appear to offer an abundant source of parasites for sandflies. Man-to-man transmission would seem unlikely for the same reason; it remains very likely that some hitherto undiscovered wild animal host is involved.

Recorded sandfly hosts — *Lutzomyia peruana* and *Lu. verrucarum* are strongly suspected as vectors, on epidemiological grounds. Transmission appears to be peri-domestic.

Known geographic distribution — The western slopes of the Peruvian Andes and the Argentinian highlands. Probably more widely distributed in the Andean countries than till now indicated.

Differential characters — The idea that the causative agent of "uta" is simply "*L. tropica*" introduced into the New World in recent times can now be dismissed, for the development in sandflies is that of a typical peripylarian. The infection produced in hamster skin and the small size of the amastigotes are characters associated with subspecies of *L. braziliensis* and, although comparative biochemical studies have still to be completed, I am following the example of Hommel[76] in including the organism as a subspecies of that parasite.

Unidentified parasites, possibly subspecies of L. braziliensis

In Pará State, north Brazil, such organisms have been recorded in the rodents *Proechimys guyanensis, Rattus rattus* and *Rhipidomys leucodactylus;* the opossum *Didelphis marsupialis;* the sloth *Choloepus didactylus;* the armadillo *Dasypus novemcinctus;* and man.[92,103,104] In Mato Grosso State, Brazil, in the rodent *Oryzomys concolor* and man.[87] In São Paulo State, Brazil, in the rodents *O. capito, O. nigripes* and *Akodon arviculoides,* and man.[57,59] A parasite, very similar to *L. b. panamensis* and *L. b. guyanensis,* has recently been isolated from soldiers carrying out jungle-warfare exercises in Belize,[133a] suggesting that the geographic range of subspecies of *L. braziliensis* extends throughout South and Central America. Walton et al.,[178] have indicated the presence of another member of the *L. braziliensis* complex, other than *L. b. panamensis,* infecting man in the Caribbean coastal region of Panama.

Section Suprapylaria
The L. mexicana Complex

L. mexicana is very widespread among wild rodents and some other animals of the New World, in which it seems to form the counterpart of *L. major* in the Old World. In this respect, it is interesting to note that the two species have the common features of large amastigotes and promastigotes, predominantly rodent hosts, an extreme ease of culture in simple blood-agar media, and the production of large histiocytoma-like skin lesions in hamsters and mice. Serologically, too, they appear more closely related than other leishmanias. Subspecies of *L. mexicana* have nuclear and kinetoplastic DNA buoyant densities of 1.718 and 1.697—1.700 g/mℓ, respectively, and may be readily distinguished from those of *L. braziliensis* on the profiles of at least ten different enzymes — ASAT and ALAT, GPI (glucosephosphate isomerase E.C.5.3.1.9.), G6PD (glucose 6-phosphate dehydrogenase E.C.1.1.1.49.), MDH (malate dehydrogenase E.C.1.1.1.37.), ACON (aconitate hydratase E.C.4.2.1.3.), PEP (aminopeptidase [cytosol] E.C.3.4.11.1.), HK (Hexokinase E.C.2.7.1.1.), MPI (mannosephosphate isomerase E.C.5.3.1.8.) and ACP (acid phosphatase E.C.3.1.3.2.).[116]

Leishmania mexicana mexicana

The disease in man — Cutaneous leishmaniasis with strong tendency for extremely chronic lesions of the external ear. Rare cases of diffuse cutaneous leishmaniasis reported. "Ulcera de los chicleros", "chiclero's ulcer", "chiclero's ear", "Bay Sore".

Recorded mammalian hosts — The forest rodents *Ototylomys phyllotis* (primary host), *Heteromys desmarestianus, Nyctomys sumichrasti* and *Sigmodon hispidus* (secondary hosts); man (accidental host).

Recorded sandfly hosts — *Lutzomyia olmeca olmeca* is the only known vector.

Known geographic distribution — The Yucatan Peninsula, Mexico, Belize and Guatemala. Isolated cases of infection with a parasite identified as *L. m. mexicana* have been reported from Texas. In each case, however, the patients were known to have visited Mexico, and more detailed epidemiological studies are needed before it can confidently be stated that the parasite's geographic range extends into the United States.

Differential characters — Values for kinetoplastic DNA buoyant densities of *L. m. mexicana, L. m. amazonensis* and *L. m. aristedesi* are 1.700, 1.699, and 1.698 g/mℓ, respectively. These three subspecies can also be differentiated on enzyme profiles for MDH, ALAT and ASAT. There is no cross immunity between *L. m. mexicana* and *L. m. amazonensis* in experimentally infected monkeys, *Cebus apella. L. m. pifanoi* is considered to be "enzymatically quite different from *L. m. amazonensis.*"[117]

Leishmania mexicana amazonensis

The disease in man — Cutaneous leishmaniasis of the single-sore type, with the production of diffuse cutaneous leishmaniasis in up to 40.0% of cases. Not associated with classical mucocutaneous leishmaniasis, although the nasopharyngeal tissues may latterly be involved in advanced cases of DCL.

Recorded mammalian hosts — Forest rodents: *Proechimys guyannensis* (primary host), *Oryzomys capito, O. concolor, O. macconnelli, Neacomys spinosus, Nectomys squamipes,* and *Dasyprocta* sp., (secondary hosts). Marsupials: *Marmosa murina, M. cinerea, Metachirus nudicaudatus, Didelphis marsupialis,* and *Philander opossum* (secondary hosts). Carnivores: the fox *Cerdocyon thous* (secondary host); man (accidental host).

Recorded sandfly hosts — *Lutzomyia flaviscutellata* is the proven vector.

Known geographic distribution — The Amazon Basin, Brazil.

Differential characters — See under *L. m. mexicana*

Leishmania mexicana pifanoi

The disease in man — Till now only known in the form of diffuse cutaneous leishmaniasis of man, although simple, curable cutaneous leishmaniasis due to this parasite surely must exist.

Recorded mammalian hosts — Probably small forest mammals. A single specimen of the rodent *Heteromys anomalus* has been found infected with a *Leishmania,* apparently resembling *L. m. pifanoi;* in the absence of published comparative studies on this parasite and that of man, however, the significance of this finding remains obscure.

Recorded sandfly hosts — *Lutzomyia flaviscutellata?* A *Leishmania* found in this sandfly has, again, not been adequately related to *L. m. pifanoi* of man.

Known geographic distribution — Venezuela.

Differential characters — A very small sample of isolates referred to as "*L. m. pifanoi*" have been variously identified biochemically as *L. m. mexicana* or hemoflagellates even farther removed, such as *Endotrypanum.*[61] This clearly indicates a mixup of strains somewhere along the line, and the urgent necessity for the characterization of a larger sample of isolates from cases of DCL in Venezuela. In the meantime, Miles, et al.[117] have considered one stock of *L. m. pifanoi* as enzymatically quite distinct from *L. m. amazonensis,* the type locality of which is certainly very much closer to Venezuela than that of *L. m. mexicana.*

Leishmania mexicana aristedesi

The disease in man — Not yet recorded in man.

Recorded mammalian hosts — Forest rodents: *Oryzomys capito* (primary host), *Proechimys semispinosus* and *Dasyprocta punctata* (secondary hosts). Marsupials: *Marmosa robinsoni* (secondary host).

Recorded sandfly hosts — Unknown. *Lutzomyia olmeca bicolor* is most strongly suspected as the vector, due to its marked attraction to rodents.

Known geographical distribution — The Sasardi region of Panama.

Differential characters — See under *L. m. mexicana*.

Leishmania mexicana garnhami

The disease in man — Simple cutaneous leishmaniasis: no evidence of the mucocutaneous disease.

Recorded mammalian hosts — A single opossum, *Didelphis marsupialis* has been found infected; man (accidental host).

Recorded sandfly hosts — *Lutzomyia townsendi* is regarded as the vector, on epidemiological grounds.

Known geographical distribution — The Venezuelan Andes, up to 1,800 m.

Differential characters — Biochemically, the parasite has not yet been separated from *L. m. amazonensis* on enzyme profiles of ASAT, ALAT, PGM, GPI and G6PD. In hamsters the organism quickly produces large nodular skin lesions containing very abundant, large amastigotes. Growth in simple blood-agar media is luxuriant. On these criteria it is clear that the parasite is a member of the *L. mexicana* complex and that the name *garnhami* can at most only be used at subspecific level. Elongate promastigotes seen by Scorza et al.,[144] in the hindguts of experimentally infected *Lu. townsendi* probably originated from "regurgitation" of flagellates from the malpighian tubules or the midgut, and cannot be compared with the round or oval paramastigotes, spheromastigotes, and promastigotes attached to the hindgut wall by hemidesmosomes, as seen in sandflies infected with peripylarian leishmanias (e.g. *L. braziliensis*).

Leishmania mexicana enriettii

The disease in man — Not yet recorded in man.

Recorded mammalian hosts — The domestic guinea pig, *Cavia porcellus:* not yet discovered in any wild animal, although one certainly must exist.

Recorded sandfly hosts — Unknown, but *Lutzomyia monticola* is suspected in view of the good development in this fly, and its abundance in pine forests near recent foci of guinea pig infection.

Known geographic distribution — Curitiba, Paraná State, Brazil.

Differential characters — In spite of much literature to the contrary *L. m. enriettii* does infect the hamster, although the lesions are much more discrete than the large, nodular lesions produced in the guinea pig. The amastigotes and promastigotes are large, and the organism is easily maintained in simple blood-agar media. From the DNA buoyant densities (K-DNA = 1.718; N-DNA = 1.701) the parasite is obviously closely related to *L. mexicana* subspecies, although it can be separated from these by enzyme profiles for MDH. For these reasons Chance[33] felt that the organism "should probably be considered as a subspecies of *L. mexicana*..." I think this view is correct.

L. mexicana subsp. (in Trinidad)

The disease in man — Although cutaneous leishmaniasis was known in the past in Trinidad, the disease seems to have disappeared in recent times. Whether or not some past cases were due to the *L. mexicana* subspecies under discussion, is doubtful.

Recorded mammalian hosts — Forest rodents: *Oryzomys capito* (primary host), *Proechimys guyannensis*, and *Heteromys anomalus* (secondary hosts). Marsupials: *Caluromys philander*, *Marmosa fuscata*, and *M. mitis* (secondary hosts).

Recorded sandfly hosts — *Lu. flaviscutellata*.

Known geographic distribution — Trinidad, West Indies.

Differential characters — From its behavior in hamster skin and blood-agar culture, and the large size of its amastigotes, this parasite is clearly a subspecies of *L. mexicana*. It is difficult to assign it to any particular subspecies, however, in the absence of further criteria, in particular biochemical data. It was originally given the name of *L. m. amazonensis,* but as Trinidad is over 2,000 km from the type locality of this parasite, and only about 700 km from that of *L. m. pifanoi* in Venezuela, it seems better to refrain from using either name until more information becomes available.

Leishmania mexicana subsp. (Mato Grosso State, Brazil)

The disease in man — Cutaneous leishmaniasis, very often with multiple lesions and involvement of the lymphatics. No evidence of the mucocutaneous disease.

Recorded mammalian hosts — No wild animal hosts have yet been recorded; they almost certainly exist, however, as the disease was described in men clearing forested land for farming.

Recorded sandfly hosts — Unknown.

Known geographical distribution — Barra de Garças region, Mato Grosso State, Brazil.

Differential characters — A single isolate from one patient was shown to have DNA buoyant densities of N-DNA 1.718 and K-DNA 1.702, leading Chance[33] to conclude that the parasite was a subspecies of *L. mexicana.* It was differentiated from other subspecies of this parasite by enzyme profiles for MDH. Attempts to infect hamsters and sandflies have, strangely enough, failed. It may be that the parasite has lost its infectivity after prolonged maintenance in culture.

Leishmania mexicana subsp. (Minas Gerais State, Brazil)

The disease in man — Cutaneous leishmaniasis.

Recorded mammalian hosts — Dogs have been found infected in the endemic areas, but it is uncertain if they represent a reservoir of infection for man, or are merely accidental "victims", like man. It is likely that a wild animal host will eventually be found.

Recorded sandfly hosts — No information.

Known geographical distribution — Caratinga and Rio Doce valleys, Minas Gerais State, Brazil.

Differential characters — Buoyant densities for nuclear and kinetoplastic DNA have been shown to be 1.718 and 1.704, respectively, which again led Chance[33] to consider the parasite as a subspecies of *L. mexicana.* There is no available information on the behavior of the organism in hamsters or in vitro culture, or on its morphology. It is separated from the unnamed Mato Grosso parasite by enzyme profiles for MDH.

Until much more information is available on the two above-mentioned leishmanias, especially in terms of a wider range of enzyme profiles, it would seem unwise to assign any names to them.

The L. hertigi Complex
Leishmania hertigi hertigi

The disease in man — Not known to infect man. Apparently restricted to tree porcupines of the New World, in which it produces no visible signs of infection.

Recorded mammalian hosts — The porcupine, *Coendou rothschildi.*

Recorded sandfly hosts — Unknown.

Known geographical distribution — Panama and Costa Rica.

Differential characters — The nuclear DNA buoyant density of 1.714 sets *L. hertigi* apart from all other known leishmanias. Its highly individual nature can further be judged by its ready separation from *L. m. amazonensis* on the profiles of eleven different enzymes — ASAT, ALAT, PGM, G6PD, MDH, GPI, PEP, PK (pyruvate kinase E.C.2.7.1.40), PGK (phosphoglycerate kinase E.C.2.7.2.3.), MPI and ACP. Differences between the two subspecies of *L. hertigi* are given below.

Leishmania hertigi deanei

The disease in man — Not known to infect man. Apparently restricted to porcupines of the New World, in which it produces no visible signs of infection.

Recorded mammalian hosts — The tree-porcupines, *Coendou prehensilis* and an undescribed *Coendou* sp.*

Recorded sandfly hosts — Unknown. Isolation of the parasite has been made from a specimen of *Lutzomyia furcata* taken from a hollow tree in which a porcupine was living. From its poor development in *Lu. furcata,* however, it is felt that this insect is not the natural vector of *L. h. deanei.*[101a]

Known geographical distribution — Piauí and Pará States, Brazil.

Differential characters — *L. h. deanei* and *L. h. hertigi* are separated morphologically by the striking difference in their amastigotes. Those of *L. h. deanei* range from 5.1×3.1 to 6.8×4.5 μm, and probably represent the largest amastigotes of any known *Leishmania:* the kinetoplast appears as a small, curved rod, and the cytoplasm is highly vacuolated. Amastigotes of *L. h. hertigi* measure only 3.5×1.2 to 4.8×2.5 μm: they have a tiny dot-like kinetoplast, and cytoplasm containing few vacuoles. The two subspecies are further distinguished by the enzyme profiles for GPI, 6PGDH, MPI and ME (malate dehydrogenase [oxaloacetate-decarboxylating] [NADP$^+$] E.C.1.1.1.40).

Both subspecies of *L. hertigi* produce very low-grade, inapparent infections in the skin of hamsters, with parasites usually only detectable by culture. Growth in blood-agar media is prolific.

The L. tropica Complex

Leishmania tropica tropica

The disease in man — Cutaneous leishmaniasis: "oriental sore", "dry, anthroponotic, urban oriental sore", "Delhi boil", "Aleppo button", "Aleppo boil", "Bouton de Biskra", "Bouton de Crete", "Baghdad boil", "Salek", "Kokan sore", "Balkh sore", "Ashkabad sore", "Tropical sore", etc. Under exceptional circumstances *L. t. tropica* may give rise to visceral leishmaniasis in man.

Recorded mammalian hosts — Carnivores: the dog, *Canis familiaris,* and possibly the badger, *Meles meles.* Although there are numerous reports of cutaneous lesions due to *L. t. tropica* in dogs (particularly in Iraq and India), the parasite has rarely been adequately identified and the importance of the dog as a reservoir is still in doubt. A single specimen of *Meles meles* has been found with skin lesions of the legs, which contained amastigotes, in southern U.S.S.R. Again, identity of the parasite remains questionable, and it may have been *L. major.*

Failure to disclose a sufficiently common reservoir host of *L. t. tropica* has led many authorities to postulate that transmission is direct from man-to-man (anthroponotic); this seems unlikely, with the amastigotes limited to a single or few lesions of the skin, and renewed efforts are needed to settle the vexed question of a reservoir-host of *L. t. tropica,* once and for all.

Recorded sandfly hosts — *Phlebotomus perfiliewi* is suspected as a vector in Italy, with *P. papatasi* strongly indicated in other parts of Europe. The latter is considered as the vector in Israel, Jordan, Lebanon, and west Syria. To the east, in Mosul and Baghdad, Meshed, Kabul, U.S.S.R., and Delhi, there is strong evidence that the major vector is *P. sergenti.* In north Africa *P. papatasi, P. sergenti* and *P. chabaudi* are the most likely vectors.

Known geographical distribution — In Europe:** the Mediterranean and neighbor

---

* Personal communication from Dr. C. O. Handley, Smithsonian Institution, Washington, D.C. A description of this new species of *Coendou* is apparently in press.

** Considerable doubt has been raised as to the continued presence of *L. t. tropica* in Europe and North Africa, as noted earlier.

countries, including Bulgaria, Crete, southern France, Greece, Italy, Portugal, Sicily, Spain and Yugoslavia. In Asia: Israel (Jericho), Jordan, Iran (Meshed, Shiraz, Tabriz, Teheran), Iraq (Baghdad, Mosul), Libya (Tripoli), Azerbaijan Soviet Socialist Republic (Barda, Kirovabad), Turkmen Soviet Socialist Republic (Ashkhabad, Mary), Usbek Soviet Socialist Republic (Kokand, Samarkand, Tashkent), Syria (Aleppo, Damascus), Afghanistan (Kabul), and India (Delhi and Cambay). In Africa, it occurs in many of the oasis towns of Algeria, Morocco, and Tunisia (particularly Constantine). Sporadic cases of "dry, urban" forms of cutaneous leishmaniasis in other parts of Central Africa (Mali and Sudan) and southwest Africa (Namibia) are at present of doubtful etiology.

Differential characters — *L. t. tropica* is not distinguishable from *L. t. aethiopica* on N-DNA and K-DNA buoyant densities, but can be separated on enzyme profiles for MDH, GPI, and 6PGDH.

Apart from morphological, immunological and serological differences, *L. t. tropica* and *L. t. aethiopica* are readily separable from *L. major* on DNA buoyant densities alone.

Leishmania tropica aethiopica

The disease in man — Simple cutaneous leishmaniasis, and DCL. "Oriental Sore", "Cuncir", "Ghisua".

Recorded mammalian hosts — In Ethiopia, the hyraxes *Procavia habessinica* and *Heterohyrax brucei*. In Kenya, the hyraxes *Dendrohyrax arboreus* and *Procavia johnstoni*, and the "giant rat", *Cricetomys*. Man (accidental host).

Recorded sandfly hosts — *Phlebotomus longipes* and *P. pedifer* in the Ethiopian highlands. In Kenya, *P. pedifer*.

Known geographical distribution — The Ethiopian highlands, and Mount Elgon in Kenya: possibly south Yemen.

Differential characters — See under *L. t. tropica*.

Leishmania tropica subsp. (In South West Africa)

The disease in man — Simple cutaneous leishmaniasis.

Recorded mammalian hosts — The hyrax, *Procavia capensis:* man (accidental host).

Recorded sandfly hosts — *Phlebotomus rossi*.

Known geographical distribution — Namibia, southwest Africa.

Differential characters — Differentiated from *L. t. tropica* and *L. t. aethiopica* on enzyme profiles for MDH, GPI, G6PD and 6PGDH. Originally, Chance[33] considered that the parasites from the hyrax and man in Namibia were different. Further studies on a larger number of isolates, however, suggest that the parasite from the hyrax, man and *P. rossi* are the same.[133a]

Leishmania tropica subsp. (Ethiopia)

The disease in man — Not yet recorded.

Recorded mammalian hosts — The rodent *Arvicanthis* sp.

Recorded sandfly hosts — Not known.

Known geographical distribution — Ethiopia.

Differential characters — Separated from *L. t. tropica* and the Namibia subspecies by the enzyme profiles for MDH, GPI, G6PD, and 6PGDH; from *L. t. aethiopica* on enzymes GPI, G6PD, and 6PGDH.[33]

The L. major Complex

Leishmanias broadly known under this name are commonly found in rodents of desert and semi-desert regions in many parts of the Old World. Transmission to man may sometimes reach epidemic levels in some regions of the U.S.S.R. and the Middle East, while in others it remains a relatively sporadic disease; it is essentially a rural problem.

Leishmania major

The disease in man — Cutaneous leishmaniasis: "wet, rural, zoonotic oriental sore", "Pendeh sore", "Sart sore", "Jericho rose", "hab", "frina", "mard el teneur", "clou de Biskra", "clou de Gafsa", etc. Many local names are indiscriminately used for lesions due to both *L. tropica* and *L. major.*

Recorded mammalian hosts — Mainly rodents; in northwest China, Turkmenian and Usbek S.S.R., north Afghanistan and northeast Central Iran, the great gerbil, *Rhombomys opimus* is the major reservoir host, with the lesser gerbil *Meriones libycus* involved in some areas. In the U.S.S.R. the following rodents are occasionally infected: *Meriones tamariscinus, M. meridianus, Spermophilopsis leptodactylus, Citellus fulvus, Hystrix leucura, Allactaga severtzovi, A. elator, Alactagulus acontion, Dipus sagitta, Nesokia indica, Mus musculus, Cricetulus migratorius,* and *Microtus afghanus.* Non-rodents include the hedgehog, *Hemiechinus auritus,* the hare *Lepus tolai,* the mustelids *Mustela nivalis,* and *Vormela peregusna.* Elsewhere, rodent hosts include *Meriones hurrianae* in northwest India (Rajasthan) and Pakistan (Baluchistan); *Meriones* spp. in southwest Iran, east Saudi Arabia, and Iraq; *Psammomys obesus* and *Meriones* spp. in Israel and Libya; *Mastomys erythroleucus, Tatera gambiana,* and *Arvicanthis niloticus* in Senegal; *Tatera* and *Xerus* spp. in Kenya. Many infections in dogs, throughout this geographical range, are probably due to *L. major* rather than *L. tropica.* Man (accidental host).

Recorded sandfly hosts — In the U.S.S.R., where the most intensive studies have been made, *P. papatasi, P. caucasicus, P. andrejevi,* and *P. mongolensis* appear to act as the principal vectors in differing enzootic areas. Other sandflies are suspected as playing some role in the epidemiology of *L. major* infection, including *P. alexandri, P. ansarii, P. grimmi,* and *P. sergenti.* In Iran and the Jordan valley, *P. papatasi* is considered as the principal vector to man; in Senegal, *P. duboscqi* has recently been incriminated, while in Rajasthan, India, the vector appears to be *P. saheli* (at least, among the rodents).

Known geographical distribution — Northwest China; The Thar desert of northwest India and Pakistan; the deserts of Turkmenia, Usbekistan, south Tadjikistan, and Kazakhstan, S.S.R.; north Afghanistan; east Saudi Arabia; southwest Iran; Iraq; Kuwait; Jordan; Libya; Israel. In Africa, Algeria; Tunisia; United Arab Republic; The Sahara; Senegal; Sudan; Kenya; and Mali. Probably Chad; Niger; and Upper Volta.

Differential characters — *L. major* is distinguished from *L. tropica* by its larger amastigotes, which may reach 5.6×3.0 μm; serologically by the Noguchi-Adler test; immunologically by the failure of *L. tropica* to protect man against *L. major;* and differential behavior of the two parasites in laboratory mice and hamsters. Nuclear DNA buoyant densities for *L. major* and *L. tropica tropica* are 1.718 and 1.719 g/ mℓ, respectively. Enzyme profiles for MDH, G6PD, and 6PGDH serve to distinguish *L. major* from *L. t. tropica,* and those of MDH, GPI, G6PD, and 6PGDH from *L. t. aethiopica* and other presumed subspecies of *L. tropica* mentioned above.[33]

L. major subsp. (northwest India)

The disease in man — Not yet isolated from man.
Recorded mammalian hosts — Rodents (*Meriones* sp? see Reference 33).
Recorded sandfly hosts — No information.
Known geographical distribution — northwest India.
Differential characters — Differentiated on enzyme profiles of G6PD.

Leishmania gerbilli Wang, Qu and Guan, 1964

The disease in man — Not recorded in man.

Recorded mammalian hosts — The great gerbil, *Rhombomys opimus.*

Recorded sandfly hosts — No information.

Known geographical distribution — South Mongolia.

Differential characters — Amastigotes larger than those of *L. major*, reaching up to 6.4 × 2.8 μm. Unlike *L. major*, *L. gerbilli* appears to be incapable of infecting either man or the golden hamster; Chinese hamsters *(Cricetulus barabensis* are, however, susceptible). There is no available information on the biochemistry of the parasite, although preliminary studies suggest that *L. gerbilli* is readily distinguished from *L. major* on a number of enzyme profiles.[133a] Whether or not it may be regarded as a subspecies of *L. major* remains to be seen.

The L. donovani complex

Lysenko[110] suggested that visceral leishmaniasis due to parasites of the *L. donovani* complex probably had its origin in a rural enzootic focus located in Central Asia, with principal hosts in a variety of canids such as jackals, wolves, and foxes. In time the domestic dog became involved, and the disease spread into urban areas in Transcaucasia and the Mediterranean Basin, India, China, and the African continent.

In most cases the canid/man relationship has been maintained — as in the Mediterranean/Middle Asia subzone, and in China. Here, man is somewhat of a "deadend" for the parasite, for it is not commonly demonstrable in his skin or blood, and the dog remains the major source of infection for the sandfly.

In India, no canid or other animal host has been found and "kala azar" is regarded as anthroponotic, with transmission direct from man-to-man. This form of infection may be regarded as the culmination of evolution from the enzootic — zoonotic — anthroponotic situation in visceral leishmaniasis. Supporting this hypothesis is the fact that the causative parasite, *L. donovani donovani* may be demonstrated in the peripheral blood of man in 90.0% or more cases.

On the African continent, visceral leishmaniasis has retained its canid connections in many localities, in particular in North Africa. It is the dog which is principally involved, although wild canids have perhaps not been adequately examined. In addition, two apparently different situations have evolved in the general areas of Sudan and Kenya. In the Sudan, wild rodents are involved as reservoir hosts, and some carnivores *(Genetta* and *Felis);* dogs appear not to be involved, and the clinical picture of infection differs considerably from that of classical Indian and Mediterranean forms of visceral leishmaniasis in the frequent development of skin lesions.

In Kenya, the failure to find any hosts among wild mammals led to the belief by some that the disease, like Indian "kala azar", might be anthroponotic. There remained the fact, however, that the infection was frequently acquired by those entering uninhabited regions, strongly suggesting a feral reservoir. This situation remains unresolved to this day, for although a few canine infections have been recorded, the low prevalence in dogs is inconsistent with a disease which may sometimes reach epidemic proportions.

The taxonomic situation regarding the parasites causing Old World visceral leishmaniasis in the above-mentioned foci has remained confused. Adler[2] differentiated between *L. donovani* causing Indian "kala azar" and *L. infantum* associated with Mediterranean visceral leishmaniasis by serological methods (the Noguchi-Adler test), which prompted Lainson and Shaw[88] and Bray[23] to use the names of *L. donovani, L. infantum* and *L. chagasi* in subsequent publications.

It has long been appreciated by most authors, however, that the taxonomic criteria for such separation are slight. Modern biochemical methods (particularly enzyme electrophoresis) have confirmed differences between *L. donovani* and *L. infantum*, but have so far been unable to separate parasites causing human visceral leishmaniasis in the Mediterranean Basin, Africa, and Latin America.

It seems, then, that in spite of the enormous geographical spread of *L. donovani*, and the variety of sandfly vectors and mammalian hosts that have become involved, there has been surprisingly little intra-specific evolution of this viscerotropic parasite. This is in marked contrast to the wide divergence into readily distinguished subspecies shown by some other leishmanias, in particular *L. mexicana*.

Numerous authors have in the past used the subspecific names of *L. d. donovani*, *L. d. infantum* and *L. d. chagasi* (reviewed by Gardener,[60]) and, in view of current trends, it seems wisest to re-adopt this terminology. At least, in this way, any distinctive epidemiological, clinical or biological features will not be lost to us under the single name of *L. donovani*.

The name *L. d. sinensis* has been used by Nicoli,[125] in 1963, for the causative agent(s) of visceral leishmaniasis in north China. The present author tends to agree with Bray,[23] however, that most of the epidemiological and clinical features indicate association with *L. d. infantum*. Chinese authorities suspect the presence of *L. d. donovani* in some parts of China.

The use of the subspecific name *L. d. archibaldi* for the parasite responsible for Sudanese visceral leishmaniasis has been discussed early in this chapter.

Leishmania donovani donovani

The disease in man — Visceral leishmaniasis: post kala azar dermal leishmanoid. "Dum-dum fever", "kala azar", "Sikari disease", "Burdwan fever", "Sahib's disease", "Tropical splenomegaly".

Recorded mammalian hosts — Only man, as far as is known.

Recorded sandfly hosts — *Phlebotomus argentipes, P. chinensis.*

Known geographic distribution — India: Assam, Bihar, Bengal, Orissa, Tamil Nadu, Gujarat; E. Pakistan; Nepal; north China Plain* and E. China,* in Hopeh, Shansi, Shantung, Kiangsu, Anhwei, Honan, Hupeh, Szechwan, Tsinghai, and Sinkiang.

Differential characters — Separated from *L. d. infantum* and *L. d. chagasi* by the Noguchi-Adler test, EF test, and enzyme profiles for 6PGDH, ASAT, and ALAT.[97,143]

Leishmania donovani infantum

The disease in man — Chinese, Mid-Asiatic, Mediterranean, and North African infantile visceral leishmaniasis. Largely restricted to juveniles.

Recorded mammalian hosts — Primitive hosts in Central Asia are the jackal *Canis aureus*, the wolf *Canis lupus* and foxes *Vulpes vulpes*, and *V. corsak*. The dog has become the major reservoir for human infection in urban areas, extending the disease into southwest Asia, the Mediterranean region, and China. The epidemiological significance of infections in the domestic rats, *Rattus rattus* and *R. norvegicus* in Yugoslavia and Italy has still to be assessed. Man (accidental host).

Recorded sandfly hosts — In south France, west of the Rhone, the vector is *Phlebotomus ariasi*, whereas east of the Rhone (Marseille) it is almost certainly *P. perniciosus*. *P. major* is the most highly suspected sandfly in Greece, Crete, Rumania, Yugoslavia, the Lebanon, Israel, Syria, and Iran; with *P. perfiliewi, P. tobbi* and *P. chinensis* also indicated where they occur. In Italy, Portugal, Spain, Algeria, Tunisia, Malta, and Libya, *P. perniciosus* is regarded as the most likely vector, with *P. perfi-*

---

* Evidence for the presence of *L. d. donovani* in China is still inconclusive, but strongly suggested by the absence of canine infection in some endemic areas, clinical features, and the differing response of *L. d. donovani* and *L. d. infantum* to anti-leishmanial drugs.

liewi, *P. ariasi* and *P. longicuspis* also under suspicion, where they are found. In the U.S.S.R., *P. kandelaki* and *P. chinensis* have been incriminated in Transcaucasia, and *P. chinensis*, *P. mongolensis*, and *P. caucasicus* in Central Asia and Kazakhstan. In China, *P. chinensis* has been proven to be the only vector of importance.

Known geographic distribution — Central Asia: in Turkmenia, Usbekistan, Tadjikistan, Kirgizia, S. Kazakhstan, Azarbaidjan, Georgia and Armenia, S.S.R.; North and N.W. China, in Liaoning, Hopeh, Shansi, Shensi, Ningsia, N. Szechwan, N. Tsinghai, and Kansu. In southwest Asia, in Iraq, Saudi Arabia, Yemen, S. Yemen, Iran, and Afghanistan. In Africa: in north Algeria, north Tunisia, Libya, Egypt, Central African Republic, Chad, Gabon, Nigeria, Malawi, Niger, Upper Volta, Zaire, and Zambia. Canine infections, only, in Congo, Somalia, and Senegal. All countries of the Mediterranean littoral, extending into Hungary and Rumania.

Differential characters — See under *L. d. donovani.*

Leishmania donovani archibaldi

The disease in man — Sudanese cutaneous, "mucocutaneous" and visceral leishmaniasis.

Recorded mammalian hosts — Rodents: The "spiny rat", *Acomys albigens*, the "Nile grass rat", *Arvicanthis niloticus* and the domestic rat, *Rattus rattus.* Carnivores: *Genetta genetta* and *Felis serval.* The individual importance of these animals in the epidemiology of the disease remains uncertain, although the wild rodents probably represent the primary source of infection. Man commonly shows a parasitemia, but it is not clear to what extent (if any) he may serve to infect sandflies. It is particularly interesting that all attempts to find infected dogs have failed.

Recorded sandfly hosts — *Phlebotomus orientalis* has repeatedly been found infected in nature, and the parasite shown to be indistinguishable from that of man and the infected wild animals.

Known geographical distribution — Southern and Central Sudan. Visceral leishmaniasis in eastern and southern Ethiopia, Djibouti, northern Somalia, Chad, Niger, Central African Republic, and Congo may possibly represent extensions of the same general focus.

Differential characters — The epidemiological and clinical features of Sudanese visceral leishmaniasis differ considerably from those of both Indian "kala azar" and the Mediterranean disease. Biochemical techniques have till now, however, failed to separate *L. d. infantum* and Sudanese stocks of *L. d. archibaldi*,[143] and some are inclined to the view that the two parasites are identical. It may be that insufficient enzymes have been studied to separate a group of parasites which are clearly very closely related.

Leishmania donovani subsp. (Kenya)

The disease in man — Cutaneous and visceral leishmaniasis. Often in a form resembling "dermal leishmanoid", or with involvement of the lymphatic glands in the apparent absence of the visceral disease. The rate of spontaneous recovery reported to be sometimes as high as 80.0%, which contrasts strikingly with all other forms of visceral leishmaniasis.

Recorded mammalian hosts — Dogs have occasionally been found infected, but these may only represent "victims" rather than efficient reservoir hosts. Epidemiological evidence points to a feral reservoir; a number of infections with a *Leishmania* have been discovered in mongooses,[120a] but the parasite has yet to be characterized.

Recorded sandfly hosts — The sandfly *Phlebotomus martini* has been found infected in nature, and epidemiological studies strongly indicate this species as a vector. The females of two other species, *P. celiae* and *P. vansomerenae,* are morphologically indistinguishable from *P. martini*, however, which poses some questions yet to be answered.

Known geographical distribution — Kenya: possibly in south Ethiopia and Somalia.

Differential characters — See earlier paragraphs concerning *L. donovani* complex. Biochemically, the parasite has yet to be differentiated from *L. d. infantum,* with which some authorities consider the Kenyan organism to be synonymous.

Leishmania donovani chagasi

The disease in man — American visceral leishmaniasis, largely affecting juveniles; "kala azar", "calazar" (strictly speaking, these terms should be used only when referring to Indian visceral leishmaniasis due to *L. d. donovani).*

Recorded mammalian hosts — Canidae: the fox, *Lycalopex vetulus* in Ceará State, northeast Brazil; the dog is the principal source of infection for man. A parasite isolated from foxes, *Cerdocyon thous* in the Amazonian (Para) Region of Brazil may be *L. d. chagasi,* or another viscerotropic *Leishmania* of man (see below).

Recorded sandfly hosts — *Lutzomyia longipalpis* is probably the vector throughout the geographical range of the parasite. It shares coincidental distribution with the disease, has been found infected with promastigotes in highly endemic areas in Brazil, and has been shown to readily transmit the parasite experimentally.

Known geographical distribution — Argentina, Bolivia, Brazil, Colombia, Ecuador, Paraguay, Surinam (?), Venezuela; Guatemala, Honduras, Mexico, El Salvador, Guadeloupe.

Differential characters — See previous pages under *L. donovani* complex and under *L. d. donovani. L. d. chagasi* has yet to be differentiated from *L. d. infantum* biochemically.

Leishmania donovani subsp. (Pará State, north Brazil)

The disease in man — Visceral leishmaniasis, seemingly in all age groups; very sporadic, isolated cases.

Recorded mammalian hosts — The fox, *Cerdocyon thous,* would appear to be the primary host, with man and the dog rarely infected.

Known geographical distribution — Pará State, Brazil, particularly the littoral zone, including the island of Marajó. A single case in Surinam possibly was due to the same parasite. All cases associated with low forest, near open savanna.*

Differential characters — As yet, inadequate information.

Mode of Spread

The maintenance of all the known *Leishmania* species depends on an efficient and constant contact between the vertebrate and the sandfly hosts, and it is doubtful if any mode of spread other than by the bite of the infected insect plays any great role in nature. The one possible exception is transmission *per os,* which has achieved experimentally, and which could be partially responsible for infection among predators such as felids, jackals, wolves, foxes, and dogs — all of which are known as hosts of leishmanias within the *L. donovani* complex.

The vector/reservoir contact may be very intimate. Thus, the delicate sandfly is extremely susceptible to dessication and sudden climatic changes; to avoid such dangers in the hot, dry deserts of central and southeast Asia and other areas endemic for cutaneous leishmaniasis due to *L. major,* sandflies have colonized the cool, humid burrows of rodents where, at the same time, there is a readily available blood supply. Such

---

*   Since this chapter was prepared, the author and colleagues have investigated two cases on the island of Marajó, Pará. *Lu. longipalpis* was found in houses and chicken-houses; and *Leishmania* was isolated from a fox, *C. thous.* It was shown to be biochemically indistinguishable from isolates from man elsewhere in Brazil, suggesting a common etiological agent, *L. d. chagasi.*

close contact of the vertebrate and invertebrate hosts leads to a high infection rate in both, and a very efficient maintenance of the parasite.

In the shady, moist forests of south and central America, silvatic sandflies are subjected to far less dramatic environmental changes; the association with the vertebrate hosts is more often of a looser, "free-ranging" nature, with the insects seeking out small mammal hosts foraging on the forest floor at night, or larger arboreal animals such as sloths and anteaters in the tree tops. It is likely that the efficiency of spread in this case is more dependent on the sheer enormity of both the invertebrate and the vertebrate populations.

The spread of an ancient focus of infection of *L. d. infantum* among wild canids of central Asia to dogs and man, and thence to China, southeast Asia, the Mediterranean Basin and Africa, has been discussed in previous pages. In general, however, modern foci of leishmaniasis tend to remain fairly static, due to a relatively rigid sandfly/parasite specificity (at least in the Old World), which seems not easily to be broken. It was suggested by Adler and Theodor[9] that visceral leishmaniasis in the Mediterranean Basin has not been known to establish itself in new foci in recent times. These authors argued that *L. d. infantum* is transmitted by sandflies of the *P. major* group only, and the parasite has not adapted to other sandflies, in spite of ample opportunity to do so. Such facts, they felt, conflicted with the hypothesis that American visceral leishmaniasis is due to *L. d. infantum* imported into the New World as recently as post-Columbian times, for the sandflies of the Old World do not even belong to the same genus as those of the New World.

Unfortunately for this argument, it has been shown[81] that undoubted *L. d. infantum* from France will develop in *Lu. longipalpis* from Brazil, although it is to be admitted that foregut infections were not recorded and no transmissions by bite were achieved. The most convincing evidence for the introduction of *L. d. infantum* into the Americas from Europe, however, was the recent establishment of a small focus of canine visceral leishmaniasis, due to this parasite, in Oklahoma, seemingly after its importation in an infected dog from Europe. How transmission to other dogs may have been effected remains a mystery as mammal-biting sandflies are unrecorded in Oklahoma. Lainson and Shaw,[92] Killick-Kendrick et al.,[81] and Lainson et al.,[97] favor the midline view that American visceral leishmaniasis may in part be due to introduced *L. d. infantum,* but that it is very likely that other local viscerotropic parasites may also be involved. Certainly, if *all* the disease were due to *L. d. infantum,* it would indicate a most extraordinarily rapid spread, through virtually all Central and South America, in less than 300 years and in the face of very poor means of communication until relatively recently.

The distribution of cutaneous leishmaniasis due to subspecies of *L. mexicana* and *L. braziliensis* in the Americas has largely remained restricted to the forested regions, which provide the only suitable natural habitat for their various vectors. The diseases due to these parasites cannot spread, therefore, to the dry open areas which make up a great deal of the South American continent. On the other hand, *Lu. longipalpis*, the vector of American visceral leishmaniasis due to *L. d. chagasi,* is a semi-domestic sandfly inhabiting relatively arid regions; the disease thus remains principally restricted to the drier parts of Latin America, where conditions are favorable for the establishment of adequate populations of this insect.

The sandfly vector of "uta", probably *Lu. peruana* or *Lu. verrucarum*, clearly has adapted to dry conditions, and transmission seems largely to be peri-domestic. The disease appears to have remained restricted to the relatively barren slopes of the Andes, and has not established itself in the forested lowlands of Peru.

It appears that in the Americas, spread of leishmaniasis is more likely to result from the pushing back of the forested regions and the creation of those conditions which are favorable for *Lu. longipalpis* and the transmission of *L. d. chagasi.* The less robust silvatic sandflies are not so likely to survive abrupt environmental changes, although some vectors of *L. b. braziliensis* s.1. *(Lu. intermedia* and *L. pessoai)* do appear to have partially invaded human habitation in south Brazil. Their source of infection, however, is probably still derived from wild animals in nearby pockets of surviving woodland, and the disappearance of the reservoir hosts with the final destruction of this vegetation will doubtless break the chain of transmission to man.

There are many other instances in which the activities of man, or other more natural ecological upheavals, have greatly influenced the prevalence of different forms of leishmaniasis. In Belize, Guatemala, and the Yucatan Peninsula, the chicleros live in the forest for nearly six months of the year, while collecting the chewing-gum latex. This period coincides with the rainy season (when the sapodilla sap is rising), and with the maximum population density of *Lu. olmeca olmeca,* the vector of *L. m. mexicana.* It is scarcely surprising that almost no chiclero escapes infection, and "chiclero's ear" is merely looked on by these tough forest-workers as a badge of their profession.

In north Brazil and the Guyanas, *Lu. umbratilis,* the vector of "pian-bois", feeds on infected sloths and anteaters in the canopy of the forest by night, and then migrates down the tree trunks to oviposit on the forest-floor.[138a] After laying their eggs, the sandflies move back up to the canopy for their next blood-meal; at certain times during the day, therefore, there are tremendous concentrations of hungry females of *Lu. umbratilis* on lower parts of the larger tree trunks. When disturbed by nearby movements the flies swarm off in small clouds and will attack the nearest person. As up to 7.0% of females from tree trunks have been found infected, it is easy to see why the infection rate among groups of men working in the forest, *during the day,* may be near the 100.0% level. "Pian-bois" is a particularly serious problem in areas of deforestation in agricultural development and road building, and among troops engaged in jungle-warfare training.

Destruction of natural forest may eliminate some forms of leishmaniasis but actually favor others. Thus Lainson and Strangways-Dixon[96] noted a marked increase in the populations of the rodent hosts of *L. m. mexicana* after a hurricane had destroyed most of the primary forest of Belize, leaving a tangled mass of fallen trees and secondary vegetation which formed an ideal refuge for these animals. The sandfly vector, *Lu. olmeca olmeca,* is a low-flying, rodent-loving sandfly and was presumably not adversely affected by the new situation, for infection among the rodents was at high level. Ward and colleagues[180] found a similar situation regarding the epidemiology of cutaneous leishmaniasis due to *L. m. amazonensis,* again principally a parasite of rodents, in Pará, north Brazil, following deforestation. The subsequent pockets of dense secondary growth were found to still support a dense population of the vector, *Lu. flaviscutellata,* possibly even increasing the risks of human infection to greater levels than those encountered in primary forest. Finally,[138a] even reforestation of areas with a totally foreign monoculture of pine or melina (for paper pulp) has not diminished the *L. m. amazonensis* enzootic in vast areas of the River Jari region of Pará. Infected rodents and marsupials have been captured deep within the plantations, which abound with *Lu. flaviscutellata.* On the other hand, *Lu. umbratilis,* the vector of "pian-bois" due to *L. b. guyanensis* in the same geographic area, seems not to have adapted to these new "forests" — probably due to the lack of suitably large trees and the absence of the principal reservoir host, the two-toed sloth.

Recent studies have indicated that there is a natural limitation of certain species or subspecies of *Leishmania* to certain species of sandflies, even when all occur in the same area. This is particularly so for the Old World, but is also to a great extent true for the Americas.[92] In the northern Amazonian forest, for example, no evidence can be found of any vector of *L. m. amazonensis* other than *Lu. flaviscutellata,* although the infected rodents and marsupials are known to attract other sandfly species in the same forest. Transmission of *L. b. braziliensis* s.1. goes on side-by-side, in the Serra das Carajás region of Pará, but seems restricted to a completely different sandfly, *Psychodopygus wellcomei*. Transmission of *L. b. guyanensis* appears to be fulfilled principally by *Lu. umbratilis*. In Central America, transmission of *L. m. mexicana* has so far been limited to *Lu. olmeca olmeca*, although numerous other species of sandflies are known to feed on the rodent host. Finally, there is strong evidence to suggest that *Lu. longipalpisis* is the major or only vector of *L. d. chagasi* in the principal endemic areas of visceral leishmaniasis in Latin America.

Limitation of spread of a *Leishmania* to man or other animals will clearly depend on the host preference shown by the vector. In some areas, the infection rate for *L. m. amazonensis* in the rodent *Proechimys guyannensis* may be as high as 25.0%, and this animal is exceedingly abundant. Human infection remains rare, however, as the vector, *Lu. flaviscutellata*, is strictly nocturnal and generally unattracted to man.[149] On the other hand, the vectors of *L. b. braziliensis* s.1. and *L. b. guyanensis* are anthropophilic sandflies, and there is a correspondingly much higher prevalence of human leishmaniasis due to these parasites in the same forest.

Mass movements of troops or civilian populations, in times of war, may have a profound influence on the prevalence or distribution of leishmaniasis. Examples may be found in the severe outbreak of Kenyan visceral leishmaniasis among troops operating in normally uninhabited regions of the interior; and in China, where the spread of visceral leishmaniasis from its previously restricted localization north of the Yangtze River to South China was attributed to the mass migration of man (and probably infected dogs) as a result of the Japanese-Chinese war of 1937 to 1945.

Epidemiology
Zoonoses

Inevitably, much of this aspect of leishmaniasis has been progressively dealt with in previous pages. We have seen that most forms of the disease are zoonoses, the various parasites being well adapted to wild animals, among which they are transmitted by certain species of phlebotomine sandflies. Man is almost always an accidental "victim", when he intrudes into the natural habitat of the wild animal hosts. In the Americas this is most frequently the forest.

In certain instances, man's own domestic animals have become important secondary or "liaison" hosts, and transmission has now become established in human dwelling places or outhouses. Such a situation is quite possibly still maintained by an outside source in wild animals, which occasionally provide a supply of infected sandflies invading habited areas. When sandfly populations reach very high levels there may be explosive outbreaks of the human disease; this appears to be the case in visceral leishmaniasis of Latin America, where there is the cycle in foxes (and possibly other wild animals), *Lu. longipalpis*, dogs and man. Visceral leishmaniasis in central and southeast Asia, the Mediterranean Basin and north Africa has a similar epidemiology, involving sandfly vectors of the genus *Phlebotomus*. In both cases, man is generally a poor source of parasites for the vectors, and human infection is almost entirely derived, therefore, from the dog/sandfly association.

Among the cutaneous forms of leishmaniasis, Peruvian "uta" may possibly represent a similar situation; as in other forms of the disease, man-to-man transmission is probably rare, due to the restriction of parasites to the skin lesions. The one possible exception to this "rule" is true "oriental sore" due to *L. t. tropica*. No wild animal reservoir of this parasite has till now been discovered, and the role of the dog in the epidemiology of the disease remains very doubtful; many authorities consider it to be anthroponotic.

Anthroponoses: In the case of Indian "kala azar", parasites are usually readily demonstrated in the peripheral blood of patients, and the infection rate of sandflies fed on them is high; man-to-man transmission is generally regarded as the rule for *L. d. donovani,* therefore, in the absence of any other known vertebrate host.

Apart from the recent finding of a few infected dogs in Kenya, there has been no major reservoir host of visceral leishmaniasis incriminated in that country (see, however, earlier paragraphs under *L. donovani*), and some feel that here, too, the disease is an anthroponosis.

Prevention and Control

This is relatively straightforward (if somewhat expensive) when leishmaniasis is an anthroponosis or, if zoonotic, with a peridomestic epidemiology. Insecticide spraying, over many years, dramatically cut the incidence of kala azar in India[142a] and West Pakistan[142] during house-to-house antimalaria campaigns, and effectively reduced oriental sore due to *L. t. tropica* and visceral leishmaniasis due to *L. d. infantum* in the U.S.S.R.[79] In Peru, DDT spraying of houses against the sandfly vectors of "Carrion's Disease" (bartonellosis) also practically eliminated human and canine "uta", due to *L. b. peruviana,* in certain of the Andean valleys.[75] In the highly endemic areas of Brazil, a three-pronged attack employing DDT spraying of houses, wholesale slaughter of infected dogs, and the treatment of diagnosed cases, cut visceral leishmaniasis to almost zero in townships of Ceara and Bahia.[11,12,46,156,157] Finally, a rare example of complete eradication of both cutaneous *and* visceral leishmaniasis is recorded in the Dalmatian Islands, where the isolation and treatment of cases, elimination of infected dogs, and intensive DDT spraying of houses appear to have banished infection altogether.[172]

The major problem in such control, as in the antimalarial programs, is the effort and expense in subduing the vector population over a long enough period to break the epidemiological chain completely. Cessation or relaxation of large-scale spraying campaigns in many countries has encouraged the risk of sandfly populations once again ascending to sufficient levels for a renewed and dramatic return of the disease — as has recently happened in India and, to a lesser extent, in parts of Brazil.

When a wild mammalian source of infection is involved, it is much more difficult to prevent or control the disease. If the sandfly vectors and vertebrate hosts live in close association, however, there are greater hopes of control. Thus, the combined use of rodent poison and insecticides in gerbil burrows, irrigation, and ploughing of wasteland harboring gerbil colonies, has greatly reduced cutaneous leishmaniasis due to *L. major* in the U.S.S.R.[79]

The problem of controlling cutaneous and mucocutaneous leishmaniasis in the huge forested areas of South America by the above methods is seemingly insoluble, for both practical and economic reasons. The large-scale use of insecticides in tropical rain forest would not only be a waste of time and money, but also dangerous from a biological standpoint; the destruction of the many wild animal hosts involved would be equally out of the question. Small-scale control has been attempted in certain situations; thus, in French Guyana, the spraying of sandfly-infested tree trunks with insecticides was claimed to be effective in controlling the acquisition of "pian-bois" *(L. b. guyanensis)* over periods of 6 weeks in the rainy season, and for as long as 3 months in the dry season.[55] Such methods may be useful for the protection of isolated groups of men working in restricted areas of forest, but only where the vectors are known to occupy fixed resting places, such as tree trunks.

Chemoprophylaxis, for those entering danger areas, is a hopeful line of approach which appears to have been sadly neglected, and vaccination with dead leishmanial antigen has regretfully had no more success than attempts to protect against any other protozoal disease. "Vaccination" against *Leishmania* is at present limited to the protection of individuals against both *L. t. tropica* and *L. major* by prior, syringe-induced infection with the latter parasite. The injection of promastigotes of a highly virulent stock of *L. major* is made into some part of the skin where the scar of the healed lesion will be of no cosmetic importance. Infection is allowed to run its natural course, with spontaneous healing; the individual is then firmly immune against both *L. t. tropica* and *L. major,* and thus avoids natural infections which might otherwise cause unsightly scars on the face. The method has been applied to the mass-vaccination of populations in the U.S.S.R. since 1937[147] and more recently in Israel. It is really no more than a sophisticated extension of the ancient Asian practice whereby material from an active lesion was introduced directly into the skin of the nonimmune, by scarification.

The development of such methods against the highly mutilating American leishmanias would be a great step forward. Unfortunately, there is little or no cross-immunity between the different species or subspecies of neotropical leishmanias;[91] in any case, our incomplete knowledge as to which parasites could be considered "safe" to use as a live vaccine at present makes the whole procedure hazardous.

Treatment
The Antimonials
Tartar Emetic (Antimony Potassium Tartrate)

In 1906 to 1907, French and British workers independently demonstrated the usefulness of antimony compounds in the elimination of hemoflagellate infections, when they used tartar emetic in the treatment of African trypanosomiasis. The Brazilian scientist Gaspar Vianna was quick to realize the potential value of this drug against *Leishmania* and, in 1912, reported his observations on the first clinical trials with cases of severe mucocutaneous leishmaniasis. The results were impressive and, in spite of its high toxicity, tartar emetic became a standard treatment for all forms of leishmaniasis. It certainly must have been heralded as a "miracle drug" by Asia, where its use against "kala azar" reduced the mortality by about 95%. Tartar emetic was also extensively used to combat Mediterranean infantile visceral leishmaniasis *(L. d. infantum)* and "oriental sore" *(L. t. tropica)*.

Stibophen [Sodium Antimony (III) bis (catechol-3, 5-disulfonate)]

The marked toxicity of tartar emetic quickly prompted a search for less dangerous derivatives, and the trivalent antimonial Stibophen (Fouadin, Reprodral®) became widely used until the advent of the pentavalent compounds. It appeared to be much more effective against cutaneous leishmaniasis than against the visceral disease. Although a very considerable improvement compared with tartar emetic, side-effects still remained a serious problem and Stibophen is now rarely used following development of the pentavalent antimonials.

Pentostam®, Bayer 561®, Solustibosan® [Sodium antimony (V) Gluconate]

The pentavalent antimonials can be tolerated at very much higher dose levels than the trivalent drugs, and they are excreted more slowly. This discovery constituted a major breakthrough in the chemotherapy of leishmaniasis, and the pentavalent antimonials still remain the drugs of choice, for most, to this day.

The pentavalent analog of Stibophen, sodium antimony (V) gluconate, was one of the most rewarding products in this period of research and it has been found to be active against all forms of leishmaniasis, including the American cutaneous and mucocutaneous diseases. It has even proved effective against Sudanese visceral leishmaniasis, which is often stubbornly resistant to other forms of treatment.

Pentostam® has a low level of toxicity and may be given both intravenously and intramuscularly. It is produced in a relatively stable solution, with 100 mg of pentavalent antimony per ml. An initial low dose of 1.0 to 2.0 ml is advised as a sensitivity test, the dosage then being increased to 6.0 ml per day for a period of 16 days. Repeat courses may safely be given, usually with intervals of 2 to 4 weeks between courses. Reduced dosage is used for children, although they generally show a greater tolerance than do adults. Occasional side-effects have been noted, including some muscular or joint pains, pricking or itching sensations of the eyes, and mild nausea.

Clinicians in the author's laboratory have found the effectiveness of Pentostam® to be variable in the treatment of cutaneous and mucocutaneous leishmaniasis, and this variation is experienced not only with different leishmanial parasites but also in individuals infected with the same organism. The drug is usually very effective against *L. m. mexicana,* when a single course is often sufficient; lesions due to *L. m. amazonensis* respond more slowly, however, and repeated courses may be needed. Early lesions due to Amazonian *L. b. braziliensis* s.1. respond well, but repeated courses are needed for advanced cutaneous or mucocutaneous cases. The most stubborn of the American leishmanias is undoubtedly *L. b. guyanensis;* even tiny, newly acquired lesions may need from 3 to 10 courses of Pentostam® before cure, and sometimes there may be complete failure to eliminate the parasite. In such cases, coincidental heat treatment of the lesions by the local application of hot water or poultices, greatly increases the rate of cure. Pentostam® was originally developed specifically to combat oriental sore and Old World visceral leishmaniasis, in the treatment of which it still is unsurpassed.

Glucantime® (Meglumine Antimoniate)

This pentavalent antimonial is also well tolerated and has been found to resolve some cases which have resisted repeated courses of Pentostam®; it can be given intravenously, although the intramuscular route is that recommended by the makers.

Compared with Pentostam®, Glucantime® has the disadvantage of requiring much larger amounts of inoculum. It is produced in ampoules of 5.0 ml aqueous solution, each containing 1.5 g of meglumine antimonate (425 mg of antimony). An initial injection of 1.0 to 2.0 ml is stepped up to daily inoculation of 5.0 to 10.0 ml for 10 to 20 days. The final, total dose is 3 g/kg body weight; side effects may be similar to those described for Pentostam®.

In the absence of Pentostam® on the Latin American market, Glucantime® has remained the drug of choice throughout Brazil and other affected countries.

Neostibosan® (Ethylstibamine)

This derivative of stibanilic acid is again comparatively nontoxic, and has proved useful against "kala azar"; unfortunately it is not very stable in solution and must be freshly prepared for each administration.

Neostibosan® contains up to 42% antimony and may be given in 25% solution intramuscularly, or a 5.0% solution for slow intravenous administration, usually on alternate days. The initial dose for adults is 0.1g, followed by 0.2 and 0.3 g; a total of 2.7 g is recommended, given in 10 injections. The drug has been extensively used against infantile visceral leishmaniasis *(L. d. infantum).* Infants below 1 year should be given a total dose of 0.1 to 0.15 g in a course of 16 intravenous injections; children of 1 to 2 years may receive a total of 0.2 to 0.25 g; older children, 0.3 g.

Urea Stibamine (Carbostibamine, Carbantine, Stiburea)

Early trials with this pentavalent antimonial gave very good results against Indian "kala azar", but different batches seem to vary considerably in antimony content, toxicity and efficacy as an anti-leishmanial agent; the drug is often used in combination with Neostibosan®, and is given intravenously as an aqueous solution. The total amount of Urea Stibamine recommended is 3.0 g, given in doses of 100 to 200 mg, alternate days, over a period of 4 weeks.

The mode of action of antimonial drugs is still incompletely known. Interestingly, viable parasites may sometimes be isolated from the lesions of patients who have received numerous courses of treatment, before the final elimination of infection by subsequent courses.

The Aromatic Diamidines

These benzoic acid derivatives have given a frustrating mixture of success and failure in the treatment of leishmaniasis.

Stilbamidine Isethionate

Ironically, although this is one of the most efficient agents known against "kala azar", the discovery of serious trigeminal neuropathy and other neuropathological signs in treated patients has militated against further use of this drug. Nowadays it is occasionally used as a last resort in cases of antimony-resistant "kala azar", particularly of the Sudanese form. The drug is administered by slow intravenous injection of a 1.0% aqueous solution; initial adult dose is 0.025 g with the dosage increased very slowly to a total of 2.0 mg/kg body weight, over a period of 10 days.

Pentamidine Isethionate (Lomidine®, M & B 800®)

Again, although this aromatic diamidine has proved very effective against the most stubborn forms of visceral leishmaniasis, its use has regretfully been linked with reports of subsequent polyneuritis and the development of diabetes. Its use is now restricted to cases in which all other forms of treatment have failed; it is given intravenously, at a dosage of 3.0 mg/kg body weight, over a period of 14 successive days.

Other Drugs
Berberine Chloride

There is little information on the use of this derivative of the plant alkaloid, berberine. Some success has been reported, however, after infiltrating the drug into and around lesions due to *L. t. tropica* ("oriental sore"). It has proved ineffective against post kala azar dermal leishmanoid.

Cycloguanil Pamoate (Cycloguanil Embonate, Camolar®)

This is a single-dose, intramuscularly administered drug with a repository action. Its efficacy against *Leishmania* was suggested during trials on malaria prophylaxis in Latin America, but Camolar® has subsequently been shown to be ineffective against "oriental sore" due to *L. t. aethiopica* in Ethiopia.

The results of trials have in general been conflicting. There seems to be a very considerable delay in elimination of the infection, and as there is often spontaneous regression of leishmanial skin lesions without any form of treatment, this makes it extremely difficult to assess the true value of Camolar®. Indeed, its use could be hazardous in cases with lesions due to *L. b. braziliensis,* when spontaneous healing or inadequate treatment is frequently followed by the development of nasopharyngeal lesions.

Quinacrine (Mepacrine)

This acridine derivative achieved its fame, of course, as an extremely potent schizonticide in the treatment of malaria. A certain degree of success in the treatment of cutaneous leishmaniasis has been reported, largely following the infiltrating of ear lesions due to *L. m. mexicana* (chiclero's ulcer). The process is extremely painful, however, and it remains doubtful whether cure is in fact due to a direct action of the drug on the parasites or merely the sloughing away of the surrounding tissue. A popular local treatment of chiclero's ulcer in Belize is cautery with acid from old car batteries, a destructive method, possibly comparable with the use of quinacrine!

D. Antibiotics

The great majority of antibiotics, so effective against the bacteria, are useless in the treatment of leishmaniasis. Some are in fact used to avoid bacterial contamination of cultures of either amastigote or promastigote stages of *Leishmania*. The administration of penicillin to patients with large, suppurating skin lesions will usually lead to an encouraging reduction in the size and moistness of the ulcers; this is simply due to the elimination of secondary bacterial infection, although it is often mistakenly taken to indicate an anti-leishmanial action. Surprisingly, however, a limited number of antibiotics are highly effective against *Leishmania,* and it may well be that other more suitable ones may be discovered in the future.

Amphotericin B (Fungizone®)

This antibiotic is derived from the soil fungus *Streptomyces nodosus.* It has been principally used in the treatment of deep systematic mycoses, but has also proved to be a potent anti-leishmanial agent. Unfortunately, in addition to its high cost, Amphotericin B is very toxic and side effects appear to be inevitable; they include nausea, anorexia, and fever. An added disadvantage is the frequent development of impaired renal function, and the fact that patients must be hospitalized and the drug given by slow intravenous infusion. Venous thrombosis may ensue at the site of the drip, although the danger of this is said to be lessened by the addition of 25 to 50 mg of hydrocortisone sodium succinate to the drip bottle.

Treatment with Amphotericin B is clearly hazardous and best reserved, therefore, for advanced cases of leishmaniasis which do not respond to any other drugs. The antibiotic is dissolved in 500 m*l* of a 5.0% dextrose solution and given over a period of about 6 hr, on alternate days. Initially, the dose is 0.5 mg/kg body weight per day; if well tolerated the dosage is slowly raised to 1.0 mg/kg per day. As with any other treatment for leishmaniasis, there remains the difficulty of criteria for complete cure; serological studies on circulating antibody levels, as indicated by the indirect fluorescence antibody test, are the only real guide as to whether or not all parasites have been eliminated. In general the total effective dose has been found to be less than that needed for the treatment of the visceral mycoses; cure, with no relapse in follow-ups of 10 years, has been reported for mucocutaneous leishmaniasis in Brazil and for drug resistant "kala azar". It has not proved effective against diffuse cutaneous leishmaniasis.

Monomycin

Russian clinicians have reported this antibiotic to be effective against *L. major* ("wet, zoonotic cutaneous leishmaniasis"), after infiltration into and around the skin lesion. There seems to be no available literature on its use in other forms of leishmaniasis.

Rifampicin (Rifaldin®)

This antibiotic is better known as a recently developed antituberculous agent, but it has been reported as effective against "oriental sore" in Kuwait and cutaneous leishmaniasis due to *L. b. braziliensis* s.1. in Brazil. It is very expensive, and the severe side effects noted by some clinicians[22] would not appear to merit its use against *Leish-*

mania. These include renal insufficiency, hepatitis, impaired coagulation rate, and the occasional development of a peculiar type of autoimmune response.

Treatment With High and Low Temperature

Little published work has appeared in this connection, but both heat and cold treatment have been claimed to cure various forms of cutaneous leishmaniasis. It should be emphasised, however, that although such local treatment is acceptable in cases infected with nonvisceralizing and nonmetastasizing species of *Leishmania,* its *sole* use is to be condemned against cutaneous leishmaniasis in areas of South America where mucocutaneous leishmaniasis occurs. Both clinician and patient may be lulled into the false belief that complete cure has been achieved when, in reality, parasites may be lurking in the nasopharyngeal tissues.

Application of solid CO_2 has been used in the treatment of "oriental sore" — more a form of cautery, perhaps. Recent success has been reported in the treatment of East African cutaneous leishmaniasis with local application of hot water or ultra-violet and infrared rays; and the daily immersion of lesions in hot water has been found to be of undoubted value in hastening the cure of patients with American cutaneous leishmaniasis who are under treatment with the customary antimonials.

As far as this author is aware, both Old and New World forms of diffuse, "anergic" cutaneous leishmaniasis, due to *L. t. aethiopica* (Ethiopia), *L. m. pifanoi* (Venezuela) and *L. m. amazonensis* (Brazil) remain incurable by the existing methods of treatment. Initially there may be *apparent* cure, with total disappearance of the skin lesions; on all occasions, however, such cases have relapsed and the lesions reappeared, with the usual heavy parasite load. At present the best that can be done is to keep the infection subdued, and thus give the patient a somewhat less unpleasant appearance. Clinicians in the author's laboratory have for the past 10 years treated two particularly severe cases with frequent, very hot baths, which have been found to reduce the size of the nodules dramatically. The water is maintained at the highest bearable temperature by a thermostat; periodic courses of Pentostam® or Glucantime® are given when considered necessary.

Combined Drug Treatment

Peters et al.,[134] have reported a striking remission of skin lesions in a patient with diffuse cutaneous leishmaniasis due to *L. m. amazonensis,* when he was treated with rifampicin and isoniazid in combination. The lesions returned, however, when the isoniazid was withdrawn.

Liposomes

Virtually the only recent advance in the chemotherapy of leishmaniasis has been the incorporation of existing antileishmanial drugs in liposomes. Liposomes are the lipid spheres produced when phospholipids are converted to hydrated crystals in an aqueous medium, and when injected intravenously into the mammalian bloodstream they speedily become phagocytized in the liver. By incorporating the antileishmanial drugs in these liposomes it is possible, therefore, to get high concentrations directly to the site of the development of the leishmanial amastigotes. It has been shown, for example, that sodium antimony gluconate (Pentostam®) was 10 times more efficient in destroying amastigotes of *L. donovani* in experimental mice when used in this way, than the same dosage of the drug given alone;[124] and this observation has clearly opened up a whole new and promising field of study in the treatment of leishmaniasis.

Observations on the chemotherapy of South American cutaneous leishmaniasis with Pentostam®, Glucantime® and heat treatment, in this chapter, have come largely from medical colleagues in the author's laboratory; I am particularly indebted to Dr.

Fernando Silveiro for his collaboration. All other information, including drug dosage and application has been obtained from current medical literature and in no way reflects the author's views. Readers are particularly advised to consult E. A. Steck (see Recommended Reading list).

REFERENCES

1. **Adler, S.**, Differentiation of *Leishmania brasiliensis* from *L. mexicana* and *L. tropica, Rev. Inst. Salubr. Enferm. Trop. Méx.*, 23, 139, 1963.
2. **Adler, S.**, *Leishmania. Adv. Parasitol.*, 2, 35, 1964.
3. **Adler, S. and Ber, M.**, Transmission of *Leishmania tropica* by the bite of *Phlebotomus papatasii, Nature, London*, 148, 227, 1941.
4. **Adler, S. and Theodor, O.**, The experimental transmission of cutaneous leishmaniasis to man from *Phlebotomus papatasii, Ann. Trop. Med. Parasitol.*, 19, 365, 1925.
5. **Adler, S. and Theodor, O.**, Further observations on the transmission of cutaneous leishmaniasis to man from *Phlebotomus papatasii, Ann. Trop. Med. Parasitol.*, 20, 175, 1926.
6. **Adler, S. and Theodor, O.**, Identity of *Herpetomonas papatasii* and *Leishmania tropica, Nature, London*, 118, 85, 1926.
7. **Adler, S. and Theodor, O.**, The exit of *Leishmania tropica* through the proboscis of *Phlebotomus papatasii, Nature, London*, 121, 282, 1928.
8. **Adler, S. and Theodor, O.**, Attempts to transmit *Leishmania* by bite; the transmission of *L. tropica* by *Phlebotomus sergenti, Ann. Trop. Med. Parasitol.*, 23, 1, 1929.
9. **Adler, S. and Theodor, O.**, Transmission of disease agents by phlebotomine sandflies, *Ann. Rev. Entomol.*, 2, 203, 1957.
10. **Adler, S., Foner, A., and Montiglio, B.**, The relationship between human and animal strains of *Leishmania* from the Sudan, *Trans. R. Soc. Trop. Med. Hyg.*, 60, 380, 1966.
11. **Alencar, J. E.**, Profilaxia do calazar no Ceara, Brasil, *Rev. Inst. Med. Trop. São Paulo*, 3, 175, 1961.
12. **Alencar, J. E.**, Influência da dedetização sobre a incidência do calazar humana no Ceará — novos dados, *Rev. Bras. Malar. Doenças Trop.*, 15, 417, 1963.
13. **Anderson, D. C., Buckner, R. G., Glenn, B. L., and MacVean, D. W.**, Endemic canine leishmaniasis, *Vet. Path.*, 17, 94, 1980.
14. **Anon.**, The Twenty-ninth annual report of the work and operation of the Gorgas Memorial Laboratory, covering the fiscal year ended June 30, 1956, U.S. Government Printing Office, Washington, 1957.
15. **Anon.**, Thirty-first annual report of the work and operation of the Gorgas Memorial Laboratory, covering the fiscal year ended June 30, 1958, U.S. Government Printing Office, Washington, 1959.
16. **Arias, J. R. and de Freitas, R. A.**, On the vectors of cutaneous leishmaniasis in the Central Amazon of Brazil. I. Preliminary findings, *Acta Amazônica*, 7, 293, 1977.
17. **Ashford, R. W., Bray, M. A., Hutchison, M. P., and Bray, R. S.**, The epidemiology of cutaneous leishmaniasis in Ethiopia. *Trans. R. Soc. Trop. Med. Hyg.*, 67, 588, 1973.
18. **Bettini, S., Gradoni, L., and Pozio, E.**, Isolation of *Leishmania* strains from *Rattus rattus* in Italy. *Trans. R. Soc. Trop. Med. Hyg.*, 72, 441, 1978.
19. **Biagi, F. F.**, Algunos comentarios sobre las leishmaniasis y sus agentes etiológicos, *Leishmania tropica mexicana*, nueva subspecie, *Medicina (México)*, 33, 401, 1953.
20. **Biagi, F. F., Biagi, B. A. M., and Beltran, H. F.**, *Phlebotomus flaviscutellata* transmissor natural de *Leishmania mexicana, Prensa Medica Mexicana*, 30, 267, 1965.
21. **Borovsky, P. F.**, (On Sart Sore). *Voenno-Medicinskij Zurnal (Military Medical Journal)*.Part 195, No. 11 (76th year), 925, 1898 (In Russian).
22. **Boman, G., Nilsson, B. S., and Saerens, E. J.**, Ed. of Proceedings of the workshop on intermittent drug therapy and immunological implications of antituberculous treatment with rifampicin, *Scand. J. Resp. Dis. Suppl.*, 84, 1973.
23. **Bray, R. S.**, *Leishmania, Ann. Rev. Microbiol.*, 28, 189, 1974.
24. **Bray, R. S. and Lainson, R.**, Studies on the immunology and serology of leishmaniasis. V. The use of particles as vehicles in passive agglutination tests, *Trans. R. Soc. Trop. Med. Hyg.*, 61, 490, 1967.
25. **Bray, R. S., Ashford, R. W., and Bray, M. A.**, The parasite causing cutaneous leishmaniasis in Ethiopia, *Trans. R. Soc. Trop. Med. Hyg.*, 67, 345, 1973.
26. **Brumpt, E.**, *Précis de Parasitologie*, 2nd ed., Masson et Cie., Paris, 1913.

27. **Carini, A. and Paranhos, U.,** Identification de l'Ulcera de Bauru avec le bouton d'Orient, *Bull. Soc. Path. Exot.,* 2, 255, 1909.

28. **Castellani, A. and Chalmers, A. H.,** *Manual of Tropical Medicine,* 3rd ed., Baillière, Tindall and Cox, 1919, 369.

29. **Cathoire, M.,** Présentation de parasite par A. Laveran, *Bull. Acad Méd.,* 68, 247, 1904.

30. **Chagas, A. W.,** Criação de Flebótomus e transmissão experimental da leishmaniose visceral americana, *Mems. Inst. Oswaldo Cruz,* 35, 327, 1936.

31. **Chagas, E.,** Primeira verificação em individuo vivo, da leishmaniose visceral no Brasil, *Brasil-Médico,* 50, 221, 1936.

32. **Chagas, E., Cunha, A. M., Ferreira, L. C., Deane, L., Deane, G., Guimarães, F. N., Paumgartten, M. J., and Sá, B.,** Leishmaniose visceral americana. (Relatório dos trabalhos realizados pela Commissão Encarregada do Estudo da Leishmaniose Visceral Americana em 1937.) *Mems. Inst. Oswaldo Cruz,* 33, 89, 1938.

33. **Chance, M. L.,** The identification of *Leishmania,* in *Problems in the identification of parasites and their vectors, Symposia Br. Soc. Parasitol.,* 17, 55, 1979.

33a. **Chance, M. L.,** Personal communication.

34. **Chance, M. L., Gardener, P. J., and Peters, W.,** Biochemical taxonomy of *Leishmania* as an ecological tool, in *Écologie des leishmanioses,* Colloques Internationaux du Centre National de la Recherche Scientifique, No. 239, 15, quai Anatole-France, 75700 Paris, 53, 1977.

35. **Chance, M. L., Peters, W., and Shchory, L.,** Biochemical taxonomy of *Leishmania,* 1: Observations on DNA. *Ann. Trop. Med. Parasitol.,* 68, 307, 1974.

36. **Chance, M. L., Schnur, L. F., Thomas, S. C., and Peters, W.,** The biochemical and serological taxonomy of *Leishmania* from the Aethiopian zoogeographical region of Africa, *Ann. Trop. Med. Parasitol.,* 72, 533, 1978.

37. **Christensen, H. A., Herrer, A., and Telford, S. R.,** *Leishmania braziliensis* from *Lutzomyia panamensis* in Panama, *J. Parasitol.,* 55, 1090, 1969.

38. **Christophers, S. R., Shortt, H. E., and Barraud, P. J.,** The development of the parasite of Indian kala-azar in the sandfly *Phlebotomus argentipes* Annandale and Brunetti, *Indian J. Med. Res.,* 12, 605, 1925.

39. **Chung, H. L.,** A resumé of kala azar work in China, *Chinese Med. J.,* 71, 421, 1953.

40. **Coelho, M. V. and Falcão, A. R.,** Transmissão experimental de *Leishmania braziliensis,* II. Transmissão de amostra mexicana por picada de *Phlebotomus longipalpis* e de *Phlebotomus renei, Rev. Inst. Med. Trop. São Paulo,* 4, 220, 1962.

41. **Cunha, A. M. and Chagas, E.,** Nova espécie de protozoário do gênero *Leishmania* pathogenico para o homem, *Leishmania chagasi,* n. sp. Nota Prévia, *Hospital (Rio de Janeiro),* 11, 3, 1937.

42. **Cunningham, D. D.,** On the presence of peculiar parasitic organisms in the tissue culture of a specimen of Delhi boil, *Sci. Mem. Med. Off. Army India,* 1, 21, 1885.

43. **Deane, L. M. and Deane, M. P.,** Encontro de cães naturalmente infectados por *Leishmania donovani* no Ceará, *Hospital (Rio de Janeiro),* 45, 703, 1954.

44. **Deane, L. M. and Deane, M. P.,** Encontro de leishmanias nas visceras e no pele de uma raposa, em zona endemica de calazar, nos arredores de Sobral, Ceará, *Hospital (Rio de Janeiro),* 45, 419, 1954.

45. **Deane, M. P. and Deane, L. M.,** Infecção natural do *Phlebotomus longipalpis* por leptomonas, provavelmente de *Leishmania donovani,* em foco de calazar, no Ceará, *Hospital (Rio de Janeiro),* 45, 697, 1954.

46. **Deane, L. M., Deane, M. P., and Alencar, J. E.,** Observações sôbre o combate ao *Phlebotomus longipalpis* pela dedetização domiciliária em focos endemicos de calazar no Ceará, *Rev. Bras. Malar. e Doencas Trop.,* 7, 131, 1955.

47. **Deane, L. M., Silva, J. E., and Figueiredo, P. Z.,** Leishmaniae in the viscera of porcupines from the State of Piaui, Brazil, *Rev. Inst. Med. Trop. São Paulo,* 16, 68, 1974.

48. **Decker, J. E., Schrot, J. R., and Levin, G. V.,** Identification of *Leishmania* spp., by radiorespirometry, *J. Protozool.,* 24, 465, 1977.

49. **Dedet, J. P., Derouin, F., Hubert, B., Schnur, L. F., and Chance, L. M.,** Isolation of *Leishmania major* from *Mastomys erythroleucus* and *Tatera gambiana* in Senegal (West Africa), *Ann. Trop. Med. Parasitol.,* 73, 433, 1979.

50. **Disney, R. H. L.,** A trap for phlebotomine sandflies attracted to rats, *Bull. Ent. Res.,* 56, 445, 1966.

51. **Disney, R. H. L.,** Observations on a zoonosis: leishmaniasis in British Honduras, *J. App. Ecol.,* 5, 1, 1968.

52. **Feng, L. C. and Chung, H. L.,** Experiments on the transmission of kala-azar from dogs to hamsters by Chinese sandflies, *Chin. Med. J.,* 60, 489, 1941.

53. **Ferreira, L. C., Deane, L., and Mangabeira, O.,** Infecção de "*Flebotomus longipalpis*" pela "*Leishmania chagasi*", *Hospital (Rio de Janeiro),* 14, 2, 1938.

54. **Floch, H.,** *Leishmania tropica guyanensis* n. ssp., agent de la leishmaniose tégumentaire des Guyanas et de l'Amerique Centrale, *Arch. Inst. Pasteur Guyane Fr.,* 15, Publ. No. 328, 1, 1954.

55. **Floch, H.**, Epidémiologie de la leishmaniose forestiére américaine en Guyane française, *Riv. di Malar.*, 36, 233, 1957.

56. **Forattini, O. P.**, Sobre os reservatórios naturais da leishmaniose tegumentar americana, *Rev. Inst. Med. Trop. São Paulo*, 2, 195, 1960.

57. **Forattini, O. P., Pattoli, D. B. G., Rabello, E. X., and Ferreira, O. A.**, Infecções naturais de mamíferos silvestres em área endêmica de *Leishmaniose tegumentar* do estado de São Paulo, Brasil, *Rev. Saúde Públ.*, 6, 255, 1972.

58. **Forattini, O. P., Pattoli, D. B. G., Rabello, E. X., and Ferreira, O. A.**, Infecção natural de flebotomíneos em foco enzoótico de leishmaniose tegumentar no estado de São Paulo, Brasil, *Rev. Saúde Públ.*, 6, 431, 1972.

59. **Forattini, O. P., Pattoli, D. B. G., Rabello, E. X., and Ferreira, O. A.**, Nota sobre infecção natural de *Oryzomys capito laticeps* em foco enzoótico de leishmaniose tegumentar no estado de São Paulo, Brasil, *Rev. Saúde Públ.*, 7, 181, 1973.

60. **Gardener, P. J.**, Taxonomy of the genus *Leishmania:* a review of nomenclature and classification, *Trop. Dis. Bull.*, 74, 1069, 1977.

61. **Gardener, P. J., Chance, M. L. and Peters, W.**, Biochemical taxonomy of *Leishmania* II: Electrophoretic variation of malate dehydrogenase, *Ann. Trop. Med. Parasitol.*, 68, 317, 1974.

62. **Garnham, P. C. C.**, Cutaneous leishmaniasis in the New World with special reference to *Leishmania mexicana*, *Sci. Rep. Sup. San.*, 2, 76, 1962.

63. **Gentile, B., Le Pont, F., and Besnard, R.**, Dermal leishmaniasis in French Guiana: the sloth *(Choloepus didactylus)* as a reservoir host, *Trans. R. Soc. Trop. Med. Hyg.*, 75, 612, 1981.

64. **Godfrey, D. G.**, The zymodemes of trypanosomes, in Problems in the identification of parasites and their vectors, *Symp. Br. Soc. Parasitol.*, 17, 31, 1979.

65. **Grôve, S. S.**, Cutaneous leishmaniasis in South West Africa, *S. Af. Med. J.*, 44, 206, 1970.

66. **Grôve, S. S. and Ledger, J. A.**, *Leishmania* from a hyrax in South West Africa, *Trans. R. Soc. Trop. Med. Hyg.*, 69, 523, 1975.

67. **Gutteridge, W. E.**, *Trypanosoma cruzi:* recent biochemical advances, *Trans. R. Soc. Trop. Med. Hyg.*, 75, 484, 1981.

68. **Heisch, R. B.**, The isolation of *Leishmania* from a ground squirrel in Kenya, *East Afr. Med. J.*, 34, 183, 1957.

69. **Heisch, R. B., Grainger, W. E., and Harvey, A. E. C.**, The isolation of a *Leishmania* from gerbils in Kenya, *J. Trop. Med. Hyg.*, 62, 158, 1959.

70. **Herrer, A.**, Estudios sobre leishmaniasis tegumentaria en el Perú, Observaciones epidemiológicos sobre la uta, *Rev. Med. Exper.* (Lima), 8, 45, 1951.

71. **Herrer, A.**, Verruga y uta en el valle de Huaillacayán (Dpto. de Ancash). I. Determinación de los límites altitudinales de la zona endêmica y de la incidencia de ambas enfermadades, *Rev. Med. Exper. (Lima)*, 11, 40, 1957.

72. **Herrer, A.**, *Leishmania hertigi* sp. n., from the tropical porcupine, *Coendou rothschildi* Thomas, *J. Parasitol.*, 57, 626, 1971.

73. **Herrer, A., Telford, S. R., and Christensen, H. A.**, Enzootic cutaneous leishmaniasis in eastern Panama. I. Investigation of the infection among forest mammals, *Ann. Trop. Med. Parasitol.*, 65, 349, 1971.

74. **Herrer, A., Christensen, H. A., and Beumer, R. J.**, Reservoir hosts of cutaneous leishmaniasis among Panamanian forest mammals, *Am. J. Trop. Med. Hyg.*, 22, 585, 1973.

75. **Hertig, M. and Fairchild, G. B.**, The control of *Phlebotomus* in Peru with DDT, *Am. J. Trop. Med.*, 2, 207, 1943.

76. **Hommel, M.**, The genus *Leishmania:* biology of the parasites and clinical aspects, *Bull. l'Inst. Pasteur*, 75, 5, 1978.

77. **Hoogstraal, H. and Heyneman, D.**, Leishmaniasis in the Sudan Republic. *Am. J. Trop. Med. Hyg.*, 18, 1091, 1969.

78. **Johnson, P. T., McConnell, E., and Hertig, M.**, Natural infections of leptomonad flagellates in Panamanian *Phlebotomus* sandflies, *Exper. Parasitol.*, 14, 107, 1963.

79. **Kellina, O. I.**, Problem and current lines in investigations on the epidemiology of leishmaniasis and its control in the U.S.S.R., *Bull. Soc. Path. Exot.*, 74, 306, 1981.

80. **Killick-Kendrick, R.**, Biology of *Leishmania* in phlebotomine sandflies, in *Biology of the Kinetoplastida, Vol. II,* Lumsden, W. H. R. and Evans, D. A., Eds., Academic Press, New York, 395, 1979.

81. **Killick-Kendrick, R., Molyneux, D. H., Rioux, J. A., Lanotte, G., and Leaney, A. J.**, Possible origins of *Leishmania chagasi*, *Ann. Trop. Med. Parasitol.*, 74, 563, 1980.

82. **Kimber, C. D., Evans, D. A., Robinson, B. L., and Peters, W.**, Control of yeast contamination with 5-fluorcytosine in the *in vitro* cultivation of *Leishmania* spp. *Ann. Trop. Med. Parasitol.*, 75, 453, 1981.

83. Knowles, R., Napier, L. E., and Smith, R. O. A., On a *Herpetomonas* found in the gut of the sandfly, *Phlebotomus argentipes,* fed on kala-azar patients. A preliminary note, *Indian Med. Gaz.,* 59, 593, 1924.

84. Lainson, R., Leishmanial parasites of mammals in relation to human disease, *Symp. Zool. Soc. London,* No. 50, in press.

85. Lainson, R. and Shaw, J. J., Studies on the immunology and serology of leishmaniasis. III. On the cross-immunity between Panamanian cutaneous leishmaniasis and *Leishmania mexicana* infection in man, *Trans. R. Soc. Trop. Med. Hyg.,* 60, 533, 1966.

86. Lainson, R. and Shaw, J. J., Leishmaniasis in Brazil. I. Observations on enzootic rodent leishmaniasis — incrimination of *Lutzomyia flaviscutellata* (Mangabeira) as the vector in the lower Amazonian basin, *Trans. R. Soc. Trop. Med. Hyg.,* 62, 385, 1968.

87. Lainson, R. and Shaw, J. J., Leishmaniasis in Brazil. V. Studies on the epidemiology of cutaneous leishmaniasis in Mato Grosso State, and observations on two distinct strains of *Leishmania* isolated from man and forest animals, *Trans. R. Soc. Trop. Med. Hyg.,* 64, 654, 1970.

88. Lainson, R. and Shaw, J. J., Leishmaniasis of the New World: taxonomic problems, *Br. Med. Bull.,* 28, 44, 1972.

89. Lainson, R. and Shaw, J. J., Leishmanias and leishmaniasis of the New World, with particular reference to Brazil, *Bull. Pan Am. Health Org.,* 7 (4), 1, 1973.

90. Lainson, R. and Shaw, J. J., Leishmanias of neotropical porcupines: *Leishmania hertigi deanei* nov. subsp., *Acta Amazônica,* 7, 51, 1977.

91. Lainson, R. and Shaw, J. J., Leishmaniasis in Brazil. XII. Observations on cross-immunity in monkeys and man infected with *Leishmania mexicana mexicana, L. m. amazonensis, L. braziliensis braziliensis, L. b. guyanensis,* and *L. b. panamensis, J. Trop. Med. and Hyg.,* 80, 29, 1977.

92. Lainson, R. and Shaw, J. J., The role of animals in the epidemiology of South American Leishmaniasis, in *Biology of the Kinetoplastida, Vol. II,* Lumsden, W. H. R. and Evans, D. A., Eds., Academic Press, New York, 1, 1979.

93. Lainson, R. and Shaw, J. J., The leishmanial parasites, in *Medical Laboratory Manual for Tropical Countries,* Vol. I, 206, Cheesbrough, M., Ed., Stephen Austin & Sons, Ltd., Hertford, England, 1981.

93a. Lainson, R. and Shaw, J. J., Unpublished observations.

94. Lainson, R. and Strangways-Dixon, J., Dermal leishmaniasis in British Honduras: some host reservoirs of *L. braziliensis mexicana.* A preliminary note, *Br. Med. J.,* 1, 1598, 1962.

95. Lainson, R. and Strangways-Dixon, J., *Leishmania mexicana:* the epidemiology of dermal leishmaniasis in British Hondruas. *Trans. R. Soc. Trop. Med. Hyg.,* 57, 242, 1963.

96. Lainson, R. and Strangways-Dixon, J., The epidemiology of dermal leishmaniasis in British Honduras. Part II. Reservoir-hosts of *Leishmania mexicana* among the forest rodents, *Trans. R. Soc. Trop. Med. Hyg.,* 58, 136, 1964.

97. Lainson, R., Miles, M. A., and Shaw, J. J., On identification of viscerotropic leishmanias, *Ann. Trop. Med. Parasitol.,* 75, 251, 1981.

97a. Lainson, R., Shaw, J. J., and Miles, M. A., Unpublished observations.

98. Lainson, R., Ready, P. D., and Shaw, J. J., *Leishmania* in phlebotomid sandflies. VII. On the taxonomic status of *Leishmania peruviana,* causative agent of Peruvian 'uta', as indicated by its development in the sandfly, *Lutzomyia longipalpis, Proc. R. Soc. London, B.,* 206, 307, 1979.

99. Lainson, R., Shaw, J. J., and Póvoa, M., The importance of edentates (sloths and anteaters) as primary reservoirs of *Leishmania braziliensis guyanensis,* causative agent of "pian-bois" in north Brazil, *Trans. R. Soc. Trop. Med. Hyg.,* 75, 611, 1981.

100. Lainson, R., Ward, R. D., and Shaw, J. J., Cutaneous leishmaniasis in north Brazil: *Lutzomyia anduzei* as a major vector, *Trans. R. Soc. Trop. Med. Hyg.,* 70, 171, 1976.

101. Lainson, R., Ward, R. D., and Shaw, J. J., Experimental transmission of *Leishmania chagasi,* causative agent of neotropical visceral leishmaniasis, by the sandfly *Lutzomyia longipalpis, Nature, London,* 266, 628, 1977.

101a. Lainson, R., Shaw, J. J., and Ward, R. D., Unpublished observations.

102. Lainson, R., Shaw, J. J., Ward, R. D., and Fraiha, H., Leishmaniasis in Brazil. IX. Considerations on the *Leishmania braziliensis* complex: importance of sandflies of the genus *Psychodopygus* (Mangabeira) in the transmission of *L. braziliensis* in north Brazil, *Tran. R. Soc. Trop. Med. Hyg.,* 67, 184, 1973.

103. Lainson, R., Shaw, J. J., Ready, P. D., Miles, M. A., and Póvoa, M., Leishmaniasis in Brazil. XVI. Isolation and identification of *Leishmania* species from sandflies, wild mammals and man in north Para State, with particular reference to *Leishmania braziliensis guyanensis,* causative agent of "pian-bois", *Trans. R. Soc. Trop. Med. Hyg.,* 75, 530, 1981.

104. **Lainson, R., Shaw, J. J., Ward, R. D., Ready, P. D., and Naiff, R. D.,** Leishmaniasis in Brazil. XIII. Isolation of *Leishmania* from armadillos *(Dasypus novemcinctus),* and observations on the epidemiology of cutaneous leishmaniasis in north Pará State, *Trans. R. Soc. Trop. Med. Hyg.,* 73, 239, 1979.

105. **Latyšev, N. I. and Krjukova, A. P.,** On the epidemiology of the cutaneous leishmaniasis as a zoonotic disease of wild rodents in Turkmenia, *Trav. Acad. Milit. Med. Armée Ronge, U.S.S.R., Moscow,* 25, 229, 1941.

106. **Leishman, W. B.,** On the possibility of the occurrence of trypanosomiasis in India, *Br. Med. J.,* 1, 1252, 1903.

107. **Levine, N. D., Corliss, J. O., Cox, F. E. G., Deroux, G., Grain, J., Honigberg, B. M., Leesdale, G. F., Loeblich, A. R., Lom, J., Lynn, D., Merinfeld, E. G., Page, F. C., Poljansky, G., Sprague, V., Vávra, J., and Wallace, F. G.,** A newly revised classification of the protozoa, *J. Protozool.,* 27, 37, 1980.

108. **Lindenberg, A.,** L'ulcère de Bauru ou le bouton d'Orient au Brésil. Communication préliminaire, *Bull. Soc. Path. Exot.,* 2, 252, 1909.

109. **Lühe, M.,** *Handbuch der Tropenkrankheiten* Vol. 3, Mense, C., Ed., I.A. Barth, Leipzig, 203, 1906.

110. **Lysenko, A. J.,** Distribution of leishmaniasis in the Old World, *Bull. W.H.O.,* Geneva, 44 (4), 515, 1971.

111. **Mackie, F. P.,** A flagellate infection of sandflies, *Indian J. Med. Res.,* 2, 377, 1914.

112. **Mattei, D. M., Goldenberg, S., Morel, C., Azevedo, H. P., and Roitman, I.,** Biochemical strain characterisation of *Trypanosoma cruzi* by restriction endonuclease cleavage of kinetoplast DNA, *FEBS Lett.,* 74, 264, 1977.

113. **McConnell, E.,** Leptomonads of wild-caught Panamanian *Phlebotomus:* culture and animal inoculation, *Exp. Parasitol.,* 51, 336, 1963.

114. **Medina, R. and Romero, J.,** Estudio clinico y parasitologico de una nueva cepa de leishmania, *Arch. Venez. Pat. Trop. Parasitol. Med.,* 3, 298, 1959.

115. **Migone, L. E.,** Un caso de kala-azar a Assuncion (Paraguay), *Bull. Soc. Path. Exot.,* 6, 118, 1913.

116. **Miles, M. A., Lainson, R., Shaw, J. J., Póvoa, M., and de Souza, A. A.,** Leishmaniasis in Brazil. XV. Biochemical distinction of *Leishmania mexicana amazonensis, Leishmania braziliensis braziliensis* and *Leishmania braziliensis guyanensis* — aetiological agents of cutaneous leishmaniasis in the Amazon Basin of Brazil, *Trans. R. Soc. Trop. Med. Hyg.,* 75, 524, 1981.

117. **Miles, M. A., Póvoa, M. M., de Souza, A. A., Lainson, R., and Shaw, J. J.,** Some methods for the enzyme characterization of Latin-American *Leishmania* with particular reference to *Leishmania mexicana amazonensis* and subspecies of *Leishmania hertigi, Trans. R. Soc. Trop. Med. Hyg.,* 74, 243, 1980.

118. **Morel, C., Chiari, E., Camargo, E. P., Mattei, D. M., Romanha, A. J., and Simpson, L.,** Strains and clones of *Trypanosoma cruzi* can be characterised by restriction endonuclease fingerprinting of kinetoplast DNA minicircles, *Proc. Nat. Acad. Sci. U.S.A.,* 77, 6810, 1980.

119. **Muniz, J. and Medina, H.,** Leishmaniose tegumentar do cobaio *(Leishmania enriettii* n. sp.), *Hospital (Rio de Janeiro),* 33, 7, 1948.

120. **Mutinga, M. J.,** The animal reservoir of cutaneous leishmaniasis on Mount Elgon, Kenya, *E. Afr. Med. J.,* 52, 142, 1975.

120a. **Mutinga, M. J.,** at the International Center of Insect Physiology and Ecology, Nairobi, Personal communication.

121. **Napier, L. E., Smith, R. O. A., and Krishnan, K. V.,** The transmission of kala-azar to hamsters by the bite of the sandfly *Phlebotomus argentipes, Indian J. Med. Res.,* 21, 299, 1933.

122. **Neave, S.,** "*Leishmania donovani*" in the Sudan, *Br. Med. J.,* 1 (2265), 1252, 1904.

123. **Neligan, A. R.,** On the discovery by Dr. A. R. Neligan of leishmania in cutaneous lesions of dogs in Teheran, Persia, Annotation in *J. Trop. Med. Hyg.,* 16, 156, 1913.

124. **New, R. R. C., Chance, M. L., Thomas, S. C., and Peters, W.,** Antileishmanial activity of antimonials entrapped in liposomes, *Nature, London,* 272, 55, 1978.

125. **Nicoli, R. M.,** Le genre *Leishmania* R. Ross 1903, *Bull. Soc. Path. Exot.,* 56, 408, 1963.

126. **Nicolle, C.,** Culture du parasite du bouton d'Orient, *C.R. Acad. Sci.,* 146, 842, 1908.

127. **Nicolle, C. and Comte, C.,** Origine canine du Kala-azar, *Bull. Soc. Path. Exot.,* 1, 299, 1908.

128. **Paraense, L. and Chagas, A. W.,** Transmissão experimental da leishmaniose visceral americana pelo *Phlebotomus intermedius.* Nota prévia. *Brasil-Méd.,* 54, 179, 1940.

129. **Parrott, L. M. and Donatien, A. L.,** Infection naturelle et infection expérimentale de *Phlebotomus papatasii* (Scop) par le parasite de bouton d'Orient, *Bull. Soc. Path. Exot.,* 19, 694, 1926.

130. **Patton, W. S.,** The parasite of kala-azar and allied organisms, *Trans. R. Soc. Trop. Med. Hyg.,* 2, 113, 1909.

131. **Patton, W. S.,** Is kala azar in Madras of animal origin? *Indian J. Med. Res.,* 1, 185, 1913.

132. **Penna, H. A.,** Leishmaniose visceral no Brasil, *Brasil-Méd.,* 48, 949, 1934.

133. Pessôa, S. B., Classificação das leishmanioses e das espécies do gênero *Leishmania*, *Arq. Hig. Saúde Públ.*, 26, 41, 1961.

133a. Peters, W., Personal communication.

134. Peters, W., Lainson, R., Shaw, J. J., Robinson, B. L., and Leão, A. F., Potentiating action of rifampicin and isoniazid against *Leishmania mexicana amazonensis*, *The Lancet*, May 23, 1981, 1122.

135. Petrović, Z., Borjoški, A., and Savin, Z., Les résultats de recherches sur le réservoir de *Leishmania donovani* dans une région endémique du Kala-azar, *Proc. 2nd European Multicoll. Parasitol. Trogir.*, 97, 1975.

136. Pratt, D. M. and David, J. R., Monoclonal antibodies that distinguish between New World species of *Leishmania, Nature, London*, 291 (5816), 581, 1981.

137. Pressat, A., *Le paludisme et les moustiques (prophylaxie)*, Masson et Cie., Editeurs, Paris, 1905.

138. Pringle, G., Oriental Sore in Iraq. Historical and Epidemiological Problems, *Bull. Endem. Dis., Baghdad*, 2, 41, 1957.

138a. Ready, P. D., Lainson, R., and Shaw, J. J., Unpublished observations.

139. Rioux, J. A., Killick-Kendrick, R., Leaney, A. J., Young, J. C., Turner, D. P., Lanotte, G., and Bailly, M., Écologie des Leishmanioses dans le sud de la France. II. La Leishmaniose viscérale canine: succès de la transmission expérimentale "Chien-Phlébotome-Chien" par la piqûre de *Phlebotomus ariasi* Tonnoir, 1921, *Ann. Parasitol. (Paris)*, 54, 401, 1979.

140. Rogers, L., Preliminary note on the development of trypanosoma in cultures of the Cunningham-Leishman-Donovan bodies of cachexial fever and kala azar, *Lancet*, 2, 215, 1904.

141. Ross, R., (1) Note on the bodies recently described by Leishman and Donovan and (2) further notes on Leishman's bodies, *Br. Med. J.*, 2, 1261 and 1401, 1903.

142. Saf'yanova, V. M., Leishmaniasis Control, *Bull. WHO*, 44, 561, 1971.

142a. Sanyal, R. K., Resurgence of Kala-azar and its control, *Ann. Nat. Acad. Sci. (India)*, 15, 228, 1979.

143. Schnur, L. F., Chance, M. L., Ebert, F., Thomas, S. C., Peters, W., The biochemical and serological taxonomy of visceralizing *Leishmania, Ann. Trop. Med. Parasitol.*, 75, 131, 1981.

144. Scorza, J. V., Valera, M., Scorza, de C., Carnevali, M., Moreno, E., and Lugo-Hernandez, A., A new species of *Leishmania* parasite from the Venezuelan Andes region, *Trans. R. Soc. Trop. Med. Hyg.*, 73, 293, 1979.

145. Sergent, Ed., Sergent, Et., Lemaire, G., and Senevet, G., Insecte transmetteur et reservoir de virus du clou de Biskra. Hippothèse et expériences préliminaires, *Bull. Soc. Path. Exot.*, 7, 577, 1914.

146. Sergent, Ed., Sergent, Et., Parrott, L. M., Donatein A., and Béguet, M., Transmission du clou de Biskra par le phlébotome *(Phlebotomus papatasii* Scop.), *C.R. Acad. Sci.*, 173, 1030, 1921.

147. Sergiev, P. G., Beyslekhem, R. I., Moshkovsky, Sh.D., Demina, N. A., Kellina, O. I., Shuykina, E. E., Sergiev, V. P., Dukhanina, N. N., Triers, I. I., Shcherbakov, V. A., Yarmyakhamedor, M. A., Uskov, N. E., Losikov, I. N., and Nedospelova, E. I., Results of mass vaccinations against zoonotic cutaneous leishmaniasis (In Russian, English summary), *Med. Parazit. Moskva*, 39, 541, 1970.

148. Shaw, J. J., *The haemoflagellates of sloths*, London Sch. Hyg. Trop., Med. Memoirs, No. 13, 1969.

149. Shaw, J. J. and Lainson, R., Leishmaniasis in Brazil. II. Observations on enzootic rodent leishmaniasis in the lower Amazon Region — the feeding habits of the vector, *Lutzomyia flaviscutellata* in reference to man, rodents and other animals, *Trans. R. Soc. Trop. Med. Hyg.*, 62, 396, 1968.

150. Shaw, J. J. and Lainson, R., An immediate intradermal reaction to leishmanial antigen in human cutaneous leishmaniasis, *Trans. R. Soc. Trop. Med. Hyg.*, 68, 168, 1974.

151. Shaw, J. J. and Lainson, R., Leishmaniasis in Brazil. X. Some observations on intradermal reactions to different trypanosomatid antigens of patients suffering from cutaneous and mucocutaneous leishmaniasis, *Trans. R. Soc. Trop. Med. Hyg.*, 69, 323, 1975.

152. Shaw, J. J. and Lainson, R., Leishmaniasis in Brazil. XI. Observations on the morphology of *Leishmania* of the *braziliensis* and *mexicana* complexes, *J. Trop. Med. Hyg.*, 79, 9, 1976.

153. Shaw, J. J. and Lainson, R., A simply prepared amastigote leishmanial antigen for use in the indirect fluorescent antibody test for leishmaniasis, *J. Parasitol.*, 63, 384, 1977.

154. Shaw, J. J. and Lainson, R., Leishmaniasis in Brazil. XIV. Leishmanial and trypanosomal IgA antibody in patients with leishmaniasis and Chagas's Disease, *Trans. R. Soc. Trop. Med. Hyg.*, 75, 254, 1981.

155. Shaw, P. K., Quigg, L. T., Allain, D. S., Juranek, D. D., and Healy, G. R., Autochthonous dermal leishmaniasis in Texas, *Amer. J. Trop. Med. Hyg.*, 25, 788, 1976.

156. Sherlock, I. A. and Almeida, S. P., Notas sobre leishmaniose canina no Estado da Bahia, *Rev. Bras. Malar. Doenças Trop.*, 22, 231, 1970.

157. Sherlock, I. A. and Almeida, S. P., Observações sobre calazar em Jacobina, Bahia. V. Resultados de medidas profiláticos, *Rev. Bras. Malar. Doenças Trop.*, 22, 175, 1970.

158. Shortt, H. E., Transmission of *Leishmania donovani, Nature, London*, 127 (3200), 308, 1931.

159. Shortt, H. E., Barroud, P. J., and Craighead, A. C., A note on a massive infection of the pharynx of *Phlebotomus argentipes* with *Herpetomonas donovani, Indian J. Med. Res.*, 13, 441, 1926.

160. **Shortt, H. E., Craighead, A. C., Smith, R. O. A., and Swaminath, C. S.,** Third series of transmission experiments in Kala-azar with *Phlebotomus argentipes, Indian J. Med. Res.,* 17, 921, 1930.

161. **Simpson, M. H., Mullins, J. F., and Stone, O. J.,** Disseminated anergic cutaneous leishmaniasis, *Arch. Dermatol.,* 97, 301, 1968.

162. **Sinton, J. A.,** Entomological notes on field service in Waziristan, *Indian J. Med. Res.,* 9, 575, 1922.

163. **Smith, R. O. A., Lal, C., Mukerjee, S., and Halder, K. C.,** The transmission of *L. donovani* by the bite of the sandfly *P. argentipes, Indian J. Med. Res.,* 24, 313, 1936.

164. **Smith, R. O. A., Halder, K. C., and Ahmed, I.,** Further investigations on the transmission of kala-azar. Part I. The maintenance of sandflies, *P. argentipes,* on nutriment other than blood, *Indian J. Med. Res.,* 28, 575, 1940.

165. **Smith, R. O. A., Halder, K. C., and Ahmed, I.,** Further investigations on the transmission of kala-azar. Part II. The phenomenon of the blocked sandfly, *Indian J. Med. Res.,* 28, 581, 1940.

166. **Splendore, A.,** Leishmaniosi con localizzazione nella cavita mucose (nuova forma clinica), *Bull. Soc. Path. Exot.,* 5, 411, 1912.

167. **Strangways-Dixon, J. and Lainson, R.,** Dermal leishmaniasis in British Honduras: Transmission of *L. brasiliensis* by *Phlebotomus* species, *Br. Med. J.,* 1, 297, 1962.

168. **Strangways-Dixon, J. and Lainson, R.,** The epidemiology of dermal leishmaniasis in British Honduras. Part III. The transmission of *Leishmania mexicana* to man by *Phlebotomus pessoanus,* with observations on the development of the parasite in different species of *Phlebotomus, Trans. R. Soc. Trop. Med. Hyg.,* 60, 192, 1966.

169. **Strelkova, M. V.,** The duration and the character of the progress of cutaneous leishmaniasis in *Meriones meridianus* Pallas, *Parazitologiya, Leningrad,* 9, 532, 1975.

170. **Sun, C. J. and Wu, C. C.,** Notes on the study of kala-azar transmission. Part II. Further observations on the natural infection of *Phlebotomus chinensis* with *Leptomonas donovani, Chin. Med. J.,* 52, 665, 1937.

171. **Sun, C. J., Yao, Y., Chu, H. J., and Wu, C. C.,** Natural infection of *Phlebotomus chinensis* with flagellates morphologically indistinguishable from those of *Leishmania donovani, Chin. Med. J.,* 50, 911, 1936.

172. **Tartaglia, P.,** Die Ansrottung der Kala-Azar und Haut-Leishmaniase auf den Dalmatinischen Insein, *Ztschr. f. Tropenmed u. Parasit., Stuttgart,* 13, 450, 1962.

173. **Tikasingh, E. S.,** Enzootic rodent leishmaniasis in Trinidad, West Indies, *Bull. Pan Am. Health Org.,* 8, 232, 1974.

174. **Townsend, C. H. T.,** The insect vector of uta, a Peruvian disease, *J. Parasitol.,* 2, 67, 1915.

175. **Velez, L. R.,** Uta et espundia, *Bull. Soc. Path. Exot.,* 6, 545, 1913.

176. **Vianna, G. de O.,** Sôbre uma nova espécie de *Leishmania* (Nota preliminar), *Brasil-Méd.,* 25, 411, 1911.

177. **Vianna, G. de O.,** Tratamento da leishmaniose pelo tartaro emetico. Comunicação ao 7 Congresso Brasileiro de Medicina e Cirurgia, Belo Horizonte, *Arq. Bras. Méd., Rio de Janeiro,* 2, 426, 1912.

178. **Walton, B. C., Shaw, J. J., and Lainson, R.,** Observations on the *in vitro* cultivation of *Leishmania braziliensis, J. Parasitol.,* 63, 1118, 1977.

179. **Wang, J., Qu, J., and Guan, L.,** A study on the *Leishmania* parasite of the big gerbil in Northwest China, *Acta. Parasitol. Sinica,* 105, 1, 1964.

180. **Ward, R. D.,** New World leishmaniasis: a review of the epidemiological changes in the last 3 decades, *Proc. 15th Int. Congr. Ent., Washington, D.C.,* 505, 1977.

181. **Ward, R. D. and Fraiha, H.,** *Lutzomyia umbratilis,* a new species of sandfly from Brazil (Diptera: Psychodidae), *J. Med. Ent.,* 14, 313, 1977.

182. **Wenyon, C. M.,** Note on the occurrence of *Herpetomonas* in the *Phlebotomus* of Aleppo, *J. Lond. Sch. Trop. Med.,* 1, 98, 1911.

183. **Wenyon, C. M.,** Observations on *Herpetomonas muscae domesticae* and some allied flagellates, *Arch. Protistenk.,* 31, 1, 1913.

183a. **Wenyon, C. M.,** Protozoology, a manual for medical men, veterinarians and zoologists, Vol. I, Baillière Tindall & Cox, London, 1926.

184. **Wijers, D. J. B. and Linger, R.,** Man-biting sandflies in Surinam (Dutch Guiana): *Phlebotomus anduzei* as a possible vector of *Leishmania braziliensis, Ann. Trop. Med. Parasitol.,* 60, 501, 1966.

185. **Wright, J. H.,** Protozoa in a case of tropical ulcer ("Delhi sore"), *J. Med. Res.,* 10, 472, 1903.

186. **Yakimoff, W. L. and Schokhor, N. I.,** Recherches sur les maladies tropicales humaines et animales au Turkestan — II. La leishmaniose cutanée spontanée du chien au Turkestan, *Bull. Soc. Exot.,* 7, 186, 1914.

187. **Young, C. W. and Hertig, M.,** The development of flagellates in Chinese sandflies *(Phlebotomus)* fed on hamsters infected with *Leishmania donovani, Proc. Soc. Exp. Biol. Med.,* 23, 611, 1926.

188. **Zelodón, R., Ponce, C., and Murillo, J.,** *Leishmania herreri* sp. n. from sloths and sandflies of Costa Rica, *J. Parasitol.,* 65, 275, 1979.

189. Zelodón, R., Ponce, C., and Ponce, E., The isolation of *L. braziliensis* from sloths in Costa Rica, *Am. J. Trop. Med. Hyg.*, 24, 706, 1975.

RECOMMENDED READING

Deane, L. M., *Leishmaniose visceral no Brasil.* Servico Nacional de Educação Sanitária, Rio de Janeiro, Brazil, 1956.

Heyneman, D., Hoogstraal, H., and Djigounian, A., Bibliography of *Leishmania* and leishmanial diseases, *U.S. Naval Medical Research Unit Number Three (NAMRU-3) Special Publication.* Available from the U.S. Department of Commerce, National Technical Information Service, Springfield, Virginia 22161. 1980.

Manson-Bahr, P. H., *Manson's Tropical Disease, A Manual of the Diseases of Warm Climates,* Cassell & Co., Ltd., London, 1954.

Pessôa, S. B. and Barretto, M. P., *Leishmaniose tegumentar Americana* Imprensa Nacional, Rio de Janeiro, Brazil, 1948.

Steck, E. A., *The Chemotherapy of Protozoan Diseases,* Vol. 2, Section 3, 1. Publication of the Walter Reed Army Institute of Research, Washington, D.C., 1971.

Wenyon, C. M., *Protozoology, a manual for medical men, veterinarians and zoologists,* Vol. 1. Baillière Tindall & Cox, London, 1926.

Zuckerman, A. and Lainson, R., *Leishmania* in *Parasitic Protozoa,* Vol. I., Kreier, J. P., Ed., Academic Press, New York, 57, 1977.

AMERICAN TRYPANOSOMIASIS

Robert G. Yaeger

CHAGAS' DISEASE

Disease
South American trypanosomiasis, schizotrypanosomiasis.

Etiologic Agent
Trypanosoma cruzi Chagas, 1909.

Common Synonyms
Schizotrypanum cruzi Chagas, 1909; *Trypanosoma triatomae* Kofoid and Mc-Culloch, 1916; *Trypanosoma escomeli* Yorke, 1920.

Historical Notes
In 1907 Carlos Chagas travelled to a station built in the northern part of the Brazilian state of Minas Gerais for the purpose of combating malaria. It was at this locality that he heard of a dreaded blood-sucking insect known to the natives as "barbeiro" which was common in the grass huts of the poor people in the area. He reported that the insects remained hidden during the daytime in walls, ceilings, cracks, and other places. He observed that after dark these blood-suckers came out to feed on the inhabitants of the huts, preferably about the face, and upon illumination of the room the bugs "ran in great haste" to their hiding places. He identified the bugs as *Triatoma megista* and initiated a study of them. He observed flagellates in the rectal portion of the bugs and noted that they had characteristicts of the genus *Crithidia*. He immediately began a study of the flagellates by inoculating various laboratory animals such as guinea pigs, rabbits, dogs, and *Callithrix* monkeys. The monkey appeared to be the more susceptible of these hosts, and exhibited higher parasitemias. As a result of these initial studies he named the organism *Trypanosoma cruzi*. During subsequent studies in guinea pigs he observed what he considered to be schizogonic stages of the parasites in the lungs of these animals, and he then referred to the parasite as *Schizotrypanum cruzi*. His illustrations show binary fission of the amastigote (leishmania) stage but also include 8-nucleated schizont-like stages of what doubtlessly was a concomitant infection with *Pneumocystis carinii*. Portions of his description of reproduction in the lungs of guinea pigs substantiate this conclusion. Although a few investigators have continued to refer to the parasite as *Schizotrypanum cruzi*, Chagas himself withdrew the genus *Schizotrypanum* and reassigned the species to the genus *Trypanosoma*.

The existence of *T. cruzi* infection in the human inhabitants of the area was the occurrence of "a certain complex of frequent and coinciding symptoms which were most striking in children". He began to examine peripheral blood smears of children with symptoms, and after 4 days of testing he found the flagellate in the blood of a gravely ill child. Studies on animals inoculated with blood from the child confirmed that the parasite was *T. cruzi*.

Life Cycle and Morphology
T. cruzi is a pleomorphic trypanosome with one phase of its life cycle in a mammalian host and another phase in the insect vector. In mammals the parasite occurs extracellularly as the trypomastigote (trypanosome) stage which may be found in various body fluids during the acute stage of the disease. Unlike the African trypanosomes *T.*

cruzi does not undergo division in the trypomastigote stage. Instead, the trypomastigote penetrates a tissue cell where it transforms into the amastigote (leishmania) stage and then proceeds to multiply by binary fission until a large number of amastigotes are formed, depending upon the size and type of cell. After binary fission has ceased, the amastigote elongates and changes into a form which resembles a promastigote (leptomonas) stage. Transformation continues into a form resembling the epimastigote (crithidia) stage, and finally the parasite completes transition when it has assumed the trypomastigote form. Rupture of the host cell releases these highly motile trypanosomes which then spread via the blood and other body fluids to infect other cells. Occasionally premature rupture of the host cell releases the other stages.

The trypomastigote stage in the mammal measures approximately 20 μm in length. Two forms may occur, a broad form which is slightly shorter and a more slender form which usually moves more rapidly. In the broad form the nucleus is subspherical, centrally located, and stains a reddish purple with the Giemsa stain; the rather large kinetoplast is at the posterior terminal end and stains a deeper purple than the nucleus. The axoneme of the flagellum originates close to the kinetoplast and then extends outside of the body of the parasite, covered with a flagellar sheath and attached by an undulating membrane. The flagellum extends anteriorly until it reaches the anteriormost end of the organism; there is no significant length of free flagellum extending beyond the anterior end of the trypomastigote. The slender form has a rather elongate nucleus and the kinetoplast is usually subterminal, occasionally midway between the nucleus and the posterior tip of the organism. In fresh preparations the broad form is very motile but tends to remain within a circumscribed area whereas the slender form usually moves rapidly through the microscopic field in an eel-like fashion.

Triatomine bugs usually become infected by ingested blood containing the trypomastigote stage; it is also possible that other stages, released by premature rupture of an infected host cell, are occasionally ingested. Bugs may also become infected by feeding on the gut contents of another infected bug or on feces from an infected bug. In the midgut of the bug the ingested trypomastigotes undergo change to amastigotes or epimastigotes; intermediate transitional forms may also be observed. Reproduction by longitudinal binary fission occurs in both the amastigote and epimastigote stages as the gut contents move down the alimentary tract. Doubtlessly, there will be differences in the proportions of the different stages in the bug, depending upon species and strain of triatomine bug and the strain of *T. cruzi.* As the gut contents move into the rectal portion, metacyclic trypomastigotes, the infective stage, begin to appear in increasing numbers. Approximately 10 days after the infected blood meal, metacyclic trypomastigotes appear in the feces; however, more time may be required, depending upon temperature, number of ingested parasites, and strain differences. Forms seen in culture media resemble those seen in the insect vector.

Infected triatomine bugs do not usually transmit *T. cruzi* infection during the process of inserting their mouthparts into the mammalian host and withdrawing blood. There is, of course, always the possibility that a bug which is interrupted while feeding on a host with a high parasitemia, may mechanically transmit the infection if the bug inserts its contaminated mouthparts into another host. The bugs frequently defecate while feeding, and if infected feces are introduced into a mucous membrane such as the conjunctiva, into the puncture wound made by a bug, or are scratched into the skin by the person or animal, the active metacyclic trypomastigotes may succeed in penetrating tissue cells and establishing the initial infection as described above. Animals have become infected by eating infected bugs or the blood and tissues of infected animals; this may be a more efficient means of transmission, at least among animals which eat insects or other mammals, than contamination of the external body surface with infected bug feces. On numerous occasions the author has observed armadillos

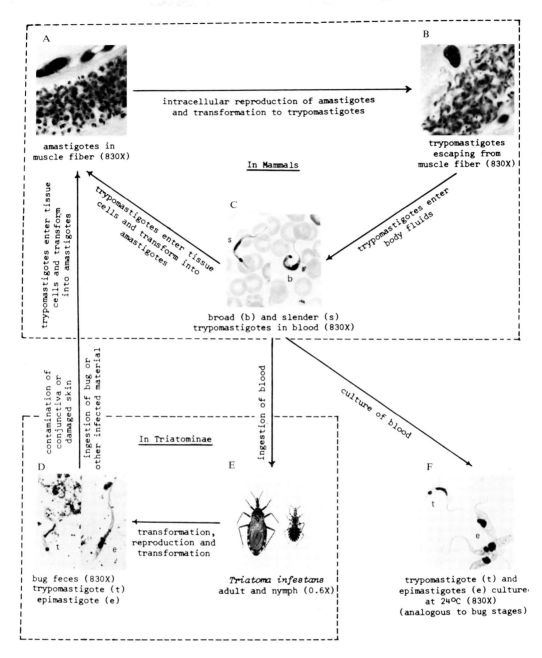

FIGURE 1.   Stages in the life cycle of *Trypanosoma crusi*. (A) Amastigotes in skeletal muscle fiber. (H.E. stain; magnification × 830.); (B) Slender trypomastigotes emerging from skeletal muscle fiber, (H. E. stain; magnification × 830.); (C) Broad (b) and slender (s) trypomastigotes in thin blood film. (Giemsa stain; magnification × 830.); (D) Trypomastigote (t) and epimastigote (e) in smear of triatomine bug feces. (Geimsa stain; magnification × 830.); (E) *Triatoma infestans*, adult and large nymph, 0.6 × natural size; (F) Trypomastigote (t) and epimastigotes (e) in smear of culture. (Giemsa stain; magnification × 830.)

ripping open dead trees riddled with insect tunnels in which triatomine bugs were se-creted. *T. cruzi* was isolated from armadillos captured in the area under observation. Bats, monkeys, puppies, kittens, and other animals frequently eat insects. There is also the possibility that a very hungry infant in a hut infested with infected triatomine bugs would eat or attempt to eat these bugs, and thus become infected via the oral route.

Transmission by ingestion of milk from infected females has been reported for man as well as other mammals. Infections have been acquired as the result of transfusion with blood from an infected individual. Careful screening of donors has apparently greatly reduced infections acquired in this manner. Congenital transmission from the females to the fetus or fetuses has been reported for man and other mammals. There have been accidental infections among laboratory workers by contact with spilled infected blood, bug feces or culture, or by being scratched or stuck with a hypodermic needle containing infected blood. Finally, there is the possibility that persons may contract infection when they skin or dress animals, particularly those wild mammals in which the prevalence of infection is higher. Although transmission of *T. cruzi* via the insect vector is primarily through contamination by infective alimentary tract contents rather than the more efficient anterior inoculative route such as occurs in African trypanosomiasis, the much higher prevalence of naturally infected insect vectors and animal reservoirs assures survival of the etiologic agent of Chagas' disease.

Hosts

Table 1 lists the Triatominae which have been reported to be naturally infected with *T. cruzi*. Similarly, the mammals listed in Table 2 are those which have been found to be naturally infected with this flagellate. However, due to the number of local publications and monographs which were not available but which may contain additional host records, the lists are probably not complete. Furthermore, it is reasonable to believe that more careful and extensive searches would reveal additional species of naturally infected triatomine bugs and mammals.

The list of bats reported as being infected with *T. cruzi* may include some species infected with a trypanosome referred to as *T. cruzi*-like by some investigators who were unwilling for one reason or another to state that the organism definitely was *T. cruzi*. This is a controversial issue which will not be discussed here, but in view of the long list of other naturally infected mammals and the opportunity for bats to become infected via the oral route because of their feeding habits, this group of mammals should be considered as an important reservoir of the disease.

Distribution

Infection with *T. cruzi* has been reported in mammals on the American continent from the temperate regions of Argentina and Chile northward to the temperate regions of the U.S.; it was also found in Trinidad. Except for Surinam, British Honduras, Guiana, and the Caribbean Islands, autochthonous human cases have been reported from countries throughout the area described. In view of the large number and wide distribution of wild mammalian hosts and insect vectors, it is probable that human infection exists in some areas where infected wild and domestic mammals occur but no human disease has yet been reported. A WHO study group estimated that at least seven million people in the Americas were infected with *T. cruzi* and furthermore, that some 35 million people were exposed to the risk of infection.

Chagas' disease is primarily a disease of rural areas where the insect vectors, animal reservoirs, and man are in close contact. In 1949 Dias estimated that from 50 to 70% of the population in the most highly endemic areas of Brazil had Chagas' disease. Of 1000 persons between the ages of 10 and 43, living in the Naranjaros Valley in Venezuela, 70.9% were positive in the complement fixation test for Chagas' disease; the parasite was isolated by xenodiagnosis in 21.3% of this group. In this same area *T. cruzi* was isolated from 42.1% of 38 dogs, 67.1% of 70 opossums, and 43.2% of 139 *Caluromys philander*. A survey of 11 rural endemic zones in Venezuela revealed that 41.3% (range: 1 to 55%) of 14,753 apparently healthy individuals had positive reactions to the complement fixation (CF) test for Chagas' disease. It was also noted that

Table 1
TRIATOMINAE REPORTED TO BE NATURALLY INFECTED WITH *TRYPANOSOMA CRUZI*

Cavernicola pilosa	*Triatoma maculata*[a]
Dipetalogaster maximus	*Triatoma neotomae*
Eratyrus cuspidatus	*Triatoma nigromaculata*
Eratyrus mucronatus	*Triatoma nitida*
Panstrongylus chinai[a]	*Triatoma leticularis*
Panstrongylus geniculatus	*Triatoma longipes*
Panstrongylus guntheri	*Triatoma oswaldoi*
Panstrongylus lignarius[a]	*Triatoma patagonica*[a]
Panstrongylus megistus	*Triatoma phyllosoma*[a]
Panstrongylus rufotuberculatus	*Triatoma phyllosoma intermedia*
Psammolestes arthuri	*Triatoma phyllosoma longipennis*
Rhodnius pallescens[a]	*Triatoma phyllosoma mazzottii*
Rhodnius pictipes	*Triatoma phyllosoma pallidipennis*
Rhodnius prolixus[a]	*Triatoma phyllosoma picturata*
Triatoma barberi	*Triatoma phyllosoma usingeri*
Triatoma brasiliensis[a]	*Triatoma platensis*
Triatoma carrioni[a]	*Triatoma protracta protracta*
Triatoma delpontei	*Triatoma protracta woodi*
Triatoma dimidiata[a]	*Triatoma rubida*
Triatoma dimidiata capitata	*Triatoma rubida sonoriana*
Triatoma dimidiata maculipennis	*Triatoma rubida uhleri*
Triatoma eratyrusiforme	*Triatoma rubrofasciata*[a]
Triatoma gerstaeckeri	*Triatoma rubrovaria*
Triatoma guasayana[a]	*Triatoma sanguisuga*
Triatoma hegneri	*Triatoma sanguisuga ambigua*
Triatoma infestans[a]	*Triatoma sordida*[a]

[a] Species reported as more or less adapted to colonization in human habitation.

the percentage of antibody carriers increased with age. A study in Guatemala revealed that 14.0% of 6126 individuals had complement-fixing antibodies for Chagas' disease. During a 10-year period in Guayaquil, Ecuador, 14.2% of 3587 human sera were found to be positive by the CF test. An epidemiological study from Chile revealed that 12% of 14,756 persons were positive for *T. cruzi* when the xenodiagnosis test was used. In the same area the CF test for Chagas' disease was positive for 14% of 10,862 persons. The same study revealed that 44% of 20,952 triatomine bugs and 10.9% of 4006 animals serving as reservoirs were infected with *T. cruzi*. Although only two indigenous cases of Chagas' disease, i.e., not acquired by a laboratory worker, have been confirmed in the U.S., serologic studies have detected antibodies in a few other individuals; however, confirmation by isolation of the parasite was not achieved. The infection rate for triatomine bugs in the U.S. is approximately 20% which is almost as high as the rates (20 to 30%) for the endemic areas of South America. One study in the southern U.S. employed cultivation of blood and revealed 13.8% of 123 opossums and 14.3% of 35 raccoons to be infected with *T. cruzi*. Using the same technique the writer found 25% of 60 armadillos, captured near New Orleans, to be similarly infected.

The numerous studies on *T. cruzi* which have been reported reveal wide ranges in the level of endemicity depending upon species and numbers of triatomine bugs, species and numbers of mammalian hosts susceptible to *T. cruzi* infection, and various environmental factors. Furthermore, some areas have been subjected to extensive surveys by investigators with much expertise whereas other areas have not been studied or the data are misleading because of inadequate diagnostic techniques or inexperienced workers.

Although Chagas' disease in man has not been found in the eastern hemisphere, *T.*

Table 2
MAMMALS REPORTED TO BE NATURALLY INFECTED
WITH *TRYPANOSOMA CRUZI*

Marsupialia

Didelphis azare (= *paraguayensis*)
Didelphis marsupialis
Didelphis marsupialis aurita
Didelphis marsupialis etensis
Didelphis marsupialis mesamericus
Didelphis virginiana
Lutreolina crassicaudata crassicaudata
Lutriolina crassicaudata paranalis

Marmosa agilis agilis
Marmosa cinerea
Marmosa mitis casta
Marmosa pallidior
Metachirus nudicaudatus
Monodelphis domestica
Caluromys philander

Chiroptera

Antrozous pallidus pacificus
Artibeus fallax lituratus
Artibeus jamaicensis jamaicensis
Artibeus jamaicensis lituratus
Carollia perspicillatus
Carollia perspicillatus azteca
Choeronyteris minor
Desmodus rotundus murinus
Eptesicus brasiliensis argentinus
Eptesicus furnalis
Eptesicus fuscus fuscus
Eumops abrasus
Eumops bonariensis beckeri
Glossophaga soricina leachi
Hemiderma perpicillatum
Histiotus macrotus laephotis
Histiotus montanus
Lonchophylla mordax

Macrotus mexicanus
Micronycteris megalotis
Molossus major major
Molossus obscurus
Myotis nigricans
Myotis occultus
Myotis velifer velifer
Noctilio labialis albiventer
Peropterix macrotis macrotis
Phyllostomus elongatum
Phyllostomus hastatus
Phyllostomus hastatus panamensis
Pipistrellus hesperus maximus
Pteronatus davyi fulvus
Saccopteryx bilineata
Tadaria brasiliensis
Tadaria mollossus
Uroderma bilobatum

Primates

Alouatta seniculus
Cebus apella
Cebus capucinus
Cebus sp.
Hapale jacchus
Homo sapiens

Hylobates pileatus
Macaca irus
Macaca mulatta
Nyciticebus coucang
Saimiri boliviensis
Saimiri sciurea

Edentata

Cabassous tatouya
Cabassous unicinctus
Chaetophractus vellerosus pannosus
Chaetophractus vellerosus vellerosus
Chaetophractus villosus
Dasypus hybridus
Dasypus novemcinctus
Dasypus novemcinctus fenestratus

Dasypus novemcinctus mexicanus
Dasypus novemcinctus texanus
Dasypus paraguayensis
Dasypus pentadactylus
Euphractus sexcinctus
Tamandua tetradactyla
Tolypeutes matacus
Zaedyus pichi caurinus

Lagomorpha

Orycytolagus cuniculus

Sylvilagus sp.

Table 2 (continued)
MAMMALS REPORTED TO BE NATURALLY INFECTED
WITH *TRYPANOSOMA CRUZI*

Rodentia

Akodon arviculoides cursor	*Neotoma alleni*
Cavia porcellus	*Neotoma fuscipes macrotis*
Cercomys cunnicularius laurentius	*Neotoma lepida lepida*
Citellus leucurus cinnamoneus	*Neotoma micropus canescens*
Coelogenus subniger	*Neotoma micropus micropus*
Coendous mexicanus laenatus	*Octodon degus degus*
Coendous prehensilis	*Peramys domesticus*
Cuniculus paca paca	*Peromyscus boylii rowlei*
Dasyprocta agouti	*Peromyscus truei gilberti*
Dasyprocta rubrata	*Peromyscus truei montipinoris*
Galea spixii spixii	*Rattus norvegicus*
Guerlinguetus gilirgularis	*Rattus rattus alexandrinus*
Leptosciurus argentinus	*Rattus rattus frugivorus*
Mus musculus	*Rattus rattus rattus*
Mus musculus brevirostris	*Sciurus gerrardi morulus*
Nectomys squamipes amazonicus	*Sciurus* sp.
Neotoma albigula albigula	*Zygodontomys pixuna*

Carnivora

Canis familiaris	*Grison vittatus*
Cerdocyon thous	*Mephitis mephitis nigra*
Dusicyon culpaeus culpaeus	*Nasua narica*
Dusicyon gracilis gracilis	*Procyon lotor*
Dusicyon griseus graislis	*Tayra barbara*
Felix domesticus	*Urocyon cinereoargenteus*
Grison cuja	

Artiodactyla

Sus scrofa domesticus	*Capra hircus*

cruzi-like parasites have been reported from nonhuman primates of southeast Asia. Flagellates indistinguishable from *T. cruzi* have been reported from *Macaca irus, Macaca mulatta, Nycticebus coucang,* and *Hylobates pileatus. T. cruzi* has been isolated several times from *M. mulatta* in the U.S. If any of these primates was housed in the open in the southern U.S. or other endemic area in the New World for a period of several weeks or longer, one cannot be certain that the animal was infected prior to entering the endemic area. Adult triatomine bugs are attracted to the animals at night and infection may be acquired by eating the infected bugs. However, in several cases, there was no possibility of infection having been acquired after being shipped from southeast Asia, and for the present we must accept the existence in southeast Asia of a trypanosome which is similar to if not identical with *T. cruzi* of the western hemisphere.

Disease in Animals

It is beyond the scope of this essay to describe the symptoms and pathology of *T. cruzi* infection in the many species of animals which have been naturally or experimentally infected. Furthermore, there is a paucity of such information for the majority of susceptible mammals. In most instances the reported pathological changes were similar to those described for man and which are described in the next section. Infections in wild mammals are usually chronic and detectable only by culture or xenodiagnosis.

Little is known about morbidity and mortality of *T. cruzi*-infected animals in the wild.

The disease in dogs has been described in more detail than any animal other than man. Infection runs a more acute course in puppies than in older dogs; a higher percentage of the younger animals die. In experimentally infected dogs trypomastigotes are readily detected in the blood in 10 days to a month, depending upon the size of inoculum, route of inoculation, and age of the dog. The Romaña sign was observed in a dog infected by introducing the inoculum into the conjunctival sac, but most dogs infected via this route did not manifest periorbital swelling. Paraplegia may occur, especially in older dogs. Hepatomegaly, splenomegaly, lymphadenopathy, anorexia, weight loss, diarrhea, hypothermia, dehydration, and other clinical signs have been reported in dogs.

Myocarditis frequently occurs in dogs and in its acute form is usually responsible for the death of most infected puppies. Chronic myocarditis in dogs is strikingly similar to that seen in man. Enlargement of the heart, especially of the right cavities, signs of congestive heart failure, ascites, edema, and various disturbances of cardiac rhythm are usually observed. ECG changes similar to those seen in humans have been reported from experimentally infected dogs.

Usually the principal pathologic lesions are seen in the heart and range from mild multifocal to diffuse necrotizing granulomatous lesions in the acute form. Anitschkow myocytes are frequently seen. Nests of amastigote forms of *T. cruzi* in the myocardial fibers may be relatively numerous in some cases. In the more chronic form there are diffuse areas of cellular infiltration, predominantly of nonspecific mononuclear type. Diffuse fibrosis, hypertrophy of cardiac fibers, vascular dilatation, and both interfibrillary and interstitial edema are usually seen. A mild granulomatous myositis is frequently seen in smooth muscle of the gastrointestinal tract and in skeletal muscle in dogs in the acute or subacute stage; occasionally nests of amastigotes may be seen. Parasites and/or a cellular reaction to their presence may occur in any of the organs during the acute phase, but occur to a much lesser degree than those already mentioned. Also, changes such as hepatic congestion and necrosis, pulmonary edema and congestion, and others, all related to the myocarditis, may be observed.

Disease in Man

Symptomatology

Although acute infection may occur at any age, the majority of such cases are seen in children. The incubation period may be as short as a week but in most instances ranges from 12 to 30 days, depending upon portal of entry, virulence of the strain, resistance of the individual, and other factors. The Romaña sign, a unilateral bipalpebral edema, occurs in one third to one half of the cases and represents the portal of entry. A nodular or occasionally ulcerative skin lesion, known as a chagoma, may be seen in about 25% of the acute cases. In the absence of these portal of entry signs, the disease may be confused with other febrile diseases, especially if it is not known that the patient had been in an endemic area and the physician is unfamiliar with the disease.

The protean symptomatology is dependent upon the variable degree of pathology which occurs in the tissues and organs. Characteristically there is fever early in the disease, a fever which may be intermittent, remitting, or continuous, and which usually subsides a month or more after the initial acute signs have disappeared. Lymphadenitis is first confined to the region of the initial lesion but may become generalized as the disease progresses. Moderate hepatosplenomegaly usually occurs. Edema may be confined to the face or may be a generalized firm and nonpitting type. Other symptoms are general malaise, muscular pains, anorexia, diarrhea, vomiting, and occasionally a rash. Encephalitis or meningoencephalitis, most often seen in infants, usually results in death of the patient. Acute myocarditis may also develop early during the disease, occasionally with a fatal outcome. It has been estimated that the overall case fatality rate is about 10% for patients with acute Chagas' disease; it is much higher in infants and children.

Most individuals who contract Chagas' disease survive the initial acute stage which may last 5 or 6 weeks, occasionally longer. Individuals who first contract the disease after they have reached maturity usually have a relatively mild acute stage which goes unrecognized; this occasionally occurs in children. Hence, the majority of persons with Chagas' disease have the chronic form, and it is believed that the infection persists for the duration of the person's life unless eradicated by treatment. Although many symptoms of the chronic form are related to damage sustained during the acute stage, there is evidence that the continued presence of the parasite at low, undetectable levels results in further pathological changes. Myocarditis occurs in the majority of chronic cases and results in premature death. Megacolon and megaesophagus are frequently associated with chronic Chagas' disease in Brazil; however, in Paraguay, Chile, Bolivia, and Argentina megacolon is frequently seen but megaesophagus is rare. Both of these manifestations of chronic Chagas' disease are rarely if ever reported from other countries where the disease is endemic.

Although myocarditis of a greater or lesser degree occurs in all acute cases of Chagas' disease, it may not be recognized in a significant number of cases. The majority of patients show enlargement of the heart shadow which is usually diffuse and variable, suggesting pericardial effusion. Tachycardia is considered to be of major significance in diagnosis. Other signs of myocarditis are abnormal ECG, prolongation of the P-R interval, primary T-wave changes, and prolongation of the QT interval. In the majority of cases the manifestations of acute Chagas' myocarditis disappear within a few months or years. The highest incidence of chronic Chagas' myocarditis occurs after the third decade of life. The ECG abnormalities seen in these patients include premature ventricular contractions, QRS abnormalities or primary T-wave changes, complete right bundle branch block, partial and complete A-V block, and abnormalities of the P waves.

Pathology

The histopathologic picture in acute Chagas' disease is better understood than that seen in the chronic phase of this disease. The parasite enters a cell where transformation and multiplication take place. These groups of intracellular parasites have been referred to as "pseudocysts". No cellular reaction to the presence of these parasites occurs as long as the host cell remains intact. Rupture of the infected cell initiates infiltration by polymorphonuclear leucocytes, lymphocytes, and plasma cells. These inflammatory and degenerative changes can be correlated with the presence of parasites which may invade any of the soft tissues during the acute phase.

In chronic Chagas' disease, however, the extensive pathological changes in the absence of parasites is not as easily explained. In most chronic cases the dominant lesion is cardiac but in some areas it may be megaesophagus or megacolon. The toxin theory is based upon the assumption that toxic substances are released when parasitized cells rupture. This is supported by a number of investigations where degeneration and inflammation were observed in hearts where no parasites could be found. The liberation of toxic substances when parasitized cells rupture has also been offered as the cause of mega disease; the denervation of the esophagus and colon results in hypertrophy and dilation. Moreover, in view of the workload of the heart, this organ is more sensitive to denervation than are the esophagus and the colon.

The chronic form of myocarditis has also been attributed to immunoallergic mechanisms. Substances produced in parasitized muscle fibers are released and these, in turn, give rise to antibodies which react with normal myocardial fibers resulting in lesions where no parasites can be found. Autoantibodies to cardiac muscle have been reported in experimentally infected animals. The discovery of EVI antibody in the sera of patients with acute Chagas cardiopathy lends support to the theory of autoimmunity; this antibody binds to the endocardium, the endothelium, and the interstitial spaces of heart tissue.

General Mode of Spread

Trypanosoma cruzi infection is primarily a disease of wild animals as is apparent from the list of mammalian hosts in Table 2. The triatomine bugs and the susceptible animal hosts are widely distributed as mentioned earlier. Spread from animal to animal may occur via infected triatomine bugs as previously described, as the result of eating infected tissue or ingestion of infected milk during nursing, or by congenital transmission. Man usually becomes involved in this cycle when certain species of triatomine bugs become established in human dwellings or enter from nearby habitats; transmission by means of the infected bug may be from man to man, from animal to man, or from man to animal, depending upon the circumstances. As infection via skin which was probably scratched or abraded and then contaminated with blood from an experimentally infected animal has been reported for man, it is possible that some human infections may have occurred in hunters, trappers, or others who have skinned or dressed an infected animal.

Geographic spread of the etiologic agent occurs to a limited extent by flight of the adult triatomine bugs. Migration of mammals, especially bats, is one mode of spread, and would be of most importance if the movement were into areas previously free of infection and in which susceptible triatomine bugs were established. The shipment of animals to zoos and laboratories has resulted in the introduction of infected animals into areas where *T. cruzi* does not naturally occur. However, the degree to which spread occurs from these animals to others is not known but, except for an occasional instance of congenital transmission, is probably insignificant. As nonhuman primates are not routinely screened for *T. cruzi* infection before or after shipment from Latin American countries, the presence of this infection in such primates used for research or establishing colonies may cause problems, especially if the animals are subjected to stress-producing conditions which may convert a low grade infection into an acute, sometimes fatal one.

Epidemiology

Transmission and life cycle of *T. cruzi* has been described in the previous sections but there are epidemiological aspects which should be introduced or emphasized at this point. The cycle involving reservoir animals and the insect vectors in nature may be maintained at a relatively high level of enzooticity, with transmission to man or domestic animals rarely occurring or not recognized as having taken place. In such areas of very low endemicity, unfamiliarity with the disease, and the lack of diagnostic facilities or expertise allows infections with *T. cruzi* to go unrecognized. The southernmost areas across the U.S. appear to fit in this category. The infectivity and virulence for man of the many *T. cruzi* strains in wild animals is debatable and was a subject of much discussion at the International Symposium on New Approaches in American Trypanosomiasis Research held in Belo Horizonte, Brazil in 1975. Human subjects cannot, for moral reasons, be employed to test strains of *T. cruzi* and the results of experiments in laboratory animals cannot be irrefutably extended to what would occur in human beings. Consideration must be given to the probability that a strain of *T. cruzi* which is transmitted from man to man via domesticated triatomine bugs is more pathogenic for man than a strain which is transmitted from another species of mammal.

Although triatomine bugs are primarily sylvatic by nature, some species have become adapted to human habitations where they may feed on both man and domestic animals. The dog and cat as well as the guinea pig where these rodents are raised for food are considered to be important domestic reservoirs. Important epidemiological factors with regard to the insect vectors are host preference, feeding, and defecation habits, suitableness for propagation of the parasite and production of the infective stages, aggressiveness, reproductive potential, and length of the life cycle. Species of bugs marked with an asterisk in Table 1 include *T. infestans* and *R. prolixus* which have a long history of adaptation to human dwellings and others which have become so adapted more recently. A number of other species have been reported as having invaded human dwellings and feeding on the inhabitants; however, these did not establish colonies in the homes. Within a species of triatomine bugs there may be geographic strain variations ranging from "no adaptation" to "well adapted" to human habitation. Other epidemiological factors are education of the inhabitants with respect to the disease and control of the vectors, construction of the dwelling, type of climate, presence of predators of the bugs, family income, and the presence of domestic animals in or close to the human dwelling.

Diagnosis

Isolation of the Parasite

During the acute phase of Chagas' disease in man and other mammals, the parasitemia may be sufficiently high to find the trypomastigotes by microscopic examination of a cover glass preparation of fresh blood, a Giemsa stained thin blood film, or a similarly stained thick blood film as employed to detect malaria parasites. In cases with meningoencephalitis, the cerebrospinal fluid should be centrifuged; the sediment is then examined for the parasite. Stained smears of the sediment, prepared in the same manner as blood smears, can be used to identify the organism more precisely.

In most instances of *T. cruzi* infection, the parasitemia will be too low to detect in thick or thin blood films. Several concentration techniques have been described for the isolation of the parasite in such cases. One rather simple method employs the use of phytohemagglutinin to agglutinate the erythrocytes in 10 mℓ of heparinized blood. The agglutinated erythrocytes are sedimented by very low speed centrifugation, sufficient only to bring down the heavier, clumped blood cells. The plasma supernate is then centrifuged at high speed to concentrate any parasites which may be present. The sediment is examined more effectively with a dark field or phase contrast microscope. Stained smears of the sediment should be prepared to identify any organisms which may be present.

Frequently the parasites are too few in the blood or other body fluids to be detected by the above methods. In such instances one must employ a technique which allows the parasite to multiply until the number is sufficiently high to detect by microscopic examination. Xenodiagnosis is one method which is widely used in the Latin American countries. It employs clean, laboratory-reared triatomine bugs which are shipped in special containers to health units or physicians. An inner container with the bugs has a gauze-covered opening through which the bugs feed when the container is fastened to the patient's arm; most bugs feed to repletion within 30 min. The container with the insects is then placed inside the shipping container for return to a central laboratory where the bugs are checked for infection after allowing sufficient time for the parasite to undergo repeated multiplication.

Culture techniques have long been employed to isolate *T. cruzi* from man and other mammals. As with xenodiagnosis, when the parasites are too few to detect by direct examination of blood, biopsied tissue, or other material, portions of the specimens are inoculated into culture medium which is then incubated at 22 to 24°C to permit the few organisms which may be present to multiply. Precautions must be taken to prevent contamination with other organisms, especially fungi. Antibiotics may be used routinely to control bacterial contamination but fungicidal drugs inhibit the growth of *T. cruzi*. The cultures should be examined at weekly intervals for up to 3 months. This lengthy period is necessary because antibodies in the inoculum may inhibit the growth of the flagellates for several weeks. Early examination of such cultures reveals occasional clumps of nonmotile amastigotes which are easily mistaken for clumps of leucocytes or other blood cells, but eventually these amastigotes transform into the motile, easily-detected epimastigote form. Such long incubation periods have frequently been observed in cultures from wild animals such as the armadillo, raccoon, and opossum which apparently had low grade chronic infections.

To verify the identity of a flagellate isolated in culture or wild-caught triatomine bugs, suckling or just-weaned mice should be inoculated. Bug fecal samples are best given subcutaneously, whereas culture material can be given subcutaneously or intraperitoneally. The inoculated animals are examined daily for the presence of trypomastigotes in the blood. When the parasitemia begins to level off, the animal should be killed and histologic sections of the various tissues should be examined for the presence of amastigotes or other intracellular forms; usually the amastigote stages predominate.

Inoculation of cultured mammalian cells with material from a patient or animal has also been employed to isolate *T. cruzi*. Organisms in the inoculum became established in the mammalian cells and undergo the cycle of reproduction and differentiation. This technique has the advantage of rapid identification of the organism as *T. cruzi* but may not be as practical, depending upon the resources of the laboratory. Also, it does not work well when the number of parasites in the inoculum is very low. When culturing blood, the technique yields better results if phytohemagglutinin is first employed to eliminate most of the blood cells, and the sediment, obtained by centrifugation of the plasma supernate, is used as inoculum.

Inoculation of blood or other material such as homogenized tissue from a mammal directly into nursing or weanling mice or other laboratory animals has been employed to isolate *T. cruzi*. However, this method has been less successful than the previously mentioned techniques. If one employs an immunosuppressive drug to lower the resistance of the animals and protects them from overwhelming bacterial infection with antibiotics, isolation of *T. cruzi* is more often achieved.

Stained impression smears, coverslip preparations of expressed fluid, and histologic examination of enlarged lymph nodes has been recommended for the detection of *T. cruzi* in man as well as other mammals. During the acute stage, the parasites may be found by examination of bone marrow or biopsied spleen.

Serologic Tests

The complement fixation test (CF) has been the most widely used quantitative serologic test for the diagnosis of *T. cruzi* infection. When properly carried out, the test has been reported to be highly sensitive and specific. However, the complement fixing antibodies may not be detectable during the first few weeks of infection. The IFA test has been employed by a number of investigators and found to be as reliable as the CF test when smears of the culture forms were used as the antigen. The IFA test was more sensitive than the CF test during the early stage of infection. The indirect hemagglutination test has also been employed for the diagnosis of Chagas' disease and, except during the early acute stage of infection, is comparable to the IFA test. Recent studies on a direct agglutination test, using trypsinized culture forms of *T. cruzi,* suggest that this may be as sensitive and reliable as the IFA and IHA tests; it detects antibodies early during the course of infection and is a relatively simple test to perform. The recently developed ELISA (enzyme-linked immunosorbent assay) was reported to compare favorably with the CF, IFA, and IHA tests. Although the precipitin reaction may be useful in detecting antibodies during the acute phase, it has not proved to be sufficiently sensitive for the diagnosis of chronic cases; furthermore, significant cross reactions with sera from infections with species of *Leishmania* were observed. A number of other tests such as the latex agglutination test, immobilization test, and the heterophile antibody reaction have been employed to diagnose Chagas' disease. However, reports in the literature suggest that the results of such tests should be confirmed by another more sensitive and specific laboratory test. Of great interest are the recent reports on the presence of a serum gamma globulin factor, the EVI antibody, in patients with chronic Chagas' cardiopathy.

Prevention and Control

As Chagas' disease is most prevalent where there is a close association between man and the insect vectors, breaking the cycle at this point would produce a significant reduction in transmission of the disease. This is primarily a socioeconomic problem which involves the elimination of the more primitive type of dwellings which afford ideal conditions for the colonization of triatomine bugs, and education of the people as to how the disease is acquired and what preventive measures must be taken. Modern residual insecticides such as BHC, DDT, Malathion, and Dieldrin have been more or less effective; however, the costs in some instances, toxicity in others, and the types of dwellings have placed limitations on the effectiveness of such control measures. Recent studies were reported on the effect of the use of insect juvenile hormone analogs which are active at very low doses, exert their effect on the triatomine bugs for many months, and have shown no observable effect on mammals. These substances were reported to block the production of fertile adults. Further investigations may reveal that synthetic juvenile hormones would be superior in several respects to the insecticides currently in use.

Transmission of *T. cruzi* infection via blood transfusion has been proved, and in highly endemic areas a significant percentage of blood donors may be infected. Individuals in the chronic stage of the disease may exhibit no overt symptoms, hence all donors should be tested serologically before their blood is transfused to a patient. It has been stated that a low concentration of crystal violet will kill any *T. cruzi* which may be present in donated blood, thus making it safe for use. However, a more recent report stated that in some studies *T. cruzi* was resistant to the crystal violet treatment, hence only blood from serologically negative donors should be used whenever possible.

At present there is no drug suitable for chemoprophylaxis for noninfected individuals going into an area in which Chagas' disease is prevalent. Moreover, there is no drug suitable for mass treatment of infected individuals. Although some protection over a limited time period has been demonstrated through the use of various vaccines in animals, a safe, effective vaccine for use in humans is not yet available.

Primaquine has been employed to produce clinical cure or improvement in acutely infected individuals. The drug appears to be effective in greatly reducing the parasitemia but apparently is ineffective against the intracellular stages. In recent years Bayer 2502® (Lampit) has been the drug of choice for treating Chagas' disease. This is a nitrofurfurylidene compound and produces toxic side effects. Fortunately, adverse side effects have been less frequently reported in children, and it is in this group where most acute infections are observed. Although a clinical cure may be attained, complete elimination of the parasites is uncertain. Complete cures with reversal of the serologic test from positive to negative have been reported. Repeated attempts to isolate the parasite from treated cases which remained serologically positive were unsuccessful. In at least one instance parasites were isolated from a treated patient whose serologic test had reverted from positive to negative.

Control of *T. cruzi* infection in domestic animals is a more difficult problem, especially if such animals are maintained outside where the triatomine bugs can feed upon them. Furthermore, in suburban and rural areas there may be a large reservoir of infected wild mammals, and transmission of the infection from these hosts to susceptible domestic animals may occur. To prevent or control *T. cruzi* infection in domestic animals, it would be necessary to utilize the same measures described above for man. Control to a limited extent may be achieved by eliminating wild mammals and their burrows or nests in the immediate areas of human dwellings; however, the adult bugs can readily fly across such cleared areas to seek a blood meal. In instances where an infected animal is considered to be of high value, chemotherapy could be used. However, in other instances, the wisest choice might be to destroy the animal to prevent the spread to others. In the case of animals used for food, thorough cooking will kill *T. cruzi* and the meat would be safe to eat.

TRYPANOSOMA RANGELI INFECTION

Etiologic Agent
Trypanosoma rangeli Tejera, 1920.

Synonym
Trypanosoma ariarii Groot, Renjifo and Uribe-Piedrahita, 1951.

T. rangeli exhibits a typical trypomastigote stage in the blood of man and other susceptible mammals. It averages 31 μm in length, and differs from *T. cruzi* in that it has a smaller subterminal kinetoplast, more undulations along the undulating membrane and a longer free flagellum at the anterior end. Only the trypomastigote stage occurs in the mammalian host, and dividing stages are rarely seen in peripheral blood. Natural infection has been reported from man, monkeys, dogs, opossums, anteaters, raccoons, and a cat. However, because the organisms are usually very scanty and detected more often by blood culture or xenodiagnosis, natural infection very likely occurs in other mammals. Experimental infections have been produced in a number of other mammalism species. It has been reported from Guatemala, Columbia, Panama, Costa Rica, Venezuela, Brazil, French Guiana, El Salvador, and Chile (questionable). The writer isolated both *T. rangeli* and *T. cruzi* from a patient who lived near San Pedro, Honduras, after he came to the U.S. for a diagnosis of his illness. Doubtlessly, the parasite exists in other countries of Latin America but further investigations are needed to demonstrate its presence.

Rhodnius prolixus, R. pallescens, Panstrongylus geniculatus, Triatoma dimidiata, T. rubrofasciata, and *T. nitida* have been reported as vectors of *T. rangeli*. The trypomastigotes in the host's blood are ingested by the bug; transformation into epimastigotes and reproduction occurs in the alimentary tract; this is followed by penetration into the hemocoel where reproduction continues. Eventually epimastigotes enter the salivary glands and transformation to the infective metacyclic trypomastigote takes place. Transmission occurs when the bug injects saliva during the feeding process. Most investigators do not believe that transmission via contamination with infected feces occurs or if so, it is of minor significance.

There is no evidence that *T. rangeli* produces pathological changes in man or other mammals. However, this parasite is transmitted by some of the same species of triatomine bugs which transmit *T. cruzi*, and mixed infections do occur. The forms which occur in culture as well as those seen in the alimentary tract of the bug are similar and an erroneous identification could result if the observer lacked the expertise essential for differentiation. Although the forms seen in blood smears differ, these may also be misidentified by an inexperienced observer. Hence, *T. rangeli* is important primarily because it may be mistakenly identified as *T. cruzi*.

REFERENCES

1. A Bibliography on Chagas' Disease, 1909—1969, Index Catalogue of Med. and Vet. Zool. Ser. Publ. No. 2, U.S. Department of Agriculture, Washington, D.C., 1972.
2. American Trypanosomiasis Research, Int. Symp. New Approaches Am. Trypanosomiasis Res., Belo Horizonte, Brazil, 1975, Pan American Sanitary Bureau, Sci. Publ. No. 318, 1976.
3. **Barretto, M. P.,** Reservatorios do *Trypanosoma cruzi* nas Americas, *Rev. Brasil. Malar.,* 16, 527, 1964.
4. **Chagas, C.,** Nova tripanosomiase humana. Estudos sôbre a morfolojia e o ciclo evolutivo do *Schizotrypanum cruzi* n. gen., n. sp., agente etiolojico de nova entidade morbida do homem, *Mem. Inst. Oswaldo Cruz,* 1, 159, 1909.
5. **Dias, E.,** Chagas-Krankheit, in *E. Rodenwaldt's Weltseuchen Atlas,* 2, 135, 1956.
6. **Fife, H. H., Jr.,** Serodiagnosis of Trypanosomiasis, in *Immunology of Parasitic Infections,* Cohen, S. and Sadun, E., Eds., Blackwell Scientific, London, 1976, 76.
7. **Goble, F. C.,** South American Trypanosomes, in *Immunity to Parasitic Animals,* Vol. 2, Appleton-Century-Crofts, New York, 1970, 597.
8. **Hutt, M. S. R., Köberle, F., and Salfelder, K.,** American Trypanosomiasis (Chagas' Disease and Chagas' Syndromes), in *Tropical Pathology,* Spencer, H., Dayan, A. D., Gibson, J. B., Huntsman, R. G., Hutt, M. S. R., Jenkins, G. C., Köberle, F., Maegraith, B. G., and Salfelder, K., Eds., Springer-Verlag, New York, 1973, 380.
9. **Laranja, F. S., Dias, E., Nobrega, G., and Miranda, A.,** Chagas' disease. A clinical, epidemiologic, and pathologic study, *Circulation,* 14, 1035, 1956.
10. Numero Comemorativo do Cinqüentenario da Descoberta da Doenca de Chagas, *Rev. Goiana Med.,* 5 (4), 1959.
11. **Pessoa, S. B.,** Reservatorios animais do *Trypanosoma cruzi.* A doença de Chagas e uma zoonose, *Ann. Congr. Int. Sôbre a Doenca de Chagas,* 4, 1155, 1963.
12. *Trypanosomiasis and Leishmaniasis,* with Special Reference to Chagas' Disease, (New series), Ciba Foundation Symp. 20, Associated Scientific Publ., Amsterdam, 1974.

AFRICAN TRYPANOSOMIASIS

J. R. Baker

DISEASE

African human trypanosomiasis; sleeping sickness.

ETIOLOGIC AGENT

A. *Trypanosoma (Trypanozoon) brucei;* (Protozoa, Mastigophora, Kinetoplastida)

There is some controversy about the nomenclature of this species. Hoare includes two subspecies — *T. brucei brucei* which does not infect man and *T. brucei gambiense* which does; within the latter he recognizes two clinical variants or nosodemes — the chronic "gambiense" and acute "rhodesiense" forms.[1] Other workers continue the "classical" usage of three species — *T. brucei, T. rhodesiense,* and *T. gambiense* — though this has little to recommend it.[2,152] The compromise used here is the acceptance of three subspecies — *T. brucei brucei* (not infective to man), *T. brucei rhodesiense* (virulent pathogen of man) and *T. brucei gambiense* (producing chronic disease in man).[3] Recently a convincing argument has been proposed for recognizing only several nosodemes and zymodemes (populations distinguished enzymatically) within the single species *T. brucei.*[149]

Morphologically all three subspecies are indistinguishable. In the vertebrate host they occur in blood, cerebrospinal fluid, and other tissue fluids as elongate organisms with a single flagellum; there are two extreme forms — long, slender trypomastigotes measuring about 30 × 1.5 μm and short, stumpy trypomastigotes (lacking a free flagellum), about 18 × 3.5 μm (Figure 1); their respective cell volumes, without the flagellum, are 11.1 and 26.6 μm.[3,4] The two forms intergrade morphologically, the former (multiplicative forms) differentiating into the latter (which are transmissive forms, infective to the invertebrate vector). They differ in their respiratory physiology, the long slender forms having functionally repressed and structurally reduced mitochondria.[4,7] At the macromolecular level, there are some differences between the subspecies — e.g., deoxyribonucleic acid buoyant densities (though this is now doubted),[8] electrophoretic mobility of certain enzymes,[9] and structure of some antigens.[10,11]

As far as is known, these trypanosomes are extracellular throughout their life in vertebrate and invertebrate hosts. Multiplication is by longitudinal (symmetrogenic) binary fission of the slender trypomastigotes; no sexual process is known though indirect evidence suggests that genetic exchange does occur.[150] Other postulated stages have not yet been confirmed.[12,13] The life cycle in the invertebrate vector hosts (*Glossina* spp.) has been comprehensively described by Hoare,[1] though there is newer evidence about routes of migration.[14-16] Morphological variants arising at different phases of the life cycle are shown in Figure 1; studies of their ultrastructure have been reviewed by Steiger.[17]

TRUE AND ALTERNATE HOSTS

The hosts of *T. brucei* subspecies fall into two major groups — vertebrate and invertebrate (vectors).

Vertebrate Hosts

Both *T. brucei gambiense* and *T. brucei rhodesiense* infect man (*Homo sapiens*).

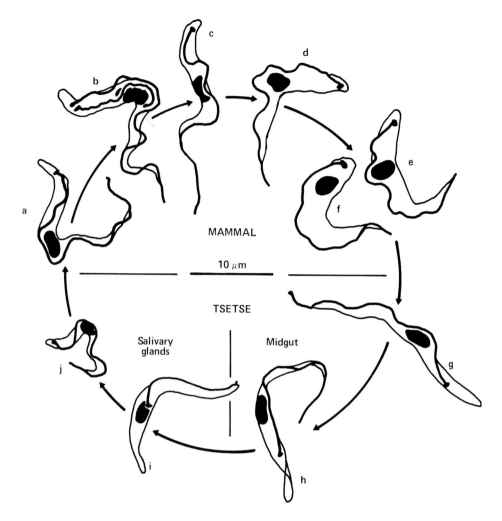

FIGURE 1.   Morphological forms of *Trypanosoma brucei* ssp. throughout its life-cycle: a to f, from blood of vertebrate host; g to j, from invertebrate host; (a) long slender trypomastigote; (b) dividing trypomastigote; (c) intermediate trypomastigote; (d,e) short stumpy trypomastigotes; (f) posteronuclear stumpy trypomastigote; (g,h) procyclic trypomastigotes (g, from stomach; h, from proventriculus); (i) epimastigote; (j) metacyclic trypomastigote.

Additional proven vertebrate hosts of the latter subspecies include *Tragelaphus scriptus* (bushbuck), *Alcelaphus buselaphus cokei* (Coke's hartebeest), *Crocuta crocuta* (spotted hyena), *Pathera leo* (lion), and *Bos taurus* (domestic cattle).[18-21] These are the only identifications based on the absolute criterion of infectivity to man. There is strong presumptive evidence, based on retention of infectivity after exposure to human serum in vitro under controlled experimental conditions (the blood incubation infectivity test),[22] that *T. brucei rhodesiense* has been isolated also from *Kobus defassa* (waterbuck).[23] Other wild ungulates and carnivores may be hosts, but adequate tests have not been made on strains of *T. brucei* ssp. indet. isolated from them.[24,25]

There is less experimental evidence for a nonhuman reservoir host of *T. brucei gambiense,* though various primates, rodents, ungulates, and carnivores are susceptible to experimental infection — as indeed are some reptiles, at least for limited periods.[26] Apparently only one proven (human-infective) isolation has been made, from a dog in Fernando Poo.[27] Domestic pigs (*Sus scrofa*) and *Cricetomys gambianus* (Gambian pouched rat) have also been suggested as possible, but unproven, hosts.[26,28,29,147,148]

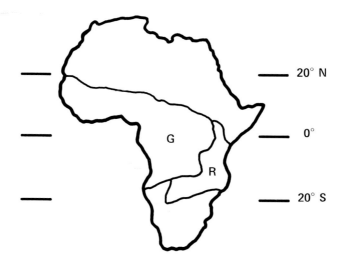

FIGURE 2. Map of Africa showing approximate limits of distribution of *Trypanosoma brucei gambiense* (G) and *T. brucei rhodesiense* (R).

Invertebrate Hosts

These are only species of the genus *Glossina* Wiedmann, 1830 (Insecta, Diptera, Muscidae).[30,31] Experimentally, both sexes and most if not all species are susceptible:[32] under natural conditions, the major vectors of *T. brucei gambiense* are *G. palpalis* and *G. tachinoides*,[33] while those of *T. brucei rhodesiense* are *G. morsitans, G. pallidipes, G. swynnertoni* and — in certain limited areas — *G. fuscipes* and possibly *G. tachinoides*.[34,35]

DISTRIBUTION

Human trypanosomiasis occurs throughout West, Central, and East Africa between latitudes 20°N and 20°S. In the east, the etiologic agent is predominantly *T. brucei rhodesiense;* in the central and western regions, it is mainly *T. brucei gambiense* (see Figure 2 and Table 1).[32,34,36]

DISEASE IN ANIMALS

Domestic Animals

In general, *T. brucei* sspp. are not important pathogens of domestic stock in Africa. Cattle, sheep, goats, and pigs, if infected, usually show mild, chronic infections; natural infections of the latter three species are rare. Indigenous breeds of cattle are particularly tolerant; but in horses and dogs infection with *T. brucei brucei* and, presumably, *T. brucei rhodesiense* is usually acute and fatal.[37] *T. brucei gambiense* produced only an asymptomatic infection in an experimentally infected dog, which apparently recovered spontaneously between 6 and 9 months after infection; the prepatent period (after infection by bite of *G. tachinoides*) was 13 days and trypanosomes could no longer be recovered from the animal's peripheral blood after 6 months; at no time did the dog appear unwell, nor was there any indication of parasite invasion of its cerebrospinal fluid (CSF).[38] Experimental infection of pigs with *T. brucei brucei* produced chronic, though ultimately fatal, infections, one animal dying after 94 days with pulmonary symptoms; trypanosomes have been detected in the CSF of infected pigs. Natural infections of pigs are rare and apparent spontaneous recovery of one

Table 1

NUMBER OF CASES OF HUMAN TRYPANOSOMIASIS REPORTED
FROM AFRICA, 1968—1975[36]

	Number of new cases[a]						
Country	1968	1969	1970	1971	1972	1973	1974
Western Africa							
Dahomey	17	18	11	22		> 157	410
Ghana	181	160	166	135		156	> 69
Guinea	379	351	357	425	38	55	31
Guinea Bissau					25	46	11
Ivory Coast	376	176	148		144	136	87
Mali	356	221	231	190	193	388	188
Niger	9	0	4	0	1	0	0
Nigeria	944	599	393	529	498	331	> 132
Senegal	43	16	16		17	10	2
Togo	36	84	14	57	23	25	21
Upper Volta	164	262	145	114	69	75	78
Central Africa							
Central African Republic	19	22	63	175	112	91	79
Chad	61	50	47	18	17	15	54
Congo	134	73	59	172	49	42	91
Gabon	86	49	59	38	413	32	47
United Republic of Cameroon	219	217	229	125	103	297	476
Zaire	3357	4957	6152	5124	4126		
Eastern and Southern Africa							
Botswana	36	37	59	272			
Burundi	65	12	78	75	144		
Ethiopia	28	173	44	12	1		
Kenya	43	20	16	26	7	13	
Malawi	1	0	0	2	0		
Rwanda	21	20	69	35	13		
Sudan			8	2	22	125	287
Uganda	90	56	81	184	160	37	
United Republic of Tanzania	403	530	564	569	612	477	488
Zambia	80	69	127	200	394	391	
Total	7148	8172	9140	8501	7151	> 2899	> 2551

[a]   The absence of an entry does not necessarily imply absence of the disease.

From *Weekly Epidemiol. Rec.*, World Health Organization, 22(4), January 23, 1976. With permission.

occurred 12 to 15 months after infection; *T. brucei gambiense* produced symptomless infections lasting for at least 2 to 3 months.[39]

The pathogenesis of *T. brucei* sspp. infections in domestic (and laboratory) animals has been reviewed by Losos and Ikede.[40] In general, the disease caused by *T. brucei brucei* in cattle, sheep, goats, horses, dogs, and probably cats resembled that produced by *T. brucei rhodesiense* in man (see below); trypanosomes were present in blood and other tissue fluids, including CSF. *T. brucei rhodesiense* produced similar symptomatology, but usually seemed less virulent to cattle and horses. *T. brucei gambiense* was less virulent to all groups, producing at the most very chronic inapparent infections sometimes resulting in spontaneous recovery, and no detailed study has been made of the pathology (if any) of the infection. A thorough study of experimental *T. brucei brucei* infection in horses emphasized the similarity of its pathogenesis to that produced in man by *T. brucei rhodesiense*, particularly when the normally very acute

Table 2
SUSCEPTIBILITY OF SOME AFRICAN MAMMALS
TO *TRYPANOSOMA BRUCEI* SPP.[24]

Group I.   Animals usually killed by infection
Thomson's gazelle (*Gazella thomsonii*)
Dikdik (*Rhynchotragus* spp.)
Blue Forest duiker (*Guevei caeruleus*)
Jackal (*Canis* spp.)
"Fox" (probably the bat-eared fox, *Otocyon megalotis*)
Ant-bear (*Orycteropus afer*)
Hyrax (*Procavia* spp.)
Serval cat (*Leptailurus serval*)
Monkey (*Cercopithecus* spp.)

Group II.   Animals usually tolerant to infection
All infectable: blood positive periods of considerable
length
Bush duiker (*Sylvicapra* spp.)
Eland (*Taurotragus oryx*)
Bohor reedbuck (*Redunca redunca*)
Spotted hyena (*Crocuta crocuta*)
Oribi (*Ourebia ourebi*)
Bushbuck (*Tragelaphus scriptus*)
Impala (*Aepyceros melampus*)
Usually infectable: trypanosomes very scanty in blood
Warthog (*Phacochoerus aethiopicus*)
Bushpig (*Potamochoerus koiropotamus*)
Porcupine (*Hystrix* spp.)
Not infectable
Baboon (*Papio* spp.)

From Ashcroft, M. T., *E. Afr. Med. J.*, 36, 289, 1959. With permission.

infection was rendered more chronic by subcurative chemotherapy.[41,42] Study of a naturally infected dog led to similar conclusions.[43] In the central nervous system, leptomeningitis, subpial gliosis, vasculitis, and perivascular cuffing (involving histiocytes, lymphocytes, morular cells and plasmocytes) were seen; these were thought to be mainly immunopathological lesions (the genesis of which has been thoroughly elucidated in experimentally infected rabbits).[44] Other changes included cellular infiltration of various organs, reticuloendothelial hyperplasia, increased hematopoesis, cardiac inflammation, and widespread occurrence of thrombi.

Wild Animals

Ashcroft and others recorded the results of attempts to initiate experimental infections of a variety of East African wild mammals with *T. brucei brucei* or *T. brucei rhodesiense* by the bite of infective *G. morsitans*.[45] They stressed the similarity of the ensuing infections, whichever subspecies was the causative organism, and classified the mammals into two groups depending on whether they were usually killed by, or usually tolerant to, the infection — the latter group including animals which apparently recovered spontaneously (warthog, bushpig, porcupine, hyena, oribi, impala, some duikers, and some reedbuck) as well as one species — the baboon — which is normally completely insusceptible (see Table 2, where the scientific names of these species are given). The course of infection in some of the mammals was described, but details of the pathology were not given. Trypanosomes were detected, however, in the CSF of experimentally infected Thompson's gazelle, dikdik, monkeys, and hyrax (and, in other work, the chimpanzee *Pan troglodytes*).[46,47] *T. brucei gambiense* produced subclinical infection in one green monkey (*Cercopithecus aethiops tantalus*) and one red monkey (*Erythrocebus patas patas*), the latter apparently recovering after about 1 year.[38] Two lions experimentally infected with *T. brucei* ssp. indet. developed anemia, hypoglycemia and hypergammaglobulinemia.[48] There are very few reports of wild animals clinically ill as a result of a naturally acquired trypanosome infection; a young lion (*Panthera leo*) infected with *T. brucei* ssp. indet. was obviously sick, possibly as a result of its trypanosomiasis,[49] and two zebra (*Equus burchelli*), with the same species demonstrable in blood and brain tissue, showed nervous symptoms suggestive of cerebral lesions resulting from the trypanosomal infection.[50] Encephalitis and myocarditis have also been reported from naturally infected lions and hartebeest.[51]

DISEASE IN MAN

Clinically, African human trypanosomiasis can be considered to evolve through three successive stages — the initial chancre, acute generalized trypanosomiasis or trypanosomal fever, and advanced cerebral trypanosomiasis or sleeping sickness.[52]

Chancre

A feeding *Glossina* may inject metacyclic trypomastigotes (Figure 1) directly into a capillary or, more usually, into the pool of extravasated blood on which it is feeding. If the latter happens, the parasites initially remain localized in the subcutaneous tissue, transform into long slender hematozoic forms (Figure 1), and multiply by longitudinal binary fission. Lymphocytic infiltration and exudation of lymph occur and a hard, painful red nodule or chancre results between 4 and 10 days after the injection of trypanosomes.[53] Gradually the parasites increase in number and invade the blood and lymphatic vessels, to give rise to the second stage of the disease.

Acute Generalized Trypanosomiasis

The incubation period depends on the numbers of metacyclic trypomastigotes introduced and the rapidity with which they enter the circulatory and lymphatic systems. It usually ranges from 7 to 10 days in the acute, rhodesiense form of the disease to perhaps 1 or 2 months in the gambiense form. There is a febrile reaction and often a characteristic frontal headache. Particularly in the gambiense disease, invasion and proliferation of trypanosomes occur in the lymphatic glands, which become enlarged and hyperplastic (swelling of the glands in the posterior triangle of the neck constitutes the well-known "Winterbottom's sign" of trypanosomiasis). Anemia and granulocytopenia ensue and the amount of immunoglobulin M (IgM) in the plasma becomes markedly increased. The spleen becomes enlarged and, like the lymph glands, hyperplastic with a change from a predominance of small lymphocytes in the germinal centers to one of plasma cells (antibody-synthesizing derivatives of lymphocytes). Myocarditis is a fairly common complication of the rhodesiense form of the disease.[54] Many of these (and later) pathological processes may be due to the release of kinins, histamine, and similar polypeptides as a result of repeated antigen-antibody reactions,[55,56] and also possibly to the accumulation of pyruvate in blood and tissue fluid[55] — the pyruvate arising as an end product of the parasites' incomplete oxidative metabolism of glucose.[57] Repeated antigen-antibody reactions occur in the blood of the infected mammal because the parasites change the molecular structure of the glycoprotein coating the external surface of the plasmalemma of the hematozoic (and metacyclic) trypomastigotes.[58] This surface coat is the antigen presented by the parasite to its host, and against which the host synthesizes antibody. Thus by changing the configuration of the antigen, some parasites evade destruction by antibody and survive to multiply until the host synthesizes antibody against the new, variant antigen; the process is then repeated. Experimentally up to 25 changes of antigen at 2 to 4 day intervals have been recorded, and no limit to the number has yet been established. The mechanism of the change is not fully understood; variants tend to arise in a similar sequence in any particular trypanosome stock during infections in different mammalian hosts, and current speculation favors sequential induction of a genetically determined program.[59,60,145,146]

There is good evidence that infection with *T. brucei* sspp. produces immunosuppression of the host with respect to other antigens, and often infected persons succumb ultimately to a secondary infection such as pneumonia.[61-64]

Advanced Cerebral Trypanosomiasis

This stage of the disease, classical "sleeping sickness," results from penetration by the trypanosomes of the so-called blood-brain barrier and their entry into the CSF and tissues of the central nervous system (CNS); they do not, however, enter any of the cells of the CNS (or of any other tissue). This stage may arise within 3 months of infection in rhodesiense disease, or not until 1½ to 2 years (or more) have elapsed if the infection is of the gambiense type. Daytime drowsiness and nocturnal insomnia often occur, but other neurological signs are varied, nonspecific, and transient.[52] IgM appears in the CSF in increasing amount, together with trypanosomes themselves. The total protein content and cell count of the fluid are both raised above the normal limits of 25 mg/100 mℓ and 7 cells/$\mu\ell$, respectively.[65] Microscopically, the brain and CNS in general show the characteristic lesion of perivascular cuffing, and infiltration of the Aschoff-Robin space surrounding the capillaries by lymphocytes, plasma cells, and morular cells.[52] The latter, the presence of which in the infiltrated areas of CSF is thought to be pathognomonic of trypanosomiasis, are probably plasma cells containing accreted immunoglobulins as a result of hyperimmunization.[66] Vacuoles in these cells contain eosinophilic globulin and are sometimes known as Russell bodies after their original describer, who mistakenly associated them with the causation of cancer.[67] Morular cells, first recorded from trypanosomiasis patients by Christy,[68] were described in more detail by Mott and hence are often known as Mott's cells.[69] Similar lymphocytic and morular cell infiltration in the meninges results in meningoencephalitis, especially marked in the arachnoid and pia mater, which become adherent. Neuroglial cells increase in number. The cuffing probably interferes with normal transport across the capillary wall of oxygen and other metabolites and leads ultimately to generalized damage of the brain and CNS, which in turn is responsible for the cerebral signs. Such damage, however, is relatively slight and usually appears to be reversible after successful treatment.[52] The pathogenesis of the CNS changes is not certainly known but is probably related to the antigen-antibody reactions and kinin release.[52,55] Death of untreated patients may ensue (often from intercurrent infection, as already mentioned) in anything from a few months (rhodesiense disease) to a few years (gambiense disease). No recorded case of spontaneous recovery is known, but so-called "healthy carriers" of infection, apparently themselves unaffected, have rarely been reported.[70,71]

GENERAL MODE OF SPREAD

By far the most common means of dissemination of human trypanosomiasis in Africa is the cyclical mode of development in *Glossina:* this is true also of *T. brucei* sspp. infection in wild and domestic mammals. Noncyclical transmission may occur, by means of *Glossina* or other hematophagous Diptera which are interrupted in the course of feeding on a parasitemic mammal and fly to another, nearby host, there to continue their meal before the blood of the first host has dried in the insect's proboscis. This type of transmission, in which the insect acts as a flying hypodermic syringe, is sometimes (inappropriately) called "mechanical transmission." It is undoubtedly rare, and cannot serve to maintain the disease in areas from which *Glossina* is absent, but it may sometimes play a significant role in epidemics (or epizootics), especially of *T. brucei rhodesiense* infection in man, where parasitemias are likely to be relatively high.[25,32,34,52]

Congenital transmission of the human disease has been rarely reported, as has transmission via human milk, though the latter is disputed.[52] Neither of these possible routes is of any epidemiological significance.

Transmission by eating infected mammals can occur experimentally, and probably contributes to the relatively high infection rates with *T. brucei* spp. amongst wild carnivores.[25,72-76] It may be of considerable epizootiological significance but is probably of little if any importance in transmitting this disease to man, since wild carnivores furnish less than 4% of the blood meals of *Glossina* and raw fresh meat forms a negligible part of the human diet in enzootic areas.[77-79]

EPIDEMIOLOGY

The epidemiologies of the two forms of the disease (gambiense and rhodesiense) are sufficiently disparate to be more easily discussed separately but comparatively. What follows is largely based on a relatively recent review,[80] and owes much to the original thought of my friend Dr. M. T. Ashcroft and others.[32,34,81-86] For a more recent discussion see Reference 149.

Gambiense Disease

The chronic nature of this disease in man has been referred to in sections on Etiologic Agents and Disease in Man; presumably related to it is the fact that parasitemias in man and in other, experimentally infected mammals, are low — often undetectable by microscopical examination. Furthermore, both *T. brucei gambiense* and *T. brucei rhodesiense* can infect only a very small percentage of those *Glossina* which ingest them in their blood meal. Even under optimum experimental conditions, in more than 90% of *Glossina* no transmissible infection becomes established in the salivary glands, and under natural conditions it is rare to find more than 0.1% of a population infected — though 4.8% has been reported.[87] This low susceptibility has been related with the development of the insect's peritrophic membrane and the biochemical adaptations to life in the invertebrate vector which the trypanosomes must undergo.[14,88,89] These two facts (low parasitemia in mammals, low susceptibility of the vector) together influence the epidemiology of the disease. Low parasitemia reduces still further the already low probability that the parasite will become established in *Glossina*. Among mammals, human beings are one of the more susceptible species; the levels of parasitemia attained in them, combined with the relatively long period of time for which infected persons survive and, because they are not acutely ill, remain ambulant and therefore available to *Glossina* as a food source, are adequate to ensure transmission to the vector. This is not true of at least most of the other possible mammalian hosts on which *Glossina* commonly feed (mainly ungulates), in which *T. brucei gambiense* often produces only a fleeting, scanty parasitemia. Thus, though such hosts presumably do occasionally become infected, it is generally thought that they cannot maintain the parasite's vertebrate-invertebrate-vertebrate cycle (Figure 3). Thus the disease can usually be maintained only where human beings and tsetse flies come into close, repeated contact, there being no nonhuman reservoir host.[86] However, this view has recently been challenged with the proposition that in some but not all endemic foci there may be a hitherto unidentified nonhuman reservoir of infection (section on Vertebrate

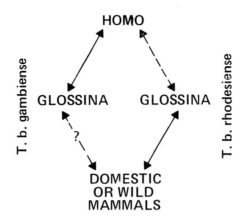

FIGURE 3. Epidemiological cycles of African human trypanosomiasis. Solid lines represent obligatory transmission cycles; broken lines show facultative ones. The query indicates an unproven facultative cycle.

Hosts);[26,147,148] the matter is at present undecided, but at least justifies the inclusion of gambiense sleeping sickness in this chapter as a potential if not actual zoonosis.

Whatever may be the outcome of this debate the disease is usually acquired "peri-domestically," near the victim's home, and therefore all of the family — men, women, and children — are equally at risk. Correlated with this is the fact that the vector species (section on Invertebrate Hosts) are those which include human blood as a major dietary component.[77,78] These species of *Glossina* (the *G. palpalis* group) generally live along forested river banks and in similar moist environments; consequently human infections are commonly acquired near fords or bridges, or at washing or water collection sites. Such sites may be of very limited extent, but at them important foci of infection may develop, with relatively high infection rates among perhaps quite a small resident population of *Glossina;* such foci may be remarkably persistent.[32,90]

Rhodesiense Disease

In contrast to the situation described above for the gambiense disease, nonhuman reservoir hosts of *T. brucei rhodesiense* definitely exist; they play an important part in the epidemiology of the disease (Figure 3), which appears to depend upon such resevoirs for its maintenance. *T. brucei rhodesiense* shares with *T. brucei gambiense* the inability to infect most of its invertebrate vectors, but differs in generally producing relatively high parasitemias in susceptible vertebrate hosts.[85] Thus probably many species of mammal can and do support the parasite under natural conditions, with no need for the intervention of human hosts. The acuteness of the disease in human beings renders them less suitable maintenance hosts, since they are all too soon removed from potential contact with tsetse (which rarely enter houses to feed) by being bedridden or dying. Probably rhodesiense sleeping sickness could not survive without its nonhuman mammalian reservoir hosts, in which the infection is less acute than it is in man but which develop parasitemias adequate to ensure transmission to a sufficient number of feeding *Glossina*. Rhodesiense trypanosomiasis is therefore generally not acquired peri-domestically, but in areas where wild mammals live and support populations of *Glossina*. Species of the *G. morsitans* group can be maintained on wild ungulates and yet will not spurn a meal of human blood when it is available, and therefore constitute the commonest and most important vectors of *T. brucei rhodesiense* (section on Invertebrate Hosts); they inhabit large areas of the East African savannah and usually retreat from areas of human settlement. The main category of persons at high risk of infection with rhodesiense trypanosomiasis is therefore those (usually men) who enter the savannah "bush" to hunt for food (or as tourists in game reserves). Thus, unlike the situation with *T. brucei gambiense,* man is not an obligate, but only a facultative host of the parasite, from whom onward transmission may not occur. Thus infection of man with *T. brucei rhodesiense* may be regarded as adventitious to the parasite's enzootic cycle, and for it to occur "sustained triple contact" between infected ungulates, *Glossina* and human beings must be inserted into the cycle.[70]

As mentioned in the section on Vertebrate Hosts, proven isolates of *T. brucei rhodesiense* have been made from only four species of wild mammals and from domestic oxen: other species may well be hosts but are yet unidentified. The carnivorous host species (hyena and lion) are probably not very important in the epidemiology of the human disease, since being rarely fed upon by *Glossina,* they presumably seldom serve as reservoirs of human infection (section on General Mode of Spread).[77-79] Wild antelope and domestic cattle are certainly important.[91,92]

The distribution of *T. brucei rhodesiense* in wild mammal populations, judged from the distribution of foci of human infection, seems to be less widespread than that of *T. brucei brucei.*[82] This may be explicable by the territorial behavior of the bushbuck (*Tragelaphus scriptus*), a known reservoir host;[18] whether this applies to other antelope reservoirs is not known. Adult bushbuck have limited "home ranges," to which they are more or less restricted, of about 25,000 to 50,000 m²; those of subadult males are larger (about 200,000 m²). Within these ranges the animals often hide in a particular thicket during the daylight.[93,94] Therefore, these animals may support a relatively small and localized population of *Glossina* with — if the bushbuck is infected with *T. brucei rhodesiense* — possibly a relatively high trypanosomal infection rate, forming a local focus of human infection. If human beings enter such a "hot spot," either regularly because bushbuck often live close to human habitations or sporadically while hunting, honey-gathering, or viewing the wildlife in a game park, the chances of their becoming infected may be considerable.[95,96] A comparable situation in schistosomiasis has been described an "an apparent continuum which may be a collection of microfoci."[97]

There are exceptions to this general picture. During epidemics *T. brucei rhodesiense* may be transmitted, like *T. brucei gambiense,* around a direct *Homo-Glossina-Homo* cycle and when this happens tsetse of the *G. palpalis* group (more usually vectors of *T. brucei gambiense*) may become vectors and the epidemiology consequently may change to one more resembling that of the gambiense disease;[98-100] but such situations probably exist for only limited periods of time.[101,102]

Bradley has attempted to classify parasitic infections in terms of their regulatory mechanisms.[97] Both rhodesiense and gambiense trypanosomiasis in man presumably belong to his type 1, "transmission-regulated" infections; *T. brucei rhodesiense* infection in man falls also into type 2, being controlled partly by the death of the human host; in contrast *T. brucei gambiense* in man, like *T. brucei rhodesiense* and *T. brucei brucei* in ungulates, is presumably controlled partly by the host's development of non-sterilizing immunity — type 3.

DIAGNOSIS

In man, as in other mammals, diagnosis of African trypanosomiasis depends ultimately on isolation of the parasites: the clinical condition can be suggestive but never conclusive.[103] Immunodiagnostic methods, a special case of demonstrating the presence of the parasite, will be discussed separately.

Parasitological Methods

In increasing order of complexity, the parasites can be sought by means of microscopical examination of fresh blood preparations, stained thick blood films, concentration from blood, fresh or stained films of lymph gland exudate, cerebrospinal fluid (fresh or stained), laboratory animal inoculation, or cultivation in vitro. Details of these procedures are available elsewhere.[104] More recent methods of concentration include the hematocrit centrifugation of blood,[105,106] separation of trypanosomes from blood cells by adsorption of the latter to diethylaminoethyl (DEAE) cellulose,[107-109,151] and removal of erythrocytes by osmotic lysis before centrifugation.[110]

In acute rhodesiense-type infections of man, parasites can usually be detected in stained thick blood films (more readily than in fresh blood preparations); failing this, and with infections of ungulates and other wild mammals, inoculation of blood to rats or mice is the most sensitive method of detection;[111,112] recourse to in vitro cultivation is seldom necessary. Trypanosomes isolated from nonhuman mammals can be morphologically identified only to the species, and identification as *T. brucei rhodesiense* must depend either on the seldom possible procedure of inoculation to human volunteers,[21] or on the retention of infectivity after controlled incubation in human blood or plasma (the blood incubation infectivity test or BIIT).[22,113-117] *T. brucei gambiense* is less easy to find in circulating blood; exudate obtained by lymph gland puncture is often a more fruitful source. This subspecies' infectivity to laboratory rodents is low; among the more susceptible hosts are Gambian pouched rats (*Cricetomys gambianus*) and suckling (8 to 10 days old) laboratory white rats.[118,119] Inoculation of blood into rabbits' scrota has also been used to isolate *T. brucei gambiense.*[120] Examination of human CSF, a valuable means of determining the progression of the disease or its response to treatment, is less often used as a confirmatory diagnostic technique though in advanced gambiense disease it might be the most likely source of parasites.

Immunodiagnostic Methods

The most widely used in diagnosing both human and nonhuman infections is the indirect fluorescent antibody test (IFAT).[121] It is a very sensitive means of detecting *T. brucei gambiense* infection in human beings,[122,123] and if carefully performed can differentiate, at least to some extent, between the three subspecies of *T. brucei;*[124] it has also been used to survey domestic ruminants.[125]

More recently, an enzyme linked immunosorbent assay (ELISA) has shown promise in detecting human infection with *T. brucei rhodesiense,* using *T. brucei brucei* antigen.[126] Cross-reaction occurred with *T. cruzi,* suggesting that, though the test is probably insufficiently specific to distinguish between *T. brucei rhodesiense* and *T. brucei gambiense,* it might be useful in detecting the latter also; it is suitable for use in mass surveys.

PREVENTION AND CONTROL

Ultimately, prevention and control of African trypanosomiasis depend upon control or elimination of the insect vector (*Glossina*). In the shorter term, they can be attempted in three ways: mass prophylaxis, individual prophylaxis, and treatment. Biological control of the vector has often been proposed but never satisfactorily practiced.[127,128]

Vector Control

This aim has been pursued by hand catching and trapping, vegetation clearing, elimination of the larger mammalian fauna, and use of insecticides.[129-133] All these methods have achieved success, though the first is applicable to only very small scale control.[134] Vegetational clearing, partial or complete, can, when correctly applied, so alter the habitats of *Glossina* that their microclimate becomes inimical to survival. Notable successes in control have been achieved by total clearing, and it is probably the oldest method of attempted control: "the aim is to replace bush or woodland by treeless grassland."[130] It is a drastic method, labor-intensive and therefore becoming increasingly expensive (though the cost can be reduced by using machinery);[135] it can be effective to make available an area of land for human settlement and farming — for which the vegetational clearing is a prerequisite anyway. Subsequent farming maintains the clearance and is a useful adjunct to this and other methods of tsetse control.[134] Partial clearing of vegetation has had its successes, but depends upon skilled local knowledge to decide what vegetation to remove and, because of the lack of this expertise, has had notorious failures too; it is cheaper than total clearing.

The effectiveness in eradicating the tsetse population of destruction of the larger mammalian fauna was first demonstrated by a natural experiment — the rinderpest panzootic in Rhodesia in 1895—6,[131] and it has subsequently been deliberately practiced mainly in that country. It is an ecologically drastic measure (as is total vegetational clearing), and in these (rightly) conservation-minded days, an unpopular one. Increased knowledge of the food preferences of *Glossina*[77,78] may permit more discriminative applications of this technique.

The use of insecticides is the commonest control measure at present, though this too has its dangers (both ecological and toxicological) and can be expensive. Local applications can be made from portable "knapsack" sprayers, or when the target is a riverine species such as *G. palpalis*, from a sprayer carried in a small boat. Larger scale application, for example in the East African savannah, is usually made from a light aeroplane.[133] The earliest compounds to be used in this way were dichlorodiphenyl trichloroethane (DDT) and benzene hexachloride (BHC). Subsequently dieldrin (hexachloro-epoxyoctohydro-dimethanonaphthalene) and a few organochlorine compounds have been used. An everpresent threat is the development of insecticide resistance by *Glossina*, but so far this seems to have been more hypothetical than actual.[132]

Any form of vector control should, ideally, be followed by human settlement of the reclaimed area since this consolidates the achievement by discouraging reinvasion by *Glossina*. With adequate medical and veterinary surveillance, settlement can safely occur before complete elimination of the vector has been achieved and this can result in considerably reduced costs.[134] Ford has written, "Much of the difficulty in effecting control of tsetse populations is logistic,"[136] and the whole problem of integrating trypanosomiasis control and land-use in the total ecology of Africa has been fully considered by the same author elsewhere.[84]

Mass Prophylaxis

In areas of gambiense trypanosomiasis where there is no, or only an unimportant, nonhuman reservoir of infection, treatment of the entire population with a prophylactic drug will reduce the prevalence of the infection and abolish parasitemia in those already infected; this results in a drastic reduction in transmission to the vector and, hence, a drastic reduction in incidence in the human population. There is no doubt the method is effective in terms of overall infection rates, and it was widely applied in the erstwhile Belgian Congo (now Zaire) under the colonial regime. However, at the personal level, there is the risk of suppression of a patent early infection and consequent failure to diagnose the disease until after involvement of the CNS, when treatment is much more difficult. In areas of rhodesiense infection the presence of reservoir hosts negates the procedure's main value and it was never adopted. The element of personal risk has now led to its general disfavor in all areas. The drug used was pentamidine [1,5-di(4-amidinophenoxy)pentane di(2-hydroxymethane-sulphonate)], either the isethionate or dimethylsulphonate ("Lomidine") salt usually being given intramuscularly at 4 mg/kg (maximum dose 300 mg) every 6 months.[137]

Table 3
SUMMARIZED TREATMENT SCHEDULES FOR AFRICAN HUMAN TRYPANOSOMIASIS[140]

Drug	Presentation	Administration	Schedule[a]
Suramin	10% w/v aqueous solution, freshly made	Intravenous	Test dose 0.2 g; then 5 doses, 1 g each, at intervals of 5—7 days
Melarsoprol	3.6% w/v solution in propylene glycol	Intravenous	Day 1, 0.5 m*l*; days 3 and 5, 1.0 m*l* each; 5—7 day rest period; 2.5 m*l* daily for 3 days; 7 day rest period; 3.0—5.0 m*l* daily for 3 days; 7 day rest period; 5.0 m*l* daily for 3 days.

[a]   Schedule given is for adults of average weight; melarsoprol dosage should be adjusted if patient's condition deteriorates; see Reference 140 for details of treatment of children and undernourished adults, and for necessary precautions, etc.

From Apted, F.I.C., in *The African Trypanosomiases*, Mulligan, H. W., Ed., George Allen and Unwin Ltd., London, 1974, 684. With permission.

Individual Prophylaxis

Generally, because of the risk of suppression mentioned above, chemoprophylaxis on an individual basis is not recommended though pentamidine is sometimes so used in areas of gambiense trypanosomiasis.[137] The only other available method of personal prophylaxis is avoidance of the bite of potentially infective tsetse; except by not entering endemic or enzootic areas, this is not easy to achieve, though the use of insect repellents and adequate clothing covering arms and legs can reduce the frequency of biting (*Glossina* can probe through thin cloth). The infection rate of *Glossina* is usually so low that, statistically, the risk of infection is not great in persons only briefly exposed. It is important to consider the possibility of trypanosomiasis if an illness develops after visiting an infected area, and to make sure that a doctor is consulted and made aware of this possibility.

Chemoprophylaxis is commonly used among herds of domestic cattle and sheep, using isometamidium chloride at 0.5 to 1.0 mg/kg, quinapyramine prophylactic, or pyrithidium bromide.[138,139] Drug-resistance may become a problem during continued chemoprophylaxis.[139]

Treatment

Early infections of both *T. brucei rhodesiense* and *T. brucei gambiense* in man are usually treated with suramin, with cure rates approaching 100%; for the latter subspecies, pentamidine is sometimes used but has no advantage. Advanced sleeping sickness is treated with melarsoprol, 2-*p*-(4,6-diamino-1,3,5-triazin-2-ylamino) phenyl-4-hydroxymethyl-1,3,2-dithiarsolan. Melarsoprol is toxic and must be given under careful supervision. It gives cure rates of only about 50 to 70%, but no other available compound approaches it for efficiency.[140] Treatment schedules are summarized in Table 3.[140]

Domestic animals infected with *T. brucei* sspp. are usually treated with quinapyramine sulphate (one dose of 4.4 mg/kg subcutaneously) or suramin (7 to 10 mg/kg, two doses 1 week apart).[139,141] Diminazene aceturate, which is widely used in treating cattle and sheep infected with *T. congolense* or *T. vivax* (more serious pathogens in these animals than *T. brucei*), is effective also (though perhaps slightly less so) against *T. brucei* (5 mg/kg, single intramuscular dose).[139] This compound is equally effective against early human infections with *T. brucei rhodesiense,* but toxicological doubts at present inhibit its widespread use.[142,143]

The chemotherapeutic outlook for human and nonhuman African trypanosomiasis is bleak, since no effective drug has been introduced into general use for over 20 years and the commercial production of some of those in use (e.g., suramin) is being increasingly limited.[144]

Note: This manuscript was submitted December, 1976.

REFERENCES

1. **Hoare, C. A.,** *The Trypanosomes of Mammals,* Blackwell Scientific, Oxford, 1972, 512.
2. **Kudo, R. R.,** *Protozoology,* 5th ed., Charles C Thomas, Springfield, Ill., 1966, 410.
3. **Baker, J. R.,** *Parasitic Protozoa,* 2nd ed., Hutchinson, London, 1975, 58.
4. **Böhringer, S. and Hecker, H.,** Quantitative ultrastructural investigations of the life cycle of *Trypanosoma brucei:* a morphometric analysis, *J. Protozool.,* 22, 463, 1975.
5. **Vickerman, K.,** Morphological and physiological considerations of extracellular blood protozoa, in *Ecology and Physiology of Parasites,* Fallis, A. M., Ed., University of Toronto Press, 1971, 58.
6. **Vickerman, K. and Preston, T. M.,** Comparative cell biology of the kinetoplastid flagellates, in *Biology of the Kinetoplastida,* Vol. 1, Lumsden, W. H. R. and Evans, D. A., Eds., Academic Press, London, 1976, 35.
7. **Bowman, I. B. R. and Flynn, I. W.,** Oxidative metabolism of trypanosomes, in *Biology of the Kinetoplastida,* Vol. 1, Lumsden, W. H. R. and Evans, D. A., Eds., Academic Press, London, 1976, 435.
8. **Newton, B. A.,** Biochemical approaches to the taxonomy of kinetoplastid flagellates, in *Biology of the Kinetoplastida,* Vol. 1, Lumsden, W. H. R. and Evans, D. A., Eds., Academic Pess, London, 1976, 405.
9. **Godfrey, D. G. and Kilgour, V.,** Enzyme electrophoresis in characterizing the causative organism of Gambian trypanosomiasis, *Trans. R. Soc. Trop. Med. Hyg.,* 70, 219, 1976.
10. **Le Ray, D., Afchain, D., Jadin, J. B., Capron, A., and Famerée, L.,** Interrelations immuno-taxonomiques de *T. brucei, T. rhodesiense* et *T. gambiense, Ann. Parasitol. Hum. Comp.,* 46, 523, 1971.
11. **Patif, B. M. A. and Adam, K. M. G.,** Differentiation of *Trypanosoma brucei, T. rhodesiense,* and *T. gambiense* by the indirect fluorescent antibody test, *Bull. WHO,* 48, 401, 1973.
12. **Ormerod, W. E. and Venkatesan, S.,** The occult visceral phase of mammalian trypanosomes with special reference to the life cycle of *Trypanosoma (Trypanozoon) brucei, Trans. R. Soc. Trop. Med. Hyg.,* 65, 722, 1971.
13. **Ormerod, W. E. and Venkatesan, S.,** An amastigote phase of the sleeping sickness trypanosome, *Trans. R. Soc. Trop. Med. Hyg.,* 65, 737, 1971.
14. **Harmsen, R.,** The nature of the establishment barrier for *Trypanosoma brucei* in the gut of *Glossina pallidipes, Trans. R. Soc. Trop. Med. Hyg.,* 67, 364, 1973.
15. **Freeman, J. C.,** The penetration of the peritrophic membrane of the tsetse flies by trypanosomes, *Acta Trop.,* 30, 347, 1975.
16. **Evans, D. A. and Ellis, D. S.,** Penetration of midgut cells of *Glossina morsitans morsitans* by *Trypanosoma brucei rhodesiense, Nature, London,* 258, 231, 1975.
17. **Steiger, R. F.,** On the ultrastructure of *Trypanosoma (Trypanozoon) brucei* in the course of its life cycle and some related aspects, *Acta Trop.,* 30, 64, 1973.
18. **Heisch, R. B., McMahon, J. P., and Manson-Bahr, P. E. C.,** The isolation of *Trypanosoma rhodesiense* from a bushbuck, *Br. Med. J.,* 2, 1203, 1958.
19. **Geigy, R., Kauffmann, M., Mayende, J. S. P., Mwambu, P. M., and Onyango, R. J.,** Isolation of *Trypanosoma (Trypanozoon) rhodesiense* from game and domestic animals in Musoma district, Tanzania, *Acta Trop.,* 30, 49, 1973.
20. **Geigy, R., Jenni, L., Kauffmann, M., Onyango, R. J., and Weiss, N.,** Identification of *T. brucei*-subgroup strains isolated from game, *Acta Trop.,* 32, 190, 1975.
21. **Onyango, R. J., van Hoeve, K., and de Raadt, P.,** The epidemiology of *Trypanosoma rhodesiense* sleeping sickness in Alego Location, Central Nyanza, Kenya. I. Evidence that cattle may act as reservoir hosts of trypanosomes infective to man, *Trans. R. Soc. Trop. Med. Hyg.,* 60, 175, 1966.
22. **Rickman, L. R. and Robson, J.,** The testing of proven *Trypanosoma brucei* and *T. rhodesiense* strains by the blood incubation infectivity test, *Bull. WHO,* 42, 911, 1970.

23. Geigy, R., Mwambu, P. M., and Onyango, R. J., Additional animal reservoirs of *T. rhodesiense* sleeping sickness, *Acta Trop.*, 29, 199, 1972.

24. Ashcroft, M. T., The importance of African wild animals as reservoirs of trypanosomiasis, *E. Afr. Med. J.*, 36, 289, 1959.

25. Baker, J. R., Trypanosomes of wild mammals in the neighbourhood of the Serengeti National Park, *Symp. Zool. Soc. London*, 24, 147, 1969.

26. Molyneux, D. H., Animal reservoirs and Gambian trypanosomiasis, *Ann. Soc. Belg. Med. Trop.*, 53, 605, 1973.

27. Denecke, K., Menschenpathogene Trypanosomen des Hundes auf Fernando Poo. Ein Beitrag zur Epidemiologie der Schlafkrankheit, *Arch. Hyg. Bakteriol.*, 126, 38, 1941.

28. van Hoof, L. M. J. J., Observations on trypanosomiasis in the Belgian Congo, *Trans. R. Soc. Trop. Med. Hyg.*, 40, 728, 1947.

29. Molyneux, D. H., Observations on naturally occurring mammals as reservoir hosts of *Trypanosoma brucei gambiense*, Proc. 13th Meet. of Int. Sci. Committee Trypanosomiasis Res. Lagos, 1971, 81.

30. Buxton, P. A., *The Natural History of Tsetse Flies*, H. K. Lewis, London, 1955, 10.

31. Potts, W. H., Systematics and identification of *Glossina*, in *The African Trypanosomiases*, Mulligan, H. W., Ed., George Allen and Unwin Ltd., London, 1970, 243.

32. Scott, D., The epidemiology of Gambian sleeping sickness, in *The African Trypanosomiases*, Mulligan, H. W., Ed., George Allen and Unwin Ltd., London, 1970, 614.

33. Nash, T. A. M., The ecology of the West African riverine species of tsetse in relation to man-fly contact, in *The African Trypanosomiases*, Mulligan, H. W., Ed., George Allen and Unwin Ltd., London, 1970, 602.

34. Apted, F. I. C., The epidemiology of Rhodesian sleeping sickness, in *The African Trypanosomiases*, Mulligan, H. W., Ed., George Allen and Unwin Ltd. London, 1970, 645.

35. McConnell, E., Hutchinson, M. P., and Baker, J. R., Human trypanosomiasis in Ethiopia: the Gilo river area, *Trans. R. Soc. Trop. Med. Hyg.*, 64, 683, 1970.

36. *Weekly Epidemiol. Rec.* 4, 22, January 23, 1976.

37. Stephen, L. E., Clinical manifestation of the trypanosomiases in livestock and other domestic animals, in *The African Trypanosomiases*, Mulligan, H. W., Ed., George Allen and Unwin Ltd., London, 1970, 774.

38. Yesufu, H. M., Experimental transmission of *Trypanosoma gambiense* to domestic animals, *Ann. Trop. Med. Parasitol.*, 65, 341, 1971.

39. Stephen, L. E., *Pig Trypanosomiasis in Africa*, Commonwealth Agricultural Bureaux, Farnham Royal, England, 1966, 46, 57.

40. Losos, G. J. and Ikede, B. O., Review of pathology of diseases in domestic and laboratory animals caused by *Trypanosoma congolense*, *T. vivax*, *T. brucei*, *T. rhodesiense* and T. gambiense, Vet. Pathol., 9(Suppl.), 23, 1972.

41. Neitz, W. O. and McCully, R. M., Clinicopathological study on experimental *Trypanosoma brucei* infections in horses. I. Development of clinically recognizable nervous symptoms in nagana-infected horses treated with subcurative doses of Antrypol and Berenil, *Onderstepoort J. Vet. Res.*, 38, 127, 1971.

42. McCully, R. M. and Neitz, W. O., Clinicopathological study on experimental *Trypanosoma brucei* infections in horses. II. Histopathological findings in the nervous system and other organs of treated and untreated horses reacting to nagana, *Onderstepoort J. Vet. Res.*, 38, 141, 1971.

43. Ikede, B. O. and Losos, G. J., Spontaneous canine trypanosomiasis caused by *T. brucei*: meningo-encephalomyelitis with extra-vascular localization of trypanosomes in the brain, *Bull. Epizoot. Dis. Afr.*, 20, 221, 1972.

44. Goodwin, L. G., The pathology of African trypanosomiasis, *Trans. R. Soc. Trop. Med. Hyg.*, 64, 797, 1970.

45. Ashcroft, M. T., Burtt, E., and Fairbairn, H., The experimental infection of some African wild animals with *Trypanosoma rhodesiense*, *T. brucei* and *T. congolense*, *Ann. Trop. Med. Parasitol.*, 53, 147, 1959.

46. Godfrey, D. G. and Killick-Kendrick, R., Cyclically transmitted infections of *Trypanosoma brucei*, *T. rhodesiense* and *T. gambiense* in chimpanzees, *Trans. R. Soc. Trop. Med. Hyg.*, 61, 781, 1967.

47. Baker, J. R. and Taylor, A. E. R., Experimental infections of the chimpanzee (*Pan troglodytes*) with *Trypanosoma brucei brucei* and *Trypanosoma brucei rhodesiense*, *Ann. Trop. Med. Parasitol.*, 65, 471, 1971.

48. Mortelmans, J. and Kageruka, P., Experimental *Trypanosoma brucei* infection in lions, *Acta Trop.*, 28, 329, 1971.

49. Sachs, R., Schaller G. B., and Baker, J. R., Isolation of trypanosomes of the *T. brucei* group from lion, *Acta Trop.*, 24, 109, 1967.

50. McCulloch, B., Trypanosomes of the brucei subgroup as a probable cause of disease in wild zebra (*Equus burchelli*), *Ann. Trop. Med. Parasitol.*, 61, 261, 1967.

51. **Losos, G. J. and Gwamaka, G.**, Histological examination of wild animals naturally infected with pathogenic African trypanosomes, *Acta Trop.*, 50, 57, 1973.

52. **Ormerod, W. E.**, Pathogenesis and pathology of trypanosomiasis in man, in *The African Trypanosomiases*, Mulligan, H. W., Ed., George Allen and Unwin Ltd., London, 1970, 587.

53. **Fairbairn, H. and Godfrey, D. G.**, The local reaction in man at the site of infection with *Trypanosoma rhodesiense*, *Ann. Trop. Med. Parasitol.*, 51, 464, 1957.

54. **de Raadt, P.**, Immunity and antigenic variation: clinical observations suggestive of immune phenomena in African trypanosomiasis, in *Trypanosomiasis and Leishmaniasis, with Special Reference to Chagas' Disease*, Elliott, K., O'Connor, M., and Wolstenholme, G. E. W., Eds., Associated Scientific Publishers, Amsterdam, 1974, 199.

55. **Goodwin, L. G.**, The African scene: mechanisms of pathogenesis in trypanosomiasis, in *Trypanosomiasis and Leishmaniasis, with Special Reference to Chagas' Disease*, Elliott, K., O'Connor, M., and Wolstenholme, G. E. W., Eds., Associated Scientific Publishers, Amsterdam, 1974, 107.

56. **Boreham, P. F. L.**, Kinin release and the immune reaction in human trypanosomiasis caused by *Trypanosoma rhodesiense*, *Trans. R. Soc. Trop. Med. Hyg.*, 64, 394, 1970.

57. **Bowman, I. B. R. and Flynn, I. W.**, Oxidative metabolism of trypanosomes, in *Biology of the Kinetoplastida*, Vol. 1, Lumsden, W. H. R. and Evans, D. A., Eds., Academic Press, London, 1976, 435.

58. **Cross, G. A. M.**, Identification, purification and properties of clone-specific glycoprotein antigens constituting the surface coat of *Trypanosoma brucei*, *Parasitology*, 71, 393, 1975.

59. **Vickerman, K.**, Antigenic variation in African trypanosomes, in *Parasites in the Immunized Host: Mechanisms of Survival*, Porter, R. and Knight, J., Eds., Associated Scientific Publishers, Amsterdam, 1974, 53.

60. **Gray, A. R. and Luckins, A. G.**, Antigenic variation in salivarian trypanosomes, in *Biology of the Kinetoplastida*, Vol. 1, Lumsden, W. H. R. and Evans, D. A., Eds., Academic Press, London, 1976, 493.

61. **Murray, P. K., Jennings, F. W., Murray, M. and Urquhart, G. M.**, Immunosuppression in trypanosomiasis, in *Parasitic Zoonoses: Clinical and Experimental Studies*, Soulsby, E. J. L., Ed., Academic Press, New York, 1974, 133.

62. **Schwab, J. H.**, Suppression of the immune response by microorganisms, *Bacteriol. Rev.*, 39, 121, 1975.

63. **Terry, R. J. and Smithers, S. R.**, Evasion of the immune response by parasites, *Symp. Soc. Exp. Biol.*, 29, 453, 1975.

64. **Ogilvie, B. M. and Wilson, R. J. M.**, Evasion of the immune response by parasites, *Br. Med. Bull.*, 32, 177, 1976.

65. **Robertson, D. H. H.**, Chemotherapy of African trypanosomiasis, *Practitioner*, 188, 80, 1962.

66. **Burns, R. B.**, Plasma cells in the avian Harderian gland and the morphology of the gland in the rook, *Can. J. Zool.*, 53, 1258, 1975.

67. **Russell, W.**, An address on a characteristic organism of cancer, *Br. Med. J.*, 2, 1356, 1890.

68. **Christy, C.**, The cerebro-spinal fluid in sleeping sickness (trypanosomiasis). 104 lumbar punctures, *Liverpool School Trop. Med. Memoirs*, 13, 57, 1904; reprinted in *Thomson Yates and Johnston Laboratories Reports*, 6, 57, 1905.

69. **Mott, F. W.**, Histological observations on sleeping sickness and other trypanosome infections, *Rep. Sleeping Sickness Comm. R. Soc.*, 7, 3, 1906.

70. **Apted, F. I. C., Ormerod, W. E., Smyly, D. P., Stronach, B. W., and Szlamp, E. L.**, A comparative study of the epidemiology of endemic Rhodesian sleeping sickness in different parts of Africa, *J. Trop. Med. Hyg.*, 66, 1, 1963.

71. **Blair, D. M., Smith, E. B., and Gelfand, M.**, Human trypanosomiasis in Rhodesia: a new hypothesis suggested for the rarity of human trypanosomiasis, *Cent. Afr. J. Med.*, 14 (Suppl.), 1, 1968.

72. **Duke, H. L., Mettam, R. W. M., and Wallace, J. M.**, Observations on the direct passage from vertebrate to vertebrate of recently isolated strains of *Trypanosoma brucei* and *Trypanosoma rhodesiense*, *Trans. R. Soc. Trop. Med. Hyg.*, 28, 77, 1934.

73. **Heisch, R. B.**, Presence of trypanosomes in bush babies after eating infected rats, *Nature, London*, 169, 118, 1963.

74. **Sachs, R., Schaller, G. B., and Schindler, R.**, Untersuchungen uber das Vorkommen von Trypanosomen bei Wildkarnivoren des Serengeti-Nationalparks in Tanzania, *Acta Trop.*, 28, 323, 1971.

75. **Bertram, B. C. R.**, Sleeping sickness survey in the Serengeti area (Tanzania) 1971. III. Discussion of the relevance of the trypanosome survey to the biology of large mammals in the Serengeti, *Acta Trop.*, 30, 36, 1973.

76. **Moloo, S. K., Losos, G. J., and Kutuza, S. B.**, Transmission of *Trypanosoma brucei* to cats and dogs by feeding on infected goats, *Trans. R. Soc. Trop. Med. Hyg.*, 67, 287, 1973.

77. **Weitz, B.**, The feeding habits of *Glossina*, *Bull. WHO*, 28, 711, 1963.

78. **Weitz, B. G. F.**, Hosts of *Glossina*, in *The African Trypanosomiases*, Mulligan, H. W., Ed., George Allen and Unwin Ltd., London, 1970, 317.
79. **Moloo, S. K., Steiger, R. F., Brun, R., and Boreham, P. F. L.**, Sleeping sickness survey in Musoma district, Tanzania. II. The role of *Glossina* in the transmission of sleeping sickness, *Acta Trop.*, 28, 189, 1971.
80. **Baker, J. R.**, Epidemiology of African sleeping sickness, in *Trypanosomiasis and Leishmaniasis, with Special Reference to Chagas' Disease*, Elliott, K., O'Connor, M., and Wolstenholme, G. E. W., Eds., Associated Scientific Publishers, Amsterdam, 1974, 29.
81. **Ashcroft, M. T.**, A critical review of the epidemiology of sleeping sickness, *Trop. Dis. Bull.*, 56, 1073, 1959.
82. **Ashcroft, M. T.**, Some biological aspects of the epidemiology of sleeping sickness, *J. Trop. Med. Hyg.*, 66, 133, 1963.
83. **Onyango, R. J.**, New concepts in the epidemiology of Rhodesian sleeping sickness, *Bull. WHO*, 41, 815, 1969.
84. **Ford, J.**, *The Role of the Trypanosomiases in African Ecology*, Clarendon Press, Oxford, 1971.
85. **Soltys, M. A.**, Epidemiology of trypanosomiasis in man, *Tropenmed. Parasitol.*, 22, 120, 1971.
86. **Willett, K. C.**, Some principles of the epidemiology of human trypanosomiasis in Africa, *Bull. WHO*, 28, 645, 1963.
87. **Rogers, A., Kenyanjui, E. N., and Wiggwah, A. K.**, A high infection rate of *Trypanosoma brucei* subgroup in *Glossina fuscipes*, *Parasitology*, 65, 143, 1972.
88. **Willett, K. C.**, Development of the peritrophic membrane in *Glossina* (tsetse flies) and its relation to infection with trypanosomes, *Exp. Parasitol.*, 18, 290, 1966.
89. **Baker, J. R.**, Development of salivarian trypanosomes in the insect vector, in *Les Moyennes de Lutte contre les Trypanosomes et leurs Vecteurs*, supplement to *Revue d'Elévage et de Médecine Vétérinaire des Pays Tropicaux*, Office international des Epizooties, Paris, 1974, 143.
90. **Duggan, A. J.**, An historical perspective, in *The African Trypanosomiases*, Mulligan, H. W., Ed., George Allen and Unwin Ltd., London, 1970, xli.
91. **Wijers, D. J. B.**, The complex epidemiology of Rhodesian sleeping sickness in Kenya and Uganda. III. The epidemiology in the endemic areas along the lake shore between the Nile and the Yala swamp, *Trop. Geogr. Med.*, 26, 307, 1974.
92. **Wijers, D. J. B.**, The complex epidemiology of Rhodesian sleeping sickness in Kenya and Uganda. IV. Alego and the other [G]. *fuscipes* areas north of the endemic belt, *Trop. Geogr. Med.*, 26, 341, 1974.
93. **Allsopp, R.**, *The Population Dynamics and Social Biology of Bushbuck (Tragelaphus scriptus Pallas)*, M.Sc. thesis, University of East Africa, Nairobi, Kenya, 1970.
94. **Allsopp, R.**, personal communication.
95. **Allsopp, R.**, The role of game animals in the maintenance of endemic and enzootic trypanosomiases in the Lambwe valley, South Nyanza district, Kenya, *Bull. WHO*, 47, 735, 1972.
96. **Allsopp, R., Baldry, D. A. T., and Rodrigues, C.**, The influence of game animals on the distribution and feeding habits of *Glossina pallidipes* in the Lambwe valley, *Bull. WHO*, 47, 795, 1972.
97. **Bradley, D. J.**, Regulation of parasite populations. A general theory of the epidemiology and control of parasitic infections, *Trans. R. Soc. Trop. Med. Hyg.*, 66, 697, 1972.
98. **Willett, K. C.**, Some observations on the recent epidemiology of sleeping sickness in Nyanza region, Kenya, and its relation to the general epidemiology of Gambian and Rhodesian sleeping sickness in Africa, *Trans. R. Soc. Trop. Med. Hyg.*, 59, 374, 1965.
99. **McConnell, E. and Baker, J. R.**, Human trypanosomiasis in Ethiopia, *Ethiopian Med. J.*, 12, 157, 1975.
100. **Hutchinson, M. P.**, Human trypanosomiasis in Ethiopia, *Ethiopian Med. J.*, 9, 3, 1971.
101. **Wijers, D. J. B.**, The complex epidemiology of Rhodesian sleeping sickness in Kenya and Uganda. I. The absence of the disease on Mfangano island (Kenya), *Trop. Geogr. Med.*, 26, 58, 1974.
102. **Wijers, D. J. B.**, The complex epidemiology of Rhodesian sleeping sickness in Kenya and Uganda. II. Observations in Samia (Kenya), *Trop. Geogr. Med.*, 26, 182, 1974.
103. **Apted, F. I. C.**, Clinical manifestations and diagnosis of sleeping sickness, in *The African Trypanosomiases*, Mulligan, H. W., Ed., George Allen and Unwin Ltd., London, 1970, 661.
104. **Baker, J. R.**, Techniques for the detection of trypanosome infections, in *The African Trypanosomiases*, Mulligan, H. W., Ed., George Allen and Unwin Ltd., London, 1970, 67.
105. **Bennett, G. F.**, The haematocrit centrifuge for laboratory diagnosis of haematozoa, *Can. J. Zool.*, 40, 124, 1962.
106. **Woo, P. T. K.**, Evaluation of the haematocrit centrifuge and other techniques for the field diagnosis of human trypanosomiasis and filariasis, *Acta Trop.*, 28, 298, 1971.
107. **Lanham, S. M.**, Separation of trypanosomes from the blood of infected rats and mice by anion-exchanger, *Nature, London*, 218, 1273, 1968.

108. **Lanham, S. M. and Godfrey, D. G.**, Isolation of salivarian trypanosomes from man and other mammals using DEAE-cellulose, *Exp. Parasitol.*, 28, 521, 1970.

109. **Lanham, S. M., Williams, J. E., and Godfrey, D. G.**, Detection of low concentrations of trypanosomes in blood by column-separation and membrane-filtration, *Trans. R. Soc. Trop. Med. Hyg.*, 66, 624, 1972.

110. **Leeflang, P., Blotkamp, C., Godfrey, D. G., and Kilgour, V.**, A convenient hypotonic lysis method for concentrating trypanosomes from infected blood, *Trans. R. Soc. Trop. Med. Hyg.*, 68, 412, 1974.

111. **Killick-Kendrick, R.**, The diagnosis of trypanosomiasis of livestock; a review of current techniques, *Vet. Rec.*, 58, 191, 1968.

112. **Robson, J. and Ashkar, T. S.**, The efficiency of different diagnostic methods in animal trypanosomiasis; based on surveys carried out in Nyanza province, Kenya, *Bull. Epizoot. Dis. Afr.*, 20, 303, 1972.

113. **Rickman, L. R. and Robson, J.**, The blood incubation infectivity test: a simple test which may serve to distinguish *Trypanosoma brucei* from *T. rhodesiense, Bull. WHO,* 42, 650, 1970.

114. **Rickman, L. R.**, An evaluation of the blood incubation infectivity test (BIIT) as a method for differentiating *Trypanosoma brucei* from *T. rhodesiense,* OAU STRC Publ. No. 105 Proc. 15th Meet. Int. *Sci. Committee Trypanosomiasis Res. Lagos,* 1971.

115. **Rickman, L. R. and Robson, J.**, Some supplementary observations on the blood incubation infectivity test, *Bull. WHO,* 46, 403, 1972.

116. **Targett, G. A. T. and Wilson, V. C. L. C.**, The blood incubation infectivity test as a means of distinguishing between *Trypanosoma brucei brucei* and *T. brucei rhodesiense, Int. J. Parasitol.,* 3, 5, 1973.

117. **Hawking, F.**, The differentiation of *Trypanosoma rhodesiense* from *T. Brucei* by means of human serum, *Trans. R. Soc. Trop. Med. Hyg.,* 67, 517, 1973.

118. **Larivière, M.**, Réceptivité du *Cricetomys gambianus* (rat de Gambie) au *Trypanosoma gambiense, C. R. Séances Soc. Biol.,* 151, 1349, 1957.

119. **Gray, A. R.**, Variable agglutinogenic antigens of *Trypanosoma gambiense* and their distribution among isolates of the trypanosome collected in different places in Nigeria, *Trans. R. Soc. Trop. Med. Hyg.,* 66, 263, 1972.

120. **Molyneux, D. H.**, Isolation of *Trypanosoma (Trypanozoon) brucei gambiense* in rabbits by the intratesticular inoculation technique, *Ann. Trop. Med. Parasitol.,* 67, 391, 1973.

121. **Molyneux, D. H.**, Diagnostic methods in animal trypanosomiasis, *Vet. Parasitol.,* 1, 5, 1975.

122. **Wéry, M., Wéry-Paskoff, S., and van Wettere, P.**, The diagnosis of human African trypanosomiasis (*T. gambiense*) by the use of [the] fluorescent antibody test. I. Standardization of an easy technique to be used in mass surveys, *Ann. Soc. Belg. Méd. Trop.,* 50, 613, 1970.

123. **Wéry, M., van Wettere, P., Wéry-Paskoff, S., van Meirvenne, N., and Mesatewa, M.**, The diagnosis of human African trypanosomiasis (*T. gambiense*) by the use of the fluorescent antibody test. II. First results of field application, *Ann. Soc. Belg. Méd. Trop.,* 50, 711, 1970.

124. **Latif, M. and Adam, K. M. G.**, Differentiation of *Trypanosoma brucei, T. rhodesiense* and *T. gambiense* by the indirect fluorescent antibody test, *Bull. WHO,* 48, 401, 1975.

125. **Zwart, D., Perie, N. M., Keppler, A., and Goedbloed, E.**, A comparison of methods for the diagnosis of trypanosomiasis in East African domestic ruminants, *Trop. Anim. Health Prod.,* 5, 79, 1973.

126. **Voller, A., Bidwell, D., and Bartlett, A.**, A serological study on human *Trypanosoma rhodesiense* infections using a micro-scale enzyme linked immunosorbent assay, *Tropenmed. Parasitol.,* 26, 247, 1975.

127. **Nash, T. A. M.**, Control by parasites and predators of *Glossina,* in *The African Trypanosomiases,* Mulligan, H. W., Ed., George Allen and Unwin Ltd., London, 1970, 521.

128. **Dame, D. A.**, Control by sterilization of *Glossina,* in *The African Trypanosomiases,* Mulligan, H. W., Ed., George Allen and Unwin Ltd., London, 1970, 533.

129. **Glasgow, J. P. and Potts, W. H.**, Control by hand-catching and traps, in *The African Trypanosomiases,* Mulligan, H. W., Ed., George Allen and Unwin Ltd., London, 1970, 456.

130. **Ford, J., Nash, T. A. M., and Welch, J. R.**, Control by clearing of vegetation, in *The African Trypanosomiases,* Mulligan, H. W., Ed., George Allen and Unwin Ltd., London, 1970, 543.

131. **Ford, J.**, Control by destruction of the larger fauna, in *The African Trypanosomiases,* Mulligan, H. W., Ed., George Allen and Unwin Ltd., London, 1970, 557.

132. **Burnett, G. F.**, Control by insecticides: general considerations, in *The African Trypanosomiases,* Mulligan, H. W., Ed., George Allen and Unwin Ltd., London, 1970, 464.

133. **Burnett, G. F.**, Control by insecticides (continued): residual deposits, aerial and ground application, pyrethrum aerosols, in *The African Trypanosomiases,* Mulligan, H. W., Ed., George Allen and Unwin Ltd., London, 1970, 490.

134. **Potts, W. H.**, An appraisal of methods for the control of *Glossina,* in *The African Trypanosomiases,* Mulligan, H. W., Ed., George Allen and Unwin Ltd., London, 1970, 564.

135. **Willett, K. C.**, Administrative and organizational aspects of control progammes, in *The African Trypanosomiases,* Mulligan, H. W., Ed., George Allen and Unwin Ltd., London, 1970, 572.

136. **Ford, J.**, Introduction to control measures, in *The African Trypanosomiases,* Mulligan, H. W., Ed., George Allen and Unwin Ltd., London, 1970, 453.

137. **Waddy, B. B.**, Chemoprophylaxis of human trypanosomiasis, in *The African Trypanosomiases,* Mulligan, H. W., Ed., George Allen and Unwin, Ltd., London, 1970, 711.

138. **Maclennan, K. J. R.**, Practical application of measures for the control of tsetse-borne trypanosomiases of livestock, in *The African Trypanosomiases,* Mulligan, H. W., Ed., George Allen and Unwin Ltd., London, 1970, 799.

139. **Williamson, J.**, Review of chemotherapeutic and chemoprophylactic agents, in *The African Trypanosomiases,* Mulligan, H. W., Ed., George Allen and Unwin Ltd., London, 1970, 125.

140. **Apted, F. I. C.**, Treatment of human trypanosomiasis, in *The African Trypanosomiases,* Mulligan, H. W., Ed., George Allen and Unwin Ltd., London, 1970, 684.

141. **Stephen, L. E.**, Care and treatment of animals suffering from trypanosomiases, in *The African Trypanosomiases,* Mulligan, H. W., Ed., George Allen and Unwin Ltd., London, 1970, 795.

142. **Temu, S. E.**, Summary of cases of human early trypanosomiasis treated with Berenil at E.A.T.R.O., *Trans. R. Soc. Trop. Med. Hyg.,* 69, 277, 1975.

143. East African Trypanosomiasis Research Organization, The treatment of early human trypanosomiasis cases with Berenil, *Trans. R. Soc. Trop. Med. Hyg.,* 69, 278, 1975.

144. **Williamson, J.**, Chemotherapy of African trypanosomiasis, *Trop. Dis. Bull.,* 73, 531, 1976.

145. **Cross, G. A. M.**, Antigenic variation in trypanosomes, *Am. J. Trop. Med. Hyg.,* 26, 240, 1977.

146. **Anon.**, Antigenic variation in African trypanosomiasis: a memorandum, *Bull. WHO,* 55, 703, 1977.

147. **Mehlitz, D.**, The behaviour in the blood incubation infectivity test of four *Trypanozoon* strains isolated from pigs in Liberia, *Trans. R. Soc. Trop. Med. Hyg.,* 71, 86, 1977.

148. **Gibson, W., Mehlitz, D., Lanham, S. W., and Godfrey, D. G.**, The identification of *Trypanosoma brucei gambiense* in Liberian pigs and dogs by isoenzymes and by resistance to human plasma, *Tropenmed. Parasitol.,* 29, 335, 1978.

149. **Gibson, W. C., Marshall, T. F. de C., and Godfrey, D. G.**, Numerical analysis of enzyme polymorphism: a new approach to the epidemiology and taxonomy of trypanosomes of the subgenus *Trypanozoon, Adv. Parasitol.,* 18, 175, 1980.

150. **Tait, A.**, Evidence for diploidy and mating in trypanosomes, *Nature, London,* 287, 536, 1980.

151. **Lumsden, W. H. R., Kimber, C. D., Evans, D. A., and Doig, S. J.**, *Trypanosoma brucei:* miniature anion-exchange centrifugation technique for detection of low parasitaemias: adaptation for field use, *Trans. R. Soc. Trop. Med. Hyg.,* 73, 312, 1979.

152. **de Raadt, P. and Seed, J. R.**, Trypanosomes causing disease of man in Africa, in *Parasitic Protozoa,* Vol. 1, Kreier, J. P., Ed., Academic Press, New York, 1977, 175.

SIMIAN MALARIA

William E. Collins

Etiologic Agents

Plasmodium cynomolgi Mayer, 1907; *P. knowlesi* Sinton and Mulligan, 1932; *P. schwetzi* Brumpt, 1939; *P. brasilianum* Gonder and von Berenberg-Gossler, 1908; *P. inui* Halberstaedter and von Prowazek, 1907; *P. simium* Fonseca, 1951; *P. eylesi* Warren, Bennett, Sandosham, and Coatney, 1965. (Haemosporina, Plasmodiidae).

Other species of simian malaria which have a potential for transmission to man are *P. coatneyi* Eyles, Fong, Warren, Guinn, Sandosham, and Wharton, 1962; *P. fieldi* Eyles, Laing, and Fong, 1962; *P. fragile* Dissanaike, Nelson, and Garnham, 1965; *P. gonderi* Sinton and Mulligan, 1933; *P. hylobati* Rodhain, 1941; *P. jefferyi* Warren, Coatney, and Skinner, 1966; *P. pitheci* Halberstaedter and von Prowazek, 1907; *P. reichenowi* Sluiter, Swellengrebel, and Ihle, 1922; *P. simiovale* Dissanaike, Nelson, and Garnham, 1965; *P. sylvaticum* Garnham, Rajapaksa, Peters, and Killick-Kendrick, 1972; *P. youngi* Eyles, Fong, Dunn, Guinn, Warren, and Sandosham, 1964.

Life Cycle

The cycle of malaria in the primate host is initiated by the inoculation of sporozoites by the female mosquito when she feeds. The sporozoites rapidly leave the blood stream and enter the parenchymal cells of the liver to initiate the exoerythrocytic cycle. After a developmental period within the liver of from 5 to 15 days (depending on the species of *Plasmodium*), the exoerythrocytic schizont matures and releases thousands of merozoites to initiate the erythrocytic cycle.

Merozoites of some species display a marked predilection to invade reticulocytes; some prefer mature red cells and others are nonselective. Within the red cell, the young trophozoite assumes various shapes depending on the species of *Plasmodium*. Nearing maturity, the parasite nucleus undergoes mitotic division producing from 8 to 30 more merozoites. These are released as the red cell ruptures. Unless destroyed by the host's immune mechanisms, these new merozoites rapidly invade other erythrocytes, thus initiating another erythrocytic cycle. The length of time required for completion of the erythrocytic cycle varies from approximately 24 hr (quotidian cycle) to approximately 72 hr (quartan cycle). Only one species, *P. knowlesi,* has a quotidian cycle. Those with a quartan cycle are *P. inui* and *P. brasilianum*. All of the other species have a tertian cycle (48 hr). The morphology of the erythrocytic stages and the length of time required for completion of the erythrocytic cycle are the primary bases for species identification.

During the course of the infection in the primate host, two types of sexual forms (male and female gametocytes) are produced. When the anophiline mosquito feeds, these gametocytes are ingested. In the midgut of the mosquito, the mature gametocytes shed their red cell envelopes and transform into gametes. The microgamete is produced by a process called exflagellation. The nucleus of the microgametocyte divides, giving rise to eight nuclei. These migrate to the periphery and enter long cytoplasmic processes projecting from the surface of the parasite. The microgamete lashes about and separates from the parent body. The microgamete enters the macrogamete to form the zygote which shortly develops into the ookinete. The motile ookinete moves to the midgut wall of the mosquito where a cyst wall is formed. The oocyst rapidly develops, projecting into the hemocoele of the mosquito. Development requires from 10 to 17 days, depending on the species and incubation temperature. Upon maturity, the oocyst ruptures, releasing large numbers of sporozoites into the hemocoele. Many sporozoites enter the acinal cells of the mosquito's salivary glands. When the mosquito feeds again, some of the sporozoites enter the salivary duct and are introduced into the bloodstream of the primate host, thus initiating a new infection.

True and Alternate Hosts

Of the 20 species of nonhuman primate malarias, two, *P. girardi* and *P. lemuris* are found in members of the family Lemuridae. These two parasites of lemurs are not thought to have a potential for human transmission. Eight species, *P. coatneyi, P. cynomolgi, P. fieldi, P. fragile, P. gonderi, P. inui, P. knowlesi,* and *P. simiovale,* are found in Old World monkeys of the family Cercopithecidae. Two, *P. brasilianum* and *P. simium,* are found in New World monkeys of the family Cebidae. Four, *P. pitheci, P. reichenowi, P. schwetzi,* and *P. sylvaticum,* are from the great apes, family Pongidae, and four, *P. eylesi, P. hylobati, P. jefferyi,* and *P. youngi,* are from gibbons, family Hylobatidae.

Many species have been reported from more than one host and have been experimentally transmitted to a number of primates used in laboratory studies. In Table 1 are listed the known natural and experimental hosts of the seven species reported transmissible to man. In Table 2 are listed the natural and experimental hosts for the other nonhuman primate malarias which have yet to be shown infectious to man.

Distribution

The geographic distributions of the nonhuman primate malarias are presented in Tables 1 and 2 of the previous section. Three are from Africa, two from South America, and thirteen from tropical Asia. Although these parasites are probably present in most of the areas inhabited by monkeys and anthropoid apes, there are many gaps in their distribution. There are some areas with high monkey populations which are known to be free of parasites. For example, in north-central India, the *Macaca mulatta* monkeys have no malarial infections due to the absence of a suitable mosquito vector. The same species of monkey in southern and northeastern India is infected, which coincides with the presence of *Anopheles leucosphyrus* group mosquito vectors.[27] Malaysian monkeys appear to have the highest prevalence of malaria whereas *P. brasilianum* appears to have the widest reported distribution among different primate species.

Disease in Animals

Prepatent periods in monkeys have a considerable range due primarily to the size of the sporozoite inoculum and the species of *Plasmodium.* Those parasites with a shorter exoerythrocytic cycle develop detectable parasitemias in a shorter period. *P. knowlesi* has a mean prepatent period of 7.1 days (range of 5 to 9 days) whereas *P. inui* has a mean prepatent period of 16.1 days (range of 10 to 28 days). Parasitemias rise rapidly, depending primarily on the length of the erythrocytic cycle (quotidian, tertian, or quartan).

The pathology of the infection varies remarkably with the host species. In *M. mulatta,* for example, *P. knowlesi* produces a fulminating infection with death often occurring within a week after the first appearance of parasites in the peripheral blood. Other monkey species, such as *M. fascicularis,* infected with the same parasite, have only moderate parasitemias and little overt signs of disease. Other species may be refractory or have very low level transient infections. The animals which are most susceptible become listless and irritable and soon stop eating. Body temperature is noticeably elevated. As the disease progresses, there is a marked anemia and rapid weight loss with evident dehydration. With fulminating infections, the animals often die with little advance signs of illness whereas chronic infections result in a marked debilitation of the animal over a period of several weeks. If the animal's immune mechanisms are allowed to control the infection or the animal is treated with drugs, recovery is rapid, although weight loss may persist for many months.

Of the seven parasites reported to infect man, *P. knowlesi, P. cynomolgi,* and *P. inui,* readily infect rhesus monkeys. Infection with the former parasite is usually fatal; with the last two, chronic infections are the rule. *P. brasilianum* produces long-term chronic infections whereas *P. simium* produces relatively transient infections in susceptible host animals. *P. schwetzi* and *P. eylesi* are parasites of the higher apes. The former produces a mild infection in chimpanzees whereas the latter produces relatively high parasitemias in gibbons which may require treatment.

Disease in Man

Information on the response of man following infection with the nonhuman malarias has been obtained as a result of a series of studies involving attempts to transmit certain of these parasites to volunteers. Infections were first established by the natural route of feeding infected mosquitoes. Subsequent infections were obtained either by the passage of infected blood from man to man or via the bites of infected mosquitoes.

P. cynomolgi (55 Volunteers — 24 Sporozoite-Induced and 31 Blood-Induced Infections)[1,7,11,13,14,26]

Prepatent periods ranged from 15 to 37 days with a mean of 19 days. Clinical symptoms consisted of cephalgia, anorexia, myalgia, and nausea. Symptoms were usually present during febrile episodes and were of moderate severity. Tertian fever patterns were not the rule but were prominent in some patients. A maximum temperature of 105.2°F was reported. The major physical findings were splenomegaly and hepatomegaly. Maximum parasitemias averaged from 150 to 300/mm^3 although a count as high as 8000/mm^3 was seen in one volunteer. Negroes as well as some Caucasians were refractory to infection.

P. knowlesi (20 Volunteers — 8 Sporozoite-Induced and 12 Blood-Induced Infections)[3,4,11]

Prepatent periods ranged from 9 to 12 days. Clinical symptoms consisted of malaise, cephalgia, and anorexia. Nausea and vomiting occurred but were uncommon. Febrile response during the first 3 or 4 days of patent infection was of the remittent type. After this, intermittent fevers with maximums up to 106°F were observed. Parasitemias as high as 21,000/mm^3 were encountered. Upon serial blood passage in man, higher parasitemias and more severe infections have been reported.[6] Both Caucasians and Negroes were susceptible to infection.

P. schwetzi (11 Volunteers — 2 Sporozoite-Induced and 9 Blood-Induced Infections)[16,11]

Prepatent periods for the two volunteers with sporozoite-induced infections were 24 and 104 days. Clinical symptoms consisted of cephalgia, generalized malaise, anorexia, and nausea. Vomiting and frank chills were frequently observed. The fever patterns were variable with a tertian pattern only occasionally evident. Paroxysms often occurred daily indicating an asynchronous infection. The maximum temperature observed was 105.6°F. The maximum parasitemia was 2750/mm^3 although parasite counts of 1000/mm^3 or higher were frequently observed. Only Caucasians were susceptible to infection.

P. brasilianum (7 Volunteers — 2 Sporozoite-Induced and 5 Blood-Induced Infections)[11,14,15]

Prepatent periods ranged from 29 to 64 days. Clinical manifestations were mild con-

Table 1
NATURAL AND EXPERIMENTAL PRIMATE HOSTS FOR THE NONHUMAN PRIMATE MALARIAS KNOWN TO INFECT MAN

Species	Natural hosts	Experimental hosts	Geographic distribution
P. cynomolgi	*Macaca cyclopis, M. fascicularis, M. mulatta, M. nemestrina, M. radiata, M. sinica, Presbytis cristatus, P. entellus*	*Aotus trivirgatus* *Cebus capucinus* *Cercopithecus aethiops* *Papio doguera, P. papio* Man	India, Sri Lanka, Malaysia, Taiwan, Indonesia (Java and the Celebes)
P. knowlesi	*Macaca fascicularis, M. nemestrina* *Presbytis melalophus* Man	*Aotus trivirgatus* *Callithrix jacchus* *Cercocebus fuliginosus* *Cercopithecus cephus,* *C. griso viridis,* *Cynocephalus papio* *Hylobates hoolock, H. lar* *Macaca arctoides, M. mulatta,* *M. radiata* *Papio doguera, P. jubilaeus,* *P. papio* *Presbytis cristatus* *Saimiri sciureus* *Semnopithecus entellus*	Malaysia Philippines
P. schwetzi	*Pan troglodytes* *Gorilla gorilla*	Man	Cameroons, Sierra Leone, Zaire, Liberia, Dem. Rep. of the Congo
P. brasilianum	*Alouatta belzebul, A. caraya,* *A. fusca, A. palliata,* *A. seniculus, A. villosa,* *Ateles fusiceps, A. geoffroyi,* *A. paniscus, A. variegatus* *Brachyteles arachnoides* *Cacajoa calvus, C. rubicundus* *Calicebus moloch, C. torquatus* *Cebus albifrons, C. apella, C. capucinus*	*Aotus trivirgatus* Man	Brazil, Venezuela, Colombia, Peru, Panama

P. inui	*Chiroptes satanas, C. albinasus* *Lagothrix lagotricha* *Pithecia monachus* *Saimiri sciureus, S. geoffroyi* *Cynopithecus niger* *Macaca cyclopis, M. fascicularus,* *M. mulatta, M. nemestrina,* *M. radiata, M. sinica* *Presbytis cristatus, P. obscurus*	*Cercopithecus mitis* Man	Sri Lanka, India, Malaysia, Philippines, Indonesia, Taiwan
P. simium	*Alouatta fusca* *Brachyteles arachnoides* Man	*Aloutta villosa* *Aotus trivirgatus* *Ateles fusiceps, A. geoffroyi,* *A. paniscus* *Callithrix jacchus* *Cebus capucinus* *Lagothrix legotricha* *Saguinus geoffroyi* *Saimiri sciureus* Man	Brazil
P. eylesi	*Hylobates lar*	Man	Malaysia

Table 2

NATURAL AND EXPERIMENTAL PRIMATE HOSTS FOR THE NONHUMAN PRIMATE
MALARIAS NOT KNOWN TO INFECT MAN

Species	Natural hosts	Experimental hosts	Geographic distribution
P. coatneyi	*Macaca fascicularis*	*Macaca mulatta, M. nemestrina,* *M. arctoides* *Presbytis cristatus*	Malaysia, Philippines
P. fieldi	*Macaca fascicularis, M. nemestrina*	*Macaca mulatta, M. radiata* *Papio doguera*	Malaysia
P. fragile	*Macaca radiata, M. sinica*	*Macaca fascicularis, M. mulatta*	Sri Lanka
P. gonderi	*Cercocebus aterrimus, C. atys,* *C. galeritis agilus* *Mandrillus leucophaeus*	*Cercopithecus aethiops* *Macaca mulatta, M. radiata* *Papio anubis, P. jubilaeus*	Cameroons, Zaire
P. hylobati	*Hylobates moloch*	*Macaca fascicularis, M. mulatta, M. nemestrina*	East Malaysia
P. jefferyi	*Hylobates lar*		Malaysia
P. pitheci	*Pongo pygmaeus*	*Pan troglodytes* *Hylobates lar*	East Malaysia
P. reichenowi	*Pan troglodytes* *Gorilla gorilla*		Cameroons, Zaire, Sierra Leone, Dem. Rep. of the Congo
P. simiovale	*Macaca sinica*	*Macaca mulatta*	Sri Lanka
P. sylvaticum	*Pongo pygmaeus*	*Pan troglodytes*	East Malaysia
P. youngi	*Hylobates lar*	*Symphalangus syndactylus*	Malaysia

sisting mainly of cephalgia and anorexia. Fevers were present, the maximum being 103.8°F. The quartan fever pattern was seldom observed, but appeared more consistently in the sporozoite-induced infections than those induced by blood inoculation. Parasite counts rarely exceeded 50/mm³, the maximum being 200/mm³. The duration of the parasitemia did not exceed 27 days. Both Caucasians and Negroes were susceptible to infection.

P. inui (7 Volunteers — 2 Sporozoite-Induced and 5 Blood-Induced Infections)[8,11]
Prepatent periods were 31 and 56 days. Major complaints were cephalgia, malaise, myalgia, and anorexia. When chills occurred, they were mild and of short duration. The quartan fever pattern was well marked in only two of the volunteers. The maximum fever was 103.2°F. Maximum parasite count was 2520/mm³. Both Caucasians and Negroes were susceptible to infection.

P. simium[17,18] and *P. eylesi*[11]
Only single infections with these parasites have been reported. They appeared to be mild and of short duration. Parasite counts were low. Both infections were in Caucasians.

General Mode of Spread
Transmission of plasmodial infection is obtained either by the bite of infected mosquitoes or by the inoculation of parasitized blood. If man and primate co-inhabit the same environment and mosquitoes susceptible to infection feed on both man and animal, transmission may occur.[9,10,28] Two such transmissions of *P. knowlesi* in nature have been reported, both from Malaysia.[3,24] Laboratory acquired infections of *P. cynomolgi* have also been reported.[22,26] A field acquired infection with *P. simium* has been reported from Brazil.[17,18] Since human malaria species are often present in these tropical areas, it is quite likely that infections with nonhuman primate malarias have been mistakenly identified as human malaria.

A potential for transmission occurs when feral animals infected with these parasites are used for experimental studies. Accidental or intentional introduction of infected erythrocytes from these animals may cause infection in man. Although only seven of these parasites are known to infect man, studies on the infectiousness of other species of *Plasmodium* are incomplete.

Epidemiology
The epidemiology of the simian malarias has been studied extensively in Malaysia, Brazil, Sri Lanka, and India. Over a period of many years, Deane and his co-workers[17,18-21] in Brazil were able to identify the simian hosts of *P. simium* and *P. brasilianum* and to identify their mosquito vectors. In the New World, high prevalence of monkey malaria is associated with humid, tall, primitive forests with dense monkey populations. In drier, bushy areas, with low populations of monkeys, the parasites are not found. The mosquito vectors are those which feed in the high canopy of the rain forest. In eastern and southern Brazil, the most abundant acrodendrophilic species is *Anopheles cruzi*. Infected mosquitoes were collected and transmission to malaria-free monkeys obtained. Malaria parasites were found in monkeys inhabiting the coastal forested mountains with abundant bromeliads. Infection rates, especially with *P. simium*, were higher during the late summer and early autumn than in other parts of the year. During the rainy summer months, the bromeliads are full of water, increasing the breeding places for the vector.

In the northern region (Amazonia) of Brazil, *A. cruzi* is not found. Here, *A. neivai* is suspected of being the vector. In still other areas, neither of these two species is present and the vectors are unknown.

In Malaysia, mosquitoes of the *A. leucosphyrus* group (*A. leucosphyrus, A. hackeri, A. introlatus,* and *A. dirus*) have been shown to be vectors of the simian malarias.[2,23,27-32] These mosquitoes are essentially primate feeders, most of the species being forest dwellers. They are attracted to man and capable of transmitting the infection if man invades the jungle environment.

In southern India and Sri Lanka, *A. elegans* has been shown to be the natural vector of *P. fragile* and *P. shortti* (= *P. inui shortti*).[5,25]

Anopheline mosquitoes which feed on monkeys in the forest canopy are seldom likely to feed on man on or near the ground. In turn, mosquitoes which normally transmit human malaria do not normally feed in the forest canopy where infected monkeys abound. It is thus a rare condition where man occupies, even temporarily, the environment in which he is fed upon by mosquitoes infected with simian malaria. This may occur, as it does in yellow fever, when deforestation or lumbering operations are being performed by man. Many mosquitoes are also restricted in their host feeding preferences. However, *A. cruzi* in Brazil is attracted to and feeds upon both man and howler monkeys.[21] In Malaysia, both *A. introlatus* and *A. leucosphyrus,* proven vectors of simian malaria, are attracted to man and monkey.[29]

Diagnosis

Diagnosis of *Plasmodium* infection in animals and man is based upon the presence of detectable parasites in the peripheral blood. Usually, this is made by the examination of a Giemsa-stained blood film. Since, in man, parasitemias of the simian malarias are usually low, thick films are examined; if parasites are found in sufficient numbers, species identification is made by examination of a Giemsa-stained thin blood film. Confirmation of human infection with a simian malaria can be made by subpassage into a malaria-free monkey (preferably splenectomized). The choice of the susceptible primate depends on the suspected agent.

The absence of parasites in the blood film of a feral animal does not guarantee a malaria-free state. Serologic tests, primarily fluorescent antibody, have been developed for the examination of monkeys to determine the presence of past or present malaria infection.[12] Many of these infections persist at patent or subpatent levels for many years and will rise to higher levels if the animal is splenectomized.

Prevention and Control

Since human malaria is often coexistent with the nonhuman simian malarias, the recommended malaria prophylaxis for a given area is sufficient to protect against these parasites. Treatment of simian malaria infections in man has been successful using a 4-aminoquinoline, such as chloroquine. There have been no reports in man of relapse after such treatment.

Simian malaria infections in nonhuman primates are cured by treatment with a 4-aminoquinoline, such as chloroquine, in combination with an 8-aminoquinoline, such as primaquine. The exact dosage depends upon the size of the animal. A 4 kg rhesus monkey is given 150 mg chloroquine base stat followed by the same dose 48 hr later. Primaquine is given at a dose of 7.5 mg base daily for 7 days. In a smaller primate, such as an *Aotus* monkey (0.8 kg), treatment is usually with 10 mg chloroquine base daily for 3 days and primaquine 2.5 mg base for 7 days. Blood-induced infections are cured by administration of chloroquine alone.

REFERENCES

1. **Beye, H. K., Getz, M. E., Coatney, G. R., Elder, H. A., and Eyles, D. E.,** Simian malaria in man, *Am. J. Trop. Med. Hyg.,* 10, 311, 1961.
2. **Cheong, W. H., Warren, McW., Omar, A. H., and Mahadevan, S.,** *Anopheles balabacensis balabacensis* identified as a vector of simian malaria in Malaysia, *Science,* 150, 1314, 1965.
3. **Chin, W., Contacos, P. G., Coatney, G. R., and Kimball, H. R.,** A naturally acquired quotidian-type malaria in man transferable to monkeys, *Science,* 149, 865, 1965.
4. **Chin, W., Contacos, P. G., Collins, W. E., Jeter, M. H., and Alpert, E.,** Experimental mosquito-transmission of *Plasmodium knowlesi* to man and monkey, *Am. J. Trop. Med. Hyg.,* 17, 355, 1968.
5. **Choudhury, D. S., Wattal, B. L., and Ramakrishnan, S. P.,** Incrimination of *Anopheles elegans* James (1903) as a natural vector of simian malaria in the Niligiris, Madras state, India, *Ind. J. Malariol.,* 17, 243, 1963.
6. **Ciuca, M., Chelarescu, M., Sofletea, A., Constantinescu, P., Teriteanu, E., Cortez, P., Balanovschi, G., and Ilies, M.,** Contribution experiméntale á l'etude de l'immunité dans le paludisme, *Editions Acad. Rep. Pop. Roumaine,* 1955.
7. **Coatney, G. R., Elder, H. A., Contacos, P. G., Getz, M. E., Greenland, R., Rossan, R. N., and Schmidt, L. H.,** Transmission of the M strain of *Plasmodium cynomolgi* to man, *Am. J. Trop. Med. Hyg.,* 10, 673, 1961.
8. **Coatney, G. R., Chin, W., Contacos, P. G., and King, H. K.,** *Plasmodium inui,* a quartan-type malaria parasite of Old World monkeys transmissible to man, *J. Parasitol.,* 52, 660, 1966.
9. **Coatney, G. R.,** Simian malarias in man: facts, implications, and predictions, *Am. J. Trop. Med. Hyg.,* 17, 147, 1968.
10. **Coatney, G. R.,** The simian malarias: zoonoses, anthroponoses, or both?, *Am. J. Trop. Med. Hyg.,* 20, 795, 1971.
11. **Coatney, G. R., Collins, W. E., Warren, McW., and Contacos, P. G.,** The Primate Malarias, U.S. Government Printing Office, Washington, D.C., 1971.
12. **Collins, W. E., Skinner, J. C., Guinn, E. G., Dobrovolny, C. G., and Jones, F. E.,** Fluorescent antibody reactions against six species of simian malaria in monkeys from India and Malaysia, *J. Parasitol.,* 51, 81, 1965.
13. **Contacos, P. G., Elder, H. A., Coatney, G. R., and Genther, C.,** Man to man transfer of *Plasmodium cynomolgi* by mosquito bite, *Am. J. Trop. Med. Hyg.,* 11, 186, 1962.
14. **Contacos, P. G. and Coatney, G. R.,** Symposium on simian malaria — experimental adaptation of simian malarias to abnormal hosts, *J. Parasitol.,* 49, 912, 1963.
15. **Contacos, P. G., Lunn, J. S., Coatney, G. R., Kilpatrick, J. W., and Jones, F. E.,** Quartan-type malaria parasite of New World monkeys transmissible to man, *Science,* 142, 676, 1963.
16. **Contacos, P. G., Coatney, G. R., Orihel, T. C., Collins, W. E., Chin, W., and Jeter, M. H.,** Transmission of *Plasmodium schwetzi* from the chimpanzee to man by mosquito bite, *Am J. Trop. Med. Hyg.,* 19, 190, 1970.
17. **Deane, L. M., Deane, M. P., and Ferreira Neto, J. A.,** A naturally acquired human infection of *Plasmodium simium* of howler monkeys, *Trans. R. Soc. Trop. Med. Hyg.,* 60, 563, 1966.
18. **Deane, L. M., Deane, M. P., and Ferreira Neto, J. A.,** Studies on transmission of simian malaria and on a natural infection of man with *Plasmodium simium* in Brazil, *Bull. WHO,* 35, 805, 1966.
19. **Deane, L. M., Ferreira Neto, J. A., Deane, M. P., and Silveira, I. P. S.,** *Anopheles (Kertesia) cruzi,* a natural vector of the monkey malaria parasites *Plasmodium simium* and *Plasmodium brasilianum,* *Trans. R. Soc. Trop. Med. Hyg.,* 64, 647, 1970.
20. **Deane, L. M., Deane, M. P., Neto, J. A., and Almeida, F. B.,** On the transmission of simian malaria in Brazil, *Rev. Inst. Med. Trop. Sao Paulo,* 13, 311, 1971.
21. **Deane, L. M.,** Epidemiology of simian malaria in the American continent, *1st Inter-American Conf. Conservation Utilization of American Nonhuman Primates in Biomed. Res.,* Pan American Health Organization, Washington, D.C., 1976, 144.
22. **Eyles, D. E., Coatney, G. R., and Getz, M. E.,** Vivax-type parasite of macaques transmissible to man, *Science,* 132, 1812, 1960.
23. **Eyles, D. E., Warren, McW., and Guinn, E. G.,** Identification of *Anopheles balabacensis introlatus* as a vector of monkey malaria in Malaya, *Bull. WHO,* 28, 134, 1963.
24. **Fong, Y. L., Cadigan, F. C., and Coatney, G. R.,** A presumptive case of naturally occurring *Plasmodium knowlesi* malaria in man in Malaysia, *Trans. R. Soc. Trop. Med. Hyg.,* 65, 839, 1971.
25. **Nelson, P.,** *Anopheles elegans,* a natural vector of simian malaria in Ceylon, *Trans. R. Soc. Trop. Med. Hyg.,* 65, 695, 1971.
26. **Schmidt, L. H., Greenland, R., and Genther, C. S.,** The transmission of *Plasmodium cynomolgi* to man, *Am. J. Trop. Med. Hyg.,* 10, 679, 1961.
27. **Warren, McW. and Wharton, R. H.,** Symposium on simian malaria — the vectors of simian malaria: identity, biology, and geographical distribution, *J. Parasitol.,* 49, 892, 1963.

28. **Warren, McW.**, Simian and anthropoid malarias — their role in human disease, *Lab. Anim. Care,* 20, 368, 1970.

29. **Warren, McW., Cheong, W. H., Fredericks, H. K., and Coatney, G. R.**, Cycles of jungle malaria in West Malaysia, *Am. J. Trop. Med. Hyg.,* 19, 383, 1970.

30. **Wharton, R. H. and Eyles, D. E.**, *Anopheles hackeri,* a vector of *Plasmodium knowlesi* in Malaya, *Science,* 134, 279, 1961.

31. **Wharton, R. H., Eyles, D. E., Warren, McW., and Moorhouse, D. E.**, *Anopheles leucosphyrus* identified as a vector of monkey malaria in Malaya, *Science,* 137, 758, 1962.

32. **Wharton, R. H., Eyles, D. E., and Warren, McW.**, The development of methods for trapping the vectors of monkey malaria, *Ann. Trop. Med. Parasitol.,* 57, 32, 1963.

BABESIOSIS*

Miodrag Ristic and G. R. Healy

Disease

Babesiosis is a tick-transmitted disease of animals which is manifested by anemia, occasional hemoglobinuria, and the appearance of infecting protozoa in the host erythrocytes.[1,2] As in most hemotropic infections, the acute and clinically apparent form of babesiosis is less frequently observed than the latent or subclinical form. The acute stage of the infection lasts for a few days, and it is usually during this stage only that the parasites can be detected by examination of stained blood smears. Animals that have recovered from acute babesiosis usually become carriers of *Babesia*. This state of the infection is frequently and more accurately termed babesiasis and refers to a dynamic equilibrium between the *Babesia* and the defenses of the host. The parasite is not easily demonstrated in blood films of carrier animals. From outside appearance, carrier animals ordinarily cannot be distinguished from normal, susceptible animals. Although there is no single reliable serological test for diagnosis of the carrier form of babesiosis, much work was recently done on the immunodiagnostic aspects of babesiosis caused by various species of *Babesia*.[3]

Post-mortem findings are characterized by splenomegaly, with dark red soft pulp and hepatomegaly. Kidneys are usually enlarged and yellowish, and histologic examination frequently reveals the presence of nephrosis and nephritis. Minute petechial hemorrhages are usually found on the pleura and pericardium, and variable amounts of serous fluid may be present in the pleural, pericardial, and peritoneal cavities. Icterus is a prominent feature in acute cases.[4] Cerebral forms of the disease due to clogging of brain capillaries with parasitized erythrocytes, cell debris, and free parasites have been described, and these are invariably fatal.[5]

Etiologic Agent

In 1888, Babes[6] first observed *Babesia* parasites in the blood of African cattle showing signs of hemoglobinuria. In 1893, Smith and Kilbourne demonstrated tick transmission of *B. bigemina,* the causative agent of bovine babesiosis, or "Texas fever". This was the first pathogenic protozoan shown to be transmitted by an arthropod vector.[7] Since then, 71 distinct species of *Babesia* have been described from various vertebrate hosts.[8] The organism may be transmitted by various blood-sucking arthropods such as tabanids, but ticks are the main vectors. Recent microscopic and electron microscopic studies of ovine, canine, and equine species of *Babesia,* including erythrocytic and tick stages, have shown that the organism is structurally similar to sporozoa.[1,9-12] Unlike *Plasmodium,* however, *Babesia* does not leave residual hemozoin pigment following the ingestion of food vacuole-stored hemoglobin.[13] Today, some 80 years after the discovery of the first infection in cattle, babesiosis remains one of the most important bovine hemotropic diseases occurring in tropical and semitropical regions of the world.

Babesial Infections in Domestic Animals and Laboratory Rodents
Cattle

B. bigemina is found throughout tropical and subtropical areas, including parts of Europe, Africa, Australia, and South America. The organism is a large piroplasm measuring approximately 4 to 5 μm long × 2 to 3 μm wide. *B. bovis* is a small piroplasm

* This study was supported in part by research grants RF-44-44-30-377 from the Rockefeller Foundation.

measuring approximately 2.4 μm long × 1.5 μm wide and occurs in southern Europe, Africa, Asia, and South America. Babesiosis caused by this parasite is most severe and, consequently, economically most important. *B. divergens* occurs in western and central Europe; it is often confused with *B. bovis,* being a pyriform, paired, or club-shaped organism about 1.5 μm long × 0.4 μm wide. A number of other babesial species have been described in cattle.

Sheep and Goats
B. motasi and *B. ovis* are found in sheep and goats in southern Europe, the Middle East, the U.S.S.R., Indo-China, Africa, and in many parts of the tropics. *B. ovis* is much smaller than *B. motasi,* being 1.0 to 2.5 μm in length.

Horses
B. caballi appears in erythrocytes as pyriform bodies 2.5 to 4.0 μm in length and about 2.0 μm wide. *B. equi* is relatively small, being less than 2.0 μm long. Both agents have been reported from many tropical and subtropical areas of the world, and infections with these agents were diagnosed in the U.S.[2]

Swine
B. trautmani has been observed in domestic pigs in southern Europe, the U.S.S.R., and central and southern Africa. It has also been seen in certain wild pigs in Africa. The pyriform parasites frequently occur in pairs and measure 2.5 to 4.0 μm in length.

Dogs
B. canis has been observed in dogs in southern Europe, the U.S.S.R., Asia, Africa, North and South America, and Australia. The parasite is one of the largest of the *Babesia* spp., measuring as much as 5.0 μm in length. *B. gibsoni* occurs in Asia.

Cats
B. felis is a small piroplasm, 1.5 to 2.0 μm in diameter, found in the domestic cat, wild cats, and certain wild Felidae in Africa and India.

Rodents
B. rodhaini was isolated from a wild rodent in Africa and subsequently established in the laboratory rat and mouse. This species has become a useful tool in experimental babesiosis. More recently, *B. microti,* a natural parasite of *Peromyscus* and *Microtus* spp.,[14] was isolated in hamsters from the blood of a human case of babesiosis.[15]

Life Cycle and Vectors
Development of *Babesia* spp. in vertebrate and tick hosts has been studied by a number of investigators.[13,16-21] Although various forms of the organisms have been found in host's erythrocytes and various organs of host ticks, and various theories have been proposed regarding the possible life cycle of the parasite, further studies are still necessary.

According to one investigator, *Babesia* multiply in bovine erythrocytes primarily by a budding process, probably a reduced form of schizogony rather than a modification of binary fission.[22] There may be an intraerythrocytic developmental cycle, with production of forms that are infective to tick vectors. Most erythrocytic forms ingested with blood die, and apparently only certain forms can initiate the developmental cycle in the tick.

Little is known about the early stages of parasitic development in the tick, but various bodies have been detected and designated as sexual stages. Although these stages have not been seen united, the various forms seen in tick gut contents could be gametes that unite to form a zygote. There is enough circumstantial evidence available to suggest that such fusion of gametes may occur.

The subsequent "zygotic" development is thought to occur by multiple fission, giving rise to numerous vermicules.[12,22] If a sexual union occurs, then sporogonic multiplication ensues, primarily in epithelial cells of gut diverticula. Vermicules are distributed to the ovaries of the replete female tick via the hemolymph and they may infect her mature ova.[20] In the gut cells of developing larvae, a further process of multiplication occurs, giving rise to similar vermicules. This appears to be the case with *B. bigemina,* although there are apparently some differences with *B. bovis.*[22] Vermicules of the first generation are equivalent to sporoblasts, and those of the second generation may be the sporozoites. Another multiple fission initiates the final developmental cycle and is probably the equivalent of erythrocytic schizogony. This multiple fission occurs in the lymph and larval salivary gland cells in *B. bigemina* and *B. bovis* infections, respectively. The resulting forms are pear-shaped, resemble the pyriform bodies in bovine erythrocytes, and are infective to the vertebrate host.

From results of electron microscopic examination of *B. ovis* in ticks, it was concluded that this *Babesia* is structurally similar to sporozoa and toxoplasma.[20]

Transmission

Babesiosis is transmitted by ticks of the genera *Rhipicephalus, Ixodes, Boophilus, Haemaphysalis, Hyalomma,* and *Dermacentor.* The hereditary transmission of *B. caballi* with *D. nitens* has been demonstrated.[23,24] Bloodsucking flies such as *Stomoxys* and *Tabanus* spp. have been implicated as mechanical vectors.[25,26]

Protective Immunity

Persistence of solid resistance to clinical babesiosis depends upon continuous maintenance of the causative agent in the blood. Presence of the organism in tissue in a metabolically active state apparently supplies the necessary antigenic stimulus for continuous maintenance of humoral and cellular defense mechanisms.[27] Sera from convalescing animals are active in precipitation, agglutination, complement-fixation (CF), and fluorescent antibody (FA) tests. Presence of specific serum antibodies indicates protective immunity of the host as long as it represents the existence of the infection. The possible role of serum antibodies in protection is indicated by the following observations: (1) the concentration of specific antibodies usually falls below detectable levels before immunity wanes, (2) passive transfer of immunity to *B. bovis* from mother to offspring does take place, presumably via colostral antibody, and (3) a delay in the onset of parasitemia occurs if the recipient animal was given the antiserum at the time of infection.[28]

The protective role of antibody in babesiosis is probably similar to that of malaria, where the parasite actively invades erythrocytes and, in the sequence, is subjected to antibody effects while in the plasma.[29] Under the circumstances, the antibody that coats the naked parasite may slow down its ability to attach and penetrate host erythrocytes. Studies of malaria indicate that complement participation is not needed for protective antibody activity in vitro and in vivo.[30,31] A decrease in serum complement level was, however, observed in rats infected with *B. rodhaini,* and deposits of IgG and the third component of complement in glomeruli of affected animals was demonstrated.[32] Recent vaccination studies using cell culture-derived surface coat antigen of *B. bovis* have shown that the resulting antibodies have a strong protective effect against virulent challenge (see below).

Studies of cell-mediated immunity (CMI) in babesiosis are fragmentary and confined principally to laboratory animals. Adoptive transfer of immunity to *B. rodhaini* was made in rats by the use of splenic homogenates.[33] The author suggested that functional elements were phagocytes and antibody-producing lymphocytes. Wolf[34] caused a relapse of babesiosis in hamsters infected with *B. microti* following treatment with anti-lymphocyte serum. He suggested that both CMI and humoral immunity are involved in protection. Perez and co-workers[35] studied groups of hamsters infected with *B. microti,* originally isolated from a human babesiosis case,[35,36] during a 5-month period and showed that CMI response persisted the entire time. Upon challenge, the animals demonstrated a rise in CMI response and were clinically protected.

Serodiagnosis

Soluble and corpuscular antigens derived from the blood of infected animals have been used in various serologic tests for diagnosis of babesiosis. These tests include complement fixation (CF), indirect hemagglutination (IHA), capillary and slide agglutination, indirect fluorescent antibody (IFA), and precipitation in gel tests. A review by Todorovic[37] describes specificity, performance, and accuracy of these tests. Early studies chose the CF test mainly because of suitability of crude antigen preparations for use in the test. In recent years, more refined antigens have been used in various types of passive agglutination and precipitation in gel tests. A capillary tube agglutination test was successfully applied to diagnosis of a human case of babesiosis in the U.S.[36]

Recent Research Developments in the Study of Babesiosis

A major breakthrough in a century-long struggle against babesiosis was the development of a microaerophilous stationary phase procedure (MASP) for continuous in vitro propagation of *B. bovis,* one of the most important agents of bovine babesiosis.[38] This agent was responsible for the first human case of babesiosis which terminated fatally.[39] The cultural procedure ingeniously utilized the apparent requirement of *B. bovis* for low oxygen tension and provided a system capable of generating massive quantities of babesial antigens on a continuous basis.

The above achievement which signifies a new era in the study of babesiosis has opened a vast horizon of possibilities for easier and more accurate studies of biologic properties of the organism and for development of modern and more effective immunoprophylactic and serodiagnostic methods for control of the disease. The highlight of a series of important findings which followed development of the MASP culture system is the abundant quantities of soluble *B. bovis* antigens continuously generated in the culture medium. These soluble antigens which apparently originate from the surface of the *B. bovis* merozoites are being shed in the culture medium at the time the organism enters erythrocytes. Investigations over the past year have demonstrated an excellent degree of protection against *B. bovis* challenge in cattle immunized with cell culture-derived soluble antigens.[40] These soluble antigens were identified as glycoproteins, having molecular weight between 40,000 and 50,000, being relatively heat stable, and consisting of three distinct antigens.

Babesiosis in Man

Until 1957, *Babesia* infections had not been reported in man. Since then, studies of 34 human cases of babesiosis have been published, indicating the zoonotic potential of the organisms. Several other infections have been diagnosed but not yet published. In 30 of the published cases, patients developed an acute form of the disease, with the organism demonstrated by microscopic examination of their blood and, in several instances, isolation in laboratory animals (Figure 1). In the remaining four cases, individuals showed no clinical signs of babesiosis, and diagnosis was made by serologic means, isolation of the organism in hamsters, or microscopic observation of *Babesia* in stained blood films.

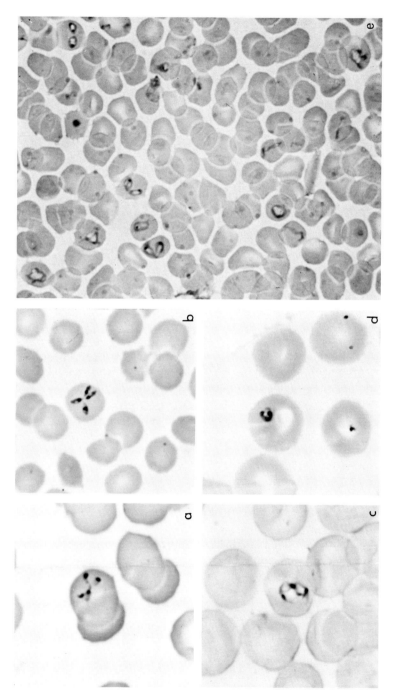

FIGURE 1. Intraerythrocytic *Babesia* organisms in peripheral blood smears of infected human beings. (a) Multiple infections. (From Anderson, A. E., Cassaday, P. B., and Healy, G., *Am. J. Clin. Pathol.*, 62, 395, 1975. With permission).(b) Multiple infections. (From Scholtens, R. G., Braff, E. H., Healy, G. R., and Gleason, N., *Am. J. Trop. Med. Hyg.*, 17, 811, 1968. With permission.) (c) Quadranucleated basket form of the organism. (From Healy, G. R., Walzer, P. D., and Sultzer, A. J., *Am. J. Trop. Med. Hyg.*, 25, 377, 1976. With permission.) (d) Singly occurring parasite. (From Healy, G., unpublished photograph. With permission.) (e) *Babesia microti* of human origin in the blood of an experimentally infected hamster. (From Ristic, M., unpublished photograph. With permission.)

Eleven of the patients had been splenectomized prior to onset of the disease; four of these individuals died. Based on identification of *Babesia* spp. in the infected persons, 5 isolates were of bovine origin, 2 of apparent equine origin, and the remaining 27 of rodent (*B. microti*) or unknown origin (Table 1).

Babesiosis in Splenectomized Individuals

There have been eleven cases of clinical babesiosis in individuals lacking a spleen. In 1957, Skrabalo and Deanovic[39] reported the first asplenic case of acute babesiosis in man. A 33-year-old farmer living on the outskirts of Zagreb, Yugoslavia, had suffered internal injuries in a car accident 11 years earlier, and his spleen had been removed. In June 1956, he was admitted to a hospital with fever, anemia, jaundice, and hemoglobinuria. His blood contained numerous intraerythrocytic "rings", which were later identified as *B. bovis*. The patient died 8 days later. Cattle in pastures where the patient tended his animals were infected with *Babesia*.

The second asplenic case occurred in 1966, in California, in a 46-year-old man who, because of hereditary spherocytosis, was splenectomized 2 years earlier.[41] The patient had visited remote coastal areas near San Francisco during the months preceding illness. He was admitted to a hospital with chills and fever, diagnosed as having malaria, placed on 250 mg of chloroquine per week for about 15 weeks, and recovered. The case was later diagnosed as babesiosis when "Maltese-cross"-type intraerythrocytic organisms were observed in his blood. The organism in question was suspected of having an equine origin. The IFA test of the patient's serum was negative to *Plasmodium* antigens, but *Babesia* antibodies were demonstrated in both CF and latex tube agglutination tests.

The third asplenic case occurred in Ireland in 1967.[42,43] A deep-sea fisherman became ill with fever, jaundice, and anemia. Intraerythrocytic parasites found in his blood (shortly before death) were later identified as *B. divergens*. The patient was splenectomized 4 months before the onset of illness. Epidemiologic investigation showed that the patient had presumably contracted the disease during a holiday from bites of infected ticks.

The fourth fulminating asplenic case of babesiosis occurred in 1969 in the same geographic location as case number one and involved a 27-year-old male factory worker.[44] This individual was splenectomized 3 years earlier, developed illness 15 to 21 days after being bitten by a tick, and died 5 days after onset of symptoms. Based on microscopic examination of stained blood smears, the organism was identified as *B. divergens*.

The fifth asplenic babesiosis case was reported in 1974 from New York state.[45] The patient, a 64-year-old male, was splenectomized a year earlier due to complications of hiatal hernia repair. The patient resided on Shelter Island where later a few other cases of babesiosis in individuals with intact spleen were reported. Specific identification of the causative agent was not made and the patient recovered without antibabesial therapy.

In 1976, the sixth asplenic human case of babesiosis was reported in France in a 61-year-old female resident of Cherbourg,[46] who had been splenectomized in 1972. The woman suddenly developed high fever, chills, headache, and pain in the left side of the back on September 20, 1975; other symptoms included hemoglobinuria and icterus. She was taken to the hospital 2 days later, where, on September 25, it was determined that 50% of her erythrocytes contained what was presumed to be *Plasmodium falciparum*. Subsequent careful examination of stained blood films revealed that the organism in question was *Babesia* spp. rather than *Plasmodium*. Following prolonged treatment with chloroquine, the patient gradually recovered and was released from the hospital on November 15. Further cytologic and immunologic studies with the *Babesia* spp. and sera collected from this patient were in progress.

Table 1
PUBLISHED CASES OF HUMAN BABESIOSIS

Clinical form	Year	Age	Sex	Outcome of infection	Country	*Babesia* sp.	Inoculation of animals	Ref.
Symptomatic								
Splenectomized	1957	33	M	Died	Yugoslavia	*B. bovis*	–	39
	1966	46	M	Recovered	U.S. (Calif.)	"Equine"	–	41
	1967	47	M	Died	Ireland	*B. divergens*	–	42, 43
	1969	27	M	Died	Yugoslavia	*B. divergens*	–	44
	1974	64	M	Recovered	U.S. (N.Y.)	*Babesia* sp.	–	45
	1975	61	F	Recovered	France	*Babesia* sp.	–	46
	1975	53	M	Recovered	France	*B. divergens*	–	47
	1978	34	M	Died	Scotland	*B. divergens*	+	48, 49
	1978	50	F	Recovered	U.S.(Cape Cod, Mass.)	*B. microti*	+	50
	1978	46	M	Recovered	U.S.(Long Island, N.Y.)	*B. microti*	+	50
	1979	36	M	Recovered	U.S. (Calif.)	*B. equi*	–	51
Intact spleen[a]	1969	59	F	Recovered	U.S.(Nantucket, Mass.)	*B. microti*	+	57
	1973	48	F	Recovered	U.S.(Nantucket, Mass.)	*B. microti*	+	54
	1975	72	F	Recovered	U.S.(Nantucket, Mass.)	*B. microti*	+	55
	1975	73	M	Recovered	U.S.(Nantucket, Mass.)	*B. microti*	+	55
	1975	56	F	Recovered	U.S.(Nantucket, Mass.)	*B. microti*	+	55
	1975	66	M	Recovered	U.S.(Nantucket, Mass.)	*B. microti*	+	55
	1975	52	M	Recovered	U.S.(Nantucket, Mass.)	*B. microti*	+	55
Asymptomatic	1976	51	M	Recovered	U.S.(Ga.)	*Babesia* sp.	–	60
	1977	49	M	Recovered	Mexico	*Babesia* sp.	+	61
	1977	31	M	Recovered	Mexico	*Babesia* sp.	+	61
	1977	29	M	Recovered	Mexico	*Babesia* sp.	+	61

[a] Additional clinically proven cases of *B. microti* infection reported since the above table was prepared were as follows: 7 Nantucket Island and 2 Martha's Vineyard Island, Mass., 2 Shelter Island and 1 Long Island, N.Y.[56]

The seventh published asplenic case of babesiosis was also reported in France in 1976 in a 53-year-old farmer in the Sorthe region of eastern France.[47] He had been splenectomized 36 years previously as the result of a traffic accident. Epidemiologic investigation disclosed that the patient's cattle had been affected periodically by babesiosis. The authors were of the opinion that the parasite was *B. divergens.*

The eighth case occurred in a 34-year-old man in Scotland.[48] Four years prior to contracting babesiosis caused by *B. divergens,* the patient had developed Hodgkin's disease and had been treated by splenectomy and cobalt irradiation. In August 1978 the patient was admitted to the hospital with extreme tiredness, malaise, vomiting, and diarrhea. Clinicopathologic symptoms of the patient included normochromic anemia, intense hemolysis, and intraerythrocytic inclusions resembling malaria parasites. In spite of treatment with chloroquine and pyrimethanime and blood transfusion, the patient died.

Inoculation of patient's blood into gerbils (*Meriones unguiculatus*) and into a splenectomized calf resulted in a patent *B. divergens* infection.[49] The latter animal provided a serum for serologic identification of the organism. In addition, adult *Ixodes ricinus* ticks were fed on the calf during the patent phase of the disease and the larvae resulting from transovarial infections were shown to cause *B. divergens* infections in gerbils and a splenectomized calf.[49]

The ninth asplenic babesiosis case occurred in 1978 in a 50-year-old woman resident of Sandwich, Mass.[50] On November 2 she developed severe headache, chills, temperature of 104°F, laryngitis, nausea, and vomiting. On November 11 she noted dark urine and two days later *B. microti* was diagnosed by microscopic examination of stained blood smears. The diagnosis was further substantiated by isolation of the organism from hamsters inoculated with patient's blood. She was treated with chloroquine phosphate and pentamidine, but in the opinion of the authors, these drugs did not have curative effect. This was the first human babesiosis case in mainland New England.

The tenth case of babesiosis in an asplenic patient occurred in a 46-year-old man, resident of Islip, Long Island.[50] The patient's backyard was heavily tick-infested and bordered on a nature preserve heavily populated by deer and rodents. The first symptoms of sluggishness, fever, headache, back and neck pain, anorexa, and scratchy throat were noted in early July 1978. It was not until the patient developed the onset of the hemolytic anemia that *B. microti* was identified in his peripheral blood sample and later recovered from hamsters inoculated with patient's blood. The patient was given chloroquine on July 26, his fever disappeared, and he was discharged July 29.

The eleventh and the most recent case of babesiosis in an immunosuppressed, asplenic patient with Hodgkin's disease occurred more recently in California.[51] A 36-year-old male was admitted in a local hospital in Panorama City, Calif. on September 1, 1979 with signs of fever, hemolytic anemia, headache, myalgia, anorexia, and prostration. While the patient does not recall tick bites, he was vacationing in Mexico and went deer hunting in central California a month and 3 weeks prior to admission, respectively. On admission, 30 to 40% of patient's erythrocytes were found infected with a protozoan organism which was initially identified as *P. falciparum.* Four days later the erythrocytic parasites were accurately identified as a *Babesia* sp. Based on the presence of characteristic "maltese cross" forms, it was indicative that the organism in question was *B. equi.*

As in most other cases, the initial therapy using antimalarial chloroquine was not successful. Chloroquine was discontinued and quinine sulphate therapy was initiated using 650 mg every 8 hr for 3 days followed by 650 mg every hr for 7 days. Pyrimethamine 240 mg twice a day for 3 days was given concurrently. Within 24 hr of the above combination therapy the patient became afebrile and there was a rapid clearance of parasites from his peripheral blood smears. The patient gradually improved and fully recovered within 3 months.

Babesiosis in Persons with a Spleen

Individuals with Clinical Babesiosis

The first human case occurred on Nantucket Island, off the coast of Massachusetts, in a previously healthy 59-year-old widow whose spleen had not been removed. Thus, this was the first spleen *in situ* case of babesiosis.[52] The patient was admitted to a New Jersey hospital on July 13, 1969, with a 2-week history of fever, headache, and crampy abdominal pain. A Wright-stained peripheral blood smear obtained on admission showed numerous ring-like structures within erythrocytes that resembled *P. falciparum* trophozoites. A diagnosis of babesiosis was made on the third hospital day.

Epidemiologic investigations revealed that, before her illness, the patient's dog was frequently infested by ticks, and it often chased, killed, and returned mice and other small rodents to the house. In mid-May, the patient found a tick deeply embedded in her own suprasternal notch and removed it with some difficulty.

A *Babesia* strain was isolated in hamsters and splenectomized monkeys from the blood of this patient.[15,36] Van Peenen and Healy[53] studied infections with the organism in laboratory-reared prairie voles. Three consecutive passages of the parasite were made in splenectomized monkeys, and it was transmitted from the monkeys to hamsters, but not to dogs. Intraerythrocytic parasites appeared as spherical, ameboid, or elongated bodies and were 1.5 to 2.5 μm in length (Figure 1). The parasite was limited by a single membrane, and its ultrastructural features were similar to those described for *B. microti*. IFA tests showed that the strain was serologically related but not identical to *B. canis*. A capillary tube agglutination test, using an antigen prepared from the blood of a dog infected with *B. canis,* reacted with antibody in sera of infected monkeys, of the patient, and of her dog; there was no reaction with sera of her horse or donkey.[36]

The second case of acute babesiosis with spleen *in situ* occurred in a 48-year-old woman also residing on Nantucket Island.[54] Medical history of the patient showed that she had received a tick bite in mid-August of 1973. On August 17, the patient's physician excised the local abscess which developed at the bite site; excised tissues also contained the tick head. The patient was admitted to the hospital on September 6 with a temperature of 104°F, symptoms of chills and myalgia in her legs and side, and depression. Intraerythrocytic parasites identified as *B. microti* were found upon examination of the patient's Giemsa-stained blood smears. The patient's serum was positive at a titer of 1:1024 to *B. microti* antigen in an IFA test. The organism was recovered in gerbils and hamsters inoculated with the blood of the patient. As in the case of the other patient with spleen *in situ,* this person had not traveled outside of the U.S. since 1971 and had lived on southeast Nantucket Island with her son since June 1973. She had no history of recent blood transfusion or parenteral drug use. Rats and ticks were abundant on the island.

Between July and October of 1975, five additional human cases of babesiosis were clinically suspected on Nantucket.[55] Organisms were identified microscopically in blood films, and isolations were made by inoculation of whole blood from the patients into splenectomized or intact hamsters at the Center for Disease Control, Atlanta. The patients, three males and two females, ranged from 52 to 73 years of age. Some, but not all infected persons exhibited symptoms such as drenching sweats, myalgia, arthralgia, nausea, and vomiting, etc. Common symptoms exhibited by all five persons were fever and fatigue.

In addition to the individual cases described in Table 1, twelve more clinical cases of human babesiosis caused by *B. microti* occurring on the east coast of the U.S. have been described in a recent review by Ruebush.[56] These were distributed as follows: seven from Nantucket Island and two from Martha's Vineyard Island, state of Massachusetts, two from Shelter Island and one from Long Island, state of New York.

The course of illness in the above patients generally started with a gradual onset of anorexia and fatigue followed by fever, sweating, rigors, and generalized myalgia. The levels of parasitized erythrocytes ranged from 1 to 10%. The organism resembled swan rings of *Plasmodium* but no pigmentation was observed. As the disease progressed a mild to moderately severe anemia developed, primarily due to hemolysis.

Three of the patients recovered from their illness with only symptomatic therapy. Most other patients received chloroquine phosphate orally. Most patients noted some symptomatic improvement; however, parasitemia persisted in all cases.

Healy et al.[57] demonstrated the existence of a reservoir of human infections in the rodent genera *Microtus* and *Peromyscus,* which are prevalent on Nantucket Island. Spielman et al.,[58] continuing studies on the epizootiology of human babesiosis on Nantucket Island, identified the deer tick *Ixodes dammini* (which resembles *I. scapularis*) as the prinicpal vector of *B. microti.* It has been shown that *I. dammini* is indiscriminate in its guesting and feeding behavior, that both larva and nymph may bite and infect mice, deer, or man. It was estimated that 5% of nymphal *I. dammini* collected from Nantucket Island were infected with *B. microti.*[59]

Individuals with Asymptomatic Babesiosis

A case of asymptomatic human babesiosis was reported from Georgia.[60] Diagnosis was made following an epidemiologic investigation of donors in a purported transfusion-acquired malaria infection. A 51-year-old black male resident of Georgia, one of the blood donors, was asymptomatic at the time organisms were detected in Giemsa-stained blood films. This individual was not splenectomized, gave no history of tick bite, and expressed an aversion to picnicking, camping, or otherwise venturing into the woods. Attempts to isolate the organism by subinoculation of blood into hamsters and mice were unsuccessful; the species of *Babesia* was not identified.

In an effort to determine if human *Babesia* infections might be present in Mexico, researchers at the National Center for Animal Study at Palo Alto selected as a testing ground an endemic rural area along the Gulf Coast, where continuous epizootics of equine, bovine, ovine, and canine babesiosis were known to occur. Of 101 individuals examined serologically by the IFA test, using *B. canis* as antigen, 38 reacted at titers from 1:10 to 1:80. Blood from these reactors was injected into splenectomized hamsters,[61] and those animals inoculated with blood from three of the individuals showed the organism in their peripheral blood. Growth of the organism was established by subpassages into additional hamsters. The pathogenesis of babesiosis in hamsters infected with *B. microti* of human origin was described by Lykins et al.,[62] (Figure 1,e).

On the basis of morphologic features alone, *Babesia* spp. were suspected as being of rodent origin.[61] Persons from whom the organisms were isolated were asymptomatic for babesiosis: Caucasian males, a 49-year-old construction worker, and 31- and 29-year-old animal caretakers. None of the 29 individuals residing in Mexico City, which represented the urban population in the survey, reacted in the IFA test.

Possible Factors Determining Frequency of Human Babesia Infections

In the first nine cases of human babesiosis, absence of a spleen was recognized as an important factor in enhancement of susceptibility to the infection (Figure 2). Susceptibility of splenectomized chimpanzees to infection with *B. divergens* offers further support to this hypothesis.[63] The remaining babesiosis cases occurred in individuals with spleen *in situ,* thus suggesting that elements other than splenectomy may have contributed to susceptibility. Conditions affecting these patients, i.e., concomitant infections, noninfectious disease syndromes, or metabolic, endocrinologic, and other disorders, could be considered as possible *Babesia* virulence-enhancing factors. With these stipulations in mind, babesiosis may present a hazard to numerous splenectom-

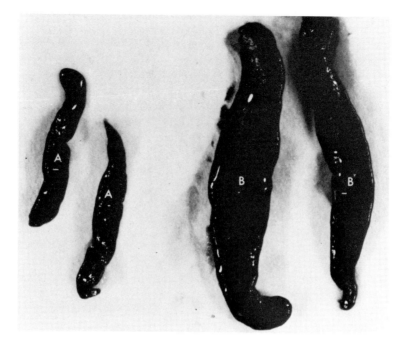

FIGURE 2.   (A) Spleens removed from normal hamsters. (B) Spleens removed from hamsters infected with *Babesia microti* isolated from an infected person. All hamsters weighed approximately 150 g. B-labeled spleens were removed 113 days after primary infection. (From Lykins, J. D., Ristic, M., and Weisiger, R., *Exp. Parasitol.*, 37, 395, 1975. With permission).

ized persons and to an unknown number of those whose splenic function is deficient or who possess "disease-precipitating co-factors."

The fact that the 19 published cases occurred in the same geographic region (four islands along Massachusetts and New York coasts) and involved persons who had not been splenectomized raises speculation regarding the role of the virulence of certain *Babesia* spp. in the pathogenesis of human babesiosis. In all instances, the organism was identified as *B. microti,* a species of rodent origin. It is well established that differences exist among various tick species with respect to their ability to feed on man. Certain ticks, such as the *Boophilus* spp. (which attack cattle), are extremely host-specific and rarely, if ever, attack man. Others, such as the *Dermacentor* spp. found on Nantucket Island (where most of the above human cases occurred), are known to readily attack man and a wide range of other animals, but Spielman's studies[58] implicate *Ixodes dammini.*

Another factor that could have relevance to the frequency of human exposure is the known ability of *Babesia* to undergo antigenic changes in vertebrate hosts.[64,65] These changes are believed to allow the parasite to persist in an immunologically hostile environment of the vertebrate host. The reported morphologic changes of *Babesia* during multiplication in tick tissues are a further indication of such antigenic changes.[9,19-21] These morphologic forms, with their associated biochemical and immunologic variations, may represent a heterogeneous pool of parasites from which variants, virulent for human beings, may arise. Thus, occurrence of clinical or latent infections in human beings may be related to the chance of exposure to a virulent babesial population able to fully or partially overcome constitutional host species resistance. Under these circumstances, frequency and chance of infection would be considerably greater in endemic areas.

Public Health Impact of Babesiosis

The human health impact of babesiosis may be greater than is indicated by the number of confirmed cases described above. Data from the study in Mexico revealed 38 serologic *Babesia* reactors in 101 persons residing in an endemic area. In similar serologic studies conducted from August 1975 to July 1976 on sera collected from 710 tourists and residents of Nantucket Island, 21 had *B. microti* antibody titers higher than 1:64. Of the seropositive persons 6 of 19 had experienced recent illness resembling babesiosis caused by *B. microti*.[56]

Information obtained from studies of babesiosis in domestic animals indicates that for every clinically demonstrable case there are hundreds of cases of latent infection.[1,2] Inapparent or latent infections are a common feature in many microbial infections of man and can be detected by using various microbiologic techniques.

Aside from the frequency of latent babesial infections, acquisition of knowledge about manifestations of this form of babesiosis is medically important. Latent human babesiosis may be manifested by symptoms not commonly ascribed to this disease. On this subject, Garnham and Bray[63] suggested that *Babesia* may be the etiologic agent of multiple sclerosis, particularly among farm workers. Babesial infections are known to affect nervous and other extravascular tissues; therefore, symptoms may be variable and numerous.[1]

There are only a few places in the world that are free of babesiosis. In many tropical and subtropical regions, babesiosis is endemic. Undoubtedly, agricultural workers and persons who spend much time in rural endemic areas frequently come into contact with *Babesia*-infected ticks. Various babesial species have been incriminated as potential human pathogens. At least four species of *Babesia* have caused babesiosis in the human cases reported above. Under these circumstances, one may speculate that the latent form of human babesiosis occurs frequently in endemic areas. Medical histories of the three persons in Mexico from whose blood *Babesia* spp. were isolated did not show any abnormalities that could be related to latent *Babesia* infections. In the absence of any knowledge regarding the time that infections were acquired by these three individuals, one could not predict long-term effects of persisting infections. Consequences resulting from one of the carriers being a blood donor are obvious.

In most of the above-described cases, the initial diagnosis was falciparum malaria, since the trophozoites of *P. falciparum* morphologically resemble certain forms of *Babesia* parasites. Serologic diagnosis is even more complicated, particularly in view of suggested cross-reactions between certain *Babesia* antigens and antibodies to malaria parasite antigens present in both *P. falciparum* and *P. vivax*.[66]

Treatment

Antimalaria chemotherapeutics, i.e., chloroquine phosphate was used in most clinical cases of human babesiosis. Generally, the drug was not effective in asplenic patients. In patients with intact spleen, as was the case with those infected with *B. microti*, some symptomatic improvement was noted; however, there appeared to be no relationship between chloroquine therapy and the duration of the patients' parasitemia.[55] Similarly it is true for a combination of chloroquine and primaquine therapy in patients with intact spleen. One such patient was treated with a 3-day course of diminazene (Ganaseg®, Berenil®), an aromatic diamidine known to be highly effective for treatment of animal babesiosis. There was a rapid reduction of parasitemia and general improvement in the patient's clinical condition. The infection, however, was not eradicated in this patient and 2 weeks after termination of the treatment he developed severe polyneuritis diagnosed as Guillain-Barre syndrome.

Berenil® was used for treatment of one asplenic babesiosis case in Yugoslavia apparently caused by bovine *B. divergens*.[44] The patient failed to respond and died as a result of the disease. The only notably successful treatment of babesiosis in an asplenic patient was in the most recent case from California. A combination therapy consisting of quinine sulphate and pyrimathamine caused reduction of parasitemia in clinical improvement within days after initiation of treatment.[51] Quinine sulfate was also employed in combination with chloroquine in a case of asplenic babesiosis in France with apparently good results. The authors, however, attributed the beneficial effect to chloroquine.[46] Prompted by failure of various drugs to treat human babesiosis, Miller et al.[67] conducted studies of the effect of various drugs in hamsters infected with *B. microti* isolated from a patient with an intact spleen, who contracted babesiosis in Martha's Vineyard. The antimalarial compounds, i.e., chloroquine, sulfadiazine, and pyrimethamine showed little effect. The antibotics, i.e., minocycline and tetracycline and berenil were effective only in high lethal dose ranges. Similar studies using mice infected with *B. rodhaini* showed antityrpanosomal berenil effective, but not so the antimalarials, chloroquine, and pyrimethamine.[68]

REFERENCES

1. **Ristic, M.,** Babesiosis, in *Bovine Medicine and Surgery,* Gibbons, W. J., Catcott, E. J., and Smithcors, J. F., Eds., American Veterinary Publications, Wheaton, Ill., 1970, 208.
2. **Ristic, M.,** Babesiosis, in *Equine Medicine and Surgery,* Catcott, E. J. and Smithcors, J. F., Eds., American Veterinary Publications, Wheaton, Ill., 1972, 137.
3. **Todorovic, R.,** Bovine babesiosis in Colombia, in Symp. Immunol. Anim. Dis. Caused by Blood Protista, *Vet. Parasitol.,* 2, 97, 1976.
4. **Almejew, H. S.,** Piroplasmose bei Hunde, *Btsch. Tieraerztl. Wochenschr.,* 66, 99, 1959.
5. **Purchase, H. S.,** Cerebral babesiosis in dogs, *Vet. Rec.,* 59, 269, 1947.
6. **Babes, V.,** Sur l'hemoglobinurie bacterinne de boeufs, *C. P. Acad. Sci.,* 107, 692, 1888.
7. **Smith, T. and Kilborne, F. L.,** Investigation into the Nature, Causation, and Prevention of Texas or Southern Cattle Fever, Bureau of Animal Industries Bull. No. 1, U.S. Department of Agriculture, Washington, D.C., 1893, 301.
8. **Levine, N. D.,** Taxonomy of the piroplasma, *Trans. Am. Microsc. Soc.,* 90, 2, 1971.
9. **Simpson, C. F., Bild, C. E., and Stoliker, H. E.,** Electron microscopy of canine and equine babesia, *Am. J. Vet. Res.,* 24, 408, 1963.
10. **Simpson, C. F., Kirkham, W. W., and Kling, J. M.,** Comparative morphologic features of *Babesia caballi* and *Babesia equi, Am. J. Vet. Res.,* 28, 1693, 1967.
11. **Friedhoff, K. T. and Scholtyseck, E.,** Fine structure of *Babesia ovis* trophozoites in *Rhipicephalus bursa* ticks, *J. Parasitol.,* 54, 1246, 1968.
12. **Holbrook, A. A., Anthony, D. W., and Johnson, A. J.,** Observations on the development of *Babesia caballi* (Nuttall) in the tropical horse tick *Dermacentor nitens* (Neumann), *J. Protozool.,* 15, 391, 1968.
13. **Rudzinska, M. A. and Vickerman, K.,** The fine structure, in *Infectious Blood Diseases of Man and Animals,* Vol. 1, Weinman, D. and Ristic, M., Eds., Academic Press, New York, 1968, 217.
14. **van Peenen, P. J. D. and Duncan, J.,** Piroplasms (Protozoa: Sarcodina) of wild mammals in California, *Bull Wildl. Dis. Assoc.,* 4, 3, 1968.
15. **Gleason, N. N., Healy, G. R., and Western, K. A.,** The "Gray" strain of *Babesia microti* from a human case established in laboratory animals, *J. Parasitol.,* 56, 1256, 1957.
16. **Dennis, E.,** The life cycle of *Babesia bigeminum* of Texas cattle fever in the tick *Margaropus annulatus,* with notes on the embryology of Margaropus, *Univ. Calif. Berkeley Publ. Zool.,* 36, 263, 1932.
17. **Li, P. N.,** Developmental forms of *Babesiella ovis* in the larvae and nymphae *Rhipicephalus bursa, Nauchn. Tr. Ukr. Nauchno Issled. Inst. Eksp. Vet.,* 24, 283, 1958.
18. **Muratov, E. A. and Cheissin, E. M.,** Development of *Piroplasma bigeminum* in the tick *Boophilus calcaratus* (transl.), *Zool. J.,* 38, 970, 1959.
19. **Riek, R. F.,** The life cycle of *Babesia bigemina* (Smith and Kilborne, 1893) in the tick vector *Boophilus microplus* (Canestrini), *Aust. J. Agric. Res.,* 15, 802, 1964.

20. **Friedhoff, K. and Scholtyseck, E.,** Feinstructuren von *Babesia ovis* (Piroplasmidae) in *Rhipicephalus bursa,* (Ixodoidea). Transformation spharoider Formen Zu Vermiculaformen *Z. Parasitenkd.,* 30, 347, 1968.

21. **Holbrook, A. A., Johnson, A. J., and Madden, D. A.,** Equine piroplasmosis: intraerythrocytic development of *Babesia caballi* (Nuttall) and *Babesia equi* (Laveran), *Am. J. Vet. Res.,* 29, 297, 1968.

22. **Riek, R. F.,** Babesiosis, in *Infectious Blood Diseases of Man and Animals,* Vol. 2, Weinman, D. and Ristic, M., Eds., Academic Press, New York, 1968, 219.

23. **Roby, T. O. and Anthony, D. W.,** Transmission of equine piroplasmosis by *Dermacentor nitens* (Neumann), *J. Am. Vet. Med. Assoc.,* 142, 768, 1963.

24. **Roby, T. O., Anthony, D. W., Thornton, C. W., and Holbrook, A. A.,** The hereditary transmission of *Babesia caballi* in the tropical horse tick, *Dermacentor nitens* (Neumann), *Am. J. Vet. Res.,* 25, 494, 1964.

25. **Neitz, W. O.,** Classification, transmission and biology of prioplasms of domestic animals, *Ann. N.Y. Acad. Sci.,* 64, 56, 1956.

26. **Abramov, I. V.,** Summary of the 36th plenary session of the U.S.S.R. Lenin Agricultural Academy, veterinary section on protozoan diseases, *Veterinaria Moscow,* 29, 55, 1952.

27. **Ristic, M.,** Babesiosis and theoleriosis, in *Immunity to Parasitic Animals,* Vol. 2, Jackson, G. J., Herman, R., and Singer, I., Eds., Appleton-Century-Crofts, New York, 1970, 831.

28. **Mahoney, D. F.,** Immune response to hematoprotozoa. II. *Babesia* spp., in *Immunity to Animal Parasites,* Soulsby, E. J. L., Ed., Academic Press, New York, 1972, 301.

29. **Hamburger, J. and Kreier, J. P.,** Antibody-mediated elimination of malaria parasites *(Plasmodium berghei)* in vivo, *Infect. Immun.,* 12, 339, 1975.

30. **Cohen, S. and Buchter, G. A.,** Properties of protective malaria antibody, *Immunology,* 14, 127, 1970.

31. **Diggs, C. L., Shin, H., Briggs, N. T., Laudenslayer, K., and Weber, R. M.,** Antibody-mediated immunity to *Plasmodium berghei* independent of the third component of complement, *Proc. Helminthol. Soc. Wash.,* 39, 456, 1972.

32. **Annable, C. R. and Ward, P. A.,** Immunopathology of the renal complications of babesiosis, *J. Immunol.,* 112, 1, 1974.

33. **Roberts, J. A.,** Adoptive transfer of immunity to *Babesia rodhaini* by spleen cells from immune rats, *Aust. J. Exp. Biol. Med. Sci.,* 46, 807, 1968.

34. **Wolf, R. E.,** Effects of antilymphocyte serum and splenectomy on resistance to *Babesia microti* infection in hamsters, *Clin. Immunol. Immunopathol.,* 2, 381, 1974.

35. **Perez, M., Ristic, M., and Carson, C. A.,** Cell-mediated immune response in hamsters infected with *Babesia microti, Vet. Parasitol.,* 3, 161, 1977.

36. **Ristic, M., Conroy, J. D., Siwe, S., Healy, G. R., Smith, A. R. and Huxsoll, D. L.,** *Babesia* species isolated from a woman with clinical babesiosis, *Am. J. Trop. Med. Hyg.,* 20, 14, 1971.

37. **Todorovic, R. A.,** Serological diagnosis of babesiosis, review, *Trop. Anim. Health Prod.,* 7, 1, 1975.

38. **Levy, M. G. and Ristic, M.,** *Babesia bovis:* continuous cultivation in a microaerophilous stationary phase culture, *Science,* 207, 1218, 1980.

39. **Skrabalo, Z. and Deanovic, Z.,** Piroplasmosis in man. Report on a case, *Doc. Med. Geogr. Trop.,* 9, 11, 1957.

40. **Ristic, M. and Levy, M. G.,** A new era of research toward solution of bovine babesiosis, in *Babesiosis,* Ristic, M. and Kreier, J. P., Eds. Academic Press, New York, 1981, 509.

41. **Scholtens, R. G., Braff, E. H., Healy, G. R., and Gleason, N. N.,** A case of babesiosis in man in the United States, *Am. J. Trop. Med. Hyg.,* 17, 810, 1969.

42. **Fitzpatrick, J. E. P., Kennedy, C. C., McGeon, M. G., Oreopouldous, D. G., Robertson, J. H., and Soyannwo, M. A.,** Human case of piroplasmosis (babesiosis), *Nature: London,* 217, 861, 1968.

43. **Fitzpatrick, J. E. P., Kennedy, C. C., McGeown, M. G., Oreopouldous, D. G., Robertson, J. H., and Soyannwo, M. A.,** Further details of a third recorded case of redwater (babesiosis) in man, *Br. Med. J.,* 4, 770, 1969.

44. **Skrabalo, Z.,** Babesiosis, in Pathology of Protozoal and Helminthic Diseases, *Marcial-Rojas, R. A.,* Ed., *Williams & Wilkins,* Baltimore, 1971, 232.

45. **Grunwaldt, E.,** Babesiosis on Shelter Island, *N.Y. State J. Med.,* 77, 1320, 1977.

46. **Bazin, C., Lamy, C., Piette, M., Gorenflot, A., Duhamel, C., and Valla, A.,** Un nouveau cas de babesiose humaine, *Nouv. Presse Med.,* 5, 799, 1976.

47. **Gorenflot, A., Piette, M., and Marchand, A.,** Babesiosis animales et sante humaine. Premier cas de babesiose humaine observe en France, *Rec. Med. Vet.,* 152, 289, 1976.

48. **Entrican, J. H., Williams, H., Cook, J. A., Lancaster, W. M., Clark, J. C., Joyner, L. P., and Lewis, D.,** Babesiosis in man: report of the case from Scotland with observations on the infecting strain, *J. Infect.,* 1, 227, 1979.

49. **Lewis, D. and Young, E. R.,** The transmission of a human strain of *Babesia divergens* by *Ixodes ricinus* ticks, *J. Parasitol.,* 66, 359, 1980.

50. Teutsch, S. M., Etkind, P., Burwell, E. L., Sato, K., Dana, M. M., Fleishman, P. R., and Juranek, D. D., Babesiosis in post-splenectomy hosts, *Am. J. Trop. Med. Hyg.*, 29(5), 738, 1980.

51. Bredt, A. B., Weinstein, W. M., and Cohen, S., Treatment of babesiosis in asplenic patients, *JAMA*, 245, p. 1938, 1981.

52. Western, K. A., Denson, G. D., Gleason, N. N., Healy, G. R., and Schultz, M. G., Babesiosis in a Massachusetts resident, *N. Engl. J. Med.*, 283, 854, 1970.

53. van Peenen, P. F. D. and Healy, G. R., Infection of *Microtus ochrogaster with piroplasms isolated from women, J. Parasitol.*, 56, 1029, 1970.

54. Anderson, A. E., Cassaday, P. B., and Healy, G. R., Babesiosis in man. Sixth documented case, *Am. J. Clin. Pathol.*, 62, 612, 1974.

55. Ruebush, T. K., Cassaday, P. B., Marsh, H. J., Lisker, S. A., Vorhees, D. B., Mahoney, E. B., and Healy, G. R., Human babesiosis on Nantucket Island. Clinical features, *Ann. Intern. Med.*, 86, 6, 1977.

56. Ruebush, T. K., Human babesiosis in North America, *Trans. R. Soc. Trop. Med. Hyg.*, 74, 149, 1980.

57. Healy, G. R., Spielman, A., and Gleason, N., Human babesiosis: reservoir of infection on Nantucket Island, *Science*, 192, 479, 1976.

58. Spielman, A., Clifford, C. M., Piesman, T., and Corwin, M. D., Human babesiosis on Nantucket Island, U.S.A.: description of the vector, *Ixodes* (Ixodes) *dammini*, n. sp. (Acarina: Ixodidae), *J. Med. Entomol.*, 15, 218, 1979.

59. Piesman, J. and Andrew Spielman, Human babesiosis on Nantucket Island: prevalence of *Babesia microti* in ticks, *Am. J. Trop. Med. Hyg.*, 29(5), 742, 1980.

60. Healy, G. R., Walzer, P. D., and Sulzer, A. J., A case of asymptomatic babesiosis in Georgia, *Am. J. Trop. Med. Hyg.*, 25, 376, 1976.

61. Osorno, B. M., Vega, C., Ristic, M., Robles, C., and Ibarra, S., Isolation of *Babesia* spp. from asymptomatic human beings, *Vet. Parasitol.* 2, 111, 1977.

62. Lykins, J. D., Ristic, M., and Weisiger, R. M., *Babesia microti:* pathogenesis of parasite of human origin in the hamster, *Exp. Parasitol.*, 37, 388, 1975.

63. Garnham, P. C. C. and Bray, R. S., The susceptibility of the higher primates to piroplasms, *J. Protozool.*, 6, 352, 1959.

64. Phillips, R. S., The role of the spleen in relation to natural and acqured immunity to infections of *Babesia rodhaini* in the rat, *Parasitology*, 59, 637, 1969.

65. Thoohgsuwan, S. and Cox, H. W., Antigenic variants of the *haemosporidian* parasite, *Babesia rodhaini*, selected by *in vitro* treatment with immune globulin, *Ann. Trop. Med. Parasitol.*, 67, 373, 1973.

66. Ludford, C. G., Hall, W. T. K., Sulzer, A. J., and Wilson, M., *Babesia argentina, Plasmodium vivax* and *P. falciparum:* antigenic cross-reactions, *Exp. Parasitol.*, 32, 317, 1972.

67. Miller, L. H., Neva, F. A., and Gill, F., Failure of chloroquine in human babesiosis (*Babesia microti*): case report and chemotherapeutic trials in hamsters, *Ann. Intern. Med.*, 88, 200, 1978.

68. Taylor, A. E. T., Terry, R. J., and Godfrey, D. G., The action of some trypanocidal and antimalarial compounds in *Babesia rodhaini* (Piroplasmidea) *Br. J. Pharmacol.*, 11, 71, 1956.

TOXOPLASMOSIS

Leon Jacobs and J. K. Frenkel

Common Clinical Descriptives

Toxoplasma abortion, lymphadenopathic toxoplasmosis, toxoplasmic (or toxoplasmal) chorioretinitis, encephalomyelitis, or myositis.

Etiologic Agent

Toxoplasma gondii Nicolle and Manceaux, 1909

T. gondii is a protozoan parasite belonging to subphylum Apicomplexa[1] and classified in the family Eimeriidae. It is related to the genus *Isospora* in that, as a result of a sexual cycle in the intestinal epithelium of the cat, it produces an oocyst with two sporocysts, each of which contains four sporozoites. In other respects it differs from the other *Isospora* species. It is unique in that it is indiscriminate in the type of cell it will parasitize. It has been found in the intestinal epithelium, hepatocytes, alveolar cells of the lung, skeletal, and cardiac muscle, adrenal cortical cells, testicular cells, lymphocytes and macrophages, retinal cells of the eye, uterine muscle and endothelium, neurons of the brain, and in red blood cells of birds. Because of its wide host cell range, *T. gondii* produces disease manifestations of a protean nature (*vide infra*). It is obligately intracellular and exists in a number of different stages in its various hosts.

The form of the parasite found during acute infection of the host is a slender arc-shaped organism, approximately 2 to 4 μm in width and 4 to 7 μm long. One end is more tapered than the other. The parasite moves in a gliding motion, apparently the result of contraction and expansion of small fibers in its cell wall. It lacks other types of locomotor organelles such as cilia or flagella. In Giemsa-stained preparations, it resembles the merozoite of malarial parasites in having a reddish-purplish nucleus and light blue cytoplasm with darkly staining cytoplasmic granules. Electron photomicrographs show a highly complicated set of organelles, and the parasite is enclosed in a double-unit membrane. The inner membrane is continuous around the organism except for a slight thickening (a polar ring) at the narrow anterior end which surrounds a conoid, and a similar thickening at the posterior end. The conoid is a truncated conical organelle which appears to be made up of rods or tubules wound in a spiral. It seems to be protrusible because in some micrographs it extends out from the anterior end more than it does in others. Subpellicular fibrils extend longitudinally from the membrane thickenings around the conoid to the posterior thick inner membrane; these are probably contractile and responsible for the gliding movements of the parasite.

The posterior end of the conoid appears to be open and from it extend posteriorly a number of structures. Arising from the conoid are the rhoptries or paired organelles, numbering from four to eight, which are club-shaped structures with a narrow, dense neck and a posterior vesicular part that increases in size as the organelle extends posteriorly. The rhoptries terminate in the area of the Golgi apparatus, just anterior to the nucleus which lies in the anterior part of the posterior half of the cell. The most likely function of rhoptries is to assist the parasite in the penetration of the host cells. This has been shown in photomicrographs of recently parasitized cells where the rhoptries appear to be depleted; their posterior parts appear less dense and are shrunken. Associated with the paired organelles and also arising from the inner end of the conoid are a number of elongate micronemes of about the same diameter as the neck of the rhoptries. These micronemes extend posteriorly in a tortuous path towards and up to the nucleus, while some extend beyond the nucleus. The nucleus is surrounded by a double membrane with pores which are covered by a single thin membrane. Within the cytoplasm is a rough-surfaced endoplasmic reticulum with associated ribosomes, free ribosomes, mitochondria with numerous cristae, and glycogen vacuoles. At the level of the anterior end of the nucleus there is a micropyle, formed by interruption of the inner cell membrane and invagination of the outer membrane. The micropyle may function as a cytostome but this has not yet been demonstrated.

Life Cycle and Morphological Variations

The definitive hosts of *T. gondii* are the domestic cat and a number of other members of the family Felidae. It is only in these animals that the sexual stages of the parasite occur. After cats ingest the infective forms of *Toxoplasma* in the flesh of prey animals, these forms invade the epithelial cells of the intestine and grow into large ellipsoid or round trophozoites. The trophozoites multiply first by endodyogeny (*vide infra*) and later by schizogony, with the formation of numerous organelles and membrane structures into which nuclear material produced by multiple nuclear divisions is distributed. After further extension of the membranes and further development of the organelles, the process of schizogony results in the production of 5 to 32 merozoites[2,3] which lie in rosette-formation within the host cell. These are released into the lumen of the intestine and in turn invade other epithelial cells. At least five generations of such propagative stages have been described.[2] These are then followed by the process of gametogony, leading to the development of microgametocytes and macrogametocytes.

Microgametogony occurs in a manner similar to schizogony. The microgametocyte measures 7×10 μm. The nucleus divides many times and a large number of protuberances form on the surface of the gametocyte, into each of which a single nucleus migrates. Within each protuberance two flagella develop from each basal body. The flagella are 6 to 10 μm long. The microgametocytes are 2 to 3 μm in size. As they are formed, they are in turn shed sequentially into the vacuole surrounding the gametocyte and, presumably, eventually become extracellular when the host cell degenerates.

The development of the macrogametocytes involves principally the growth of the trophozoite. The earliest recognizable macrogametocyte measures 5×7 μm. It contains many PAS-positive granules. The mature macrogamete measures about 13 μm.

Fertilization of the macrogamete by the microgamete results in the formation of a zygote which measures 10×12 μm. The zygote is unsporulated when shed but, after a period of incubation in the external environment, a sporoblast is formed. The sporoblast gives rise to two sporocysts, each containing four sporozoites. The sporocysts measure 6 to 8×5 to 7 μm. This form is indistinguishable from the "small race" of *Isospora bigemina*.

The ingestion of sporulated oocysts by a new host is followed by the appearance of the asexual forms of the parasite which proliferate in many tissues. *T. gondii* is not only indiscriminate in the types of cells it will parasitize, but also in the hosts which it can infect. There is no order of mammals in which toxoplasmosis has not been found. It has been reported also in a wide variety of birds. Although most of these reports are based solely on morphological evidence, there are enough substantiated reports of isolations of *T. gondii* from pigeons, chickens, and other birds to assure us that birds can easily be infected. Reptiles and amphibia have also been infected. When the ambient temperature is raised to about 37°C, there is evidence that *T. gondii* can replicate in these animals;[5] but this is not quite clear in amphibia. Levine[6] has recently described a new species *T. ranae*, from frogs. The basis for its speciation was based solely on morphology, and the description was published for documentation purposes. In the absence of serological and transmission data, the speciation of the parasite described in the frog cannot really be accepted as *sui generis.*

The first asexual form of *T. gondii* to appear in the acute infection of its numerous intermediate hosts (i.e., hosts in which the sexual cycle does not occur) has been described (*vide supra*). It has been referred to as the proliferative form or trophozoite. However, the term ''trophozoite'' is now reserved for the first intestinal stage in the cat and should no longer be used for the asexual stage. Other terms proposed by Hoare and Frenkel, respectively, are *endozoite* and *tachyzoite;* the former is merely descriptive of its location inside host cells while the latter is descriptive of a rapid rate of multiplication within the cells.

The mode of replication is a process termed endodyogeny by Goldman et al.[7] This process is characterized by the formation of two conoids and their associated membranes within an original growing organism. The nucleus of the organism buds out into each of these two cytoplasmic structures, and eventually the newly formed membranes enclose the nuclear buds and the other organelles, the mitochondria, Golgi apparatus, cytoplasmic reticulum, and ribosomes which are replicated and partitioned between the two daughter cells. The initial membrane formed around the daughter cells is single. As they break out of the depleted mother organism, they acquire the outer membrane. This process of endodyogeny appears to be a special form of schizogony, in that only two *merozoites* are formed from the parental organism. The repetitive reproductive cycles of endodyogeny within a parasitized cell result in the production of rosettes of organisms, which distend the cell and eventually cause it to rupture. The heavily parasitized cell was originally called a terminal colony and later a pseudocyst.

As the acute infection subsides, perhaps mediated by the appearance of humoral antibodies, a new asexual form appears in the tissues of the intermediate host. This is the cyst. It has a dense wall formed by the deposition of material from the parasite on the vacuolar membrane in which it is contained. It is likely that the host cell contributes to this deposition, because in electron photomicrographs of developing cysts a heavy concentration of mitochondria and host cell endoplasmic reticulum lines the outside of the parasitophorous vacuole. Division of the parasite within the cyst goes on by endodyogeny, but at an apparently slower rate than in the proliferative forms. This has prompted Frenkel[8] to suggest the term *bradyzoite* for these cyst forms. Hoare[9] suggests the term *cystozoite.* The dense material which forms the cyst wall is also distributed among the parasites in the cyst, which become tightly packed as reproduction continues and the wall becomes thicker. Eventually, the cysts may reach a diameter of 100 μm or more and may contain many parasites.

A unique feature of the cystozoite or bradyzoite is that, while one cannot easily distinguish it morphologically from the endozoite or tachyzoite, it is resistant to the action of gastric juice. The endozoite is immediately destroyed by gastric juice, while the cystozoite is released rapidly from the cyst when exposed to gastric juice, but is able to survive in it for at least 3 hr.[10] Thus the cyst form is adapted to transmission to carnivores. Cystozoites serve as the special infective agent for the cat, in which animal the sexual cycle is completed in 3 to 10 days, rather than the 19 to 48 days required after ingestion of tachyzoites or oocysts (Figure 1). In other carnivorous animals, the asexual cycle is repeated.

Distribution

Toxoplasmosis has been found all over the world. It is more prevalent in the temperate and moist tropical regions of the world than in the arctic zones or in hot arid regions. Other reports relate low altitude to high prevalence.[14] Feldman[15] has reported higher prevalence rates of antibodies in army conscripts from the east and south of

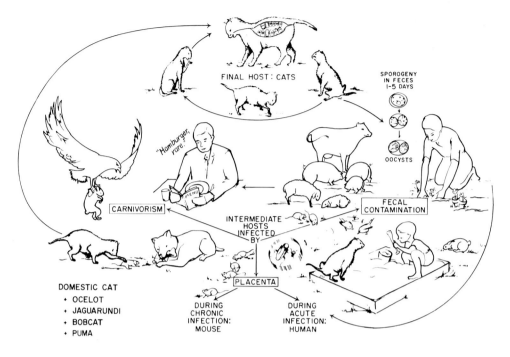

FIGURE 1.   Postulated transmission of toxoplasmosis.

the U.S. than from the mountain and Pacific zones. In some countries with temperate climates, such as the U.S., the prevalence of *T. gondii* antibody in the general population increases with increasing age.[16] In England, this phenomenon may not always be seen after age 20 years.[17] In some tropical countries, antibody is acquired mainly by adults.[18] In others, there is a high rate in young children[19] and, in either pattern, practically the entire population develop antibody titers after 50 years of age.[20] The variation in the prevalence rates from country to country is probably related to different customs, food habits, climate, and the cat population. Reports on the occurrence of toxoplasmosis in animals indicate that the infection is widespread in many countries.[21] High rates of infection occur in sheep in New Zealand[22] and England.[23] Pigs surveyed in the U.S. were also found heavily infected; 22% of pork samples were found to contain *T. gondii* cysts.[24] Similar findings have been reported from Japan.[25] In contrast to these food animals, infection in cattle is much less. In two surveys conducted, one in the U.S. and one in New Zealand,[26,27] no success was obtained in the isolation of *T. gondii* from beef specimens. However, Mayer[28] reported the isolation of the parasite from the retina of 18% of 597 cattle. Zardi et al.[29] also reported isolation of *T. gondii* from the eyes of eight cattle, as well as from swine, sheep, horses, and cats. Feldman and Miller[30] serologically tested various herds of cattle in upper New York state and found a spotty distribution; some herds were completely negative, while others had low percentages of low dye test antibody titers. Sogandares-Bernal et al.[31] used the dye test to examine beef and dairy cattle in the northwest U.S. They found a lower prevalence of antibodies in the beef cattle (27 to 35%) than in dairy cattle (62%). They speculate that the difference in prevalence found was due to the fact that beef cattle are allowed to range and therefore have little contact with cats, while the dairy cattle are kept close to and in the barn and thus have more contact with cats. Cats sometimes defecate in ground animal feed, increasing the chances of farm animals becoming infected, as opposed to range cattle.[32]

Catar et al.[33] in Czechoslovakia reported the isolation of *T. gondii* from 11 of 15

(73.3%) pools of diaphragms from 75 pigs and from the diaphragm and brain of 13 of 30 (43.3%) swine examined individually. They performed similar isolation trials on 85 cattle and obtained eight positives (9.4%). Janitschke et al.[34] isolated *T. gondii* from 6 of 50 seropositive sheep in Germany, but not from 74 healthy calves. Work[35] isolated *T. gondii* from the diaphragm of 7 of 31 sheep and 10 of 29 swine, but not from 30 cattle in Denmark. Berengo et al.[36] obtained isolates from 18 of 60 (30%) pigs from Siena, Italy. Amaral and Macrus[37] reported isolation of the parasite from 8 of 25 hog diaphragms slaughtered in Sao Paulo, Brazil. Jamra et al.[38] found *T. gondii* in (6.8%) of 73 pork specimens, but none in 73 beef specimens in Sao Paulo. This is not an all-inclusive list of studies on the prevalence of toxoplasmosis in meat animals, but it is indicative of the extent and distribution of the infection.

Surveys conducted on chickens in the U.S. have indicated a high prevalence of infection. Pools of tissues from the ovaries and oviducts of apparently healthy hens were examined by Jacobs and Melton.[39] Each pool was derived from ten birds. Twelve of sixty-six such pools yielded isolates of *T. gondii*. In a much earlier study, Jacobs et al.[40] did a survey of pigeons trapped in Washington, D.C., and found 12.5% positive. There are other reports of relatively high rates of infection in pigeons.[41]

Epidemics of toxoplasmosis have occurred in rabbit colonies, mink and chinchilla farms, and in other small animals bred for commercial purposes.[42,43,44] Prevalence figures in wild animals are rare. A serological survey, using the dye test, of 95 rabbits, 77 racoons, and 24 squirrels at the Patuxent Wildlife Refuge in Maryland revealed prevalence rates of *T. gondii* antibodies in these species of 22.1%, 23.4%, and 8.3%, respectively.[45] Berengo et al.[36] found that 42% of 50 foxes and 24% of 21 rabbits in the area of Siena, Italy were positive for toxoplasmosis by the dye test. There are enough reports of the presence of *T. gondii* in zoo animals to indicate that infection is widespread in many species.[46]

Dogs have high rates of infection in all parts of the world. In cats, the occurrence of toxoplasmosis is likewise high in many parts of the world.[21] Jones et al.[47] isolated *T. gondii* from the brains of 34 (24.3%) of 140 cats that they examined in Memphis, Tennessee. Similarly, 4 out of 35 Columbia, S.C. cats were shown to be infected. The isolates were of the tissue form, presumably cysts, indicating chronic infection. More recently, some data on the prevalence of oocysts in the feces of cats have become available. Jacobs[48] reported the occurrence of infective forms in 2 of 53 stray cats. Wallace[49] isolated *T. gondii* from 12 of 1604 cats in Hawaii. Janitschke and Kuhn[50] identified the oocysts in cats. Dubey et al.[51] reported that 0.7% of 1000 cats in the Columbus, Ohio area passed *T. gondii* oocysts in their feces.

Definitive and Intermediate Hosts

The hosts of *T. gondii* are numerous (*vide supra*). The host in which the sexual cycle occurs is considered the definitive host and includes several members of the family Felidae. The domestic cat seems to be the true host of *T. gondii*. The jaguarundi and ocelot, bobcat, Asian leopard cat, and mountain lion[11,12] have been experimentally infected with cysts and have shed oocysts. It is likely that other Felidae can support the sexual cycle of *T. gondii*.

In addition to being able to support the enteroepithelial proliferative cycle and the formation of gametes leading to oocyst formation, cats also support the proliferation of tachyzoites and bradyzoites as in the other intermediate hosts. Cats are thus considered complete hosts of *T. gondii*.

The hosts in which only the asexual cycle of *T. gondii* occurs are considered the intermediate hosts. The asexual stages appear to be capable of infecting all warm-blooded animals, mammals, marsupials, and birds. Poikilothermic vertebrates can also be infected if their body temperature is raised high enough. The number of intermediate hosts of *T. gondii* is so extensive that a listing would be as extensive as a zoological catalogue. This has been reviewed by Jira and Kozojed.[13]

Disease in Animals

Toxoplasmosis in animals is usually asymptomatic. *T. gondii* can live in the cytoplasm of a large variety of cells of several species of mammals including man, birds, some reptiles, and perhaps amphibians. The actively multiplying organisms called tachyzoites (endozoites, the proliferative forms) reproduce, and groups of 8 to 32 tachyzoites are often seen by the time the infected host cell is destroyed. If cells of the host regenerate at a reasonably fast rate so that little or no cell loss occurs as a result of the destruction of the parasitized cells, the infection may remain asymptomatic. Whenever the parasitized cells are destroyed faster than they can be replaced, disease results, and the manifestations depend on the tissues and organs involved.[58]

It is useful to discuss the disease in relation to three sequential stages of infection. In the acute stage, the parasites multiply and spread via the blood stream to the various tissues in which they can grow. In infection of more than 1 or 2 weeks duration, the subacute stage ensues. Parasitemia diminishes, and it is rare that organisms continue to be found in the blood. There is a diminution in the extent to which the extraneural tissues harbor the proliferating organisms. Cysts containing bradyzoites (cystozoites) usually develop whch sometimes persist for months or years. This chronic stage is usually asymptomatic. However, rupture of the cysts sometimes may give rise to symptoms due to the accompanying hypersensitivity.

Acute Toxoplasmosis

This form is generally acquired by ingestion, in carnivores usually by cysts from another infected animal, and in herbivores by oocysts from cat feces. The small intestine is the first site of acute infection with tachyzoites (endozoites). The organism multiplies in the mucosa. The epithelial lining is sometimes destroyed leading to flattening of villi and occasionally ulceration. But in cats, a special cyclic development occurs in the epithelial cells. This developmental sequence appears to be synchronized with the production of new enteroepithelial cells since in spite of millions of oocysts developing, few or no lesions are ordinarily present. Nevertheless, diarrhea has been observed clinically.

From the intestine, the organisms spread via the bloodstream and the lymphatics to other organs. Intense proliferation by tachyzoites may lead to lymphadenitis and splenitis with necrosis. The liver may show focal, and rarely extensive, necrosis with groups of organisms in the adjacent hepatocytes. The lungs provide a good substrate for the multiplication of organisms leading to interstitial and alveolar pneumonia which is the most common cause of death during the acute stage of the infection. Small focal lesions may occur in the brain, eye, myocardium, and skeletal muscle.

As a rule, however, immunity develops after a week to 10 days, with subsidence of lesions. Immunity depends on the antibody which affects the extracellular organisms, and on cellular immunity which affects the intracellular organisms. Because most of the organisms are in an intracellular location and they migrate directly from one cell to another, cellular immunity in toxoplasmosis is most important. Lymphocytes that are specifically sensitized mediate cellular immunity. However, they are usually insufficient to eliminate all the organisms from a host, and *T. gondii* cysts generally persist leading to the chronic latent infection.

Subacute Toxoplasmosis

This stage of infection is characterized by progressive encephalitis with subsiding lesions in the extraneural viscera. The infection continues to progress because immunity develops more slowly in the brain than in the extraneural tissues. Similarly, ocular lesions usually of the retina may also be progressive. Occasionally there are progressive adrenocortical lesions since the presence of local hypercorticism inhibits the expression of immunity.[58]

Chronic Toxoplasmosis

This is usually without symptoms because cysts persist for months or years, and even their slow attrition may not lead to symptoms. Occasionally, with heavy infections, clinically significant lesions do result from cyst-rupture in the brain, eye, and myocardium. Although in many animal species chronic infection is the rule, in cattle it is short-lived, lasting sometimes only from 2 to 6 months based on subinoculation of tissues.[59,60]

Reactivation

With the disappearance of immunity either due to advancing age, or as a consequence of treatment with corticosteroids and cytostatic agents, tachyzoites may resume proliferation generally giving rise to more advanced lesions than are seen in the fatal acute disease.[61] Depending on the animal species, encephalitis, pneumonia, pancreatitis, or other lesions may be most prominent.

Disease in Specific Animals

In cats and other felines, little or no disease has been attributed to the enteroepithelial cycle other than diarrhea. However, young kittens may develop symptoms of generalized disease with fever, dyspnea, pneumonia, bilirubinemia, hepatitis, mesenteric adenitis, and encephalitis. In old cats, the syndrome of enteric myositis with intestinal obstruction has been described.[62,63,64] Iritis and chorioretinitis have been observed occasionally.[65,66] In cats treated with corticosteroids, pancreatitis, intestinal myositis and pneumonia and hepatitis were prominent.[67,68]

Dogs (and foxes) infected with *T. gondii* most frequently show disease manifestations such as pneumonia, hepatitis, and encephalitis.[69] Enteritis with ulceration and mesenteric adenitis have also been observed. Congenital infection is usually associated with central nervous system symptoms.[70] Abortion has rarely been ascribed to toxoplasmosis in dogs.[71] Concomitant infection with the virus of canine distemper appears to occur frequently, giving rise to prolonged illness characterized by encephalitis and pneumonia.[70,72] Also, concurrent infection with hookworm larvae may accentuate the severity of toxoplasmosis.[73] Toxoplasmosis has been observed in some dogs submitted for rabies examination.[74]

Sheep have most frequently been found infected after intrauterine transmission occurring in an endemic or epidemic situation.[75,76,77] Although in the ewe the infection is asymptomatic, abortion consequent to *T. gondii* placentitis and encephalitis of lambs is common in certain herds presumably exposed to cat feces contaminated with oocysts.[32,78] Chronically infected sheep do not transmit the infection.[77] The placental lesions consist of necrotic cotyledons appearing as white flecks containing actively multiplying *T. gondii* organisms.[79] Occasionally, ewes may succumb to secondary bacterial infection following abortion where parts of the fetal membranes are retained. The lambs have an unsteady gait, and histologically show leukoencephalitis. Lesions of lesser importance, such as pneumonia, are also observed. Some lambs may survive the infection.

Pigs, especially young or suckling pigs, develop fever, pneumonia, hepatitis, and ulcerative enteritis when infected transplacentally or after the ingestion of oocysts. The illness may be prolonged with fever, loss of weight, weakness, and respiratory symptoms, leading to ataxia and sometimes paralysis with encephalitis as cause of death.[80,81,82] Chorioretinitis has also been observed.[83]

Horses have been erroneously diagnosed as suffering from toxoplasmic encephalitis,[84,85,86] the causative organism being apparently a stage of another sporozoan. No illness from bona fide toxoplasmosis in horses is known to us. However, a low prevalence of antibody has been described.[87]

Cattle generally have asymptomatic infections. Rarely, fever, apathy, and failure to gain weight have been described,[59] and encephalitis has been reported after neonatal infection.[88] The duration of chronic infection appears to be limited. In one sequential study, organisms have been recovered from six out of six calves up to 38 days, but in only 1 out of 11 calves between 49 and 230 days; while in another, for over 100 days.[59,60] Antibodies have been observed to reach a peak titer in the third week (by dye test) or fourth week (by IFA test). But they were reported to fall to low levels or become negative after 3 to 4 months, at which time no organisms could be isolated from some cows.

Rabbits and hares have been observed with toxoplasmic hepatitis, lymphadenitis, and pneumonia, often accompanied by encephalitis. In more slowly progressing disease, encephalitis may be the prominent lesion which is accompanied by lymphoreticular hyperplasia.[89,90,91]

Chinchillas have been observed infected with *T. gondii* in an endemic situation.[92] Some animals died with generalized symptoms of pneumonia and hepatitis, others with encephalitis.

Mink develop generalized fatal toxoplasmosis, and abortion has been linked with this disease.[44] Ferrets inoculated with tissues from dogs with distemper sometimes develop generalized toxoplasmosis.[93]

Kangaroos and wallabies, mostly in zoos, but occasionally in the wild, develop clinical toxoplasmosis with symptoms of rhinitis, apathy, dyspnea, and paralysis. Pneumonia, encephalitis, and adrenal necrosis were the main lesions observed at necropsy.[91,94-96]

Neotropical monkeys, such as *Lagothrix, Saguinus, Ateles,* and *Callithrix,* have been reported to die with generalized toxoplasmosis after a brief illness.[97] Hepatitis and pneumonia were the most prominent lesions observed. In experimental infections with oocysts, incubation periods of as short as 9 days have been observed in *Saguinus* with the formation of very numerous tachyzoites. In Old World monkeys, on the other hand, infection rarely leads to illness. When it does, the disease tends to be more prolonged with the development of encephalitis.[98,99]

Hyrax appear to be prone to develop illness when they become infected with *T. gondii* causing generalized lesions.[100,101]

Pigeons initially develop disseminated infection with advanced lesions occurring in the brain, choroid, and conjunctiva.[102] Epidemics have been observed in carrier pigeons, although asymptomatic infection is more frequent.

Chickens infected with *T. gondii* rarely develop illness. However, a few instances of encephalitis have been reported.[103,39]

Sporadic outbreaks of toxoplasmosis have been described in many birds.[13] In many of these, the nature of the infecting organism is uncertain since hemogregarines and tissue stages resembling those of *Isospora serini*[104] and others have been mistaken for *T. gondii*. Isolation of the infectious agent in a laboratory animal and experimental reproduction of the disease may be necessary to establish that the original illness was caused by *T. gondii*. However, the presence of asymptomatic infection may provide a source of confusion, making it necessary to relate organisms to the lesion observed in sections. The fact that some birds do not develop dye test or IFA antibody is a source of frustration if one attempts to depend on a serologic diagnosis of lesions associated with small sporozoa.[12] Subinoculation to small rodents, however, permits the use of antibody development as a diagnostic aid, if the infection does not follow an acute, fatal course.

Zoo animals have been found infected with *T. gondii* not infrequently. This may be manifest merely by the presence of antibody.[105] Reports of sporadic illness or deaths from toxoplasmosis in zoo animals have been summarized by Hilgenfeld.[46]

Mice, hamsters, rabbits, young rats, multimammate rats, and canaries often develop acute fatal toxoplasmosis. Adult rats and guinea pigs more often develop an asymptomatic infection. But there has been limited work conducted employing standardized methods of infection such as the use of different *T. gondii* isolates and controlled dose of inoculum. The intraperitoneal inoculation of mice and hamsters still appears to be the most practical laboratory technique for demonstration of the parasite; often the animals will show *T. gondii* in their peritoneal fluid after 4 to 5 days. If negative, the animals are serologically tested after one month for *T. gondii* antibody. It has been claimed that some strains of mice, gerbils, multimammate rats, and canaries are especially susceptible to small inocula.[106] Certain strains of mice appear to be more susceptible than others.[107]

Of special interest are animal models of human disease. Retinochoroiditis develops in some hamsters after peripheral inoculation[108] and in rabbits after direct inoculation into the eye.[109] Immunosuppression with corticosteroids, cyclophosphamides, and other agents leads to relapsing toxoplasmosis in hamsters.[61] Adrenal necrosis and the equivalent of Addison's disease have been observed in hamsters with chronic toxoplasmosis.[110,111]

Cold-blooded animals have been reported to be hosts for *T. gondii*. Experimentally infected amphibia and reptiles usually remained asymptomatic, except for skinks, *Eumeces anthracinus,* which died of the infection.[112] Reports of experimental infections in amphibia have been negative. However, natural infections described from amphibia showed the presence of large cysts with lesions in the brain. Such parasites have been classified as *T. gondii* on the basis of morphology and for purposes of documentation. Nothing is known about their life cycles. There is no evidence, however, that they are biologically related to *T. gondii.*

Disease in Man

T. gondii infection is usually asymptomatic in adult humans and often so in children. As in animals, clinical illness results if destruction of affected cells is not compensated by regeneration and leads to anatomic or functional lesions. The manifestations of clinical toxoplasmosis depend on the tissues or organs involved. As in animal toxoplasmosis, it is useful to classify human toxoplasmosis into an acute, subacute, and a chronic form of infection which may either be asymptomatic or accompanied by illness. In addition, the illness may result from relapse.[58]

Acute Toxoplasmosis

In acute primary infection there is an active, generalized proliferation of tachyzoites (endozoites) which may be accompanied by such symptoms as fever, malaise, rash, pneumonia, myocarditis, hepatitis, lymphadenopathy, and rarely encephalitis. Necrosis of parasitized cells and a mononuclear reaction are characteristically present. Pneumonia and encephalitis are most likely to be fatal. Symptoms of acute infection are usually terminated by the development of immunity. Lymphocytosis and lymph node enlargement sometimes occur at this time as a result of the hyperplasia of lymphoreticular cells that are concerned wih immunity. Persistance of *T. gondii* cysts leading to a chronic latent stage of infection is common. Women who acquire the infection during pregnancy may transmit it to their infant in utero although they themselves are asymptomatic. According to Desmonts and Couvreur,[113] 34% of mothers who became infected during pregnancy transmitted the infection to their babies. Acute congenital infection in the newborn may be characterized by all of the signs described (*vide supra*) and is designated as congenital toxoplasmosis of the visceral type. It is usually, however, accompanied by encephalomyelitis and retinochoroiditis as well.

Subacute Toxoplasmosis

This clinical form of toxoplasmosis is frequently seen in the newborn. Infection of the fetus is accompanied, or soon followed, by the passive transfer of antibody which delays the hematogenous dissemination of the *T. gondii* organism. The development of active immunity by the fetus and the newborn is slow because of immaturity of their immunologic mechanism. As a consequence, illness in the neonate tends to be prolonged, affecting especially the brain and eye where expression of immunity is more difficult. Pneumonia, jaundice, and hepatitis have been observed in 21 to 54% of 152 infected newborn children and signs of encephalitis (abnormal spinal fluid) and retinochoroiditis in 69 to 80%.[114] Convulsions have been observed in 34%, hydrocephalus in 14%, and intracerebral calcifications in 27%. The extraneural lesions are similar to those seen in acute toxoplasmosis, but possibly less severe. Lesions observed in the brain of children affected with neonatal toxoplasmosis are usually of four types: (1) formation of microglial nodules as a result of the destruction of individual cells by the tachyzoites; (2) scattered areas of infarction necrosis resulting from thrombosis of cortical blood vessels which are usually involved by proliferating parasites; (3) ependymal ulceration with periaqueductal and periventricular vasculitis and infarction necrosis resulting in the occlusion of the aqueduct of Sylvius and the development of an internal hydrocephalus; and (4) tissue necrosis associated with delayed hypersensitivity following rupture of a *T. gondii* cyst.[58,115]

Chronic Toxoplasmosis

Chronic infection with *T. gondii* cysts generally persists for months or years. This is suggested by the persistent antibody titer, by occasional clinical symptoms and reactivated disease, and by analogy with experimental infection in animals. Usually, chronic infections are asymptomatic and accompanied by adequate immunity of the premunition type. Intact cysts are not harmful, but rupture of a cyst is usually accompanied by tissue necrosis as consequential to a delayed hypersensitivity reaction which occurs in most infected individuals. Rupture of a cyst in the retina especially is likely to be accompanied by symptoms because of necrosis of the retina and the inflammatory reaction in the vitreous obscuring the infected individual's vision. Most of the retinal lesions are self-limiting, leaving small scars, and all of the liberated organisms are destroyed. Occasionally, lesions become progressive, and this is believed to be due to a deficient local immunity with tachyzoites resuming proliferation.[108] Such lesions in the retina may progress to blindness if untreated.[117,118] Occasional instances of myocarditis, myositis, and encephalitis have been attributed to cyst rupture and, perhaps, to limited proliferation of *T. gondii*.[119-122]

Reactivated Toxoplasmosis

This form of toxoplasmosis occurs usually in immunosuppressed patients such as those receiving organ transplants, or being treated for lymphomas, leukemias and other neoplasms, or lupus erythematosus.[123] Encephalitis is the most common manifestation, and also the most life-threatening, with myocarditis, myositis, and pneumonia also being observed.[124] Recently, multifocal retinochoroiditis was observed to arise in a patient with an undiagnosed hematologic disease treated systematically with 4 to 35 replacement doses of corticosteroids over a 9-month period.[125] Under local immunosuppressive treatment with respiratory corticoids injected under the Tenon's capsule, retinitis progressed to loss of vision. At autopsy, tachyzoites of *T. gondii* were found to give rise to focal retinal necrosis with little inflammatory reaction. Cysts were scattered throughout the normal retina. Focal *T. gondii* encephalitis has been observed also in immunosuppressed humans and hamsters, some of which also showed focal pneumonia.[61] These lesions are of interest for their focal nature, suggesting that they have originated from a single cyst that disintegrated, liberating the organisms which then entered and multiplied in adjacent cells, eventually forming a grossly visible necrotic focus with a peripheral swarm of tachyzoites. The immunosuppression apparently abolishes local cellular immunity. However, antibody effects probably remain intact inasmuch as there are usually no lesions at a distance which can be ascribed to hematogenous dissemination.

Mode of Spread

The most general mode of spread of toxoplasmosis depends on the presence of the oocysts, which are produced only by the intestinal stages in the cat and the other members of the family Felidae. It is important to note that the intestinal cycle in the cat produces a million-fold increase in the number of infective forms. Oocysts can infect the cat and its relatives, and also all of the hosts in which only the asexual stages of the parasite develop.

There is a method of spread which does not involve the oocyst. Toxoplasmosis can be perpetuated among carnivorous and omnivorous animals by cannibalism or by poor animal husbandry practices, similar to those which occur in *Trichinella spiralis* and *Capillaria hepatica* infections. Cannibalism in rodents would keep the asexual cycle of *T. gondii* going not only in rodents but also in dogs and other animals, including hawks, etc. that prey on rodents. The practice of feeding garbage to swine would undoubtedly maintain toxoplasmosis in swine in the absence of oocysts. The occurrence of toxoplasmosis in human beings could be the result of the ingestion of infected pork.[57] Indeed, the existence of the sexual cycle in the cat, with the production of oocysts, is inadequate to explain all of the transmission of toxoplasmosis in human beings.

Infected cat feces are a durable source of infection and difficult to dispose of adequately. Depending on humidity, the oocysts in the soil persist for weeks or months to a year and a half.[141] Oocysts have been shown to survive two Kansas winters and a summer.[55] The habit of cats to defecate near their natural habitat increases the concentration of oocysts in yards and sandpiles near houses. The feline habit of covering their feces enhances the survival of oocysts since the humidity is greater underground than on the surface.

Epidemiology

It is clear that the entire life cycle of *T. gondii* requires the cat. In areas where cats are nonexistent, such as certain Pacific Islands, toxoplasmosis is also lacking.[126-128] Where the cat is present, a variety of factors affect the distribution of *T. gondii* in animals and man. For example, in New Zealand and in England, abortion due to *T. gondii* occurs in ewes which are brought in from the fields and kept close to the farmstead prior to the lambing season.[129,130] The opportunity for fecal contamination of feed by cats is enhanced by this type of husbandry. The occurrence of toxoplasmosis among human beings differs from one country to another depending on customs. Desmonts et al.[131] have associated a rapid rate of seroconversion from dye test negative to positive in a group of hospitalized tubercular children with the fact that these patients were fed undercooked meat, such as mutton. They believe that the high incidence of toxoplasmosis in France is connected with the common practice of eating rare meat. In the U.S. the increasing prevalence of *T. gondii* antibodies in the population with increasing age suggests also that rare meat may be a source of infection; this same pattern formerly occurred in trichinosis. On the other hand, in England, where the prevalence rate beyond age 20 levels off, one can assume that infection probably results more frequently from contact with soil contaminated with *T. gondii* oocysts. The same is probably true in many tropical countries where meat is usually eaten well done, and where sanitation may well leave something to be desired. The practice in some European countries, and in some parts of the U.S., of eating raw pork sausage is certainly a possible source of toxoplasmosis.

The characteristics of the oocyst are of great importance in the epidemiology of toxoplasmosis. Like those of the other coccida, *T. gondii* oocysts are quite resistant to the external environment, but they are sensitive to drying and heat. Hutchison[53] originally reported that the infective forms of the parasite could survive for up to 17 months in water after separation from cat feces. In untreated fecal material, the infectivity of the oocysts persisted for 14 days at a relative humidity ranging from 22 to 44% and for 18 days at 80% relative humidity. After being dried completely over concentrated sulfuric acid, oocysts may remain viable for about 2 days. However, clean oocysts, washed out of fecal material, were destroyed by drying in less than 24 hr. Oocysts of *T. gondii* remained infectious for as long as 51 weeks in three shaded areas, one relatively dry and two moist. The shortest persistence of infectivity was 8 weeks in a partially sunny area, and 10 weeks in a moist forest shade. Fecal deposits from cats placed in exposed soil in Kansas remained infectious for at least 18 months. Slugs and sow bugs may move *T. gondii* oocysts out of the soil onto vegetation. Earthworms may acquire oocysts because they ingest soil. Thus there appear to be ample means by which oocysts can be acquired by herbivorous animals, birds, and man either from contaminated soil, plants contaminated by various invertebrates, or from invertebrates that are attracted to fecal deposits.

Cold inhibits sporulation of oocysts and unsporulated oocysts are killed in from 1 to 7 days of constant freezing. Sporulated oocysts can survive constant freezing at −20°C for 28 days.

Diagnosis

Diagnosis of toxoplasmosis must be made by a consistent pattern of findings appropriate to the stage of infection, viz. acute, subacute, chronic, or reactivated. These findings usually consist of two or more of the following: serology, isolation, microscopic demonstration of the organisms in smear or section, or demonstration of the oocyst in the feces of cats. Serologic examination is best carried out by means of paired serum specimens taken one or more weeks apart which are compared in parallel series in a single serologic test. The indirect fluorescent antibody (IFA) test[132] is sensitive and specific, but requires the appropriate fluorescein-labeled antispecies globulin free of antibody to *T. gondii*.[136] The dye test (DT)[133,134] is more versatile, and requires human serum without antibody as accessory factor, but has an added disadvantage of requiring the use of live organisms. An agglutination test[135] requires large numbers of organisms but no additional serum. The indirect hemagglutination test (IHA)[132] is widely used but does not become positive as early as the DT or IFA. Complement-fixation tests and a precipitin test in agar have been described. Recently, an enzyme-linked immunosorbent assay (ELISA) has been perfected which can be quantitated more sensitively than the IFA test.[136] For the best available tests, current literature should be consulted.

Typical serologic findings can be interpreted as follows. If the antibody titers in paired serum specimens rise by three or four tubes, this can be taken as presumptive evidence of concurrently active toxoplasmosis. If antibody is absent in both specimens, *T. gondii* can be excluded as an etiologic agent in the disease process observed. Likewise, in the presence of a stable antibody titer, toxoplasmosis can be excluded if the symptoms of the illness are acute. Subacute toxoplasmosis is associated with high stable or rising titers in a newborn infant; however, maternal antibody transferred passively has a half-life of 1 month, and a tenfold drop in titer can be expected every 3 months in the absence of infection.[137] Because IgM is not placentally transferred, the IgM-IFA test demonstrates the antibody developed by an infant, indicating infection rather than passively transferred antibody. Chronic toxoplasmosis is typically accompanied by a stable low antibody titer; retinochoroiditis is usually found in this category.[138] In reactivated toxoplasmosis, the antibody titer tends to rise probably because antibody-forming B-cells are less affected by immunosuppression than T-cells mediating cellular immunity.

Of great interest are infants with possible subclinical infections because they can be treated in an attempt to prevent retinal and brain damage. A febrile, respiratory illness in a pregnant woman, premature birth, low birth weight, and an increase in cells and protein of the spinal fluid are indications for serologic testing in an effort to detect subclinical infection.

For the proper interpretation of antibody titers in animals, the serologic responses of the various animal species should be known from experimental infections. For example, dogs develop antibody titers similar to those in humans. However, peak titers developed by cats are much lower, and the antibody appears later.[52] Some birds such as chickens, crows, Japanese quail, and bluejays do not develop bivalent antibody, and therefore the DT and IFA test are not useful.[12] A complement fixation inhibition test was devised to measure *T. gondii* antibody in infected chickens.[139] Pigeons, however, develop a good antibody response.

Isolation of *T. gondii* is carried out best by the inoculation of mice. After intraperitoneal injection, exudate may be formed in which the crescentic tachyzoites (endozoites) may be seen after 4 to 6 days. If no organisms are found, the exudate together with portions of spleen, liver, lungs, and lymph nodes can be subinoculated every 4 days into fresh mice (before immunity develops) to raise the level of organisms to one that is visible on smears and sections. Mice that die after 10 days should be examined for the presence of cysts in the brain using both fresh squash preparations or permanently stained smears or sections. Cysts are easily seen after about 4 to 8 weeks, and the periodic acid-Schiff technique facilitates their recognition.

Usually after 14 days infected mice would have developed antibody. The demonstration of the appearance of antibody in a group of mice (that was seronegative before, or that came from seronegative stock) is presumptive evidence of isolation. Since many *T. gondii* isolates are nonpathogenic to mice, serodiagnosis is the most practical diagnostic method to use. This should be complemented by the demonstration of cysts. Cysts can frequently be identified microscopically in seropositive mice in preparations of snips of brain crushed in saline by pressure of a coverslip on a slide. Microscopic demonstration of the organisms can also be based on smears stained with Giemsa, or sections stained with hematoxylin and eosin.

Demonstration of the *T. gondii* oocyst in cat feces is carried out by one of the flotation methods, using a solution of sp gr 1.15 (53 g cane sugar, 100 m*l* water, and 0.8% wt/vol of phenol as a preservative). A zinc sulfate solution of sp gr 1.1 can also be used. Fecal material is mixed with the flotation solution and then centrifuged. Most of the fecal material will sink to the bottom of the tube, while the oocysts, if present, will float to the surface.[140] Sporulation can then be carried out in the 2% sulfuric acid.[140]

Prevention and Control

As shown in Figure 2, toxoplasmosis is transmitted *principally* via the feces of cats deposited in soil, by the ingestion of meat of infected animals, and *more rarely,* by placental transfer, blood transfusion, and *possibly* through the infected mother's milk. The common mode of transmission is by ingestion, either of oocysts or of meat. Be-

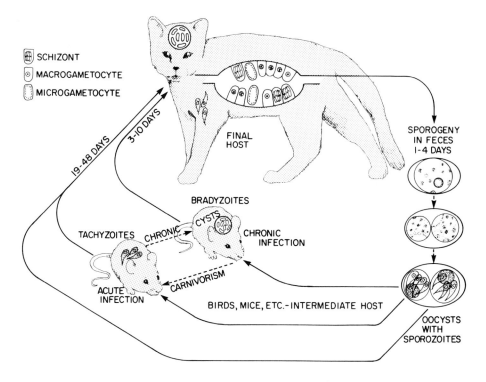

FIGURE 2.   *Toxoplasma gondii* life cycle.

cause cats can shed several million oocysts capable of infecting a similar number of animals or humans, cats are of pivotal importance in the dissemination of toxoplasmosis. Much of the prevention is directed toward avoidance of the infection of cats to preclude their contaminating the environment with large numbers of oocysts.

Cats are infected mainly by the ingestion of *T. gondii* cysts from infected intermediate hosts. After an interval of 3 to 10 days, oocyst shedding begins which lasts usually 1 or 2 weeks. Prevention of infection in cats depends on the control of the cat's diet. Cats kept indoors and fed dried, canned, or cooked food have little opportunity to become infected. Stray and free-roaming cats usually acquire infection from preying on rodents and birds, and because they defecate, unobserved, in sand or soil, contamination is not easily controlled.

Many types of meat, most frequently pork and mutton, have been found to contain *T. gondii* cysts, and the opportunity for exposure depends on the frequency with which raw meat is handled and raw or undercooked meat is eaten. Hands should be washed after handling raw meat. Meat should be cooked throughout to over 60°C to ensure that *T. gondii* is killed. Although freezing causes a sharp reduction of viable organisms, it cannot be depended upon to kill all cysts.

Flies and cockroaches have served as experimental vectors of oocysts and should be controlled. Destruction of oocysts in cat feces or on the soil, could be achieved using boiling water or dry heat which are the only quick, dependable means for disinfection. Chemicals are not effective enough in destroying oocysts. However, most chemical disinfectants, such as alcohol and even soap and water may destroy the cyst forms of *T. gondii* that may be encountered in handling raw meat.

Preventive methods can be summarized as follows:

1.   Feed cat only dried, canned, or cooked meat.
2.   Keep cat from hunting birds and mice.

3. Change litter boxes daily; disinfect them with boiling water.
4. If pregnant, wear plastic gloves or delegate maintenance of cat to someone else.
5. Use work gloves when working in soil contaminated by cat feces.
6. Cover children's sandboxes when not in use.
7. Control of stray cats.
8. Control of flies and cockroaches.
9. Avoid eating raw meat; heat all meat to over 66°C, or until color changes.
10. Wash hands before meals; do not put dirty hands to the face or mouth.

REFERENCES

1. **Levine, N. D.**, *Protozoan Parasites of Domestic Animals and of Man*, 2nd ed., Burgess, Minneapolis, 1973.
2. **Dubey, J. P. and Frenkel, J. K.**, Cyst-induced toxoplasmosis in cats, *J. Protozool.*, 19, 155, 1972.
3. **Piekarski, G., Pelster, B., and Witte, H. M.**, Endopolygeny in *Toxoplasma gondii*, *Z. Parasitenkd.*, 36, 122, 1971.
4. **Pelster, B. and Piekarski, G.**, Elektronenmikroskopische Analyse der Mikrogametenentwicklung bei *Toxoplasma gondii*, *Z. Parasitenkd.*, 37, 267, 1971.
5. **Jacobs, L. and Melton, M.**, *Toxoplasma* and toxoplasmosis, *Ann. Rev. Microbiol.*, 17, 429, 1963.
6. **Levine, N. D. and Nye, R. R.**, *Toxoplasma ranae* sp. n. from the leopard frog *Rana pipiens* Linnaeus, *J. Protozool.*, 23(4), 488, 1976.
7. **Goldman, M., Carver, R. K., and Sulzer, A. J.**, Reproduction of *Toxoplasma gondii* by internal budding, *J. Parasitol.*, 44(2), 161, 1958.
8. **Frenkel, J. K.**, Toxoplasmosis: parasite life cycle, pathology, and immunology, in *The Coccidia, Eimeria, Isospora, Toxoplasma, and Related Genera*, Hammond, D. M. and Long, P. L., Eds., University Park Press, Baltimore, 1973, 343.
9. **Hoare, C. A.**, The developmental stages of Toxoplasma, *J. Trop. Med. Hyg.*, 75, 56, 1972.
10. **Jacobs, L., Remington, J. S., and Melton, M. L.**, The resistance of the encysted form of *Toxoplasma gondii*, *J. Parasitol.*, 46(1), 11, 1960.
11. **Jewell, M. L., Frenkel, J. K., Johnson, K. M., Reed, V., and Ruiz, A.**, Development of *Toxoplasma* oocysts in neotropical Felidae, *Am. J. Trop. Med. Hyg.*, 21, 512, 1972.
12. **Miller, N. L., Frenkel, J. K., and Dubey, J. P.**, Oral infections with *Toxoplasma* cysts and oocysts in felines, other mammals, and in birds, *J. Parasitol.*, 58(4), 928, 1972.
13. **Jira, J. and Kozojed, V.**, *Toxoplasmosis 1908—1967*, Vol. 1,2, Fischer Verlag, Stuttgart, 1970.
14. **Walton, B. C., Arjona, I., and Benchoff, B.**, Relationship of *Toxoplasma* antibodies to altitude, *Am. J. Trop. Med. Hyg.*, 15(4), 492, 1966.
15. **Feldman, H. A.**, A nationwide serum survey of United States military recruits, *Am. J. Epidemiol.*, 81(3), 385, 1965.
16. **Feldman, H. A. and Sabin, A. B.**, Skin reactions to *Toxoplasma* antigens in people of different ages without known history of infection, *Pediatrics*, 4, 798, 1949.
17. **Beverley, J. K. A., Beattie, C. P., and Roseman, C.**, Human *Toxoplasma* infection, *J. Hyg.*, 52, 37, 1954.
18. **Wallace, G. D.**, The prevalence of toxoplasmosis on Pacific islands, and the influence of ethnic group, *Am. J. Trop. Med. Hyg.*, 25(1), 48, 1976.
19. **Remington, J. S., Efron, B., Cavanaugh, E., Simon, H. J., and Trejos, A.**, Studies on toxoplasmosis in El Salvador: prevalence and incidence of toxoplasmosis as measured by the Sabin-Feldman dye test, *Trans. R. Soc. Trop. Med. Hyg.*, 64(2), 252, 1970.
20. **Lunde, M. and Jacobs, L.**, Results of dye and hemagglutination tests for toxoplasmosis in a survey of Trinidad natives, *Am. J. Trop. Med.*, 7, 523, 1958.
21. **Siim, J. C., Biering-Sorensen, U., and Moller, T.**, Toxoplasmosis in domestic animals, *Adv. Vet. Sci.*, 8, 335, 1963.
22. **Jacobs, L.**, Toxoplasmosis in man and animals, *N. Z. Vet. J.*, 9, 85, 1961.
23. **Beverley, J. K. A. and Watson, W. A.**, Ovine abortion and toxoplasmosis in Yorkshire, *Vet. Rec.*, 73(1), 6, 1961.
24. **Jacobs, L. and Melton, M. L.**, A procedure for testing meat samples for *Toxoplasma* with preliminary results of a survey of pork samples, *J. Parasitol.*, 43, 38, 1957.

25. Nobuto, K., Hanaki, T., Koizumi, T., and Yonemochi, K., Some aspects of natural infection of toxoplasmosis in pigs, *Natl. Inst. Anim. Health Q.*, 9, 136, 1969.

26. Jacobs, L., Remington, J. S., and Melton, M. L., A survey of meat samples from swine, cattle, and sheep for the presence of encysted *Toxoplasma, J. Parasitol.*, 46(1), 23, 1960.

27. Jacobs, L., Moyle, G. G., and Ris, R. R., The prevalence of toxoplasmosis in New Zealand sheep and cattle, *Am. J. Vet. Res.*, 24(101), 673, 1963.

28. Mayer, H. F., Primeros aislamientos de *Toxoplasma gondii* de retina de bovinos, *Ann. Inst. Med. Reg.*, 6(1/2), 25, 1962/63.

29. Zardi, O., Sulli, E., and Venditti, G., Studi epidemiologici sulla toxoplasmosi. Isolamento de stipiti di *Toxoplasma gondii* da animali domestici, *Nuovi Ann. Ig.*, 15, 545, 1964.

30. Feldman, H. A. and Miller, L. T., Serological study of toxoplasmosis prevalence, *Am. J. Hyg.*, 64, 320, 1956.

31. Sogandares-Bernal, F., Marchiondo, A. A., Duszynski, D. W., and Ward, J. K., Prevalence of *Toxoplasma* antibodies in range vs. dairy cattle from the Bitterroot Valley of Montana, *J. Parasitol.*, 61(5), 965, 1975.

32. Penkert, R. A., Possible spread of toxoplasmosis by feed contaminated by cats, *J. Am. Vet. Assoc.* 162(11), 924, 1973.

33. Catar, G., Bergendi, L., and Holkova, R., Isolation of *Toxoplasma gondii* from swine and cattle, *J. Parasitol.*, 55(5), 952, 1969.

34. Janitschke, L., Weiland, G., and Rommel, M., Untersuchungen uber den Befall von Schlachtkalbern und schafen mit *Toxoplasma gondii, Die Fleischwirtschaft*, 47(2), 135, 1967.

35. Work, K., Isolation of *Toxoplasma gondii* from the flesh of sheep, swine, and cattle, *Acta. Pathol. Microbiol. Scand.*, 71(2), 296, 1967.

36. Berengo, A., de Lalla, E., Cavallini-Sampieri, L., Bechelli, G., and Cavallini, F., Prevalence of toxoplasmosis among domestic and wild animals in the area of Siena, Italy, *Am. J. Trop. Med. Hyg.*, 18(3), 391, 1969.

37. de Amaral, V. and Macrus, R., *Toxoplasma gondii:* isolamento de amostras a partir de diafragmas de suinos clinicamente sadios, abatidos em matadouros de Sao Paulo, Brazil, *Arq. Inst. Biol. Sao Paulo*, 36, 47, 1969.

38. Jamra, L. F., Deane, M. P., and Guimaraes, E. C., Isolation of *Toxoplasma gondii* from human food of animal origin. Partial results in the city of Sao Paulo, Brazil, *Rev. Inst. Med. Trop. Sao Paulo*, 11, 169, 1969.

39. Jacobs, L. and Melton, M. L., Toxoplasmosis in chickens, *J. Parasitol.*, 52(6), 1158, 1966.

40. Jacobs, L., Melton, M. L., and Jones, F. E., The prevalence of toxoplasmosis in wild pigeons, *J. Parasitol.*, 38(5), 457, 1952.

41. Johnson, C. M., Immunological and epidemiological investigations, *Ann. Rep. Gorgas Memorial Lab.*, p. 15, 1943.

42. Wiktor, T. J., Toxoplasmose animale; sur une épidémie des lapins et des pigeons a Stanleyville (Congo Belge), *Ann. Soc. Belge Med. Trop. (Bruxelles,)* 30(1), 97, 1950.

43. Hulland, T. J., Toxoplasmosis in Canada, *J. Am. Vet. Med. Assoc.*, 128, 74, 1956.

44. Fish, N. A., Toxoplasmosis: diagnosis by serological and cultural methods, *Can. J. Pub. Health*, 52, 107, 1961.

45. Jacobs, L. and Stanley, A. M., Prevalence of *Toxoplasma* antibodies in rabbits, squirrels, and raccoons collected in and near the Patuxent Wildlife Research Center, *J. Parasitol.*, 48(4), 550, 1962.

46. Hilgenfeld, M., Toxoplasmose bei Zootieren, *D. Zoolog. Garten*, 30(5), 262, 1965.

47. Jones, F. E., Eyles, D. E., and Gibson, C. L., The prevalence of toxoplasmosis in the domestic cat, *Am. J. Trop. Med. Hyg.*, 6(5), 820, 1957.

48. Jacobs, L., *Toxoplasma* and toxoplasmosis, *Adv. Parasitol.*, 5, 1, 1967.

49. Wallace, G. D., The role of the cat in the natural history of *Toxoplasma gondii, Am. J. Trop. Med. Hyg.*, 22(3), 313, 1973.

50. Janitschke, K. and Kühn, D., *Toxoplasma*-Oozysten im Kot naturlich infizierter Katzen, *Berl. Muench. Tierärztl. Wochenschr.*, 85, 46, 1972.

51. Dubey, J. P., Christie, E., and Pappas, P. W., Characterization of *Toxoplasma gondii* from the feces of naturally infected cats, *J. Infect. Dis.*, 136, 432, 1976.

52. Frenkel, J. K. and Dubey, J. P., Toxoplasmosis and its prevention in cats and man, *J. Infect. Dis.*, 126, 664, 1972.

53. Hutchison, W. M., The nematode transmission of *Toxoplasma gondii, Trans. R. Soc. Trop. Med. Hyg.*, 61(1), 80, 1967.

54. Dubey, J. P., Miller, N. L., and Frenkel, J. K., Characterization of the new fecal form of *Toxoplasma gondii, J. Parasitol.*, 56, 447, 1970.

55. Frenkel, J. K., Ruiz, A., and Chinchilla, M., Soil survival of *Toxoplasma* oocysts in Kansas and Costa Rica, *Am. J. Trop. Med. Hyg.*, 24, 439, 1975.

56. Frenkel, J. K. and Dubey, J. P., Effects of freezing on the viability of *Toxoplasma* oocysts, *J. Parasitol.*, 59(3), 587, 1973.

57. Weinman, D. and Chandler, A. H., Toxoplasmosis in man and swine — an investigation of the possible relationship, *JAMA*, 161(3), 229, 1956.

58. Frenkel, J. K., Toxoplasmosis. Mechanisms of infection, laboratory diagnosis and management, *Curr. Topics Pathol.*, 54, 28, 1971.

59. Rommel, M., Sommer, R., Janitschke, K., and Müller, I., Experimentelle *Toxoplasma* Infektionen bei Kälbern, *Berl. Muench. Tierarztl. Woschrschr.*, 79, 41, 1966.

60. Costa, A. J., Araujo, F. G., Costa, J. O., and Lima, J. D., Experimental infection of bovines with oocysts of *Toxoplasma gondii*, *J. Parasitol.*, 63, 212, 1977.

61. Frenkel, J. K., Nelson, B., and Arias-Stella, J., Immunosuppression and toxoplasmic encephalitis: clinical and experimental aspects, *Human Pathol.*, 6, 97, 1975.

62. Meier, H., Holzworth, J., and Griffiths, R. C., Toxoplasmosis in the cat — fourteen cases, *J. Am. Vet. Med. Assoc.*, 131(9), 395, 1957.

63. Petrak, M. and Carpenter, J., Feline toxoplasmosis, *J. Am. Vet. Med. Assoc.*, 146, 728, 1965.

64. Hirth, R. S. and Nielsen, S. W., Pathology of feline toxoplasmosis, *J. Small Anim. Pract.*, 10, 213, 1969.

65. Vainisi, S. J. and Campbell, L. H., Ocular toxoplasmosis in cats, *J. Am. Vet. Med. Assoc.*, 154(2), 141, 1969.

66. Piper, R. C., Cole, C. R., and Shadduck, J. A., Natural and experimental ocular toxoplasmosis in animals, *Am. J. Ophthalmol.*, 69, 662, 1970.

67. Smart, M. E., Downey, R. S., and Stockdale, P. H. G., Toxoplasmosis in a cat associated with cholangitis and progressive pancreatitis, *Can. Vet. J.*, 14(12), 313, 1973.

68. Dubey, J. P. and Frenkel, J. K., Immunity to feline toxoplasmosis: modification by administration of corticosteroids, *Vet. Pathol.*, 11(4), 350, 1974.

69. Capen, C. C. and Cole, C. R., Pulmonary lesions in dogs with experimental and naturally occuring toxoplasmosis, *Pathol. Vet.*, 3, 40, 1966.

70. Koestner, A. and Cole, C. R., Neuropathology of canine toxoplasmosis, *Am. J. Vet. Res.*, 21(84), 831, 1960.

71. Chamberlain, D. M., Docton, F. L., and Cole, C. R., Toxoplasmosis. II. Intra-uterine infection in dogs, premature birth, and presence of organisms in milk, *Proc. Soc. Exp. Biol. Med.*, 82, 198, 1953.

72. Campbell, R. S. F., Martin, W. B., and Gordon, E. D., Toxoplasmosis as a complication of canine distemper, *Vet. Rec.*, 67, 708, 1955.

73. Jacobs, L., Melton, M. L., and Cook, K., Observations on toxoplasmosis in dogs, *J. Parasitol.*, 41, 353, 1955.

74. Sanmartin, C. and Ayala, S. C., Toxoplasma in animals submitted for rabies diagnosis in Cali, Colombia, *Trans. Roy. Soc. Trop. Med. Hyg.*, 66, 799, 1972.

75. Hartley, W. J. and Marshall, S. C., Toxoplasmosis as a cause of ovine perinatal mortality, *N.Z. Vet. J.*, 5(4), 119, 1957.

76. Watson, W. A. and Beverley, J. K. A., Epizootics of toxoplasmosis causing ovine abortion, *Vet. Rec.*, 88, 120, 1971.

77. Hartley, W. J. and Moyle, G. G., Further observations on the epidemiology of ovine *Toxoplasma* infection, *Aust. J. Exp. Biol. Med. Sci.*, 52, 647, 1974.

78. Plant, J. W., Richardson, N., and Moyle, G. G., *Toxoplasma* infection and abortion in sheep associated wtih feeding of grain contaminated with cat feces, *Aust. Vet. J.*, 50(1), 19, 1974.

79. Hartley, W. J., Jebson, J. L., and McFarlane, D., Toxoplasmosis as a cause of perinatal mortality and abortion in sheep, *Aust. Vet. J.*, 30, 216, 1954.

80. Nobuto, K., Suzuki, K., Omuro, M., and Ishii, S., Studies on toxoplasmosis in domestic animals. Serological response of animals to experimental infection and successful application of complement fixation test for exposure of infected herds, *Bull. Natl. Inst. Anim. Health*, 40, 29, 1960.

81. Koestner, A. and Cole, C. R., Neuropathology of porcine toxoplasmosis, *Cornell Vet.*, 50, 362, 1960.

82. Møller, T., Fennestad, K. L., Eriksen, L., Work, K., and Siim, J. C., Experimental toxoplasmosis in pregnant sows. II. Pathological findings, *Acta. Pathol. Microbiol. Scand. A*, 78, 241, 1970.

83. Hansen, H-J. and Mostafa, I. E., Chorioretinitis in porcine toxoplasmosis, *Acta, Vet. Scand.*, 10, 292, 1969.

84. Cusick, P. K., Sells, D. M., Hamilton, D. P., and Hardenbrook, H. J., Toxoplasmosis in two horses, *J. Am. Vet. Med. Assoc.*, 165(3), 249, 1974.

85. Dubey, J. P., Davis, G. W., Koestner, A., and Kiryu, K., Equine encephalomyelitis due to a protozoan parasite resembling *Toxoplasma gondii*, *J. Am. Vet. Med. Assoc.*, 165(3), 249, 1974.

86. Beech, J. and Dodd, D. C., *Toxoplasma*-like encephalomyelitis in a horse, *Vet. Pathol.*, 11(1), 87, 1974.

87. **Riemann, H. P., Smith, A. T., Stormont, C., Ruppanner, R., Behymer, D. C., Suzuki, Y., Franti, C. E., and Verma, B. B.,** Equine toxoplasmosis: a survey for antibodies to *Toxoplasma gondii* in horses, *Am. J. Vet. Res.,* 36(12), 1797, 1975.

88. **Sanger, V. L., Chamberlain, D. M., Cole, C. R., and Farrell, R. L.,** Toxoplasmosis. V. Isolation of *Toxoplasma* from cattle, *J. Am. Vet. Med. Assoc.,* 123, 87, 1953.

89. **Møller, T.,** Toxoplasmosis cuniculi. Verificering af diagnosen, patologiskanatomiske og serologiske undersogelser, *Nord. Vet. Med.,* 10, 1, 1958.

90. **Møller, T.,** Toxoplasmosis. Studies on the route of infection and pathogenesis in domestic animals, *Acta Pathol. Microbiol. Scand.,* 51, 235, 1961.

91. **Møller, T.,** Three casuistic reports of toxoplasmosis in zoo animals (*Macropus benneti, Marmota marmota, Lepus timidus*), *Nord. Vet. Med.,* 14, 233, 1962.

92. **Keagy, H. F.,** *Toxoplasma* in the chinchilla, *J. Am. Vet. Med. Assoc.,* 114(862), 15, 1949.

93. **Coutelen, F.,** Existence d'une toxoplasmose spontanee et generalisee chez le furet. Un toxoplasme nouveau, *Toxoplasma laidlawi* n. sp., parasite de *Mustela (Putoris) putoris* var. *furo, C. R. Soc. Biol. (Paris),* 111, 284, 1932.

94. **Cook, J. and Pope, J. H.,** *Toxoplasma* in Queensland: a preliminary survey of animal hosts, *Aust. J. Exp. Biol. Med. Sci.,* 37, 253, 1953.

95. **Hilgenfeld, M.,** Zur pathologischen Anatomie und Histologie der Toxoplasmose beim Kanguruh, *Abh. Dtsch. Akad. Wiss. Berl. Med.,* 1, 113, 1966.

96. **Munday, B. L.,** Laboratory investigation of specimens from diseased and apparently normal free-living wild animals in Tasmania, *Tasm. Dept. Agr. Res. Bull.,* 5, 1, 1966.

97. **McKissick, G. E., Ratcliffe, H. L., and Koestner, A.,** Enzootic toxoplasmosis in caged squirrel monkeys *Saimiri sciureus, Pathol. Vet.,* 5(6), 538, 1968.

98. **Araumo, F. G., Wong, M. M., Theis, J., and Remington, J. S.,** Experimental *Toxoplasma gondii* infection in a nonhuman primate, *Am. J. Trop. Med. Hyg.,* 22, 465, 1973.

99. **Wong, M. M. and Kozek, W. J.,** Spontaneous toxoplasmosis in macaques: a report of four cases, *Lab. Anim. Sci.,* 24(2), 273, 1974.

100. **Ratcliffe, H. L. and Worth, C. B.,** Toxoplasmosis of captive wild birds and mammals, *Am. J. Pathol.,* 27(4), 655, 1951.

101. **Guillon, J. C., Mollaret, H., and Destombes, P.,** Constatation fortuite d'une infestation par *Toxoplasma gondii* chez un daman (Dendrohyrax), *Bull. Soc. Pathol. Exot.,* 54, 706, 1961.

102. **Jacobs, L., Melton, M. L., and Cook, M. K.,** Experimental toxoplasmosis in pigeons, *Exp. Parasitol.,* 2(4), 403, 1953.

103. **Nobrega, P., Trapp, E., and Giovannone, M.,** Toxoplasmose espontanea de galinha (Spontaneous toxoplasmosis in the domestic fowl), *Arquivos do Instit. Biol. Sao Paulo,* 22(6), 43, 1955.

104. **Box, E. D.,** Exogenous stages of *Isospora serini* (Aragao) and *Isospora canaria* sp. n. in the canary (*Serinus canarius Linnaeus*), *J. Protozool.,* 22(2), 165, 1975.

105. **Riemann, H. P., Behymer, D. E., Fowler, M. E., Schulz, T., Lock, A., Orthoefer, J. G., Silverman, S., and Franti, C. E.,** Prevalence of antibodies to *Toxoplasma gondii* in captive exotic mammals, *J. Am. Vet. Med. Assoc.,* 798, 1974.

106. **Lainson, R.,** Toxoplasmosis in England. II. Variation factors in the pathogenesis of *Toxoplasma* infections: the sudden increase in virulenceof a strain after passage in multimammate rats and canaries, *Ann. Trop. Med. Parasitol.,* 49, 397, 1955.

107. **Araujo, F. G., Williams, D. M., Grumet, F. C., and Remington, J. S.,** Strain-dependent differences in murine susceptibility to *Toxoplasma, Infect. Immun.,* 13(5), 1528, 1976.

108. **Frenkel, J. K.,** Pathogenesis of toxoplasmosis with a consideration of cyst rupture in *Besnoitia* infection, *Sur. Ophthalmol.,* 6(6), 799, 1961.

109. **Nozik, R. A. and O'Connor, G. R.,** Studies on experimental ocular toxoplasmosis in the rabbit. II. Attempts to stimulate recurrences by local trauma, epinephrine and corticosteroids, *Arch. Ophthalmol.,* 84, 788, 1970.

110. **Frenkel, J. K.,** Pathogenesis of toxoplasmosis and of infections with organisms resembling *Toxoplasma, Ann. N.Y. Acad. Sci.,* 64, 215, 1956.

111. **Frenkel, J. K.,** Adrenal infection, necrosis, and hypercorticism. Animal model: chronic besnoitiosis of golden hamsters (*Mesocricetus auratus*), *Am. J. Pathol.,* 86(3), 749, 1977.

112. **Stone, W. B. and Manwell, R. D.,** Toxoplasmosis in cold-blooded hosts, *J. Protozool.,* 16(1), 99, 1969.

113. **Desmonts, G. and Couvreur, J.,** Toxoplasmosis in pregnancy and its transmission to the fetus, *Bull. N.Y. Acad. Med.,* 50(2), 146, 1974.

114. **Eichenwald, H. F.,** A study of congenital toxoplasmosis, in *Human Toxoplasmosis,* Siim, J. C., Ed., Munksgaard, Copenhagen, 1960, 41.

115. **Frenkel, J. K.,** Pathology and pathogenesis of congenital toxoplasmosis, *Bull. N.Y. Acad. Med.,* 50, 182, 1974.

116. Alford, C. A., Stagno, S., and Reynolds, D. W., Congenital toxoplasmosis. Clinical, laboratory, and therapeutic considerations, with special reference to subclinical disease, *Bull. N.Y. Acad. Med.,* 50(2), 160, 1974.

117. Wilder, H. C., *Toxoplasma* chorioretinitis in adults, *AMA Arch. Opthalmol.,* 48, 127, 1952.

118. Zimmerman, L. E., Ocular pathology of toxoplasmosis, *Sur. Ophthalmol.,* 6(6), 832, 1961.

119. Kass, E., Andrus, S., Adams, R., Turner, F., and Feldman, H., Toxoplasmosis in the human adult, *AMA Arch. Intern. Med.,* 89, 759, 1952.

120. Bobowski, S. J. and Reed, W. G., Toxoplasmosis in an adult, presenting as a space-occupying cerebral lesion, *AMA Arch. Pathol.,* 65, 460, 1958.

121. Koeze, T. H. and Klingon, G. H., Acquired toxoplasmosis, *Arch. Neurol.,* 11, 191, 1964.

122. Cespedes, F., Mullner, F., Segura, J., Ruiz, P., Ingianna, M., and Acuna, R., Miositis toxoplasmica aguda en un adulto, *Acta Medica Cost.,* 16(1), 75, 1973.

123. Ruskin, J. and Remington, J. S., Toxoplasmosis in the compromised host, *Ann. Intern. Med.,* 84(2), 193, 1976.

124. Vietzke, W. M., Gelderman, A. H., Grimley, P. M., and Valsamis, M. P., Toxoplasmosis complicating malignancy, *Cancer,* 21(5), 816, 1968.

125. Nicholson, D. H. and Wolchok, E. B., Ocular toxoplasmosis in an adult receiving long-term corticosteroid therapy, *Arch. Ophthalmol.,* 94(2), 248, 1976.

126. Wallace, G. D., Marshall, L., and Marshall, M., Cats, rats, and toxoplasmosis on a small Pacific island, *Am. J. Epidemiol.,* 95, 475, 1972.

127. Wallace, G. D., Zigas, V., and Gajdusek, D. C., Toxoplasmosis and cats in New Guinea, *Am. J. Trop. Med. Hyg.,* 23(1), 8, 1974.

128. Munday, B. L., Serological evidence of *Toxoplasma* infection in isolated groups of sheep, *Res. Vet. Sci.,* 13, 100, 1972.

129. Hartley, W. J., Some investigations into the epidemiology of ovine toxoplasmosis, *N.Z. Vet. J.,* 14(7), 106, 1966.

130. Watson, W. A. and Beverley, J. K. A., Ovine abortion due to experimental toxoplasmosis, *Vet. Rec.,* 88, 42, 1971.

131. Desmonts, G., Couvreur, J., Alison, F., Baudelot, J., Gerbeaux, J., and Lelong, M., Étude épidémiologique sur la toxoplasmose: de l'influence de la cuisson des viandes de boucherie sur la fréquence de l'infection humaine, *Rev. Franc. Etudes Clin. Biol.,* 10(9), 952, 1965.

132. Center for Disease Control, PHS/DHEW, Serodiagnosis of: Toxoplasmosis, Rubella, Cytomegalic Inclusion Disease, Herpes Simplex, Immunology Series No. 5, Procedural Guide, Atlanta, Georgia, 1974.

133. Frenkel, J. K. and Jacobs, L., Ocular toxoplasmosis, *AMA Arch. Ophthalmol.,* 59, 260, 1958.

134. Wallace, G. D., Sabin-Feldman dye test for toxoplasmosis, *Am. J. Trop. Med. Hyg.,* 18(3), 395, 1969.

135. Couzineau, P., Baufine-Ducrocq, H., Peloux, Y., and Desmonts, G., Le serodiagnostic de la toxoplasmose par agglutination directe, *Nouv. Presse Med.,* 2(23), 1604, 1973.

136. Voller, A., Bidwell, D. E., Bartlett, A., Fleck, D. G., Perkins, M., and Oladehin, B., A microplate enzyme-immunoassay for *Toxoplasma* antibody, *J. Clin. Pathol.,* 29, 150, 1976.

137. Desmonts, G. and Couvreau, J., Congenital toxoplasmosis. A prospective study of 378 pregnancies, *N. Engl. J. Med.,* 290(20), 1110, 1974.

138. Jacobs, L., Cook, M. K., and Wilder, H., Serologic data on adults with histologically demonstrated toxoplasmic chorioretinitis, *Trans. Am. Acad. Ophthalmol. Otolaryngol.,* p. 193, 1954.

139. Harboe, A. and Reenaas, R., The complement fixation inhibition test with sera from chickens experimentally infected with toxoplasma, *Acta Pathol. Microbiol. Scand.,* 41, 511, 1957.

140. Frenkel, J. K., Toxoplasmosis, in *Current Veterinary Therapy V.,* 5th ed., Kirk, R. N., Ed., W. B. Saunders Co., Philadelphia, 1974, 775, (6th ed., 1977, 1318.)

141. Yilmaz, S. M. and Hopkins, S. H., Effects of different conditions on duration of infectivity of *Toxoplasma gondii* oocysts, *J. Parasitol.,* 58, 938, 1972.

OTHER PROTOZOA: *EIMERIA, ISOSPORA, CYSTOISOSPORA, BESNOITIA, HAMMONDIA, FRENKELIA, SARCOCYSTIS, CRYPTOSPORIDIUM, ENCEPHALITOZOON,* AND *NOSEMA*

Ronald Fayer

INTRODUCTION

Within the protozoan subphylum Apicomplexa is a unique and interesting group of parasites collectively referred to as the coccidia. The genera *Eimeria, Isospora, Cystoisospora, Besnoitia, Hammondia, Frenkelia, Sarcocystis, Cryptosporidium* and *Toxoplasma* comprise this group. The life cycle of each genus follows a common basic pattern involving both asexual and sexual phases. The stages within each phase possess structures common to the group. Genera are distinguished from one another by their unique variations from the basic life cycle in the size, shape, and number of parasites found at each phase of the cycle; by the location of parasites within the host; and by their host specificity. *Toxoplasma* and *Cryptosporidium* are the only coccidia known to be zoonotic (see "Toxoplasmosis" chapter). The intramuscular cyst stage of *Sarcocystis* in humans is probably zoonotic (explanation to follow). Serologic evidence alone suggests that *Hammondia* may also infect humans. However, neither clinical nor experimental nor serologic evidence exists to implicate any of the remaining coccidian genera as zoonotic agents.

EIMERIA, ISOSPORA, AND *CYSTOISOSPORA*

The simplest, most direct life cycles among the coccidia are found within the genus *Eimeria* (Figure 1). With few exceptions, *Eimeria* complete their life cycle within the intestine of a single host and have a host range limited to that host species alone. Unsporulated oocysts are passed in the feces and sporulate aerobically outside the body. Sporulated oocysts are tetrasporic (four sporocysts) and sporocysts are dizoic (two sporozoites). After oocysts are ingested, fusiform cells called sporozoites excyst (leave the oocyst), enter gut epithelium, and develop asexually by formation of numerous nuclei; the latter process is called merogony or schizogony. Each nucleus is incorporated into another fusiform cell called a merozoite, which enters another host cell and initiates a subsequent asexual generation. Two, three, or more asexual generations may be initiated by merozoites of the preceding generation. Eventually, merozoites enter cells and initiate the sexual phase of the cycle (gametogony). Merozoites develop into either biflagellate sperm-like microgametes or egg-like macrogametes. Fertilized macrogametes form a wall around their cytoplasm and become oocysts. Oocysts leave the host cell, enter the intestine, and leave the body via the feces.

Eimerians are common parasites of nearly all species of livestock and poultry but do not parasitize dogs, cats, or man. Because ingested oocysts may pass through the intestine unchanged, the presence of oocysts in the feces is not always indicative of an active infection: *Eimeria bovis* oocysts have reportedly been found in the feces of a human given a folk medicine remedy for tuberculosis, consisting of bovine feces and milk; oocysts of two *Eimeria* of fish were found in human feces and incorrectly described as human parasites; oocysts of an *Eimeria* of rabbits were found in the feces of a mental hospital patient who ate raw rabbit livers; and oocysts of an *Eimeria* of pigs were found in feces of people who probably acquired them from sausage casings.[23]

The oocysts of *Isospora* and *Cystoisospora* are passed unsporulated in the feces and sporulate aerobically outside the body. Sporulated oocysts are disporic and both spo-

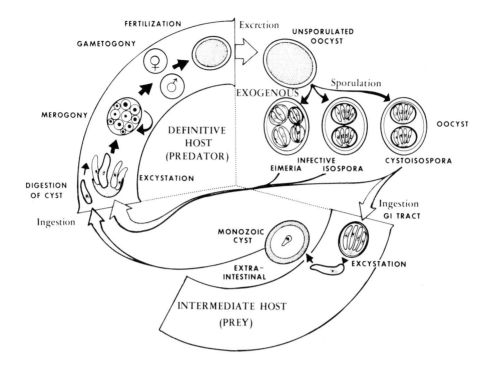

FIGURE 1.   Life cycle of *Eimeria, Isospora, Cystoisospora.*

rocysts are tetrazoic (four sporozoites). These oocysts are morphologically similar to oocysts of *Toxoplasma, Hammondia,* and *Besnoitia.*

The life cycles of *Isospora* species are basically the same as those of *Eimeria* species. Isosporans parasitize songbirds, dogs, cats, swine, and humans. Humans have been reported to harbor four named species of *Isospora: I. natalensis, I. chilensis, I. hominis,* and *I. belli* [23a] and an undescribed species with *Isospora*-like oocysts,[3] *Isospora belli* is probably the only named species that is valid. Although *I. belli* is distributed worldwide it is not highly prevalent. Our perception of its prevalence, however, may in part reflect the difficulty of diagnosis. Diagnoses are usually based on stool examinations, and if these are initially negative for oocysts, one or more reexaminations may be necessary to confirm their presence. Occasionally it becomes necessary to obtain a mucosal biopsy of small intestine from patients to complete a diagnosis; from such specimens, portions of the life cycle have been described.[6] An unusual aspect of the life cycle is the finding of both unsporulated and sporulated oocysts in the lumen of the duodenum. Reinfection by such sporulated oocysts may explain some of the unusually long chronic infections. Because the ultimate source of human infection is not known and nonhuman reservoirs have not been identified, infection is assumed to result from contamination of food or water with oocysts from human feces. The pathogenicity is not well known, but illness and death have been reported. Acute illness is characterized by fever, headache, asthenia, nausea, diarrhea, steatorrhea, weight loss, and abdominal pain. Treatment regimens have been attempted but none are predictably successful. Two combinations of drugs that have been effective in eliminating the parasite are pyrimethamine and sulfadiazine[32] and trimethoprim and sulfamethoxazole.[30,35] The latter combination is marketed as either Septrin® or Cotrimoxazole.®*

---

* Mention of a trademark, proprietary product, or vendor does not constitute a guarantee or warranty by the U.S. Department of Agriculture and does not imply its approval to the exclusion of other products or vendors that may also be suitable.

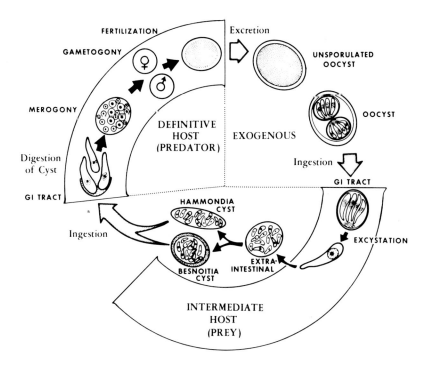

FIGURE 2.   Life cycle of *Besnoitia* and *Hammondia*.

The life cycles of *Cystoisospora* species differ from those of *Eimeria* species in that cystoisosporans have the additional ability to infect intermediate hosts (Figure 1). After sporulated *Cystoisospora* oocysts are ingested by the intermediate host, sporozoites excyst from oocysts in the intestine, become extraintestinal, enter cells in the viscera, and remain dormant until the intermediate host is eaten by the final host whereupon the sporozoites are released, enter the intestinal epithelium, and initiate merogony and then gametogony and oocyst-formation.

Only four species of *Cytoisospora* have been identified; two have cats as definitive hosts (*C. felis* and *C. rivolta*) and two have dogs as definitive hosts (*C. canis* and *C. ohioensis*). Experimental intermediate hosts for both cat species include mice, rats, dogs, hamsters, chickens, and cattle.[11,14,36] Experimental intermediate hosts for the dog species include mice for *C. canis* and cats and mice for *C. ohioensis*, respectively.[11] Although infection in humans is not known, the high prevalence of *Cystoisospora* species in cats and dogs, the recently discovered multihost potential for development of monozoic cysts of *Cystoisospora* in intermediate hosts, and the close association between humans and their pets suggest that a zoonotic potential may exist.

BESNOITIA AND HAMMONDIA

Besnoitia and *Hammondia* have historically been characterized by their distinctive tissue cyst stages in their respective intermediate hosts. In other respects, the life cycles of these two genera are quite similar (Figure 2). Both have an obligatory two-host (predator-prey) life cycle with cats serving as the final host (predator). Transmission is not known to occur between intermediate hosts or between final hosts. Cats ingest cysts in the organs of the intermediate host. Fusiform cells within the cysts called cystozoites, bradyzoites, merozoites, or just zoites, are released from the cysts following ingestion. They initiate merogony and then gametogony and oocyst-formation in the feline small intestine, and unsporulated oocysts are passed in the feces. Intermediate hosts become infected by ingesting sporulated oocysts. The fusiform cells called spo- rozoites excyst from the oocyst in the lumen of the small intestine and find their way to extraintestinal tissues where they become intracellular and multiply asexually into clusters of fusiform cells which initiate cyst development. Zoites within cysts remain in a hypobiotic or dormant state, perhaps for the life of the host.

Naturally infected intermediate hosts of *Besnoitia* spp. include reptiles, mice, kang- aroo rats, opossum, and a variety of domestic and wild ruminants.[11] Cysts are found principally in connective tissue. *Besnoitia* has not been found in man.

Naturally infected and laboratory infected intermediate hosts of *Hammondia ham- mondi* include almost all the voles and field mice species, hamsters, rats, multimam- mate rats, guinea pigs, rabbits, pigs, dogs, and monkeys, but not pigeons, quail, or chickens.[10,12,13,18,33] Cysts are found principally in striated muscles and are morpholog- ically similar to cysts of *Toxoplasma*. It is not known if humans become infected with *Hammondia*. Of 97 human sera collected from apparently normal people in Hawaii, 15 sera reacted with *Hammondia* antigen in an indirect fluorescent antibody test; 12 of these were also positive in the *Toxoplasma* dye test;[33] and two sera were *Toxo- plasma*-positive but *Hammondia*-negative. Serologic cross-reaction between *Hammon- dia* and *Toxoplasma* may explain the cases in which antibody titers to both parasites were found. However, infection with both *Hammondia* and *Toxoplasma* is a reasona- ble alternative explanation. Infection with *Hammondia* alone may explain the three cases that were *Hammondia*-positive and *Toxoplasma*-negative. Further circumstantial support for the possibility of human infection with *Hammondia* comes from the close association of humans with cats and the infectivity of *Hammondia* oocysts from cats for a primate: *Saguinus nigricollis*, the white-lipped marmoset.[12] However, infectivity for primates generally appears to be low; although 2×10^6 *Hammondia* oocysts were fed to each of four monkeys, only one became infected.[12]

FRENKELIA AND *SARCOCYSTIS*

Frenkelia and *Sarcocystis* have historically been characterized by their distinctive tissue cyst stages in their respective intermediate hosts. In other respects, the life cycles of these two genera are quite similar (Figure 3). Both have an obligatory two-host (predator-prey) life cycle with carnivorous birds serving as the final hosts for *Frenkelia*, and a variety of carnivorous reptiles, birds, and mammals serving as final hosts for *Sarcocystis* spp. Transmission is not known to occur between final hosts and has been completed only via blood transfusion between intermediate hosts of *Sarcocystis* spp.[17] Carnivores ingest cysts in the brain or striated muscles of the intermediate host. Fusi- form cells within the cysts called cystozoites, bradyzoites, merozoites, or just zoites are released from the cysts following ingestion. They initiate gametogony and then oocyst-formation in the carnivore small intestine. Unlike those of most other coccidia, oocysts of *Frenkelia* and *Sarcocystis* sporulate in the small intestine, and sporulated oocysts or sporocysts are passed in the feces. Intermediate hosts become infected by ingesting the oocysts or sporocysts. Fusiform cells called sporozoites excyst from the sporocysts in the lumen of the small intestine and find their way to extraintestinal tissues where they become intracellular and multiply asexually, producing schizonts. Schizonts of *Sarcocystis* spp. develop in the endothelium of arteries and capillaries and produce merozoites. Merozoites enter the bloodstream and multiply by endodyogeny either in leukocytes or extracellularly. Tissue cyst development is initiated when mero- zoites from the bloodstream enter brain cells (*Frenkelia*) or cardiac, and skeletal muscle cells (*Sarcocystis*). In these sites merozoites appear to dedifferentiate into a rounded, noninfectious, reproductive stage called a metrocyte. Metrocytes increase in number

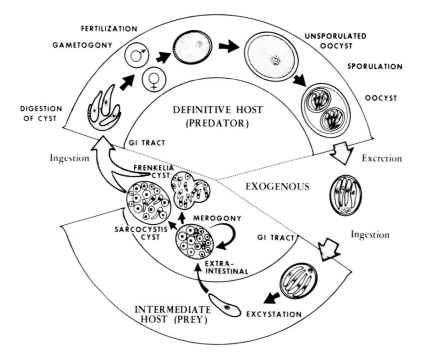

FIGURE 3. Life cycle of *Sarcocystis* and *Frenkelia*.

and some give rise to infectious zoites that remain in a hypobiotic or dormant state, perhaps for the life of the host. As a wall forms around the increasing mass of parasites a cyst is formed.

Frenkelia spp. are found only in rodent intermediate hosts and have never been found in man.

Two species of *Sarcocystis* are known in which humans serve as the final host: *S. hominis*, which has a bovine intermediate host, and *S. suihominis*, which has a porcine intermediate host. Humans become infected by eating raw beef or pork containing infectious cysts. Infection in humans is limited to the intestine and sporocysts are passed in the feces. The sporocysts of both species have historically been incorrectly identified as *Isospora hominis*.

Of 20 human volunteers in five studies who ate raw beef infected with *S. hominis*, 12 became infected and began to pass oocysts or sporocysts in their feces 9 to 39 days later.[2,19,21,27,31] Acute clinical symptoms were reported for only one volunteer who developed low grade nausea, stomach ache, and diarrhea within 3 to 6 hr after eating the beef; these clinical symptoms lasted from 24 to 36 hr.[19] There appears to be no immunity to repeated infection as evidenced by repeated passage of sporocysts in feces following ingestion of raw beef.[2] Nonhuman primates also serve as final hosts of *S. hominis*. Six rhesus monkeys and four baboons passed sporocysts after eating infected beef; no clinical signs were reported.[20,31]

Of 15 human volunteers in three studies who ate raw pork infected with *S. suihominis*,[19,26,27] 14 became infected and began to pass oocysts and sporocysts in their feces 10 to 17 days later. Acute clinical symptoms were reported for 12 of the volunteers beginning at 6 hr and lasting as long as 48 hr after eating the infected pork. Symptoms were varied but included: bloating, nausea, inappetance, stomach ache, vomiting, dry heaves, diarrhea, coldness and sweating, dyspnea, rapid pulse, and fever. Well-cooked pork from the same pigs used in one of the studies did not cause any clinical problems when eaten by nine control volunteers.[19] Other primates were also found to serve as final hosts of *S. suihominis.* One chimpanzee, two rhesus and two cynomolgus monkeys passed sporocysts after eating infected pork but had no clinical signs of infection; the rhesus and cynomolgus monkeys developed no immunity to reinfection.[15]

Illness in humans who eat raw beef or pork containing *S. hominis* and *S. suihominis* may be caused by the parasites, by their metabolic products which are toxic or stimulate a hypersensitivity reaction, or by both. This conclusion is suggested by the study of Hiepe et al.[21] who fed naturally infected raw pork to seven human volunteers and *Sarcocystis* cysts from the pork to four grass monkeys. Although the species of *Sarcocystis* in the pork was not infectious for either the human volunteers or the monkeys (sporocysts were not produced), indirect fluorescent antibody test titers became elevated in all recipients; one volunteer had gastrointestinal complaints a day after eating the pork, and the two monkeys receiving the most cysts had severe intestinal or central nervous system disorders.

Although *S. hominis* and *S. suihominis* have been transmitted to nonhuman primates experimentally, natural infections have not been described. However, the opportunity for such cycles to occur in nature clearly exists. Chimpanzees have been observed attacking and killing fairly large animals; chimpanzees and baboons have been observed eating meat from carcasses of a variety of animals; and wild pigs have been observed eating the remains of nonhuman primates.[15] In areas where such predator-prey relations exist, humans could become final hosts by eating raw meat from an intermediate host (prey) that acquired *Sarcocystis* via a nonhuman primate.

No treatment is known for intestinal infection with *Sarcocystis* spp.

About 40 human cases have been reported in which intramuscular cysts of *Sarcocystis* were found in the heart, larynx, pharynx, foot, neck, arm, calf, and in a hemangioma.[5] The actual number of species in humans is unknown. The only named species in humans is *Sarcocystis lindemanni* and this must be considered invalid because of the poor description of the cyst. Based on morphologic differences among the cysts, such as overall size, thickness of the cyst wall, presence or absence of septa, and size of zoites within the cyst, at least seven morphologic types of *Sarcocystis* have been observed, each possibly representing one or more species.[5] In such cases where intramuscular cysts were found, based on our present knowledge of an obligatory two-host *Sarcocystis* life cycle, humans were serving as intermediate hosts (prey). Their infections originated from ingestion of sporocysts from the feces or the intestine of the final host. Because the eating of humans by predators is not a common occurence anywhere in the world, accidental zoonotic infection related to a nonhuman primate-carnivore cycle as described above is currently the most reasonable explanation for such human infections. Carnivorous mammals, reptiles, or birds could also serve as the final hosts. Indeed, as documented in 30 of the 40 reports, human infections were probably acquired in the tropics where nonhuman primate cycles may be found.

Most of what is known of the pathology due to *Sarcocystis* infection comes from experimental studies and natural outbreaks of sarcocystosis in livestock.[11] Acute illness in livestock is characterized by the rapid onset of fever, anemia, inappetence, weight loss, and abortion in pregnant females, and death is associated with the presence of schizonts in vascular endothelium throughout the body and the liberation of merozoites into the bloodstream. Hemorrhage occurs in the skeletal musculature, serosa, and most notably throughout the heart. Interstitial mononuclear cell infiltrates in the heart, kidneys, lungs, and striated muscles are often massive and striking. Immune complexes are found in the basement membranes in glomeruli of kidneys. Chronic infections in livestock are characterized by atrophy of skeletal muscles, stiff-legged gait, loss of hair or wool, and to a lesser extent terminal central nervous system signs.

Acute sarcocystosis has not been diagnosed in humans. However, clinical manifestations observed in four cases may have been the result of early stages of infection (schizonts).[5] There is no conclusive evidence that the cyst stage induces pathology in either humans or animals.

In those humans in which clinical manifestations appeared to be related to *Sarcocystis* infection, muscle weakness, soreness, or wasting was noted in seven cases, subcutaneous swelling in five cases, eosinophilia in two cases, periarteritis or polyarteritis nodosa in two cases and cardiopathy in one case.[5]

No treatment is known for intramuscular *Sarcocystis* infection in man. The anticoccidial drugs amprolium and salinomycin have been effective for treating precystic stages during acute experimental sarcocystosis in ruminants.[16,22]

CRYPTOSPORIDIUM

Cryptosporidia differ from all other coccidia because they are extracellular organisms that inhabit the microvillous border of enterocytes in the small intestine. Like other coccidia they undergo asexual development as schizonts and then sexual development as micro- and macrogamonts. Fertilized macrogametes develop into tiny oocysts (approximately 4 to 5 μm in diameter) that pass in the feces. Oocysts may be infectious immediately upon passage.[30] Oocysts contain four sporozoites but no sporocysts. Cryptosporidia have been reported in snakes, mice, rats, guinea pigs, rabbits, chickens, turkeys, calves, lambs, piglets, foals, monkeys and humans. Reports of *Cryptosporidium* in foxes and dingos are erroneous; the organisms identified in the feces were *Sarcocystis* sporocysts. There are about five named species of *Cryptosporidium* based on the assumption that each exhibits host specificity.[24] However, recent transmission studies suggest that *Cryptosporidium* is a single-species genus. Tzipori and colleagues[39] obtained oocysts from calf feces and established infections in seven other animal species. Reese and colleagues[31] produced indistinguishable infections in mice and rats inoculated with oocysts of human and calf origin.

Severe watery diarrhea, sometimes leading to death, has been reported for neonatal calves, lambs and other animals with cryptosporidiosis. Similar clinical signs are reported for humans.

In the first eight reported human cases of cryptosporidiosis all patients had developing, suppressed or deficient immune systems.[27,28,35,42] Recently, two human cases have been reported from immunologically normal adults.[40]

Although initial diagnosis in humans were made by histologic examination of intestinal and rectal biopsies, a better method of diagnosis is identification of oocysts in fecal flotations by phase-contrast microscopy.[31]

There is no known effective treatment for crytosporidiosis in animals or humans.

MICROSPORIDIA

Nearly 700 species of microsporidia are known, with hosts throughout all the invertebrate phyla and within all five classes of vertebrates.[9] Microsporidia are intracellular parasites with a distinctive thick-walled spore stage that contains a polar filament and an infective sporoplasm. These spores are among the smallest found within the Protozoa. Spores in vertebrate hosts are simple in outline. They are ovoid or piriform, and measure about 2 to 12 μm long.

All known microsporidia have direct life cycles (Figure 4). Spores contaminate the environment and are ingested by a host. Within the host the polar filament everts from the spore and the sporoplasm squeezes through the hollow filament and is injected into a host cell. Sporoplasms usually infect gut epithelium and then migrate to other viscera where they undergo asexual multiplication by schizogony or binary fission.

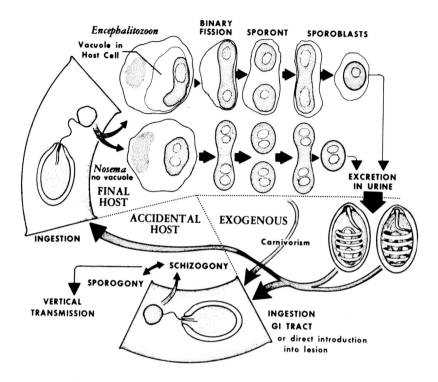

FIGURE 4.   Life cycle and hypothetical transmission of *Microsporidia*.

Eventually sporogony begins; it is characterized by the division of the sporont into sporoblasts and by the addition of layers external to the plasmalemma. Cytoplasmic reorganization within the sporoblasts results in the formation of the characteristic spore. In the final stages of development the spore coat is formed by compression of loosely arranged polaroplast membranes and deposition of electron dense material. Variations of this life cycle constitute a basis for generic separation.

In addition to transmission via spores contaminating the environment, microsporidia have been transmitted congenitally[1] and from prey to predator via carnivorism.[9]

Diagnosis and accurate classification of microsporidia are difficult and confusing because of the small size of the spores, the thick spore wall that obscures critical observation of the sporoplasm, and often the lack of representative material from other life cycle stages. Based on careful light microscopy by Cali[8] and electron microscopy by Sprague and Vernick[29] *Nosema* and *Encephalitozoon* are considered distinct valid genera. Although both genera have two spores derived from each sporont, i.e., they are disporous; *Nosema* has double nuclei (diplokarya) whereas *Encephalitozoon* has only a single nucleus during most of the life cycle.

These two genera of microsporidia have each been identified in association with a single human infection. *Encephalitozoon* was identified in urine and cerebrospinal fluid by Matsubayashi et al.;[25] its identity was verified by Weiser,[34] *Nosema* was identified in histologic sections of numerous organs by Margileth et al.;[24] its identity was verified by Sprague.[28] In a third report of human microsporidiosis, organisms were found in histologic sections and smears of a biopsied lesion by Ashton and Wirasinha;[4] however, the classification of the parasite has not been accurately determined.[7] Although several other claims of human infection by microsporidia have been recorded they either have not been verified or have been disclaimed.

In the three reports of human infection the symptoms differed markedly. *Encephalitozoon* infection in a 9-year-old boy in Japan was associated with fever, convulsions,

unconsciousness, vomiting, and headaches,[25] *Nosema* infection in a 4-month-old immunologically defective male was associated with diarrhea, malabsorption syndrome,
and thymic alymphoplasia.[24] Microsporidian infection in an 11-year-old boy in Ceylon
was associated with a localized infection of the eye.[4] The source of infection is not
known with certainty for any of the three cases. The boy with the eye lesion gave a
history of having been gored by a goat 6 years previously after which the right upper
eyelid was sutured.

No effective treatment is known for human microsporidiosis. The boy with *Encephalitozoon* was first treated with penicillin and then sulfisoxazole but the efficacy of
either cannot be determined.

ACKNOWLEDGMENT

The author wishes to acknowledge the help of Robert Ewing in preparing the figures
for this chapter.

REFERENCES

1. **Anver, M. R., King, N. W., and Hunt, R. D.**, Congenital encephalitozoonosis in a squirrel monkey *(Saimiri sciureus), Vet. Pathol.,* 9, 475, 1972.
2. **Aryeetey, M. E. and Piekarski, G.**, Serologische *Sarcocystis-Studien an Menschen und Ratten, Z. Parasitenk.,* 50, 109, 1976.
3. **Ashford, R. W.**, Occurrence of an undescribed coccidian in man in Papua New Guinea, *Ann. Trop. Med. Parasitol.,* 73, 497, 1979.
4. **Ashton, N. and Wirasinha, P. A.**, Encephalitozoonosis (Nosematosis) of the cornea, *Br. J. Ophthal-mol.,* 57, 669, 1973.
5. **Beaver, P. C., Gadgil, R. K., and Morera, P.**, *Sarcocystis* in man: a review and report of five cases, *Am. J. Trop. Med. Hyg.,* 28, 819, 1979.
6. **Brandborg, L. L., Goldberg, S. B., and Breidenbach, W. C.**, Human coccidiosis — a possible cause of malabsorption. The life cycle in small bowel mucosal biopsies as a diagnostic feature, *N. Eng. J. Med.,* 283, 1306, 1970.
7. **Bywater, J. E. C.**, Is encephalitozoonosis a zoonosis?, *Lab. Anim.,* 13, 149, 1979.
8. **Cali, A.**, Morphogenesis in the genus *Nosema,* Proc. 4th Int. Colloq. Insect Pathol., College Park, Md., 25 to 28 August 1970, 431, 1970.
9. **Canning, E. U.**, Microsporidia, in *Parasitic Protozoa,* Vol. 4, Kreier, J. P., Ed., Academic Press, New York, 1977, 155.
10. **Dubey, J. P.**, Experimental *Hammondia hammondi* infection in dogs, *Br. Vet. J.,* 131, 741, 1975.
11. **Dubey, J. P.**, *Toxoplasma, Hammondia, Besnoitia, Sarcocystis,* and other tissue cyst-forming coc-cidia of man and animals, in *Parasitic Protozoa,* Vol. 3, Kreier, J. P., Ed., Academic Press, New York, 1977, 101.
12. **Dubey, J. P. and Wong, M. M.**, Experimental *Hammondia hammondi* infection in monkeys, *J. Parasitol.,* 64, 551, 1978.
13. **Eydelloth, M.**, Experimentelle Untersuchungen uber das Wirtsspektrum von *Hammondia hammondi,* Inaugural Dissertation, Ludwig-Maximillians University, Munich, Germany, 46, 1977.
14. **Fayer, R. and Frenkel, J. K.**, Comparative infectivity for calves of oocysts of feline coccidia: *Bes-noitia, Hammondia, Cystoisospora, Sarcocystis,* and *Toxoplasma, J. Parasitol.,* 65, 756, 1979.
15. **Fayer R., Heydorn, A. O., Johnson, A. J., and Leek, R. G.**, Transmission of *Sarcocystis suihominis* from humans to swine to nonhuman primates *(Pan troglodytes, Macaca mulatta, Macaca irus), Z. Parasitenk.,* 59, 15, 1979.
16. **Fayer, R. and Johnson, A. J.**, Effect of amprolium on acute sarcocystosis in experimentally infected calves, *J. Parasitol.,* 61, 932, 1975.
17. **Fayer, R. and Leek, R. G.**, *Sarcocystis* transmitted by blood transfusion, *J. Parasitol.,* 65, 890, 1979.
18. **Frenkel, J. K. and Dubey, J. P.**, *Hammondia hammondi* gen. nov., sp. nov., from domestic cats, a new coccidian related to *Toxoplasma* and *Sarcocystis, Z. Parasitenk.,* 46, 3, 1975.
19. **Heydorn, A. O.**, Sarkosporidieninfiziertes Fleisch als-mogliche Krankheitsurasche fur den Menschen, *Arch. Lebensmittelhyg.,* 28, 27, 1977.

20. **Heydorn, A. O., Gestrich, R., and Janitschke, K.,** Beitrage zum Lebenszyklus der Sarkosporidien VIII. Sporozysten von *Sarcocystis bovihominis* in den Fazes von Rhesusaffen *(Macaca rhesus)* und Pavianen *(Papio cynocephalus), Berl. Muench. Tieraerztl. Wochenschr.,* 89, 116, 1976.

21. **Hiepe, F., Hiepe, Th., Hlinak, P., Jungmann, R., Horsch, R., and Wiedauer, B.,** Experimentelle Infektion des Menschen und von Tierraffen *(Cercopithecus callitrichus)* mit Sarkosporidien-Zysten von Rind und Schwein, *Arch. Exp. Vet. Med. Leipzig,* 33, 819, 1979.

22. **Leek, R. G. and Fayer, R.,** Experimental *Sarcocystis ovicanis* infection in lambs: salinomycin chemoprophylaxis and protective immunity, Proc. and Abstr. 55th Ann. Meet. Am. Soc. Parasitol., Berkeley, Calif., Aug. 4-8, 1980, 43, 1980.

23. **Levine, N. D.,** *Protozoan Parasites of Domestic Animals and of Man,* Burgess Publ., Minneapolis, 1961, 242.

24. **Levine, N. D.,** *Protozoan Parasites of Domestic Animals and of Man,* 2nd ed., Burgess Publ., Minneapolis, 1973, 406.

25. **Margileth, A. M., Strano, A. J., Chandra, R., Neafie, R., Blum, M., and McCully, R. M.,** Disseminated nosematosis in an immunologically comprised infant, *Arch. Pathol.,* 95, 145, 1973.

26. **Matsubayashi, H., Koike, T., Mikata, I., Takei, H., and Hagiwara, S.,** A case of encephalitozoon-like body infection in man, *AMA. Arch. Pathol.,* 67, 181, 1959.

27. **Meisel, J. L., Perera, D. R., Meligro, C., and Rubin, C. E.,** Overwhelming watery diarrhea associated with a cryptosporidium in an immunosuppressed patient, *Gastroenterol.,* 70, 1156, 1976.

28. **Nime, F. A., Burek, J. D., Page, D. L., Holscher, M. A., and Yardley, J. H.,** Acute enterocolitis in a human being infected with the protozoan cryptosporidium, *Gastroenterol.,* 70, 592, 1976.

29. **Piekarski, G., Heydorn, A. O., Aryeetey, M. E., Hartlapp, J. H., and Kimmig, P.,** Klinische, parasitologische und serologische Untersuchungen zur Sarkosporidiase *(Sarcocystis suihominis)* des Menschen, *Immun. Infekt.,* 6, 153, 1978.

30. **Pohlenz, J., Moon, H. W., Cheville, N. F., and Bemrick, W. J.,** Cryptosporidiosis as a probable factor in neonatal diarrhea in calves, *J. Am. Vet. Med. Assoc.,* 172, 452, 1978.

31. **Reese, N. C., Current, W. L., Ernst, J. V., and Bailey, W. S.,** Human and calf cryptosporidiosis: a case report and results of comparative infections in mice and rats, *Am. J. Trop. Med. Hyg.,* In press.

32. **Rommel, M. and Heydorn, A. O.,** Beitrage zum Lebenszyklus der Sarkosporidien. III. *Isospora hominis* (Railliet und Lucet, 1891) Wenyon, 1923 eine Dauerform der Sarkosporidien des Rindes und des Schweins, *Berl. Muench. Tieraerztl. Wochenschr.,* 85, 143, 1975.

33. **Sprague, V.,** *Nosema connori* n. sp., a microsporidian parasite of man, *Trans. Am. Microsc. Soc.,* 93, 400, 1974.

34. **Sprague, V. and Vernick, S. H.,** The ultrastructure of *Encephalitozoon cuniculi* (Microsporida, Nosematidae) and its taxonomic significance, *J. Protozool.,* 18, 560, 1971.

35. **Stemmermann, G. N., Hayashi, T., Glober, G. A., Oishi, N., and Frankel, R. I.,** Cryptosporidiosis report of fatal case complicated by disseminated toxoplasmosis, *Am. J. Med.,* 69, 637, 1980.

36. **Syrkis, I., Fried, M., Elian, I., Petrushka, D., and Lengy, J.,** A case of severe human coccidiosis in Israel, *Isr. J. Med. Sci.,* 11, 373, 1975.

37. **Tadros, W. and Laarman, J. J.,** Studies on sarcosporidiosis and sarcocystis-induced coccidiosis in man, monkeys and other animals, No. 137, 5th Int. Congr. Protozool., New York, June 26 to July 2, 1977.

38. **Trier, J. S., Moxey, P. C., Schimmel, E. M., and Robles, E.,** Chronic intestinal coccidiosis in man: intestinal morphology and response to treatment, *Gastroenterol.,* 66, 923, 1974.

39. **Tzipori, S., Angus, K. W., Campbell, I., and Gray, E. W.,** Cryptosporidium: evidence for a single-species genus, *Infect. Immun.,* 30, 884, 1980.

40. **Tzipori, S., Angus, K. W., Gray, E. W., and Campbell, I.,** Vomiting and diarrhea associated with cryptosporidial infection, *N. Eng. J. Med.,* 818, 1980.

41. **Wallace, G. D.,** Observations on a feline coccidium with some characteristics of *Toxoplasma* and *Sarcocystis, Z. Parasitenk.,* 46, 167, 1975.

42. **Weisburger, W. R., Hutcheon, D. F., Yardley, J. H., Roche, J. C., Hillis, W. D., and Charache, P.,** Cryptosporidiosis in an immunosuppressed renal-transplant recipient with IgA deficiency, *Am. Soc. Clin. Pathol.,* 72, 473, 1979.

43. **Weiser, J.,** To the identity of the microsporidia affecting man, *Vest. Cs. Spol. Zool.,* 40, 157, 1976.

44. **Westerman, E. L. and Christensen, R. P.,** Chronic *Isospora belli* infection treated with co-trimoxazole, *Ann. Intern. Med.,* 91, 413, 1979.

45. **Wolters, E., Heydorn, A. O., and Laudahn, C.,** Das Rind als Zwischenwirt von *Cystoisospora felis, Berl. Muench. Tieraerztl. Wochenschr.,* 93, 207, 1980.

PNEUMOCYSTOSIS

D. D. Juranek

Common Synonyms

Common synonyms are *Pneumocystis carinii* pneumonia, pulmonary pneumocystosis, interstitial plasma cell pneumonia, infantile pneumocystosis, hypoergic pneumocystosis, hypoimmune pneumocystosis, epidemic pneumocystosis, pneumocystis pneumonitis.

Etiologic Agent *Pneumocystis carinii* Delanöe and Delanöe, 1912

Pneumocystis is an extracellular organism most frequently found in the pulmonary alveoli of infected animals and humans. It was first described in 1909 by Chagas, who observed the organism in the lungs of guinea pigs infected with *Trypanosoma cruzi*.[16] Carini and Maciel[15] observed the organism in rats infected with *T. lewisi* and believed that the cyst represented a developmental stage in the trypanosome life cycle. Professor and Madame Delanoe[22] were the first to describe the organism in rats without trypanosomes, naming it *P. carinii* in 1912. Ammich[1] and Benecke[5] are credited with the first descriptions of *Pneumocystis* in humans. Although the organism found in humans is also referred to as *P. carinii* in most literature, some scientists believe that the organism in man is a different species.[41]

The taxonomic position of *P. carinii* is uncertain.[51,52,69,93,94] It is regarded as a protozoan by some investigators and as a fungus by others.[20,61] The developmental stages of *P. carinii* have been observed to lack definitive morphologic characteristics that would compel the placement of the organism in either taxonomic group. A serious obstacle to further taxonomic study of the organism has been its failure to grow in vitro. Culture of *P. carinii* might allow the observation of morphologic stages that have not been previously seen, such as mycelial elements or protozoan-type division. While recent reports indicate that it is now possible to culture *Pneumocystis,* there is no indication that definite morphologic characteristics which would lay the taxonomic controversy to rest have been observed.[59,70] However, the recent finding of microtubules in an intracystic body of *P. carinii* by Vossen et al.[96] strongly supports the protozoan nature of *Pneumocystis.*

P. carinii has been extensively studied in tissue sections and smears by light,[51,93] phase-contrast,[6] fluorescent,[71] and electron microscopy.[7,10,14,89,95,99] Five morphologic entities in lung tissue have been described: trophozoites, precysts, cysts, intracystic bodies, and empty cysts.

Trophozoites measure 1 to 5 μm in length and are ovoid to ameboid. The nucleus is usually the only structure seen by light microscopy. Cytoplasmic inclusions and organelles are clearly visible only in electron-microscopic preparations. Precysts measure about 5 μm, are ovoid, have no pseudopodia, and are limited by a thin, semirigid cell wall. These are probably the "thin-walled cysts" visible in specimens stained with PAS or methenamine silver stains. Cysts measure between 3.5 and 5 μm in diameter and are surrounded by a thick, rigid wall. Cyst cytoplasm typically contains several nuclear masses or separate intracystic bodies, easily seen by light microscopy. Eight intracystic bodies, each measuring 1 to 2 μm in diameter, are usually formed in mature cysts. Empty cysts are irregular in shape but often appear crescentic because of the collapse of the cyst wall. Such cysts may contain cytoplasmic remnants recognizable by electron microscopy and occasionally may contain a few intracystic bodies.

Distribution

P. carinii infection occurs world-wide. Infections in humans have been reported in the U.S., Canada, Uruguay, Chile, Brazil, England, most European countries, the U.S.S.R., China, Japan, India, Iran, Israel, South Africa, Congo, Melanesia, Australia, and New Zealand.[13,32,61]

True and Alternate Hosts

P. carinii infection has been reported in man, guinea pigs,[16,22] rats, mice, rabbits,[83] hares,[74] fox,[36] dogs,[19,37,91,92] cats,[102] horses,[85] cattle,[50] sheep,[50,81] goats,[64] pigs,[50,57] and a variety of zoo animals,[18,63,75] including the red kangaroo, common tree shrew, Senegal-galago, Demidoff's galago, brown howler monkey, woolly monkey, long-haired spider monkey, white-eared marmoset, owl monkey, chimpanzee, three-toed sloth, palm squirrel, red panda, fennec fox, tree hyrax, and large-tooth hyrax. *P. carinii* has been found neither in hamsters[40] nor in several hundred birds obtained from the Amsterdam Artis Zoo.[75]

Latent pulmonary infection with *P. carinii* is widespread in apparently healthy laboratory, domesticated, and wild animals.[31,33,39,58,83] There is also evidence of the existence of latent infection in man.[29,31,33,41,42,82]

Disease in Animals

The clinical and histopathologic picture of *Pneumocystis* pneumonitis in animals closely resembles hypoergic pneumocystosis of humans, but it is usually less severe. Naturally acquired pneumocystosis is rarely fatal in animals, but deaths in swine, dogs, foals, and a goat have been reported.[63,85] Experimental illness in mice and rabbits may be produced with *P. carinii* by the administration of high doses of corticosteroids. In rats, on the other hand, experimental disease may be produced by the administration of corticosteroids or cyclophosphamide.[39,83] Plasma-cell infiltrates are rarely seen in the lungs of animals with experimental or naturally acquired disease.[40,83,84] Radiographic changes in the lungs of domesticated animals with *P. carinii* pneumonia have not been studied because ante-mortem diagnosis is rarely made.

Disease in Man

P. carinii pneumonia is usually seen in patients whose immunologic mechanisms are impaired. Based on epidemiologic, clinical, and histologic grounds, two patterns of disease can be distinguished: (1) epidemic pneumocystosis (infantile pneumocystosis), seen in premature, malnourished, and debilitated infants between 2 and 6 months of age, and (2) a sporadically occurring form of pneumocystosis, seen in hypoergic or hypoimmune children and adults.

Epidemic Pneumocystosis of Infants

Epidemic pneumocystosis was first recognized in infants in nurseries for newborns in Europe following World War II. Incubation periods of 1 to 2 months have been estimated from retrospective studies of institutional outbreaks. The onset of disease is insidious and is characterized by anorexia, weight loss, and diarrhea. Tachypnea and a dry, nonproductive cough are the first signs of respiratory involvement. Full development of clinical disease takes 1 to 4 weeks. During this period, tachypnea, dyspnea, and cyanosis become progressively worse. Additional signs include sternal retraction and flaring of the nasal alae. Chest sounds are normal on auscultation and percussion. Fever is not a prominent feature of the disease but may be present.[31,46] The radiographic appearance of the lungs varies with the stage of clinical disease.[72] Chest roentgenograms may show hyperinflated lungs with a bilateral, diffuse, interstitial pulmonary infiltrate that originates at the hilus and extends peripherally. Lighter areas having the appearance of halos are indicative of emphysema.

Lungs appear pale gray and firm at necropsy, and they do not collapse when the chest cavity is opened. There may be gross evidence of parenchymal, interstitial, or mediastinal emphysema along the periphery of the lobes. Cut surfaces do not exude edematous or hemorrhagic fluids; however, an opaque, grayish-pink material may be scraped off the cut lung surface. On microscopic examination, this material has a "honeycombed," foamy appearance and frequently may contain numerous *P. carinii* cysts and trophozoites. Alveolar walls are greatly thickened, a response to the extensive invasion by plasma cells.[2,31,46]

Pneumocystis in the Immunocompromised Host

In hypoergic or hypoimmune pneumocystosis of children and adults, the predisposing immune defect may be caused by either congenital or acquired immunosuppressive disease, immunosuppressive drugs, or both. Disease in the immunocompromised host is clinically similar to that in debilitated infants (see above), except onset of illness is more often abrupt, the clinical course is generally more rapid, and the patient is more often febrile. Radiographic, gross pathologic, and histologic changes in the lungs are similar to those seen in the epidemic form of the disease in infants, except the cellular component of the interstitial infiltrate is predominantly made up of lymphocytes and histiocysts rather than plasma cells.[2]

Mode of Spread

The mode of spread of *P. carinii* is poorly understood, but infection is probably acquired by the respiratory route. Intrauterine, transplacental, and milk-borne (breast milk) transmission have also been implicated.[13] Although latent *Pneumocystis* infections are widespread in both wild and domesticated animals, there are no existing data to support animal-to-human transmission. On the other hand, available data are not sufficient to rule out this route of transmission.

Epidemiology

The life cycle of *P. carinii* is unknown. According to an intrapulmonary cycle hypothesis of Campbell, intracystic bodies escape through the cyst wall and develop into small trophozoites. Mature trophozoites develop directly into precysts and then into cysts. Alternatively, mature trophozoites may undergo a reproductive phase of development before becoming precysts.[14] However, reproductive stages (sexual or asexual) have never been identified in light- or electron-microscopic preparations. Further study of *Pneumocystis* in vitro is necessary to confirm the existence of an intrapulmonary cycle. While *Pneumocystis* is occasionally found in extrapulmonary sites (lymph nodes, thymus, spleen, liver, bone marrow),[3,13,49] the organism has never been found outside of the host.

Infantile *Pneumocystis* pneumonia with plasma-cell infiltrate first assumed clinical significance in the 1940s, when the disease was epidemic and endemic in European nurseries. Several thousand cases were reported, principally in debilitated and premature infants. Mortality rates for infected infants ranged between 20 and 60%.[84] Few cases have been reported since 1960, and it has been suggested that this decline is due to improved nutrition and housing following World War II.[25]

P. carinii pneumonia was first reported in the U.S. in 1956.[21] Since then, the number of cases has continued to increase.

However, the epidemiologic features of the disease in the U.S. differ markedly from those observed in Europe. Pneumonia caused by *P. carinii* in the U.S. usually occurs sporadically and generally affects only immunosuppressed hosts. The disease is more acute and has a higher case fatality ratio (90 to 100%) in untreated patients than the epidemic form of the disease in infants.[46] The incidence of *Pneumocystis* pneumonia in the U.S. is unknown. In certain high-risk groups such as children undergoing intensive chemo- and radiotherapy for acute lymphocytic leukemia, the incidence has been as high as 30 to 40%.[45] Walzer et al. studied the epidemiologic characteristics of the 194 proven cases of pneumocystosis reported to the Center for Disease Control over a 3-year period and found that the most common underlying disease was malignant neoplasia (78%); 13% of the patients had underlying primary immune-deficiency disease, 11% were organ transplant recipients, and the rest had a variety of immunosuppressive disorders or diseases that required immunosuppressive chemotherapy. The authors concluded that the age and sex characteristics of patients with *P. carinii* pneumonia primarily reflect the epidemiologic features of the patients' underlying diseases.[98]

P. carinii organisms from animals are morphologically identical to those from man. There may or may not be antigenic differences; conflicting reports concerning serologic differences between human and animal *Pneumocystis* have appeared in the literature.[53,54] Frenkel reported that he was unable to transmit *Pneumocystis* from rats to hamsters and concluded that the organism exhibited at least some host specificity and was therefore an unlikely source of human infection.[41] However, evidence of intraspecies transmission (e.g., rat-to-rat) is not convincing. A small number of experiments have been conducted, and only a few animals were used in each experiment. The major difficulty encountered by investigators is the presence of latent infection in recipient and control animals.[39,82] While the possibility of animal-to-human transmission of *P. carinii* cannot be dismissed, the many reports implicating person-to-person transmission[11,12,31,46,66,80,97] or activation of latent infection in the immunocompromised host[39,45,73,79,82] suggest that the role of animals as a source of human infection is minor.

Diagnosis

A definitive diagnosis of *P. carinii* pneumonia can be made only by demonstrating the organism in pulmonary tissues or fluids. While *Pneumocystis* has occasionally been recovered from gastric fluids,[78,90] nasopharyngeal secretions,[62,88,90] sputum,[28,30,38,88] and tracheal and bronchial secretions,[23,90] a higher rate of diagnostic success has been achieved with open-lung biopsy, percutaneous needle biopsy or needle aspiration of the lung, transbronchial lung biopsy, or endobronchial brush biopsy.[46,98] The procedure of choice depends upon the clinical status and age of the patient, equipment and facilities available, and the physician's experience with the diagnostic procedure.

Pneumocystis can be most readily detected in tissues, fluids, and secretions stained with Gomori's methamine silver nitrate.[34,35] Cysts appear as dark brown to black ovoid and cup-shaped structures that can be visualized under high, dry magnification. Trophozoites do not stain. Care must be taken to distinguish cysts of *Pneumocystis* from other organisms and cells that also stain positively with methamine silver, especially small fungi, (e.g., *Histoplasma, Candida, Cryptococcus, Torulopsis*), erythrocytes, and parasites such as *Nosema*.[55,100] Smith and Hughes[87] developed a modification of the Gomori stain that reduces the staining time from 3 hr to 10 min, but the technique is not adaptable to biopsy specimens.

Toluidine blue O stain also provides good contrast between cysts and background material.[17] Cysts stain violet or purple, while the background becomes yellow or shades of green. As with Gomori's stain, trophozoites do not stain. The major advantage of toluidine blue O stain over Gomori's stain is that it is a simpler and more rapid technique.

Viable trophozoites, precysts, and cysts can be demonstrated with Giemsa, Wright's, or polychrome methylene blue stains.[26,55] These stains do not provide good contrast between the organism and background material but do reveal morphologic detail not seen with Gomori's or toluidine blue O stains. The principal advantages of these three stains are that they stain rapidly, show morphologic characteristics of *Pneumocystis* that are not easily confused with other cells or organisms, and are readily available in most laboratories. The major disadvantage is that when few organisms are present in specimens, they are not easily detected. Many hours may be spent searching slides in order to confirm the diagnosis.

Serodiagnosis of hypoergic pneumocystosis is unreliable. The indirect immunofluorescence test (IIF) has low sensitivity; and it has been shown to detect only 40% of the proven cases.[53] Also, in one study, 25% of asymptomatic, immunosuppressed individuals had measurable antibody to *P. carinii*.[98] Elevated antibody titers have also been noted in patients with cytomegalovirus infections who did not have pneumocystosis.[46] Thus a negative IIF titer does not rule out the possibility of infection, and a positive result does not confirm that *Pneumocystis* is the cause of disease.

The complement-fixation (CF) test has been a useful diagnostic tool for epidemic *P. carinii* pneumonia of infants. In central Europe, 75 to 97% of children with *P. carinii* pneumonitis produced antibody measurable by the CF test.[4,27,31,46,65] On the other hand, the CF test has not been satisfactory for detecting *P. carinii* antibodies in sporadically occurring cases of hypoergic pneumocystosis reported in the U.S.[29,46,66-68,77,86] Serologic techniques may improve as purer antigens are prepared from organisms grown in vitro.

Prevention and Control

There are no established or universally accepted methods for preventing or controlling pneumocystosis. More information about the organism's source and mode of transmission is needed before definitive recommendations can be formulated. Preventive measures currently under investigation include respiratory isolation of high-risk patients early in the course of undiagnosed respiratory infection and chemoprophylaxis of high-risk patients with trimethoprim-sulfamethoxazole.[26,47]

Treatment

Pentamidine isethionate was once considered the drug of choice for treatment of *Pneumocystis* pneumonia, but the frequent adverse effects associated with its use prompted a search for a less toxic alternative. Recent studies in animals, children, and adults with *Pneumocystis* pneumonia have demonstrated that the oral combination antimicrobial agent, trimethoprim-sulfamethoxazole, is an equally effective and much less toxic drug than pentamidine.[43,44,47,60]

Pentamidine is administered to humans at a dose of 4 mg/kg body weight for 12 to 14 days.[24] Adverse reactions were noted in about one half of the 404 patients who were reported to the Center for Disease Control between November 1967 and January 1971. Major side effects in these patients included impaired renal function (in 24% of the patients treated), pain and swelling at the injection site (18%), liver dysfunction (10%), hypotension (10%), and hypoglycemia (6%).[98] Recovery rates in patients with confirmed pneumocystosis who are treated with pentamidine range between 43 and 75%.[47,98]

Trimethoprim-sulfamethoxazole is given orally to children and adults at the rate of 20 mg of trimethoprim and 100 mg of sulfamethoxazole daily for 12 to 14 days.[24] Toxicity appears minimal; maculopapular rash was noted in 4 of 19 patients treated by Hughes.[44] Recovery rates for patients treated with trimethoprim-sulfamethoxazole have been equivalent to rates for patients treated with pentamidine.[47,48,60]

A third combination (pyrimethamine and a sulfonamide) has also been investigated but appears to be less promising than trimethaprim-sulfamethoxazole.[39,76,102]

REFERENCES

1. **Ammich, O.**, Uber die nichtsyphilitische interstitielle Pneumonie des ersten Kinderalters, *Virchows. Arch. A*, 302, 539, 1938.
2. **Arean, V. M.**, Pulmonary pneumocystosis, in *Pathology of Protozoal and Helminthic Diseases*, Marcial-Rojas, R. A., Ed., Williams & Wilkins, Baltimore, 1971, 291.
3. **Barnett, R. N., Hull, J. G., Vortel, V., Kralove, H., and Schwartz, J.**, *Pneumocystis carinii* in lymph nodes and spleen, *Arch. Pathol.*, 88, 173, 1969.
4. **Barta, K.**, complement-fixation test for pneumocystosis, *Ann. Intern. Med.*, 70, 235, 1969.
5. **Benecke, E.**, Eigenartige Bronchiolenerkrankung im ersten Lebensjahr, *Verh. Dtsch. Ges. Pathol.*, 31, 402, 1938.
6. **Bommer, W.**, Vergleichende morphologische studien an Pneumocysten, Hefen und Zellkernen mit dem Phasenkontrastmikroskop, *Arch. Kinderheilkd.*, 163, 113, 1961.
7. **Bommer, W.**, Electronenmikroskopische Untersuchungen an *Pneumocystis carinii* aus menschlichen Lungen, *Dtsch. Med. Wochenschr.*, 86, 1309, 1961.
8. **Bommer, W.**, *Pneumocystis carinii* from human lungs under electron microscope, *Am. J. Dis. Child.*, 104, 657, 1962.
9. **Bommer, W.**, Die interstitielle plasmacellulare Pneumonie und *Pneumocystis carinii, Ergeb. Mikrobiol. Immunitaetsforsch. Exp.*, 38, 116, 1964.
10. **Bommer, W.**, Untersuchungen an *Pneumocystis carinii, Zentralbl. Bakteriol. Parasitenkd. Infektionskr. Hyg. Abt. 1: Orig.*, 192, 300, 1964.
11. **Brazinsky, J. H. and Phillips, J. E.**, *Pneumocystis* pneumonia transmission between patients with lymphoma (letter to the editor), *JAMA*, 209, 1527, 1969.
12. **de Brito, T. and Enge, L. G. H. B.**, Pneumonia intersticial plasmocclular pelo *Pneumocystis carinii, Rev. Inst. Med. Trop. Sao Paulo*, 4, 261, 1962.
13. **Burke, B. A. and Good, R. A.**, *Pneumocystis carinii* infection, *Medicine (Baltimore)*, 52(1), 23, 1973.
14. **Campbell, W. B.**, Ultrastructure of *Pneumocystis* in human lung. Life cycle in human pneumocystosis, *Arch. Pathol.*, 93, 312, 1972.
15. **Carini, A. and Maciel, J.**, Uber *Pneumocystis carinii, Centralbl. Bakteriol.*, 77, 46, 1915.
16. **Chagas, C.**, Nova tripanozomiaza humana. Estudos sobre a morfolojia e o ciclo evolutive de *Schizotrypanum cruzi* n. gen., n. sp., ajente etiologio de nova entidade morbida de homen, *Mem. Inst. Oswaldo Cruz.*, 1, 159, 1909.
17. **Chalvardjian, A. M. and Grawe, L. A.**, A new procedure for the identification of *Pneumocystis carinii* in tissue sections and smears, *J. Clin. Pathol.*, 16, 283, 1963.
18. **Chandler, F. W., McClure, H. M., Campbell, W. G., and Watts, J. C.**, Pulmonary pneumocystosis in nonhuman primates, *Arch. Pathol. Lab. Med.*, 100, 163, 1976.
19. **Copland, J. W.**, Canine pneumonia caused by *Pneumocystis carinii, Aust. Vet. J.*, 50(1), 515, 1974.
20. **Csillag, A.**, Contribution to the taxonomical classification of the so-called *Pneumocystis carinii, Acta. Microbiol. Acad. Sci. Hung.*, 4, 1, 1957.
21. **Dauzier, G., Willis, T., and Barnett, R. N.**, *Pneumocystis carinii* in an infant, *Am. J. Clin. Pathol.*, 26, 787, 1956.
22. **Delanöe, P. and Delanöe, M.**, Sur les raports des kystes de Carini du poumon des rats avec le *Trypanosoma lewisi, C.R. Acad. Sci.*, 155, 658, 1912.
23. **Drew, W. L., Finley, T. N., Mintz, L., and Klein, H. Z.**, Diagnosis of *Pneumocystis carinii* pneumonia by bronchopulmonary lavage, *JAMA*, 230, 713, 1974.
24. Drugs for parasitic infections, *Med. Lett. Drugs Ther.*, 24(601), 5, 1982.
25. **Dutz, W.**, *Pneumocystis carinii* pneumonia, *Pathobiol. Annu.*, 5, 309, 1970.
26. **Dutz, W. and Burke, B. A.**, Cytologic diagnosis of *Pneumocystis carinii, Natl. Cancer Inst. Monogr.*, 43, 157, 1976.
27. **Dymowska, Z.**, Serological investigations in children suspected of having pneumocystoses, *Med. Dosw. Mikrobiol.*, 17, 319, 1965.
28. **Esterly, J. A. and Warner, N. E.**, *Pneumocystis carinii* pneumonia — twelve cases in patients with neoplastic lymphoreticular disease, *Arch. Pathol.*, 80, 433, 1965.
29. **Esterly, J. A.**, *Pneumocystis carinii* in lungs of adults at autopsy, *Am. Rev. Respir. Dis.*, 97, 935, 1968.
30. **Erchul, J. W., Williams, L. P., and Meighan, P. O.**, *Pneumocystis carinii* in hypopharyngeal material, *N. Engl. J. Med.*, 267, 926, 1962.
31. **Gajdusek, D. C.**, *Pneumocystis carinii* etiologic agent of interstitial plasma cell pneumonitis of premature and young infants, *Pediatrics*, 19, 543, 1957.
32. **Gajdusek, D. C.**, *Pneumocystis carinii* as the cause of human disease. Historical perspective and magnitude of the problem, *Natl. Cancer Inst. Monogr.*, 43, 1, 1976.

33. Goetz, O., Die Actiologic der interstitiellen Sogenannten plasmacellulare pneumonie des jungens Sauglings, *Arch. Kinderheilkd.* (Suppl.), 163, 1, 1960.

34. Gomori, G., A new histochemical test for glycogen and mucin, *Am. J. Clin. Pathol.*, 10, 177, 1946.

35. Grocott, R. A., A stain for fungi in tissue sections and smears, *Am. J. Clin. Pathol.*, 25, 975, 1955.

36. Faust, E. C., Russell, P. F., and Jung, R. C., Other sporozoa: toxoplasma, sarcocystis, pneumocystis, in *Craig and Faust's Clinical Parasitology*, 8th ed., Lea & Febiger, Philadelphia, 1970, 229.

37. Farrow, B. R., Watson, D., and Hartley, W. J., *Pneumocystis* pneumonia in a dog, *J. Comp. Pathol.*, 82, 447, 1972.

38. Fortuny, I. E., Tempero, K. F., and Amsden, T. W., *Pneumocystis carinii* pneumonia diagnosed from sputum and successfully treated with pentamidine isethionate, *Cancer (Brussels)*, 26, 911, 1970.

39. Frenkel, J. K., Good, J. T., and Schultz, J. A., Latent *Pneumocystis* infection of rats, relapse, and chemotherapy, *Lab. Invest.*, 15, 1559, 1966.

40. Frenkel, J. K., Protozoal diseases of laboratory animals, in *Pathology of Protozoal and Helminthic Diseases*, Marcial-Rojas, R. A., Ed., Williams & Wilkins, Baltimore, 1971, 355.

41. Frenkel, J. K., *Pneumocystis jiroveci* n. sp. from man: morphology, physiology, immunology in relation to pathology, *Natl. Cancer Inst. Monogr.*, 43, 13, 1976.

42. Hamlin, W. B., *Pneumocystis carinii*, *JAMA*, 204, 173, 1968.

43. Hughes, W. T., McNabb, P. C., Makres, T. D., and Feldman, S., Efficacy of trimethoprim and sulfamethoxazole in the prevention and treatment of *Pneumocystis carinii* pneumonitis, *Antimicrob. Agents Chemother.*, 5, 289, 1974.

44. Hughes, W. T., Feldman, S., and Sanyal, S. K., Treatment of *Pneumocystis carinii* pneumonitis with trimethoprim-sulfamethoxazole, *Can. Med. Assoc. J.*, 112, 478, 1975.

45. Hughes, W. T., Feldman, S., Aur, R. J. A., Verzosa, M. S., Hustu, H. O., and Simone, J. V., Intensity of immunosuppressive therapy and the incidence of *Pneumocystis carinii* pneumonia, *Cancer (Brussels)*, 36, 2004, 1975.

46. Hughes, W. T., Current status of laboratory diagnosis of *Pneumocystis carinii* pneumonitis, *CRC Crit. Rev. Clin. Lab. Sci.*, 6(2), 145, 1975.

47. Hughes, W. T., Treatment of *Pneumocystis carinii* pneumonitis, *N. Engl. J. Med.*, 295, 726, 1976.

48. Hughes, W. T., Feldman, S., and Chaudhary, S., Comparison of trimethoprim-sulfamethoxazole (TMP-SMZ) and pentamidine (PNT) in the treatment of *Pneumocystis carinii* pneumonitis (PCP), *Pediatr. Res.*, 10, 399-A, 1976.

49. Jarnum, S., Rasmussen, E. F., Ohlsen, A. S., and Sorensen, A. W. S., Generalized *Pneumocystis carinii* infection with severe idiopathic hypoproteinemia, *Ann. Intern. Med.*, 68, 138, 1968.

50. Jecny, V., Demonstration of *Pneumocystis carinii* in calves, lambs, and piglets, *Cesk. Epidemiol. Microbiol. Immunol.*, 22(3), 135, 1973.

51. Jirovec, O. and Vanek, J., Zur morphologie der *Pneumocystis carinii* und zur pathogeneses der *Pneumocystis* pneumonie, *Zentralbl. Allg. Pathol.*, 92, 424, 1954.

52. Jirovec, O., Das problem der *Pneumocystis* pneumonie vom parasitologischen standpunkte, *Monatsschr. Kinderheilkd.*, 108, 136, 1960.

53. Kagan, I. G. and Norman, L. G., Serology of pneumocystosis, *Natl. Cancer Inst. Monogr.*, 43, 121, 1976.

54. Kim, H. K., Hughes, W. T., and Feldman, S., Studies of morphology and immunofluorescence of *Pneumocystis carinii*, *Proc. Soc. Exp. Biol. Med.*, 141, 304, 1972.

55. Kim, H. and Hughes, W. T., Comparison of methods for identification of *Pneumocystis carinii* in pulmonary aspirates, *Am. J. Clin. Pathol.*, 60, 462, 1973.

56. Kucera, K., Some new views on the epidemiology of infections caused by Pneumocystis carinii, *Proc. Int. Congr. Parasitol.*, Vol. 1, Pergamon Press, New York, 1964, 452.

57. Kucera, K., Slesinger, L., and Kadlec, A., Pneumocystosis in pigs, *Folia Parasitol. Prague*, 15, 75, 1968.

58. Kucera, K., Vanek, J., and Jirovec, O., Pneumozystose, in *Leitfaden der Zooanthroponosen*, Toppich, E. and Kruger, W., Eds., VEB Verlag Volk and Gesundheit, Berlin, 1971, 279.

59. Latorree, C. R., Sulzer, A. J., and Norman, L. G., Serial propagation of *Pneumocystis carinii* in cell line cultures, *Appl. Microbiol.*, 33, 1204, 1977.

60. Lau, W. K. and Young, L. S., Trimethoprim-sulfamethoxazole treatment of *Pneumocystis carinii* pneumonia in adults, *N. Engl. J. Med.*, 295, 716, 1976.

61. LeClair, R. A., *Pneumocystis carinii* and interstial plasma cell pneumonia, a review, *Am. Rev. Respir. Dis.*, 96, 1131, 1967.

62. Le-tan-Vinh, G. G., Cochard, A. M., Vu-Trien-Dong, and Solonar, W., Diagnostic "in vivo" de la pneumonie a "pneumocystic," *Arch. Fr. Pediatr.*, 20, 773, 1963.

63. Long, G. G., White, J. D., and Stookey, J. L., *Pneumocystis carinii* infection in splenectomized owl monkeys, *J. Am. Vet. Med. Assoc.*, 167, 651, 1975.

64. McConnell, E. E., Basson, P. A., and Pienaar, J. G., Pneumocystis in a domestic goat, *Onderstepoort J. Vet. Res.*, 38(2), 117, 1971.

65. Meidl, F., On the pathogenesis and laboratory diagnosis of so-called interstitial plasma-cell pneumonia in infants, *Zentralbl. Bakertiol. Parasitenkd. Infektionskr. Hyg. Abt. 1: Orig.,* 180, 281, 1960.

66. Meuwissen, H. J., Brzosko, W. J., Nowoslawski, A., and Good, R. A., Diagnosis of *Pneumocystis carinii* pneumonia in the presence of immunological deficiency, *Lancet,* 1, 1124, 1970.

67. Meuwissen, J. H. E. and Leeuwenberg, D., A micro-complement fixation test applied to infection with *Pneumocystis carinii, Trop. Geogr. Med.,* 24, 282, 1972.

68. Minielly, J. A., McDuffie, F. C., and Holley, K. E., Immunofluorescent identification of *Pneumocystis carinii, Arch. Pathol.,* 90, 561, 1970.

69. Mojon, M., Hommage a Jirovec, Critique de la place taxonomique de *Pneumocystis carinii, Lyon Med.,* 288, 325, 1972.

70. Murphey, M. J., Pifer, L. L., and Hughes, W. T., *Pneumocystis carinii* in vitro — a study by scanning electron microscopy, *Am. J. Pathol.,* 86, 387, 1977.

71. Opkerkuch, W. and Ricken, D., Die Fluorchromierung von *Pneumocystis carinii, Virchows Arch. A,* 332, 132, 1959.

72. Paldy, L. and Ivady, G., Roentgenologic diagnosis of interstitial plasma cell pneumonia in infancy, *Natl. Cancer Inst. Monogr.,* 43, 99, 1976.

73. Perera, D. R., Western, K. A., Johnson, H. D., Johnson, W. W., Schultz, M. G., and Akers, P. V., *Pneumocystis carinii* pneumonia in a hospital for children, *JAMA,* 214(6), 1074, 1970.

74. Poelma, F. G. and Broekhuizen, S., *Pneumocystis carinii* in hares, *Lepus europaeus pallas,* in Netherlands, *Z. Parasitenkd.,* 40, 195, 1972.

75. Poelma, F. G., *Pneumocystis carinii* infections in zoo animals, *Z. Parasitenkd.,* 46, 61, 1975.

76. Post, C., Fakouhi, T., Dutz, W., Bandarizadeh, B., and Kohout, E. E., Prophylaxis of epidemic infantile pneumocystosis with a 20:1 sulfadoxine-pyrimethamine combination, *Curr. Ther. Res. Clin. Exp.,* 13, 273, 1971.

77. Rifkind, D., Faris, T. D., and Hill, R. B., *Pneumocystis carinii* pneumonia, *Ann. Intern. Med.,* 65, 943, 1966.

78. Reisetbauer, E. and Moritsch, H., Epidemiologische and serologische Undersuchungen bei interstitieller plasma-zellularer Fruhgeburtenpneumonie, *Monatsschr. Kinderheilkd.,* 104, 41, 1956.

79. Ruebush, T. K., Weinstein, R. A., Bachner, R. L., Smith, J. W., Gonzales-Crussi, F., Wolff, D., Bartlett, M. S., Sulzer, A. J., and Schultz, M. G., An outbreak of *Pneumocystis* pneumonia in children with acute lymphocytic leukemia, *Am. J. Dis. Child.,* 132, 143, 1978.

80. Ruskin, J. and Remingron, J. S., The compromised host and infection. I. *Pneumocystis carinii* pneumonia, *JAMA,* 202(12), 96, 1967.

81. Shchetinin, A. N., *Pneumocystis* infection in sheep, *Veterinaria Moscow,* 3, 74, 1973.

82. Sheldon, W. H., Subclinical *Pneumocystis* pneumonitis, *Am. J. Dis. Child.,* 97, 287, 1959.

83. Sheldon, W. H., Experimental pulmonary *Pneumocystis carinii* infection in rabbits, *J. Exp. Med.,* 110, 147, 1959.

84. Sheldon, W. H., Pulmonary *Pneumocystis carinii* infection, *Med. Prog.,* 61, 780, 1962.

85. Shively, J. N., Dellers, R. W., Buergelt, C. D., Hsu, F. S., Kabelac, L. P., Moe, K. K., Tennant, B., and Vaughan, J. T., *Pneumocystis carinii* pneumonia in two foals, *J. Am. Vet. Med. Assoc.,* 162, 648, 1973.

86. Smith, E. and Gaspar, I. A., Pentamidine treatment of *Pneumocystis carinii* pneumonitis in an adult with lymphatic leukemia, *Am. J. Med.,* 44, 626, 1968.

87. Smith, J. W. and Hughes, W. T., A rapid staining technique for *Pneumocystis carinii, J. Clin. Pathol.,* 25, 269, 1972.

88. Stopka, E., Wunderlich, C., and Carlson, S., Morphologische and kulturelle Untersuchungen an Pneumozysten in Sputum und Lungenmaterial, *Z. Kinderheilkd.,* 79, 246, 1957.

89. Timmel, H., Morphologischer Beitrag zum *Pneumocystis*-Probleme, *Zentralbl. Allg. Pathol.,* 102, 439, 1961.

90. Toth, G., Balogh, E., and Belay, M., Tracheal smear in pentamidine-treated plasma-cell pneumonia, *Acta Paediatr. Acad. Sci. Hung.,* 7, 339, 1966.

91. Tvedten, H. W., Langham, R. F., and Beneke, E. S., Systemic *Pneumocystis carinii* infection in a dog, *J. Am. Anim. Hosp. Assoc.,* 10(6), 592, 1974.

92. van den Akker, S. and Goldbled, E., Pneumonia caused by *Pneumocystis carinii* in a dog, *Trop. Geogr. Med.,* 12, 54, 1960.

93. Vanek, J. and Jirovec, O., Parasitare Pneumonie, ''Interstitielle'' Plasmazell en Pneumonie der Fruhgeborenen, verursacht durch *Pneumonocystis carinii, Zentralbl. Bakteriol. Parasitenkd. Infektionskr. Hyg. Abt. 1: Orig. Reihe A,* 158, 120, 1952.

94. Vanek, J., Parasitare Pneumonie verursacht durch *Pneumocystis carinii* bei einer 60 jahrigen Frau, *Zentralbl. Allg. Pathol.,* 90, 424, 1953.

95. Vavra, J. and Kucera, K., *Pneumocystis carinii* Delanöe: its ultrastructure and ultrastructural affinities, *J. Protozool.,* 17, 463, 1970.

96. Vossen, M. E. M. H., Beckers, P. J. A., Meuwissen, J. H. E. T., and Stadhouders, A. M., Microtubules in *Pneumocystis carinii.* Short communications, *Z. Parasitenkd.,* 49, 291, 1976.

97. Watanabe, J. M., Chinchinian, H., Weitz, C., and McIlvaney, S. K., *Pneumocystis carinii* pneumonia in a family, *JAMA,* 193(8), 119, 1965.

98. Walzer, P., Perl, D. P., Krogstad, D. J., Rawson, P. G., and Schultz, M. G., *Pneumocystis carinii* pneumonia in the United States: epidemiologic, diagnostic, and clinical features, *Ann. Intern. Med.,* 80, 83, 1974.

99. Wessel, W. and Richen, D., Elektronenmikroskopische Untersuchung von *Pneumocystis carinii, Virchows Arch. A,* 331, 545, 1958.

100. Young, R. C., Bennett, J. E., and Chu, E. W., Organisms mimicking *Pneumocystis carinii, Lancet,* 2, 1082, 1976.

101. Young, R. C. and deVita, V. T., Treatment of *Pneumocystis carinii* pneumonia: current status of the regimens of pentamidine isethionate and pyrimethamine-sulfadiazine, *Natl. Cancer Inst. Monogr.,* 43, 193, 1976.

102. Zavala, V. J. and Rosado, E. R., *Pneumocystis carinii* en animales domesticos de la ciudad de Merida, Yucatan, *Salud Publica Mex.,* 14, 103, 1972.

PART 2. CESTODE ZOONOSES

THE CESTODE ZOONOSES

Primo Arambulo III

INTRODUCTION

The Cestode Zoonoses constitute a medically and economically important group of parasitic zoonoses. On one hand, they are medically important as a cause of serious human illness, like cysticercosis and hydatidosis, while on the other hand, they are economically important as a universal cause of condemnation of hundreds of tons of meat and livers, exacerbating the already scarce supply of animal protein and compounding the problem of human malnutrition.

Tapeworms, by virtue of their size, have been known since prehistoric times. It is perhaps the first zoonosis to be recognized. On a religious basis, the biblical edict under the Mosaic Laws prohibited the consumption of pork. In 1855, it was shown by Kuchenmeister that, by feeding cysterci from the flesh of a pig to a condemned prisoner, he was later able to recover the adult tapeworm, *Taenia solium,* from the dead man's intestine.[11] In 1861, Leuckart demonstrated the development of cysticerci in the flesh of a calf, by feeding with gravid segments of *T. saginata.* Oliver, 8 years later, completed the life cycle of the human beef tapeworm, *T. saginata,* by feeding cysterci from cattle to humans and later recovering the adult worm. Since then, these zoonoses have been extensively studied.[13]

The cestodes are taxonomically divided into two basic groups: Pseudeophyllidea and Cyclophyllidea.[9] *Diphylobothrium* and the etiologic agents of sparganosis belong to the pseudophyllidean group of tapeworms. They could be described in broad morphological terms as possessing a spatulate scolex with two opposite sucking organs without hooklets and accessory attachment structure, and their eggs are operculated and immature when laid.

The etiologic agents of taeniasis and cystcereosis, echinococcosis and hydatidosis, dipylidiasis, hymenolepiasis, and *Raillietina* and *Bertiella* infections are cyclophyllidean tapeworms. Their general morphological attributes consist of a scolex that is more or less transversely quadrate provided with a cup-like sucker at each of the four angles and, in many species, has a special organ of attachment which is armed with hooklets, except *T. saginata.* Their eggs contain a mature embryo when laid.

The tapeworms are cosmopolitan in distribution. Their geographical range is generally delimited by sociocultural determinants, much less by biological factors. The two well-known human tapeworms, *T. solium* and *T. saginata,* are cosmopolitan in their distribution. Stoll, in his now classic paper entitled, "This Wormy World", estimated in 1947 that some 39 million persons in the world were infected with *T. saginata,* while some 2.5 million were infected with *T. solium.* But since 1947, the world's population has more than doubled, while the cattle and swine populations increased by approximately twofold. Today, it would seem reasonable to assume that the number of people infected with these cestodes is more than Stoll's earlier estimates. Moreover, several other factors including intensification of animal agriculture, development of meat industries in developing countries, increase in the world meat and livestock trade, large scale migration of agricultural workers, *inter alia,* have actually contributed to the increase in prevalence of taeniasis and cysticercosis.[1]

It has been observed that one of the more important means of spread of cysticercosis in food animals is through the agricultural use of contaminated sewage for irrigation or the utilization of water from contaminated sources, like rivers and ponds, as livestock drinking water. In many areas, sewage is not treated. And even if sewage treatment facilities do exist, the widespread use of laundry detergents in recent years has promoted the survival of *Taenia* and other parasite eggs, by interfering with sedimentation, putrefaction, and oxidation.[18]

It was estimated in 1973 that some nine million persons were infected with *Diphyllobothrium*: five million in Europe, four million in Asia, and less than one tenth of a million in the Americas (see chapter on Diphyllobothriasis by Bylund).

The incidence of human infection with larval tapeworms, such as Echinococcosis (hydatidosis) and cysticercosis, is difficult to quantify due to the lack of precise diagnostic tools.[20] For instance, it was reported in 1974 in endemic areas in South America, such as in Uruguay, Argentina, and Chile, that the mean annual morbidity based on hospitalized cases and radiography was between 20.7 and 150 cases per 100,000 population. There is apparently a broad discrepancy between the true level of incidence of human infection with hydatidosis and that reflected by clinical and laboratory diagnostic results (see chapter on Echinococcosis by Schantz).

T. solium cysticercosis, especially neurocysticercosis, is a serious problem in Latin America particularly. As in hydatidosis, the diagnostic methods available for human cysticercosis are not very reliable. Recently the enzyme-linked immuno-specific assay (ELISA) was adapted for the laboratory diagnosis of human cysticercosis, and was shown to be statistically more specific than the indirect hemagglutination inhibition (IHA) test.[4] Neurocysticercosis causes hundreds of hospital admissions each year, especially in Mexico and Latin America. The incidence of neurocysticercosis based on neurosurgical diagnosis, which is a very poor reflection of its true incidence, varies from 0.03 to 2.9% in Brazil, 0.5 to 1.3% in Chile, 0.9% in Colombia, and 3.3 to 8.9% in Mexico[15] (see chapter on Taeniasis and Cysticercosis by Pawłowski).

The economic losses from the cestode zoonoses are prodigious, while their social consequences are immense and unquantifiable. It was estimated in the 1960s that the annual monetary losses from human hydatidosis in three endemic countries in South America, based on hospitalization and surgery costs alone, was $500,000 in U.S. dollars. It would seem reasonable to assume that the present losses are ten times more than this estimate, considering the drastic increase in the cost of medical care. Recent studies conducted in two hospitals in Mexico city showed that it cost an estimated $1,600 in U.S. dollars for a single human patient to be treated for cysticercosis, prognosis of which is usually unfavorable once diagnosis has been established.[15]

Pecuniary losses are in some ways better quantifiable in animals since costs could be assigned to specific direct losses in meat and carcass value. Still, the consequential losses and opportunity cost loss are difficult to quantify. It was estimated that, in the 1960s, Belgium, East Germany, Ireland, West Germany, and Yugoslavia sustained annual losses of some $4.3 million in U.S. dollars from bovine cysticercosis.[8] In the U.S., about $500,000 in U.S. dollars is lost annually from condemnation and freezing of carcasses infected with *T. saginata* cysticercus.[16] Kenya, Uganda, and Ethiopia sustain an estimated combined annual loss of some $10 million in U.S. dollars. It is estimated that, in the U.K., losses between $500,000 to $1 million in U.S. dollars are incurred every year due to bovine cysticercosis.[1]

There is a high incidence of *T. solium* cysticercosis in swine, particularly in Latin America and Asia. In fact, in these regions, *T. solium* cysticercosis in pigs is more prevalent than *T. saginata* cysticercosis in cattle. Unfortunately, the information available from most countries where *T. solium* cysticercosis is common are limited and at most sketchy. In Latin America, it was estimated that 95,747 tons of pork valued at $67,787,250 in U.S. dollars are condemned annually due to *T. solium* cysticercosis.[15] In Southeast Asia, the rate of infection with *T. solium* cysticercus has been reported to range between 0.03 to 11.67/100,000 pigs. These data are based on post-mortem inspection in the different major slaughterhouses in the Philippines.[3]

Human behavior and food habits are significantly linked to the acquisition of many parasitic zoonoses. The epidemiology of the major cestode zoonoses are perhaps influenced more by sociocultural determinants rather than biological factors. Humans are infected with the adult tapeworms by eating raw or undercooked flesh harboring the infective larval stage, the bladder-like cysticercus in meat in case of the cyclophyllidean tapeworms, or the ribbon-like sparganun in fish in case of the pseudephyllidean tapeworms.

The consumption of raw or undercooked flesh of mammals or fish is a complex human behavioral pattern. There are a number of psychological imperatives associated with this human behavior; these play the most fundamental factor in maintaining the endemicity and ensuring the transmission of food-borne cestode zoonoses. This human behavior factor plays a major role in the interaction of the various disease determinants within the classic epidemiological triad of host, causative agent, and environment. For instance, while in juxtaposition, a suitable environment and susceptible population may ensure the completion of the biological cycle of the cestode zoonoses, behavior factors may alter the pattern of infection and maintain endemicity within a racial, ethnic, or religious group, or within a geographical population. Sociocultural factors exert an overwhelming influence on the maintenance of foci of infection of some cestode zoonoses, despite the availability of knowledge and methods for their prevention and control. Deeply rooted cultural practices and traditions often defy any change, even that aimed at improving health and well-being. Food habits in all their global diversity sometimes defy any logic, and this is particularly significant in the maintenance of endemicity of the cestode zoonoses.[5]

Various types of raw or undercooked meat and fish delicacies have been linked to human infection with cestode zoonoses. Dishes like "shaslik" in the U.S.S.R. and Turkey, "tikka" in India and Pakistan, "basterma" in Egypt, "larb" in Thailand, "sinugba" and "kinilaw" in the Philippines, and various undercooked steaks or roasts consumed under different names have been associated with the different *Taenia* infections.[1,6]

In Peru and the Pacific coast of South America, a native delicacy called "ceviche", prepared by marinating bite-size morsels of marine fish in lime juice and hot pepper, and eaten raw is believed to be responsible for human infection with *D. pacificum* in those areas. The developmental cycle of this species of *Dyphyllobothrium* apparently takes place entirely in a marine habitat. In the Finnish Lake District, slightly salted fillets of various fresh water fish are customary diet. The fillets are kept in brine for 1 to 3 days and eaten without further cooking (see chapter on Dyphyllobothriasis by Bylund).

Endemic areas of taeniasis in the Philippines have been associated with the consumption of a native dish called "kinilaw", which is prepared basically like "ceviche", but using various kinds of meat or fish as the basic ingredient. Dog meat especially is a local *piéce de resistance,* although it has not been directly associated with *Taenia* infection in humans.[6]

Religious traditions and practices exert a significant influence on the maintenance of infection of cestode zoonoses. For instance, for reasons still not completely known, the pastoral Turkana people of northwestern Kenya have the highest incidence of hydatidosis of any population group in the world; it is even considerably higher than their related pastoral neighbors who share some of their cultural practices.[17] The basic reason is that, among these tribal groups, only the Turkana practice the religious custom of leaving their dead kin exposed to hyenas and dogs, thus acting as reservoirs of infection.

Traditional behaviors and customs in similar fashion exert tremendous influence on the high incidence of hydatidosis in some countries of the Eastern Mediterranean. In

Lebanon, for example, the age old surviving local practice of leather preparation by batting hides in a decoction of dog feces is believed to be responsible for the high risk of hydatid infection among Lebanese shoemakers and shoe repairers (see chapter on Echinococcosis by Schantz).

The taxonomy and epidemiology of the cestodes are in a state of constant flux. In fact, Davaine succinctly expressed the confusion that reigns in relation to the cestodes in his famous quote that: "no animal has been responsible for more hypotheses, discussions, and errors than the tapeworms." For one, the cestode as a group are prone to morphological abnormalities.

Perhaps some of the drawbacks of the present method of taxonomic classification of the cestodes is that it uses morphology as the fundamental basis. For instance, it has been shown that physiological and chemical criteria (such as electrophoretic separation of isoenzymes) could be used to distinguish the "horse strain" of *Echinococcus granulosus* prevalent in the U.K. and parts of Western Europe.[20]

The taxonomic confusion is particularly severe among the pseudophyllidean tapeworms; evidence of this is the proliferation of genera and species of agents of sparganosis (see chapter on Sparganosis by Daly). Equally, the taxonomic confusion is still unresolved with the speciation of the genus *Echinococcus,* so much so that, to avoid further confusion, a moratorium had to be imposed by research workers to the effect that minor variations within the genus should be informally designated as "strains" until their epidemiological and taxonomic status could be fully clarified.

A paradoxical situation has been described in the Philippines, of the existence of foci of *T. saginata* taeniasis, but no cysticercus of *T. saginata* was found in cattle.[6] A 5-year study on two endemic foci in the rural southern Philippines reported a prevalence of human infection with *T. saginata* of 11%. The same areas are also endemic for paragonimiasis and schistosomiasis, in addition to high prevalence of ascariasis, trichuriasis, and hookworm infection. The adult tapeworms recovered following treatment of human cases grossly and microscopically conform with the morphology of *T. saginata.* Epidemiological investigation revealed that the population consume a local delicacy called "kinilaw", prepared by soaking various meat (generally pork) in lime juice seasoned with hot pepper, and eaten without further cooking while imbibing a local alcoholic beverage made from palm tree sap. Carebeef* and dog meat are occasionally prepared into "kinilaw", but beef is rarely eaten due to unavailability and expensiveness. Only 1.6% of the cases ate beef, while 92.6% responded affirmatively to eating pork either as "kinilaw" or "sinugba".

The literature on cysticercosis in the Philippines was reviewed exhaustively which revealed that the cysticercus of *T. saginata* was reported only once in an indigenous cattle, oddly located in the liver,[14] and that it has not been encountered on routine meat inspection of carcasses of slaughtered cattle or water buffalo.[2]

In an endemic area in the Wulai District of Taiwan where there are no cattle, wild goats have been suggested to serve as the intermediate host of *T. saginata* although the cysticercus has not been demonstrated.[10]

Cestode zoonoses in which humans have traditionally been an accidental host, such as dipylidiasis, *Hymenolepis diminuta* and *H. nana* infections, and infections with *Raillietina* and *Bertiella* species (see corresponding chapters by Jueco) may actually become more of a problem in the future due to increased contact between humans and synantropic animals (particularly dogs and rodents) resulting from increased urbanization, and the alteration of human susceptibility to infections through the increasing use of immuno-suppressive drugs. Equally, other uncertain factors related to the con-

---

*   Meat from water buffalo.

tinuing and dynamic biological struggle between parasite and host may actually end in the establishment of previously innocuous tapeworms as human pathogens.

Other rare *Taenia* species have been occasionally reported in humans, such as *T. confusa* from Nebraska, Texas, Louisiana, Illinois, Tennessee, and Mississippi in the U.S. and East Africa; and *T. africana* from a native soldier in East Africa. The latter two species possess a scolex that is not armed with hooklets, like *T. saginata. T. taeniaformis,* a parasite of cats, has been reported in a 5-year-old child in Buenos Aires, Argentina.

The larva of the cestodes of the genus *Multiceps* produces coenurosis in humans, but determination of the particular species to which the coenuri in humans belong is difficult to establish. Some 51 cases of human coenurosis have been recorded in literature, distributed as follows: Nigeria—2, Congo—3, Uganda—17, Ruwanda—9, Kenya—1, South Africa—9, U.S.—1, Brazil—1, England—2, and France—6.[9]

The species of *Multiceps* in animals include *M. multiceps* (the "gid" worm producing ocular or cerebral coenurosis), *M. glomerolatus, M. serialis,* and *M. brauni.* The adult tapeworms are found in the intestine of canine definitive hosts, including dogs, foxes, and wolves. The larval coenuri occurs in various species of animals, acquired following ingestion of taeniid eggs from the feces of the definitive hosts.

Human infection with adult *Multiceps (M. longihamatus)* have been reported in Japan.[12]

The prevention and control of the different cestode zoonoses are described in detail in the respective chapters.

In dealing with the prevention and control of the cestode zoonoses, one cannot help but ponder on the strange paradoxes in human behavior, particularly that in relation to the attainment of individual health. The question as to why some deliberately engage in practices that would undermine health despite the awareness of their consequences is a psychological imperative that could not be explained by any rational process. Deep rooted cultural traditions and religious practices seem to exert an imperturbable force on individual behavior which will defy any kind of change.

The mode of transmission of most of the cestode zoonoses has been elucidated. Adequate, practical knowledge exists on how to interrupt their biological cycle to prevent further transmission. Critical points have been identified where intervention measures could be applied to prevent human infection. An example of this is the application of veterinary meat inspection procedures in slaughter places. The necessary technology is available in preventing the dissemination of infection, such as the containment of human feces and proper sewage disposal. But apparently, despite the wherewithal to prevent and control the cestode zoonoses, no dramatic reduction in prevalence has been achieved in contemporary times. New foci of infections are continuously being established and recognized. For instance, in the case of *T. saginata* taeniasis, the increasing affluence in some countries also increases the risk of infection by enabling a greater portion of the population to consume more beef, usually in the form of steak consumed rare to preserve the delicate flavor of beef.

The approach to the prevention and control of the cestode zoonoses should be viewed from the vantage point of a sociocultural perspective. Recommendations should not merely take the form of bland statements such as: "avoid eating raw foods", "avoid contact with dog feces", etc. A thorough study, especially of certain local practices, behaviors, and habits that contribute to the endemicity of infection, should be carried out. These studies should form the bases of the educational program for prevention and control which should involve community participation within the concept of Primary Health Care. For instance, education, both in schools and the community level, is believed to be the most effective method in successfully controlling hydatidosis in New Zealand and Iceland.[17]

The search for more effective drugs against the cestode zoonoses should continue. As yet, the only recourse for patients with hydatidosis is surgery. There is yet no effective treatment for neurocysticercosis. Drugs with ovicidal and anticyst properties should be developed. Likewise, better diagnostic methods for hydatidosis and cysticercosis should be continuously assessed.

REFERENCES

1. **Abdussalam, M.**, The Problem of Taeniasis — Cysticercosis, PAHO Sci. Publ. No. 295, World Health Organization, Washington, D.C., 1975, 111.
2. **Arambulo, P. V., III, Cockrill, R. W. and Borjal, A. C.**, A preliminary note on the examination of carabaos for *Cysticercus bovis, Phil. J. Vet. Med.*, 113, 1970.
3. **Arambulo, P. V., III**, A Summary of Zoonoses in the Philippines, American Veterinary Epidemiological Society, Atlanta, 1971, 11.
4. **Arambulo, P. V., III, Walls, K. W., Bullock, S., and Kagan, I. G.**, Serodiagnosis of human cysticercosis by microplate enzyme-linked immunospecific assay (ELISA), *Acta Trop.*, 35, 63, 1978.
5. **Arambulo, P. V., III and Moran, N.**, The problem of food-transmitted parasitic zoonoses, *Int. J. Zoonoses,* 7, 7, 135, 1980.
6. **Cabrera, B. D. and Arambulo, P. V., III**, Studies on the epidemiology and transmission of human taeniasis in the Philippines — a paradoxical public health problem, *J. Philipp. Med. Assoc.*, 53, 105, 1977.
7. **Cabrera, B. D.**, The treatment of Taeniasis saginata with Bithionol (Bitin) in Jaro, Leyte, *Acta Med. Philipp.*, 9, 139, 1973.
8. **Dewhirst, L. W.**, Parasitologic and Economic Aspects of Cysticercosis in the Americas, PAHO Sci. Publ. No. 295, World Health Organization, Washington, D.C., 1975, 133.
9. **Faust, E. C., Rusell, P. F., and Jung, R. C.**, *Craig and Faust's Clinical Parasitology,* 8th ed., Lea & Febiger, Philadelphia, 1977.
10. **Huang, S. W.**, Studies on *Taenia* species prevalent among the aborigines in Wulai District, Taiwan, *Bull. Inst. Zool. Acad. Sci.,* 6, 29, 1967.
11. **Kuchenmeister, I.**, Die und dem Dorper des Lebenden Menschen Vorkrommenden Parasiten, *J. Med. Hebdomad. (Vienna),* 1855.
12. **Morishita, K. and Sawada, I.**, On tapeworms of the genus *Multiceps* hitherto unrecorded in humans, *Jpn. J. Parasitol.,* 15, 495, 1966.
13. **Pawłowski, Z. and Schultz, M. G.**, Taeniasis and cysticercosis (*Taenia saginata*), *Adv. Parasitol.,* 10, 269, 1972.
14. **Refuerzo, P. G. and Albis, F. S.**, *Cyticercus bovis* and *Cysticercus cellulosae* in animals with notes on human taeniasis in the Philippines, *Philipp. J. Anim. Ind.,* 9, 123, 1947.
15. **Schenone, Hugo**, Cysticercosis as a Public Health and Animal Health Problem, PAHO Sci. Publ. No. 295, World Health Organization, Washington, D.C., 1975, 122.
16. **Schultz, M. G., Hermos, J. A., and Steele, J. H.**, Epidemiology of beef tapeworm infection in the United States, *Public Health Rep.*, 85, 169, 1970.
17. **Schwabe, C.**, *Veterinary Medicine and Human Health,* 2nd ed., William & Wilkins, Baltimore, 1969.
18. **Silverman, P. H. and Griffiths, R. B.**, A review of methods of sewage disposal in Great Britain with special reference to the epizootiology of *Cysticercus bovis,* *Ann. Trop. Med. Parasitol.*, 49, 436, 1955.
19. **WHO**, Research needs in Echinococcosis (Hydatidosis), *Bull. WHO,* 39, 101, 1968.
20. **WHO**, Parasitic Zoonoses, Tech. Rep. Ser. No. 637, World Health Organization, Geneva, 1979.

BERTIELLA INFECTION

Nonette L. Jueco

Common Synonym
Bertiellosis.

Etiologic Agent
Bertiella studeri Blanchard, 1891 (Synonyms: *B. satyri* Blanchard, 1891; *B. satyri* [Blanchard, 1891] Stiles and Hassall, 1902) and *B. mucromata* (Mayer, 1895) Stiles and Hassall, 1902; and *B. studeri* (Blanchard, 1891) Stiles and Hassall, 1902.[4,8]

The total length of these tapeworms is from 275 to 300 mm and the maximum breadth is 10 mm. The scolex is subglobose, measuring 475 μm in diameter, with four suckers and a rudimentary unarmed rostellum. The proglottids are wider than long, craspedote, the mature proglottids measuring about 6 mm broad by 0.75 mm long. There is a single set of reproductive organs per segment. The genital pores are irregularly alternating; the genital ducts dorsal to the osmoregulatory canals. Cirrus pouch is well developed. Testes are numerous, medullary; ovary multilobate, slightly poral, filling most of the medullary width. The gravid proglottid becomes filled up with the uterus while the male organ may persist for some time before it finally disappears. Gravid segments are shed off in groups. The eggs are ovoidal (45 to 46 μm by 49 to 50 μm). There is a delicate middle envelope and an inner shell with a bicornuate protrusion on one side.[4,7]

TRUE AND ALTERNATE HOST

B. studeri is a common parasite of monkeys and other primates in Asia and Africa. It was first recovered from an orangutan in Borneo. Primates and other host range where this worm had been found include: the bonnet monkey, *Macaca radiata, M. syrichta syrichta, M. syrichta fascicularis, M. mullata, Macacus rhesus, Cercopithecus aethiops pygerythus, C. nictitans schmidti, Hylobates hoolock, Simia satyris, Anthropithecus troglodytes,* and *Cynomolgus simicus.* It has been recovered from a dog in the Philippines.[1]

Distribution
Human infections have been reported in individuals who had close contacts with primates. Most of the infections have been in children in tropical and subtropical countries. The intermediate hosts are the oribatid mites which are world-wide in distribution. Six different species of oribatid mites, members of five genera and four families, were proved to be vectors of this cestode. The eggs fed to *Scheloribates laevigates* and *Galumna* sp. develop into cysticercoids after less than 2 months.

Human infections have been reported from the following countries: four from Mauritius, eight from India, one from Sumatra, two from Java, one from Borneo, two from the Philippines, one from Singapore, one from East Africa, one from Cuba, one from St. Kitts Island in the British West Indies, one each from Brazil, Argentina, and Paraguay, one from Minnesota, U.S.,[2] one from Canada (the boy had come from the Republic of Congo),[2] and one from Britain (the boy may have contracted the infection while on a holiday in East Africa).[1,2,3,5,8,9]

Disease in Animals
The disease has been inadequately described in the host animals.

Disease in Man

Infection in man apparently provokes no manifest symptoms. In rare instances, the patient may complain of severe recurrent abdominal pain with intermittent vomiting. The symptoms are usually relieved after adequate therapy.[6]

Mode of Spread

Transmission in nature involves the monkey-oribatid mites cycle. Gravid segments and eggs passed out by the definitive hosts are ingested by mites which develop into cysticercoid larvae in less than 2 months. Primates get infected by ingestion of the infected mites.

Epidemiology

Infections in man are usually accidental. In most human cases, the patients had contacts or close association with monkeys either as pets or those in the zoo. Monkeys in captivity may also transmit the infection among themselves. Most of the monkeys brought to the U.S. come from different regions in Africa, South America, and Asia. There is the danger therefore of introducing this parasite in captive animals imported for use as laboratory animals or for exhibition in zoological gardens in different parts of the world.

Diagnosis

Diagnosis is made from passage of characteristic gravid proglottids and demonstration of typical eggs in the stool.

Prevention and Control

Control and prevention of this zoonosis would be difficult since the vectors responsible for transmission, the oribatid mites, are cosmopolitan and have a wide range of distribution. Prevention of human infection could be achieved by avoidance of close contact with monkeys and other primates either in the zoos or laboratories, or kept as pets.

Treatment

Oleoresin de aspidium, quinacrine, and dichlorophen have been found effective for expelling *Bertiella*.

REFERENCES

1. **Africa, C. M. and Garcia, E. Y.,** The occurrence of *Bertiella* in man, monkey and in dog in the Philippines, *Philipp. J. Sci.,* 56, 1, 1935.
2. **Costa, H. M. de A., Correa, L., and Brener, Z.,** A new human case of parasitism by *Bertiella mucronata* (Cestoda — Anoplocephalidae), *Rev. Inst. Med. Trop. S. Paulo* , 9, 95, 1967.
3. **D'Allessandro, B. A., Beaver, P. C., and Pallares, R. M.,** *Bertiella* infection in man in Paraguay, *Am. J. Trop. Med. Hyg.,* 12, 193, 1963.
4. **Faust, E. C., Russell, P. F., and Jung, R. C.,** *Clinical Parasitology,* 8th ed., Lea & Febiger, Philadelphia, 1970.
5. **Jones, R., Hunter, H., and van Rooyen, C. E.,** *Bertiella* infestation in a Nova Scotia child formerly resident in Africa, *Can. Med. Assoc. J.,* 104, 612, 1971.
6. **Koivastik, T.,** Anoplocephalid tapeworm infection in a child, *Lancet,* 83, 63, 1963.
7. **Schmidt, G. D.,** *How to Know the Tapeworms,* Wm. C. Brown, Iowa, 1970.
8. **Stunkard, H. W., Koivastik, T., and Healy, G. R.,** Infection of a child in Minnesota by *Bertiella studeri* (Cestoda: Anoplocephalidae), *Am. J. Trop. Med. Hyg.,* 13, 402, 1964.
9. **Thompson, C. D., Jellard, C. H., and Buckley, J. J. C.,** Human infection with a tapeworm, *Bertiella* sp. probably of African origin, *Br. Med. J.,* p. 659, 1967.

DIPHYLLOBOTHRIASIS

B. Göran Bylund

Common Synonyms

Bothriocephaliasis, fish tapeworm infection, broad tapeworm infection.

Etiologic Agent

Diphyllobothrium latum (Linnaeus, 1758) Lühe, 1910 (Cestoda, Pseudophyllidea). "The Fish Tapeworm" or "The Broad Tapeworm" (Synonyms: *Taenia lata* Linnaeus, 1758, *Bothriocephalus latus* [L. 1758] Bremser, 1819, *Dibothriocephalus latus* [L. 1758] Lühe, 1899).

Several species of the cestode genus *Diphyllobothrium* are parasites of man, mammals, and birds. By far the most important and the one usually associated with the term diphyllobothriasis is *D. latum*.

D. latum is the largest parasite of man. Specimens reaching 25 m in length have been recorded[6] but usually it ranges from 5 to 10 m, the number of segments or proglottids being as large as 2000 to 4000. One patient harboring 17 specimens with a total length of 330 m has been recorded in Finland.[23] The size of the worm depends on the species of host where it is found. Also a pronounced "crowding effect" usually induces retarded growth when numerous specimens are present in the same host. The species-specific morphological features are clearly observable only if the worm is completely relaxed before being studied.

The small (1.0 to 1.5 × 2 to 3 mm) almond-shaped scolex has two deep suctorial grooves or bothridia extending its full length. An attenuated, unsegmented neck zone is followed by a series of immature proglottids which gradually mature and become gravid. The proglottids closest to the anterior end are much broader than they are long, while those at the posterior end are square or even twice as long as they are broad. The maximum width of specimens from man is about 20 mm.

When expelled from the host the worm is of a creamy white or ivory color. The brownish, rosette-formed, egg-filled uterus is seen in the center of the proglottid. The genital pores are visible to the naked eye on the ventral side, anteriorly in the median line of the segment. The inner of the segment is almost completely filled by the male and female genital organs embedded in parenchymatous tissues. The posteriormost segments have already ceased to function, they are usually without eggs, more or less completely broken up or disintegrated before expelled with the feces of the host.

Thus the ovoid, operculated egg is usually discharged with the feces, but not within the proglottid. The mean size of the yellowish-brown egg is about 45 × 65 µm but there is a considerable range concerning the dimensions. The egg is therefore of little or no value for a reliable species diagnosis.[2,10]

Life Cycle

The life cycle of *D. latum* involves two intermediate and a final host.

From the intestine of the final host the eggs are expelled with the feces. For further development the egg has to be discharged into fresh water. The first larval stage, the coracidium, containing the six-hooked oncosphere, develops inside the egg within 10 to 12 days at 18 to 20°C. Development is retarded at lower temperatures.[18] At temperatures close to 0°C the egg can remain viable for many months without developing. In the presence of light the fully developed coracidium escapes from the egg through the opercular opening.

In order to continue its development the free-swimming coracidium has to be ingested by an appropriate copepod, the first intermediate host, within the next 12 to 72 hr. In the digestive tract of the copepod the larva discards its ciliated cover, penetrates the intestinal tract of the host and enters its hemocoel. Within 2 to 6 weeks, depending on the water temperature, it develops into the next larval stage, the procercoid. A single copepod may harbor five to six procercoids measuring up to 500 μm in length.

If the copepod is eaten by a plankton-eating fish of a particular species the larva is set free, penetrates the ventricle or the intestinal wall and migrates to the muscles or various visceral organs of the fish. In these organs it grows into the plerocercoid larva, infective for the final host.

The glistening white plerocercoid, which can readily be identified on the basis of its morphological features, may reach a maximum length of 4 to 5 cm. Plerocercoids can be found in almost any organ of the fish, frequently also free in the abdominal cavity. As a rule the plerocercoids lie unencysted in the host tissues but they also occur enclosed in connective tissue cysts. If the plankton-eating fish is eaten by a larger, predatory fish, the plerocercoids once again traverse the digestive tract, migrate to the organs of the predatory fish and retain their infectivity.[19,31] The plerocercoid may survive for several years in the host fish.

If raw or insufficiently cooked fish tissues are consumed by man or another suitable host the plerocercoid is set free during digestion and attaches itself by the bothridial grooves to the mucosa of the small intestine. Within 3 to 4 weeks it develops into an adult, egg-producing tapeworm. The growth rate during this developmental phase may be as high as 22 cm/day or almost 1 cm/hr.[19] In man the adult tapeworm may survive for a very long time. Patients carrying their infection for more than 25 years have been recorded.[16]

True and Alternate Hosts

The diphyllobothriid cestodes are characterized by rather poor host specificity. An ostensible host specificity in many cases seems to be attributed to ecological segregation rather than physiological barriers.[26] This concerns all developmental stages.

Man is without doubt the most suitable *final host* of *D. latum*. Of our domestic animals dog, cat, and pig have been recorded as hosts from natural as well as experimental infections. Reports by several authors list the following animals as hosts for adult *D. latum*:[6,17] wolf (*Canis lupus*), coyote (*Canis latrans*), jackal (*Canis aureus*), puma (*Felis concolor*), tiger-cat (*Felis tigrina*), lynx (*Lynx lynx*), red fox (*Vulpes vulpes*), arctic fox (*Alopex lagopus*), polar bear (*Ursus maritimus*), brown bear (*Ursus arctos*), black bear (*Ursus americanus*), otter (*Lutra lutra*), seals (*Phoca vitullina, P. hispida, Monachus albiventer*), sea lion (*Eumetopias californianus*), walrus (*Odobaena rosmarus*), and porpoise (*Phocaena phocaena*).

Several authors dealing with *D. latum* in animals base their reports on material and observations of doubtful validity with regard to their species identifications. Nevertheless, the long host list provides evidence enough of the considerable host spectrum of this parasite.

Numerous species of fresh-water fish can serve as second intermediate hosts of *D. latum*. Those of genera *Esox, Perca,* and *Lota* must be considered as the most important transmitters of the infection to man. In endogenic regions on the Eurasian continent plerocercoids are most frequently found in pike (*Esox lucius*), perch (*Perca fluviatilis*), burbot (*Lota lota*), and ruff (*Acerina cernua*). In North America the infection is referred to pike (*Esox lucius*), wall-eyed pike (*Stizostedeon vitreum*), sand pike (*S. canadense griseum*), burbot (*Lota maculosa*), yellow perch (*Perca flavescens*), and apparently also *Onchorhynchus* species.[6] Rausch predicts that other fish species may also be involved as transmitters of the disease in Alaska.[26] In Japan plerocercoids have been recorded from four different species of the genus *Onchorhynchus*.[6] *D. latum* plerocercoids have been found also in salmon (*Salmo salar*), trout (*S. trutta*), char (*Salvelinus alpinus*), grayling (*Thymallus thymallus*), eel (*Anguilla anguilla*), pike-perch (*Lucioperca lucioperca*), bull-heads (*Cottus* sp.), ten-spined stickleback (*Pungitus pungitus*), and three-spined stickleback (*Gasterosteus aculeatus*).[6,7] In these fish the plerocercoids are incidental or rare and they seem to be of little epidemiological significance.

About 40 species of fresh-water copepods have been demonstrated to serve as first intermediate host of *D. latum:* calanoid copepods of the genera *Diaptomus, Eudiaptomus, Acanthodiaptomus, Arctodiaptomus, Eurytemora,* and *Boeckella;* in addition, some species of the genus *Cyclops* are very liable to infection.[18] Even in the same lake, infection can be transmitted by different copepod species.

Distribution

In 1973 Carneri and Vita[14] estimated the number of human *Diphyllobothrium* carriers at nine million with five million in Europe, four million in Asia, and less than one tenth of a million in America.

Infection is most prevalent in the temperate and subarctic regions of the Northern Hemisphere. A well-known focus for endemic diphyllobothriasis is the Baltic region in Northern Europe. However, the prevalence has decreased to a considerable degree in this region. Of the Finnish population 20 to 25% harbored the parasite in 1952; 20 years later, 1972, the prevalence was 1.8%.[32] In the former endemic center in northern Italy and Switzerland, diphyllobothriasis seems to be rare today. In the Danube delta in Romania and in the Volga basin of the U.S.S.R. the incidence seems to be fairly high. Diphyllobothriasis, apparently to some extent due to other *Diphyllobothrium* species than *D. latum,* is widespread over the northern parts of the European Soviet Union and Siberia. From Japan foci with a heavily infested population have never been stated, but sporadic cases have been collected.[6] In southern Japan human infection with marine diphyllobothriids have been recorded.

In North America endemic regions are found in the upper Great Lakes region and also in central and western Canada. Apparently the disease was introduced to the Great Lakes region by immigrants from the Baltic countries. Diphyllobothriasis is also a disease of high prevalence among aboriginal peoples at high latitudes in North America.[26] Although several *Diphyllobothrium* species are involved in this region, *D. latum* appears to be the species most common in man. In South America an endemic focus exists in southern Chile. Diphyllobothriasis caused by the marine species *D. pacificum* is a rather frequent disease in coastal areas of Peru and Chile.

Sporadic infections have been reported from Argentina, Venezuela, Uganda, Botswana, Madagascar, China, Korea, the Philippines, and Australia. Apparently most of these reports deal with imported cases. The existence of autochthonus infections in tropical countries must be questioned.[6]

Other *Diphyllobothrium* Species Occurring as Adults in Man

A large number of tapeworms of the genus *Diphyllobothrium* have been described in different regions of the world. The validity of several of these species must be questioned. The taxonomy of *Diphyllobothrium* species is characterized by considerable uncertainty and conflicting information. This confusion is surprising in view of the medical importance of these parasites. Until recently taxonomists working with these worms greatly underestimated the vast range of morphological variability characteristic of the group. New species have continuously been created on the basis of minor structural differences of no taxonomic significance.[10]

D. dendriticum (Nitzsch, 1824) is a species normally parasitic in birds and mammals but frequently recorded also in man.[8,15] It has a circumpolar range and has been found in more than 20 species of birds and mammals.[8] The plerocercoid larva is most frequently found in salmoniid and coregoniid fish. The wide geographical range, the poor host specificity, and pronounced instability in morphological structure has led to numerous attempts to subdivide this species and to set up new species from it. Of *Diphyllobothrium* species recorded in man *D. norvegicum* Vik, 1957, recorded in northern Europe, and *D. minus* (Cholodkovsky, 1916) and *D. strictum* Talysin, 1932, both species recorded in Siberia, are all identical with *D. dendriticum*.[8,15]

Besides *D. latum* and *D. dendriticum,* Rausch and Hilliard[26] reported two other species occurring in man and mammals in Alaska.[26] *D. ursi* Rausch, 1954 is a species usually parasitic in bears in the northwestern parts of North America. It is also an incidental parasite of man in this region. The plerocercoid larvae are most frequently found in sockeye salmon, *Onchorhynchus nerca.* The risk of human infection is low because the larvae reside in the visceral organs of the fish, not in the body musculature.

D. dalliae is a common parasite of dog and arctic fox in western Alaska but is also involved in human infections.[26] The plerocercoids occur in blackfish (*Dallia pectoralis*). This fish is frequently eaten raw or frozen by the Eskimos. The larvae of *D. dalliae* have also been recorded in eastern Siberia.[33]

D. pacificum (Nybelin, 1931) is a parasite of sea lions off the coastal area of Peru and Chile. Recent investigations have revealed that it is a rather frequent parasite also of man in the same area.[3] Apparently *D. pacificum* is a species which develops normally entirely in a marine habitat. Nobody has been able to identify with certainty the particular plerocercoid. Human infestation apparently takes place through the Peruvian national dish "ceviche", containing raw fish of marine origin.

A number of reports dealing with other *Diphyllobothrium* species in man, seem to be of doubtful validity: *D. parvum* (Stephens, 1908), *D. cordatum* (Leuckart, 1863), *D. lanceolatum* (Krabbe, 1865), *D. giljacicum* (Rutkevich, 1937), *D. luxi* (Rutkevich, 1937), *D. nenzi* (Petrov, 1938), *D. skrjabini* (Plotnikov, 1932), and *D. tungussicum* (Podyopolskaya and Gnedina, 1932) have all been reported from human infections in the northern hemisphere. In some cases these reports deal with incidental records of immature specimens. Most of these records were made at a time when the criteria for reliable species identification were insufficiently known. Without doubt redescriptions will reveal most of these species as synonyms of other diphyllobothriids.

Disease in Animals

There are few reports dealing with the pathogenic effects of adult diphyllobothriids on their animal hosts. It is apparent that in most cases the condition of the host animals is not seriously affected by the parasite. Domestic animals, when found infected, are subjected to medical care, i.e., dehelminthized, which is of course important from an epidemiological point of view. Clinical symptoms, however, are mild or absent.

As demonstrated by Rausch, however, the course of infection in some cases may be very serious or even fatal for the animal host.[25] A black bear experimentally infected with a *Diphyllobothrium* sp. succumbed to the infection. The post-mortem examination revealed two worm specimens which had migrated up the pancreatic ducts inducing extensive pathological changes in this and other organs. Undoubtedly, many graded and more subtle effects on the host animals will be demonstrated when detailed analysis of host parasite relations is performed.

The harmful effects of diphyllobothriid plerocercoid larvae on their host fish are firmly established in several reports on epizootic fish mortalities.[9]

Disease in Man

Most human *Diphyllobothrium* carriers suffer little discomfort from their infection.

In some cases, however, a wide variety of subjective symptoms have been reported to accompany the infection. An extensive field investigation carried out in Finland showed to what extent such, often vague, symptoms were related to the presence of the parasite.[27] A very significant increase in the frequency of fatigue and weakness, dizziness, diarrhea, and numbness of the extremities was noted in worm carriers. A sensation of hunger as well as a "craving for salt" was also associated with the infection. The symptoms were more pronounced in young worm carriers under 30 years of age.

Symptoms like abdominal pain, heartburn, loss of weight, etc. contrary to previous statements, could not be significantly related to the worm infection, although abdominal pain, for example, may occur in diphyllobothriasis as well as in infections with other parasites.

Vomiting of the parasite or parasite fragments may occur but is a rare condition in diphyllobothriasis. Symptoms from the central nervous system frequently accompany the disease in patients suffering serious illness from the infection, i.e., in those with manifest tapeworm anemia. Paresthesia, disturbances in motility and coordination, and impairment of sensibility are the most common neurological symptoms.[5] Also psychic disturbances and cerebral manifestations are known to occur.[6]

The most serious effect induced by the parasite is tapeworm anemia, a disease almost exclusively recorded in patients infected with *D. latum*. Contrary to earlier estimates it was recently shown that anemia is not a rare sequel in diphyllobothriasis. Manifest anemia occurs in about 2% of the worm carriers.[27] Tapeworm anemia is megaloblastic, of the pernicious type, closely resembling genuine or Addisonian pernicious anemia. The parasite causes the anemia by competing with its host for dietary vitamin B_{12}. The clinical manifestations and pathogenesis involved in tapeworm anemia have been studied by Bonsdorff and colleagues.[6]

The vitamin B_{12} is of essential importance to the human body. Apparently the vitamin is involved in DNA synthesis and maturation of cell nuclei. Normally the human organism has considerable reserves of vitamin B_{12}, a serum level between 150 and 900 pg/mℓ. If the serum level lies markedly below 100 pg/mℓ a tendency towards cytomegaly is observable in blood cells, bone marrow, and the epithelial cells of several organs. This critical level is reached in more than 50% of the carriers of *D. latum*. Thus the majority of worm carriers suffer from a latent B_{12} deficiency and are on the border of manifest pernicious anemia.

Vitamin B_{12} is absorbed in the intestine only when bound to a carrier protein, the intrinsic factor, secreted with the gastric juice. When established in the intestine the worm is in the position to interfere with the B_{12}-intrinsic factor complex. Nyberg and colleagues[20-22] demonstrated that an active principle, a releasing factor, in the worm is capable of splitting the B_{12}-intrinsic factor complex. The vitamin B_{12} split off from the complex is absorbed and utilized to a considerable extent by the parasite.

The site of the worm in the intestine has a decisive influence on the development of the anemic state.[6] In man the site of vitamin B_{12} absorption is the ileum. If the worm establishes itself high up in the intestine, in the jejunum, the metabolically most active proximal portion of the parasite utilizes large quantities of the vitamin before it reaches the absorptive zone of the intestine. In serious cases of megaloblastic anemia the parasite or parasites are usually found to reside high up in the jejunum.

Although vitamin B_{12} deficiency is the predominant metabolic disturbance associated with *D. latum* infection, recent investigations indicate that the parasite may interfere with the absorption and metabolism of other substances as well (folates and other vitamins).[6] As many of the subjective symptoms recorded from *Diphyllobothrium* carriers do not correlate with the serum B_{12} levels, it has been suggested that such symptoms may be due to a polyvalent vitamin deficiency.[6]

The clinical changes associated with tapeworm anemia are most strikingly revealed by the blood picture. The red cell count is much reduced. The diameter of the red cells is increased; poikilocytosis and anisocytosis with a preponderance of macrocytes occur in most cases. The mean corpuscle volume and the mean corpuscle hemoglobin content is increased. Nucleated erythrocytes, megaloblasts, and normoblasts occur in the peripheral blood. The number of platelets is reduced and coagulation time is prolonged. A more or less mild leucopenia may occur. Hypersegmented leucocytes occur frequently. Eosinophilia is not, however, associated with this parasite disease.

Mild hemolysis is frequently involved due to ineffective erythropoiesis. The morphology of cellular components of the, mostly hyperplastic, bone marrow is much affected. A predominating factor is the high frequency of megaloblasts and promegaloblasts.

The clinical changes in the blood picture are frequently accompanied by anemic fever, glossitis, edema, hemorrhages, etc. The basic pathologic manifestation in the central nervous system is a subacute combined spinal and peripheral nerve degeneration with demyelation and degeneration of the axis cylinder.

Very rapid remission usually follows expulsion of the worm.

General Mode of Spread

The infection is acquired by ingestion of raw or inadequately prepared fish containing infective larvae. Raw fish or fish products are highly appreciated dietary components of certain population groups. Slightly salted fillets of various fresh-water fish are a customary diet in the Finnish lake district, for example. The fillets are kept in brine for 1 to 3 days and are eaten without further preparation. In the same region slightly salted hard roe is considered a delicacy, a dangerous delicacy, however, as the roe of pike and burbot frequently contains larvae of *D. latum.* In different geographic regions the infection is attributable to different dishes and dietary habits; raw fish and fish products, however, are always a common component. Animals, especially domestic animals, frequently acquire their infection from fish offal given to them.

Epidemiology

The complicated life cycle of *D. latum* can be completed and maintained only when: (1) a water biotope suitable for the development of the larval stages and suitable intermediate hosts are present; (2) the feeding habits of the population include ingestion of raw or inadequately prepared fish products of species harboring plerocercoid larvae; and (3) sanitary habits and sewage disposal facilitate the spread of the worm eggs to natural waters.

The infection is established in an area if all these prerequisites are present. Of equal importance from an epidemiological point of view is the fact that elimination of only one of these prerequisites is enough for elimination of the infection from an area.

Water biotopes suitable for larval development exist in large parts of the temperate and subarctic regions. The embryonic development and hatching of the first larval stage takes place in fresh water at temperatures between 4 and 25°C. Shallow littorals with water temperatures of 15 to 20°C provide the most favorable conditions. As host specificity is rather poor, suitable species of intermediate hosts seem to be frequently present in most parts of the temperate and subarctic regions. The fish species most susceptible to infection by *D. latum,* pikes, perches, and burbots, have an almost circumpolar range in the northern hemisphere.

The presence of a population with dietary habits facilitating the transmission of infective larvae to man seems to be the decisive factor for the spread and establishment of diphyllobothriasis. This requirement also gives diphyllobothriasis its nature of an endemic disease. Sporadic cases occasionally occur outside the endemic areas. Usually these cases are found among immigrants; or they may be due to ingestion of fish imported from endemic regions. As the ecological conditions of water biotopes in parasite-free regions also frequently fulfill the requirements of the parasite, imported cases occasionally give rise to new, temporary tapeworm foci. Due to the high reproductive potential of the parasite, sporadic worm carriers can give rise to a high frequence of larvae in fish populations even in lakes of considerable size.[1]

Well established, new endemic foci of the disease usually originate from population transfers from infected areas due to emigration, war, etc. In such circumstances the population often retain their dietary habits, indispensable for the epidemiological cycle of the disease. This is what happened in several regions of Europe during and after the Second World War.[6]

The role of domestic and wild animals in the epidemiology of diphyllobothriasis is a question of controversy. It has been firmly established that specimens of *D. latum,* when grown in various mammals, produce considerable amounts of viable eggs.[10,19,30] Thus it seems reasonable to assume that infected animals may be a factor in the dissemination of the infection in endemic areas where human infections also occur. However, it has never been definitely demonstrated that the life cycle of the parasite is maintained without the participation of man. On the contrary, available data indicate that the infection is rare or absent in regions with all ecological prerequisites present, including fish-eating mammals, but without human population.[7]

Not only dietary habits but also sanitary habits are decisive for the maintenance of the parasite life cycle in endemic areas. The practice of flushing untreated fecal products, via water closets and sewers, into lakes and rivers, greatly facilitates the spread of the infection. In such conditions a few worm carriers may be responsible for the pollution of extensive bodies of water.[1]

Diagnosis

The diagnosis of diphyllobothriasis is based on recovery of the characteristic eggs in feces. Due to the high production of eggs the diagnosis is rapid. In suspected cases several samples should be examined as the egg production of the parasite may temporarily cease, or the eggs may be overlooked in about 5% of worm carriers.[6] The tapeworm anemia is diagnosed from changes in the blood picture and bone marrow. For differential diagnosis, genuine pernicious anemia should be considered.

Prevention and Control

The aim of preventive and control measures must be to break the life cycle of the parasite. Theoretically, any point of the life cycle can be attacked. In practice, the work has to be focused on three points: (1) treatment of persons harboring the parasite; (2) preventing contamination of lakes and rivers with viable tapeworm eggs through rational sewage disposal; and (3) preventing transmission of infective larvae from fish to man.

Expulsion of the parasite is easily achieved in diphyllobothriasis. Desaspidin and niclosamide are the recommended drugs: both drugs are without side effects. Their curative effect is about 80 to 95%. Mepacrine (Atabrine®, Quinacrine) is also used. New drugs, perhaps still more efficient are being tested.[11] In cases with anemia, substitution therapy with vitamin B_{12} should be given.

Elimination of tapeworm eggs from waste waters is an indispensable need in endemic areas. Modern purification plants, if properly dimensioned, retain 95 to 99% of the worm eggs. The resistance of the eggs to external influences is poor. Dehydration and temperatures below −5°C destroy the eggs.[4,6] In garbage piles and well aerated latrines they quickly lose their viability. Treatment of fecal products with chemicals (chlorine, formaldehyde, etc.) is recommended in hospitals with diphyllobothriasis patients and is also suggested for example in vessels in traffic on lakes and rivers in endemic areas.

It is obvious that preventive measures most efficiently should be focused on preventing the transmission of infective larvae from fish to man. Infected fish need not necessarily be avoided but should be treated, before consumption, in a manner rendering the larvae innocuous. The plerocercoid dies when exposed to temperatures over 56°C or below −10°C. The risk of infection is efficiently eliminated if the fish is eaten boiled, fried, or adequately smoked at a high temperature.[6,24,28] If the fish is frozen for a day or two the potential risk is also eliminated; this is also true of the hard roe. It is easily emphasized that a campaign against diphyllobothriasis, which presupposes changes in dietary traditions, must be based largely on educational work. Preventive and control measures should not ignore the potential role played by reservoir hosts, especially domestic animals, in the epidemiology of diphyllobothriasis.

REFERENCES

1. **Almer, B.,** Controlling the broad tapeworm (*Diphyllobothrium latum*), National Swedish Environment Protection Board, *Limnol. Sur. SNV PM 460,* 74, 3, 1974.
2. **Andersen, K. and Halvorsen, O.,** Egg size as a taxonomic criterion in *Diphyllobothrium* (Cestoda, Pseudophyllidea), *Norw. J. Zool.,* 24, 469, 1976.
3. **Baer, J. G.,** *Diphyllobothrium pacificum,* a tapeworm from sea lions endemic in man along the coastal area of Peru, *J. Fish. Res. Bd. Can.,* 26, 717, 1969.
4. **Bauer, O. N.,** Parasites of freshwater fish and the biologic basis for their control, *Isr. Progr. Sci. Transl. Jerusalem,* p. 69, 1962.
5. **Björkenheim, G.,** Neurological changes in pernicious tapeworm anemia, *Acta Med. Scand. Suppl.,* 260, 124, 1951.
6. **von Bonsdorff, B.,** *Diphyllobothriasis in Man,* Academic Press, London, 1977, 1.
7. **Bylund, G.,** Binnikemasklarver i våra fiskar, *Inf. Parasitol. Inst. Soc. Sci. Fenn.,* 8, 5, 1968.
8. **Bylund, G.,** Experimentell undersökning av *Diphyllobothrium dendriticum* (= *D. norwegicum*) från norra Finland, *Inf. Parasitol. Inst. Soc. Sci. Fenn.,* 10, 3, 1970.
9. **Bylund, G.,** Pathogenic effects of a diphyllobothriid plerocercoid on its host fishes, *Comm. Biol. Soc. Sci. Fenn.,* 58, 1, 1972.
10. **Bylund, G.,** Delimitation and Characterization of European *Diphyllobothrium* Species, Acad. dissert. Åbo Akademi, Åbo, 1975.
11. **Bylund, G., Bång, B., and Wikgren, K.,** Tests with a new compound (Praziquantel) against *Diphyllobothrium latum., J. Helminthol.,* 51, 115, 1977.
12. **Bylund, G. and Wikgren, B.-J.,** Fågelmaskar i människor, *Inf. Parasitol. Inst. Soc. Sci. Fenn.,* 8, 19, 1968.
13. **Bylund, G., Wikström, M., and Penttinen, K.,** Reningsanläggningar för avfallsvatten — Barriärer mot binnikemaskens spridning, *Inf. Parasitol. Inst. Soc. Sci. Fenn.,* 14, 1, 1975.
14. **de Carneri, I. and Vita, G.,** Drugs used in cestode diseases. In: Cavier, R., J.E.P.T., Sect. 64, 145, Pergamon Press, New York, 1973.
15. **Chizhova, T. P. and Gofman-Kadoshnikov, P. B.,** A natural focus of diphyllobothriasis in the Baikal Lake and its pattern, *Med. Parazitol. Parazit. Bolezni,* 20, 168, 1960.
16. **Dogiel, V. A.,** *Allgemeine Parasitologie,* (Überarbeitet und ergänzt von Poljanski, G. I. and Cheissin, E. M.). VEB G. Fisher Verlag, Jena, 1963, 191.
17. **Gnezdilov, V. G. H.,** Hamster (*Mesocricetus auratus*) as a potential final host of the broad tapeworm (*Diphyllobothrium latum*). *Dokl. Akad. Nauk SSSR,* 114, 1328, 1957.
19. **Kuhlow, F.,** Untersuchungen über die Entwicklung des breiten Bandwurm *(Diphyllobothrium latum), Z. Tropenmed. Parasitol.,* 6, 213, 1955.
20. **Nyberg, W.,** The influence of *Diphyllobothrium latum* on the vitamin B_{12}-intrinsic factor complex, *Acta Med. Scand.,* 167, 189, 1960.
21. **Nyberg, W., Gräsbeck, R., Saarni, M., and von Bonsdorff, B.,** Serum vitamin B_{12} levels and incidence of tapeworm anemia in a population heavily infected with *Diphyllobothrium latum, Am. J. Clin. Nutr.,* 9, 606, 1960.

22. **Nyberg, W., Wolff, R., and Nabet, P.,** Action d'un extrait de *Diphyllobothrium latum* sur la vitamin B$_{12}$ combinee, *C.R. Soc. Biol.,* 156, 1672, 1962.

23. **Ostling, G.,** Treatment of tapeworm infection with desaspidin, a new phloroglucinol derivate isolated from Finnish fern, *Am. J. Trop. Med. Hyg.,* 16, 855, 1961.

24. **Pesonen, T. and Wikgren, B.-J.,** Bandmasklarvernas salt — och temperaturtolerans, *Mem. Soc. Fauna Flora Fenn.,* 35, 112, 1960.

25. **Rausch, R.,** Unusual pathogenicity of *Diphyllobothrium* sp. in a black bear, *Proc. Helminthol. Soc. Wash.,* 22, 95, 1955.

26. **Rausch, R. and Hilliard, D. K.,** Studies on the helminth fauna of Alaska. XLIX. The occurrence of *Diphyllobothrium latum* (Linnaeus, 1758) (Cestoda, Diphyllobothriidae) in Alaska, with notes on other species, *Can. J. Zool.,* 48, 1201, 1970.

27. **Saarni, M., Nyberg, W., Grasbeck, R., and von Bonsdorff, B.,** Symptoms in carriers of *Diphyllobothrium latum* and in non-infected controls, *Acta Med. Scand.,* 173, 147, 1963.

28. **Salminen, K.,** The effect of household smoking on the infestiveness of *Diphyllobothrium latum* from fish to man, *Acta Vet. Scand.,* 11, 228, 1970.

29. **Sarelin, H.,** Undersokning av olika reningsanlaggningars effektivitet vid eliminering av binnikemaskagg ur avfallsvatten, *Inf. Parasitol. Inst. Soc. Sci. Fenn.,* 11, 3, 1970.

30. **Tarassov, V.,** Das Schwein und der Hund als endgultige Trager des *Diphyllobothrium latum, Arch. Schiffs Trop. Hyg.,* 38, 156, 1934.

31. **Wikgren, B.-J. and Muroma, E.,** Studies on the genus *Diphyllobothrium*. A revision of the Finnish finds of diphyllobothriid plerocercoids, *Acta Zool. Fenn.,* 93, 3, 1956.

32. **Wikstrom, M.,** The incidence of fish tapeworm, *Diphyllobothrium latum,* in the human population of Finland, *Comm. Biol. Soc. Sci. Fenn.,* 58, 3, 1972.

33. **Zhukow, E. V.,** Parazitofauna ryb Chukotki. Soobshchrnie II. Endoparaziticheskie chervi morskikh i presnovodnykh ryb, *Parazitol. Sb.,* 21, 96, 1963.

DIPYLIDIASIS

Nonette L. Jueco

Common Synonym
Dog tapeworm infection.

Etiologic Agent
Dipylidium caninum (Linneaus, 1758) Railliet, 1892 (Synonyms: *Taenia canina* L., 1758; *T. cucumerina* Bloch, 1782; *D. cucumerinum* [Bloch, 1782] Leuckart, 1863; *D. sexcoronatum* von Ratz, 1900).[1] "The double-pored dog tapeworm."

D. caninum is a common intestinal cestode of dogs. The length varies from 100 to 700 mm. The scolex is small, rhomboidal with four cup-like suckers, and a protrusible rostellum armed with one to seven circlets of spines. The neck is short and slender. The immature proglottids are broader than long while the mature and gravid proglottids are longer than wide and typically pumpkin-seed shaped. Each segment is provided with a double set of reproductive organs. The gravid proglottids are filled with pockets or capsules, each containing from eight to fifteen eggs. The eggs are spherical, thin-shelled, and hyaline.[3]

True and Alternate Hosts
The definitive hosts are dogs, cats, wild cats, jungle cats, civet cats, hyenas, jackals, dingos, fox, and man.[1,3,8,11,12,14]

Arthropods which serve as intermediate hosts include the following: dog flea (*Ctenocephalides canis*), cat flea (*C. felis*), human flea (*Pulex irritans*), and dog louse (*Trichodectes canis*).[3,14]

Distribution
Cosmopolitan. Human cases have been reported from Argentina, Australia, Brazil, Cape Colony, Chile (23 cases in children 6 months to 8 years old), Cuba, England, Guatemala, Italy, Japan, the Philippines, Portugal, Puerto Rico, Rhodesia, Uruguay, U.S., and Venezuela.[1-3,5,8-10]

Disease in Animals
Animal hosts do not usually manifest any severe pathology.[7] Sometimes the dog may exhibit some mild irritability or listlessness during passage of segments or strobila. In dogs with heavy infections, the disease may cause nervous or digestive troubles, emaciation, and weakness. Passage of the segments through the anus often cause itching and irritation manifested by the animal's sitting down and dragging itself forward on its haunches trying to get rid of the segments.[1]

Disease in Man
In man, pathogenicity depends on the intensity of infection and susceptibility of the patient to the absorbed metabolic wastes of the parasite. Symptoms are usually absent or slight, or may be manifested as weight loss, vague abdominal pain, general irritability, and perianal pruritus.[3,10,11]

Mode of Spread
Transmission from host to host is accomplished by the ingestion of the arthropod intermediate hosts which harbor the cysticercoid larvae.

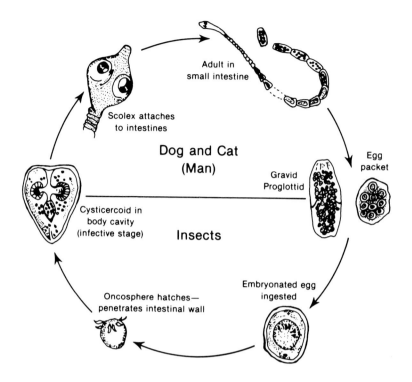

FIGURE 1. Life cycle of *Dipylidium caninum*. (From life cycle charts, Common intestinal helminths of man, Communicable Disease Center, U.S. Department of Health, Education and Welfare, Atlanta, Georgia, 1959.)

Epidemiology

The primary definitive hosts of *D. caninum* are dogs and cats. The infected animals pass gravid segments which disintegrate when deposited on the ground or while inside the intestines. The egg capsules containing the eggs are ingested by the larval flea and develop into cysticercoid larvae in about 2 weeks time. The tapeworm embryos remain in the fleas until they become adult fleas. Dogs and cats get infected by eating fleas or lice harboring the cysticercoid.

Diagnosis

Diagnosis of dipylidiasis is by recovery of gravid proglottids passed with the feces or that crawled out of the anus. Characteristic egg pockets or capsules may sometimes be demonstrated on microscopic examination of stool specimens.

Prevention and Control

Preventive and control measures include treatment of infected animals, use of insecticide dusting on dogs and cats to kill the arthropod intermediate hosts, and children should be taught proper handling of pets.

Treatment

Dipylidiasis could be treated by administration of anticestodal drugs, such as atabrine, yomesan, mepacrine, pelletierene tannate, and hetrazan.[3,4,11]

REFERENCES

1. **Bearup, M. J. and Morgan, E. L.**, The occurrence of *Hymenolepis diminuta* (Rudolphi, 1819) and *Dipylidium caninum* (Linnaeus, 1758) as parasites of man in Australia, *Med. J. Aust.,* 104, 1939.
2. **Belmar, R.**, *Dipylidium caninum* infection in children. Report of 13 cases and treatment with Salicylamide derivative, *Bol. Chil. Parasitol.,* 18, 63, 1963.
3. **Faust, E. C., Russell, P. F., and Jung, R. C.**, *Craig and Faust's Clinical Parasitology,* 8th ed., Lea & Febiger, Philadelphia, 1970.
4. **Garcia, E. Y.**, Two rare human tapeworms expelled by "Hetrazan", *Med. Rep.,* 4, 12, 1952.
5. **Goldsmid, J.**, Human infection with *Dipylidium caninum* Linnaeus (Platyhelminthes: Cestoda) in Rhodesia, *S. Afr. Med. J.,* 24, 333, 1965.
6. **Jueco, N. L.**, personal communications.
7. **Lapage, C.**, *Veterinary Parasitology,* Oliver and Boyd, Edinburgh, 1956.
8. **Marshall, A. G.**, The cat flea, *Ctonocephalides felis* (Bouche, 1935) an intermediate host for cestodes, *Parasiology,* 57, 419, 1967.
9. **Mendoza-Guazon, M. P.**, A case of infestation with *Dipylidium caninum, Philipp. J. Sci.,* 11, 19, 1916.
10. **Moore, D. V. and Connell, F. M.**, Additional records of *Dipylidium caninum* infections in children in the United States with observations on treatment, *Am. J. Trop. Med. Hyg.,* 9, 604, 1960.
11. **Moore, D. V.**, A review of human infections with the common dog tapeworm, *Dipylidium caninum,* in the United States, *Southwest. Vet.,* 15, 1962.
12. **Nelson, C. S., Pester, F. R. N., and Lichman, R.**, The significance of wild animals in the transmission of cestodes of medical importance in Kenya, *Trans. R. Soc. Trop. Med. Hyg.,* 59, 507, 1965.
13. **Rendtorff, R. C.**, Additional records of human cases of *Dipylidium caninum* infections, *J. Parasitol.,* 47, 538, 1961.
14. **Yutuc, L. M.**, The cat flea hitherto unknown to sustain the larva of *Dipylidium caninum* (Linnaeus, 1758) from the Pilippines, *Philipp. J. Sci.,* 97, 285, 1968.

ECHINOCOCCOSIS

Peter M. Schantz

Common Synonyms

Unilocular echinococcosis; echinococcus or hydatid disease (caused by *E. granulosus*); multilocular echinococcosis or alveolar hydatid disease (caused by *E. multilocularis*); polycystic echinococcosis (caused by *E. vogeli*).

Description

Echinococcosis is a condition caused by cestodes of the genus *Echinococcus* Rudolphi, 1801 (Cestoda:Taeniidae), the life cycles of which involve two mammalian hosts (figure 1). Their definitive hosts are carnivores, in which adult worms are present in the intestines. Intermediate hosts are various species of herbivorous and omnivorous animals, in which metacestodes develop. Humans and other intermediate hosts become infected by ingesting eggs passed in the feces of infected definitive hosts. The metacestode forms are referred to as hydatid cysts, and the disease caused by them is commonly referred to as hydatid disease.

Classic cystic hydatid disease is caused by *E. granulosus*. This species is adapted to dogs and a wide variety of domestic and sylvatic animal intermediate hosts. It exists throughout the world; in many regions it is a major public health and economic problem.

Alveolar hydatid disease is caused by *E. multilocularis*, whose final and intermediate hosts are foxes and their rodent prey, respectively. Human infection caused by this species is one of the most lethal parasitic infections known to exist. The greater host specificity of *E. multilocularis* and its restriction to a relatively small number of sylvatic animal hosts limit the geographic distribution of this agent and reduce potential human exposure.

The life cycles of *E. oligarthrus* and *E. vogeli* are limited to sylvatic animals. E. oligarthrus utilizes wild felids as definite hosts while *E. vogeli* has been found in a wild canid. Both use a variety of rodents as intermediate hosts. These cestodes have been reported from Central and South America, and *E. vogeli* has been demonstrated to be the cause of a polycystic form of hydatid disease in humans.

Etiologic Agents

Historical aspects of the controversy concerning speciation within the genus *Echinococcus* have been reviewed by Smyth,[279] and more recently, by Rausch[221-223] and by Rausch and Nelson,[220] and Rausch and Bernstein.[225] Awareness of the wide range of hosts, the degree of intraspecific morphologic variation, and host-induced morphologic effects has led to the understanding that (1) taxonomic characters of both larval and adult stages from the corresponding natural hosts must be described, (2) the range of susceptible hosts must be defined, and (3) ecological and physiological factors must be evaluated in order to characterize a given species.[223] At least 15 species have been described, but not more than 4 can be considered valid based on presently available evidence (Table 1).

E. granulosus (Batsch, 1786), *E. multilocularis* Leuckart, 1863, *E. oligarthrus* (Diesing, 1863), and *E. vogeli* Rausch and Bernstein, 1972 are morphologically distinct in both adult and larval stages. They are separated ecologically, although not necessarily geographically, by the nature of their respective unique host assemblages.

E. granulosus

This organism was the first *Echinococcus* sp. to be described, its larval form having

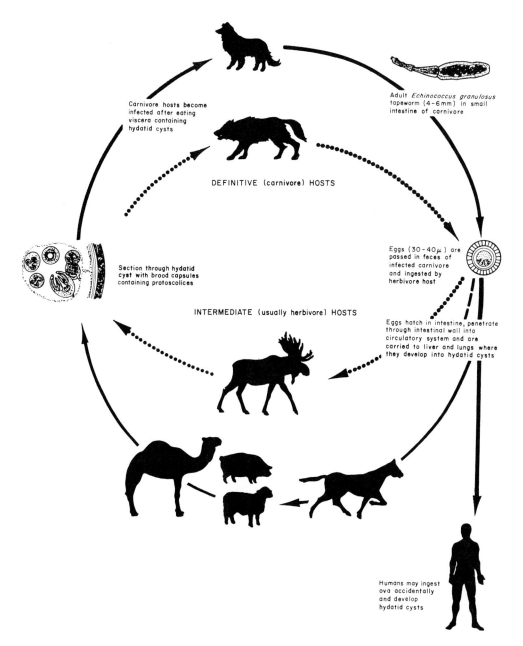

FIGURE 1.   *Echinococcus granulosus* schematic life cycle diagram showing sylvatic (dotted lines) and synanthropic cycles. (Adapted from Andersen, F. L., Everett, J. R., Barbour, A. G., and Schoenfeld, F. J., *Proc. 78 Ann. Meet. U.S. Animal Health Assoc.*, 78, 370, 1974.)

been characterized in the writings of Hippocrates. It is also the most thoroughly described member of that genus. Growth and development studies have demonstrated considerable intraspecific morphologic variation,[202,220,255,313,318] which may be partially host induced.[257] Undue emphasis on nonsignificant morphologic variation and/or the finding of cestodes in animals that are not considered to be natural hosts for *E. granulosus* led to the proposal of at least nine different species, now considered to be only synonyms of the type species (Table 1).[220,255] Morphological and biological differences among populations of *E. granulosus* have led other researchers to designate them as subspecies. However, in a recent critical review of the criteria used to define these

Table 1
SPECIES OF THE GENUS *ECHINOCOCCUS* RUDOLPHI, 1801
AND THEIR SYNONYMS

Valid species	Synonyms
E. granulosus (Batsch, 1786)	*E. cameroni* Ortlepp, 1934; *E. intermedius* Lopez Neyra and Soler, 1943; *E. longimanubrius* Cameron 1926; *E. minimus* Cameron, 1926; *E. lycaontis* Ortlepp, 1934; *E. ortleppi* Lopez Neyra and Soler, 1943; *E. felidis* Ortlepp, 1937; *E. patagonicus* Szidat, 1960; *E. cepanzoi* Szidat, 1971
E. multilocularis Leuckart, 1863	*E. sibiricensis* Rausch and Schiller, 1954
E. oligarthrus (Diesing, 1863)	*E. cruzi* Brumpt and Joyeux, 1924(?); *E. pampeanus* Szidat, 1967
E. vogeli Rausch and Bernstein, 1972	*E. cruzi* Brumpt and Joyeux, 1924(?)

subspecies, Rausch[222] rejected most as invalid because of a lack of evidence of ecological segregation or marked host specificity between the type species and the proposed subspecies. He pointed out that modern taxonomic concepts preclude the sympatric existence of more than one subspecies of a single polytypic species. In the absence of geographic or ecologic segregation, any genetic differences would disappear because, by definition, the different subspecies of a polytypic species interbreed. His suggestion that different populations be designated "strains" or "forms" until more conclusive information becomes available has gained acceptance.

Although the taxonomic and epidemiological implications are not yet resolved, evidence of morphological and biological differences between populations of *E. granulosus* is increasing. One population, currently limited to the higher latitudes of North America and Eurasia, has been designated as the northern sylvatic form. This particular form does not readily infect domestic ungulates,[49] occurs in wolves and wild ungulates (moose and wild reindeer), and probably represents the original form of the cestode.[221] Human infection is characterized by predominantly pulmonary localization, slower and more benign growth, and a less frequent occurrence of clinical complications than reported for other forms.[327]

Populations of *E. granulosus* in domestic animals are commonly referred to as the pastoral form, but recent studies have confirmed the existence of important differences among them. In Ireland, Great Britain, and Western Europe, a strain or strains of *E. granulosus* recovered from the horse/dog cycle has been found to be morphologically and biologically distinct from those recovered from the sheep/dog cycle.[121,301,326] In vitro and in vivo studies have shown different growth characteristics of the two strains, suggesting different physiological, nutritional, or metabolic requirements.[185,186,283,284] In other endemic areas, equine hosts are rarely (if ever) parasitized with *E. granulosus*. The apparent absence of infection in persons exposed to the horse/dog strain suggests that this strain may not be infective to man.[301]

In the U.S.S.R., morphological and biological differences have been demonstrated between cestodes recovered from the sheep/dog cycle and those of the pig/dog cycle.[159,340] Organisms recovered from the former were virtually noninfective to pigs. In contrast, worms recovered from the pig/dog cycle were not infective to sheep.

The differences between some of these populations appear to be strongly defined.

According to Rausch,[219] a possibility to be considered is that they are reproductively isolated and are in fact sibling species.

E. multilocularis

The causative agent of alveolar hydatid disease was first recognized by Virchow in 1855 as being the larval stage of an *Echinococcus* cestode, but the relationship of this organism to the adult form in canids and its taxonomic designation remained unresolved for more than 100 years. Some investigators believed that, under certain conditions, the larva of *E. granulosus* may develop anomalously to produce the alveolar larval form, but others thought that a distinct species was involved (reviewed by Smyth[279]). Rausch and Schiller[217] described the life cycle and morphological characteristics of an Alaskan cestode that is distinct from *E. granulosus,* and they named this organism *E. sibiricensis*. In Germany, Vogel[318] demonstrated that this cestode is identical to the causative agent of alveolar hydatid disease in Eurasia and confirmed Leuckart's earlier designation of *E. multilocularis* as having priority.

Populations of *E. multilocularis* in Eurasia, Alaska, and South Dakota are morphologically identical. However, they differ in their degree of pathogenicity for laboratory animals, suggesting that biological differences do exist.[224] Abuladze's[1] creation of a unique genus for *E. multilocularis,* which he named *Alveococcus* in 1960, appears unwarranted. This term is used widely in the U.S.S.R., but acceptance of the proposed generic criteria would require extensive reclassification of the family Taeniidae.

E. oligarthrus

E. oligarthrus was first described by Diesing in 1863 from strobilate specimens recovered from a Brazilian puma. The larval cyst from the Brazilian agouti was named *E. cruzi* by Brumpt and Joyeux in 1924. Cameron[48] considered these specimens to be identical to *E. oligarthrus,* but their taxonomic status remains uncertain. It was not until recently that the studies of Sousa and Thatcher[287,288,295-297] in Panama led to the demonstration of the life cycle in fields and their rodent prey. It is not yet known if *E. oligarthrus* from Argentina, which is morphologically somewhat different from the Panamanian variety,[252] differs biologically in important ways from the other geographic strains. No human infections due to this species have been confirmed.

E. vogeli

This species was first described by Rausch and Bernstein in 1972 as adult specimens recovered from a bush dog, *Speothos venaticus* (Lund), captured in the province of Esmeraldas, Ecuador.[225] Subsequent studies have shown that the larval form occurs in rodents and that *E. vogeli* causes a polycystic form of hydatid disease in man.[65,228]

Morphology and Biology

Literature concerning the morphology and biology of the different developmental stages of taeniid cestodes, including *Echinococcus* spp., has been reviewed by Smyth,[279,281] Freeman,[83] and Slāis.[278] Because of the presumed monophyletic origin of the taeniid cestodes, development is essentially similar in all species. However, features that distinguish the metacestode and strobilate stages of the different species of *Echinococcus* are herein discussed.

There are four developmental stages of *Echinococcus* sp. In sequence, these are (1) the ovum, which is produced by the adult and undergoes cellular differentiation when fertilized, (2) the oncosphere, or larva, which migrates to a suitable parenteral site in the intermediate host, (3) the metacestode, which possesses differntiated protoscolices when completely developed, and (4) the sexually mature adult. When ingested by a suitable definitive (final) host, the protoscolices undergo proglottidation and develop into a sexually mature adult.[83]

Development from ovum to an egg that contains the oncosphere or hexacanth embryo takes place in utero in the adult *Echinococcus* while it is in the intestine of a definitive host. The fully differentiated oncosphere is protected by four enclosing embryonic membranes or envelopes. The oncosphere measures approximately 0.018 mm and is bilaterally symmetrical, possessing three pairs of hooks (hexacanth), muscle fibers, and glands, which aid it in penetration and locomotion within the intermediate host. The embryophore, which appears as a thick, radially striated capsule, develops from the inner envelope and is the principal and most resistant protective cover of the oncosphere. The oncosphere and its surrounding membranes (diameter: 0.030 to 0.036 mm) is often referred to as the cestode egg.

Eggs are shed with the feces into the external environment, and, when ingested by a suitable intermediate host, the oncospheres hatch and become activated. Hatching refers to the complete liberation of the oncosphere from the embryonic envelope and results from digestion of the membranes from without by host enzymes, as well as from mechanical activity and lytic processes of the activated oncosphere from within.[123] Hatching and activation are facilitated by factors present in the gut environment,[222] but may also occur spontaneously in extraintestinal parenteral sites.[22,35] Lytic secretions may facilitate the passage of the motile oncosphere through the intestinal mucosa and into the host's circulatory system (via venous and lymphatic pathways).[122] They are distributed to other sites via the host's circulatory system, where postoncospheral development continues. Factors that determine the final localization of taeniid larvae in a given host are still poorly understood, but they include anatomic[53] and physiologic factors of the host, as well as the strain of cestode.[327]

Within a few days after the oncospheres reach their preferred site, cystic development begins. This process involves degeneration of the oncospheral stage and emergence of the metacestode stage. Successful in vitro culture of *E. granulosus* oncospheres showed that within 4 to 7 days the larva had changed into a typical bladder with a germinative layer.[128] In 10 days, the latter had formed acellular laminations. Growth (increase in cyst diameter) averaged 4 mm/month in vitro[128] but is much slower in vivo and varies widely from one host species to another (reviewed by Heath[123]). In general, hydatid cysts increase in diameter from 1 to 5 cm each year, depending upon factors still unknown. Protoscolex formation occurs as early as 4 months in white mice, but may require more than 1 year in sheep.

The fully developed metacestode (hydatid) of *E. granulosus* is typically unilocular and fluid filled. Structurally, the cyst consists of an inner germinative layer of cells supported externally by a characteristic acidophilic-staining, acellular, laminated membrane of variable thickness (Figure 2). Cytoplasmic extensions of the germinative layer unite to form a syncytium, which is differentiated into numerous microtriches. The microtriches project peripherally into the laminar layer toward the host tissues surrounding the cyst.[36,37,189] Surrounding the parasitic cyst is a host-produced, granulomatous, adventitial reaction of extremely variable intensity. Small secondary cysts, called brood capsules, bud internally from the germinative layer and, by polyembryony, produce multiple protoscolices. A protoscolex is a scolex with the rostellum and suckers deeply withdrawn into the post-sucker region. In humans, the slowly growing hydatid cysts may attain a volume of many liters and contain many thousands of protoscolices.

The explanation for the ability of metacestodes, including those of *Echinococcus* spp., to persist indefinitely in the tissues of immunologically competent hosts has been of great interest to parasitologists.[229,322] Recent studies prove that host serum proteins, including IgG and IgM, freely penetrate the laminated membrane and reach the germinative layer, which somehow prevents or regulates their passage into the cysts.[34,56,57,60] However, Coltorti and Varela-Diaz[57] found host IgG in nearly one third of *E. granulosus* cysts in gerbils, and Kassis and Tanner[150] found IgG and IgM on the

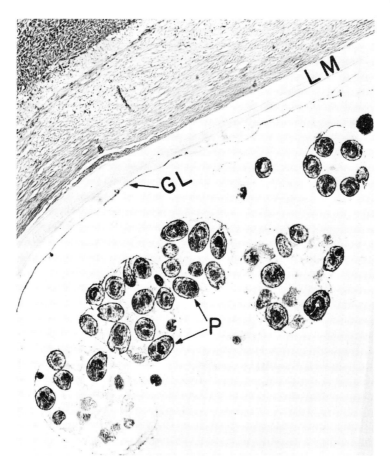

FIGURE 2.   Hydatid cyst of *Echinococcus granulosus* in liver of sheep showing protoscolices (P) in brood capsules, germinative layer (GL) and laminated membrane (LM). (H. and E.; magnification about × 500.)

surfaces of protoscolices in 100% of *E. multilocularis* cysts in cotton rats. Complement in normal human serum causes lysis of protoscolices both in vitro and in vivo.[49,131,229] Rickard et al.[237] showed that the lytic process was mediated by the alternate pathway rather than the classical pathway of complement activation. How protoscolices in the hydatid cyst evade immunologic damage mediated by antibodies and complement that enter the cyst is not completely understood, although anticomplementary substances produced by metacestodes may assist. It has been proposed that low-molecuar-weight cytotoxic factors in hydatid cyst fluid interfering with host immunocompetent cells may account for the long-term survival of the metacestode.[13]

Postoncospheral development of *E. multilocularis* is fundamentally the same as that of *E. granulosus,* except that the primary vesicle gives rise to others by continuous exogenous budding, to produce a larval mass made up of hundreds of contiguous vesicles that may occupy more than one half of the invaded hepatic lobe (Figure 3). There is no limiting membrane of host or parasitic origin. Growth of the larva from the single primary vesicle to the compound multivesicular stage with infective protoscolices may be completed in as short a period as 2 months or as long a time as 7 months, depending upon conditions for growth in the host.[78,197, 319] The rapid rate of development of *E. multilocularis* as compared with that of *E. granulosus* is an adaptation in the short-lived intermediate hosts.[217] The number of protoscolices within a

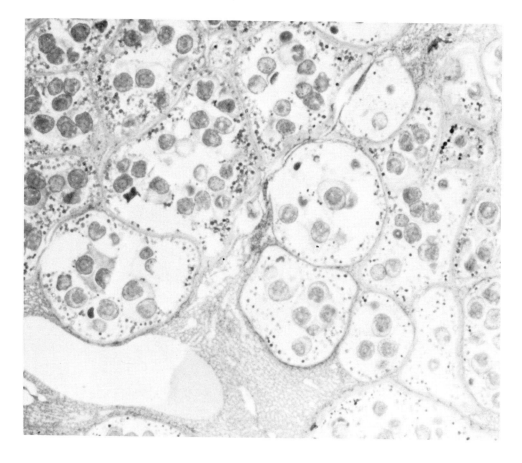

FIGURE 3.　Lesion of larval *Echinococcus multilocularis* in liver of infected rodent. Note typical alveolar-like microvesicles with protoscolices, (H. and E.; magnification about × 500.)

larval mass derived from a single embryo is highly variable within and between species of hosts, but may number to several thousand.[197,224]

E. multilocularis infection in the cotton rat has been a useful model for investigating the mechanisms which regulate the host-parasite interaction.[228] A preexisting larval infection can prevent or suppress the growth of a secondary infection, which will spread quickly if the primary infection is resolved. In addition to the effects of humoral factors (antibody and complement), nonspecific and specific cellular activity is involved. Suppression and destruction of cysts is characterized by the infiltration of large numbers of macrophages and leucocytes, although we do not yet know the functional role of these cells and how they are stimulated.[228]

Development and maturation of *E. multilocularis* larvae are closely linked to the physical and sexual maturation of the intermediate hosts. Development of protoscolices is delayed in voles during the overwintering period, when young voles are in a retarded, immature state, but larvae become infective during the subsequent period of rapid physical and sexual maturation of the voles themselves.[78]

In their natural hosts, the metacestode form of *E. oligarthrus* consists of cysts with a structure similar to that of *E. granulosus* (Figure 4). The vesicular cysts tend to become septate and form multi-chambered masses[287] that are readily distinguishable from the alveolar cysts of *E. multilocularis* by their larger size and abundant cyst fluid. Cysts become fertile (develop protoscolices) after 4 to 5 months of development.[287]

The development of *E. vogeli* in natural intermediate hosts has not yet been de-

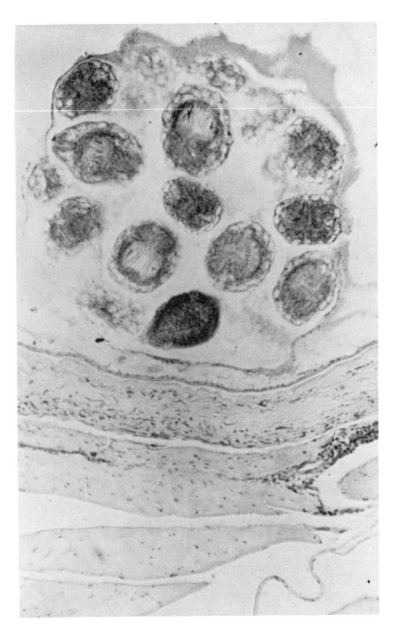

FIGURE 4.   Hydatid cyst of *Echinococcus oligarthrus* from intermuscular connective tissue of infected rodent (H. E.; magnification about × 1000.) (Specimen courtesy of O. E. Sousa.)

scribed. In humans, the larval *E. vogeli* produces multiple, relatively large fluid filled vesicles with brood capsules and numerous protoscolices.

When metacestodes of *Echinococcus* sp. are ingested by suitable definitive hosts, the protoscolices, stimulated by bile, pH, and presumably other host factors, evaginate in the upper part of the duodenum.[279] According to Smyth,[281] they then make their way between the villi and may enter the crypts of Lieberkuhn, achieving intimate contact with the host intestinal mucosa. Proglottidation is initiated, and strobilar development proceeds until the gravid adult stage is reached in approximately 32 days for *E. multilocularis*,[217] 48 days for *E. granulosus*,[89] and 80 days for *E. oligarthrus*.[287]

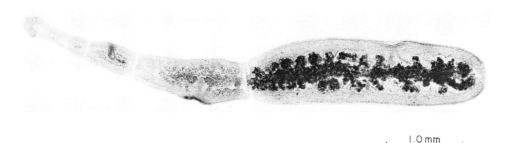

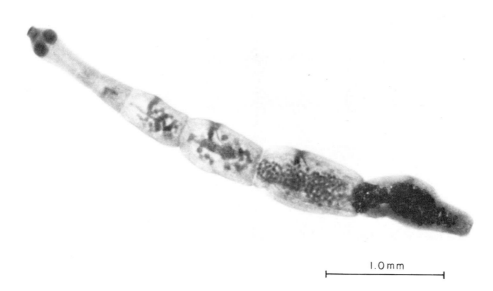

FIGURE 5. Strobila of *Echinococcus granulosus* from dog with experimental infection, 76th day.

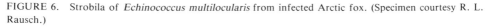

FIGURE 6. Strobila of *Echinococcus multilocularis* from infected Arctic fox. (Specimen courtesy R. L. Rausch.)

The completely developed strobilae of *Echinococcus* sp. consist of a scolex (with four suckers and a double row of rostellar hooks) and two to five proglottids (Figures 5 and 6). The entire strobila measures 2 to 6 mm. The first proglottid adjacent to the scolex is sexually immature but is usually followed by one to three hermaphroditic proglottids in different stages of maturity. The final proglottid has a gravid uterus containing between 200 and 400 eggs. In *E. granulosus,* this is detached approximately every 2 weeks, following which the penultimate proglottid becomes gravid.

The specific morphologic characteristics of *Echinococcus* sp. that are valuable for taxonomic discrimination of the adult stage have been the subject of much discussion.[220,313,318] According to Rausch and Bernstein,[225] when used in combination, the taxonomic criteria include the form of strobila, position of the genital pore in the mature and gravid segments, size of rostellar hooks, number and distribution of testes, and form of gravid uterus.

True and Alternate Hosts

E. granulosus

The occurrence of this cestode in a particular host assemblage (e.g., wolf/moose; dog/sheep; dog/horse) usually presumes a well-established host-parasite relationship, with adaptations that are reflected in the "strain" characteristics. According to

Rausch,[221] *E. granulosus* evolved and was maintained in cycles involving the wolf (*Canis lupus* Linnaeus) and wild ungulates such as swine (*Sus scrofa* L.), red deer (*Cervus elaphus* L.), and aurochs (*Bos primigenus* Bojanus).

In early Neolithic times in Europe (and perhaps elsewhere), as the wolf and several of the ungulates became domesticated, a synanthropic cycle became possible in which the dog replaced the wolf as the definitive host and domestic ungulates became the intermediate hosts. The cestode became dispersed widely with its host and adpated itself to a variety of domestic and sylvatic host species. Naturally acquired or experimentally produced larval infection has been reported in at least seven orders of mammals.[248,280] Many of the reported host associations appear fortuitous, however, and probably do not represent parts of an established and independent transmission cycle. In contemplating control, it is important to know which potential hosts have been found to be infected and whether they represent incidental infections only. It should be determined whether these hosts are of little epidemiological significance, or whether they represent the active reservoirs of infection upon which the parasite depends (locally) for its survival.[270]

Comparison of infection rates in domestic animals and man indicates that throughout the greater part of the cestode's geographic range, the sheep appears to be the most important intermediate host.[246] In some regions, nevertheless, other domestic ungulates, including goats, swine, cattle, Asian buffalo, equids, and camelids, assume dominant importance.

Both susceptibility to infection and cyst fertility rates are important considerations when ranking the importance of the different intermediate hosts. Sheep are highly susceptible, and more than 90% of the cysts become fertile in this animal. Furthermore, sheep husbandry methods almost always involve the use of dogs, thus creating possibilities for parasite transmission. Goats and swine are also highly susceptible to *E. granulosus*, and their cysts have high fertility rates.[156,272] The coprophagic habits of swine increase the possibility that cestode eggs will be ingested.

Certain other hosts are highly susceptible to *E. granulosus*, but full cyst development appears inhibited, thereby reducing their roles in continued transmission. For example, although infection rates in cattle are relatively high in most endemic areas, cyst fertility rates are low[272] in some areas. Elsewhere, however, cyst fertility rates in bovines are comparable to those in sheep.[109,313] In the epidemiological sense, humans are usually considered to be accidental hosts.

Host specificity is more strongly defined in the adult-stage *E. granulosus* than in the larval stage. Almost all known definitive hosts are members of the family Canidae,[279,280] including the domestic dog and dingo (*Canis familiaris* L.), the wolf (*C. lupus* L.), the coyote (*C. latrans* Say), the jackal (*C. aureus* L.), and the hunting dog (*Lycaon pictus* Temminck).

The suitability of foxes as definitive hosts for *E. granulosus* varies according to species and other factors. Some experimental transmission attempts with *Vulpes* and *Urocyon* spp. demonstrated that strobilar growth and development were retarded and that the organisms did not reach the gravid stage.[64,176,177,179] Other workers, however, successfully infected foxes and obtained gravid strobilae. Successful experimental infections were obtained in *V. corsac*,[274] *V. vulpes*,[42,67,113,172,290] and *V. bengalensis*.[216] These apparently conflicting results were at least partially explained by the demonstration that different populations of *E. granulosus* varied in their adaptation in the species of fox hosts. Howkins et al.[132] showed that cyst larvae from English horses were infective to *V. vulpes* and dogs and developed equally well within them. In contrast, cyst larvae from Australian sheep were established poorly in *V. vulpes*, and strobilar growth and development were retarded.

South American foxes of the genus *Dusicyon* (Molina) are highly susceptible to experimentally produced infections, and field studies have demonstrated naturally acquired infections in these animals in some parts of Argentina.[32,248,255,257]

Infected lions (*Felis leo* L.) have been observed in South Africa, Tanzania, and Uganda,[242] and the cestodes were identified as *E. granulosus.* Domestic cats sometimes permit the experimental establishment of *E. granulosus* strobilae, but development is always retarded.[87,202,290]

E. multilocularis

In contrast to *E. granulosus, E. multilocularis* is characterized by a greater degree of host specificity, particularly in the larval stages. The natural definitive and intermediate hosts, respectively, of this cestode are foxes of the genera *Alopex* and *Vulpes,* and small cricetid rodents, mainly of the subfamily Arvicolinae Gray, 1821.[227] In the comparatively simple biotic conditions of the arctic tundra zone, the cestode is maintained in cycles involving the arctic fox, *A. alopex* L., and several kinds of voles of the genera *Microtus* Schrank and *Clethrionomys* Tilesius.[217]

In more complex biomes, a greater variety of host species is involved. The red fox, *V. vulpes,* is the most important definitive host throughout most of the range of distribution outside of the Arctic Circle. In the U.S.S.R., 26 species of rodents are involved in transmission, including the muskrat, *Ondatra zibethicus* (L.), an introduced species from North America.[169] In the north central U.S., deer mice, *Peromyscus maniculatus* (Wagner), are the principal intermediate hosts. Although *Echinococcus* cysts in deer mice produce fewer protoscolices than do cysts in voles captured in the same locality, the former hosts have a higher prevalence of infection, probably resulting from their feeding behavior.[164,224]

Other carnivores that have been found naturally infected and that may occasionally play important epidemiological roles are domestic dogs and cats,[227,318] coyotes,[164] and wolves.[169] Domestic ungulates are not susceptible to *E. multilocularis.*

E. oligarthrus

E. oligarthrus is the only species that characteristically uses wild felids as definitive hosts. Naturally acquired infections have been demonstrated in the puma (*F. concolor* L.),[41,295] the jaguarundi (*F. yagouaroundi* Geoffroy),[48,295] the jaguar (*F. onca* L.),[296] the pampas cat (*F. colocolo* Molina),[293] and Geoffroy's cat (*F. geoffroyi* D'Orbigny and Gervais).[252] The cestode undergoes complete development in domestic cats. In dogs, however, growth is stunted and the strobilae do not reach maturity.[287]

A naturally acquired infection in the agouti (*Dasyprocta punctata* Gray) in Panama has been positively identified as *E. oligarthrus* by experimental transmission to a domestic cat.[288] Naturally acquired hydatid infections have been identified in *D. agouti* in Brazil, the spiny rat (*Proechimys panamensis* Tomes) in Panama,[288] *P. pialis* L. in Colombia,[297] *D. rubrata* in Venezuela,[287] and *Microcavia australis* in Argentina.[252] In most cases cited above, cysts were tentatively identified as *E. oligarthrus* on the basis of cyst morphology and protoscolex-hook size; however, experimental transmission studies were not done. The reports were made before the larval stages of *E. vogeli* had been described, and since this latter species was recorded in tropical lowland areas of northern South America, the possibility that some of the infections cited above were actually caused by *E. vogeli* cannot be ruled out.

E. vogeli

The principal definitive host of *E. vogeli* appears to be the bush dog, *Speothos venaticus* (Lund). Domestic dogs are also adequate hosts but cats are not. The paca, *Cuniculus paca* L. may be the principal intermediate host although agoutis and spiney rats have also been found infected.[65,228]

Distribution
E. granulosus

The adaptability of *E. granulosus* to a wide variety of host species and the repeated introduction of domestic animals from Europe to other parts of the world have made possible the present broad geographical distribution of this cestode and the disease it produces, from north of the Arctic Circle to as far south as Tierra del Fuego, Argentina, and Stewart Island, New Zealand. Within this cosmopolitan distribution, the cestode occurs in all major climates, in a wide variety of hosts, and at various levels of prevalence.

Several hundred articles have recorded that *E. granulosus* infection in man and other animals occurs throughout the world. This literature has been reviewed by Gemmell,[88] Simitch,[276] Rausch,[221] Schantz and Schwabe,[246] Williams et al.,[324] and Matossian et al.[184] The following account and Figure 7 are based on these reviews and have been updated to account for more recently published data and changes that have resulted from successful control programs. Specific prevalence data are not given because of the limitations of comparing prevalence data obtained in different regions; these limitations will be discussed later in this section.

In the higher latitudes of the Western Hemisphere, the sylvatic strain of *E. granulosus* occurs in wolves and wild ungulates in parts of Alaska and Canada.[221] The same or a similar strain has been reported from the northernmost regions of the Scandinavian countries[240] and the U.S.S.R. In these areas, the confinement of the organism to sylvatic animal intermediate hosts limits the risk of human exposure. In Alaska and Canada, human infection is largely limited to indigenous Eskimos and Indians, especially hunting and trapping tribes,[49,218] which feed their dogs on lungs and other offal of reindeer and moose.

Infection occurs sporadically throughout North, Central, and northern South America in cycles involving dogs and sheep (in the western U.S. and Mexico), and dogs and swine (in the southeastern U.S., Mexico, Guatemala, El Salvador, Venezuela, and Ecuador).[246] The apparent absence of *E. granulosus* from many tropical areas appears to be related to a lack of suitable intermediate hosts rather than to environmental factors per se. In the Americas, the highest infection prevalence is observed in the intensive sheep-raising areas of southern South America (i.e., Argentina, Chile, Uruguay, central Peru, Bolivia, and southern Brazil), where the simultaneous presence of sheep and dogs combines with the ignorance or irresponsibility of man, producing optimal conditions for the perpetuation of the cestode.[324]

Iceland, which a century ago had the highest human infection rate ever recorded (22%), is now free of the infection.[25] In Europe, the highest prevalence in human and animal hosts is reported from countries adjacent to the Mediterranean Sea (Spain, Italy, Yugoslavia, Greece, and Cyprus), where the dog/sheep cycle is dominant. In some parts of Western Europe, Great Britain, and Ireland, the cestode is prevalent in a dog/horse cycle but appears to account for little human morbidity.[301] A dog/pig cycle is prevalent in several eastern European countries (Poland and Hungary) and in the U.S.S.R. (Byelorussia S.S.R. and Ukrainia S.S.R.). The infection is widespread throughout the remainder of the U.S.S.R. in the dog/sheep cycle. Control programs have reduced the prevalence considerably in most Russian republics but have had limited impact in the Kazakh S.S.R. and the Central Asian republics.

In most Middle Eastern countries, infection is hyperendemic in sheep, camels, goats, and donkeys.[246] Reports indicate that the infection occurs in most Asian countries, with Iran, India, Nepal, and Pakistan reportedly having the highest prevalence. Although no published data are available concerning this infection in the People's Republic of China, it probably exists in the sheep-raising northern areas. In Southeast Asia, *E. granulosus* has been reported from North and South Vietnam, Cambodia, the Philippines, Taiwan, and Indonesia.[321]

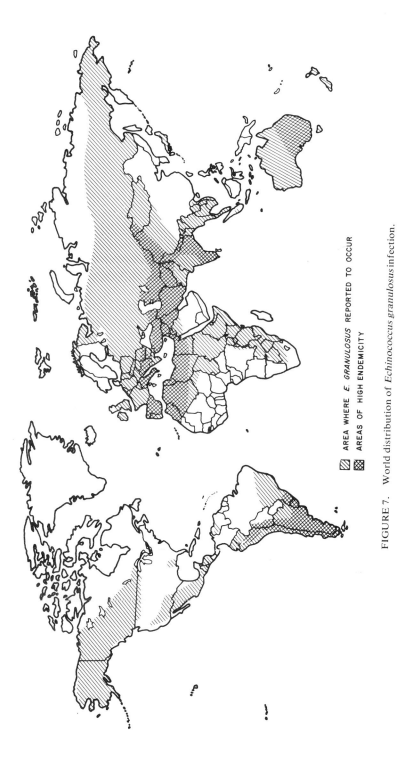

FIGURE 7.   World distribution of *Echinococcus granulosus* infection.

AREA WHERE *E. GRANULOSUS* REPORTED TO OCCUR

AREAS OF HIGH ENDEMICITY

In North Africa (Morocco, Algeria, Tunisia, Libya, and Egypt), a high prevalence is reported, and host-parasite relationships are similar to those in the Middle East. Infection is reported sporadically throughout sub-Saharan Africa. In East Africa, infection in domestic livestock is widespread, but human infection is mainly limited to certain groups in northwestern Kenya and Uganda, where a set of poorly understood environmental and cultural factors combines to produce one of the highest morbidity rates ever reported.[173,198,199]

In the 1950s, human infection rates in New Zealand caused that country to be ranked with other hyperendemic areas. However, after control efforts were intensified in 1957, the incidence of new cases dropped markedly, particularly in the younger age groups.[46] In Australia, prevalence has been considerably reduced on the island of Tasmania by control measures initiated in 1965. However, a high prevalence is still reported in most of western Australia.[24]

Comparing data on the prevalence of echinococcosis, particularly in human hosts, is a frustrating exercise. Shaded areas on the map shown in Figure 7 are regions where, according to published data, *E. granulosus* infections are probably a major public health and economic problem. This information must be regarded as an estimate because the availability of prevalence data for any disease is often a function of the presence of interested investigators, which is sometimes inversely correlated with the magnitude of the disease problems. Selection bias and differences in methodology combine in most published studies to prevent an objective comparison from one country or region to another. Some of the methods for measuring the prevalence of human infection are discussed below in order to illustrate both their usefulness and some of the pitfalls in their interpretation.

The most common index of the level of human infection in an area or region is the annual incidence of diagnosed or surgical cases. Diagnostic coverage varies from one region to another, depending upon the availability and degree of utilization of local medical services and the completeness of physician reporting. Where disease-reporting systems include hydatid disease and are reasonably complete, the annual number of cases can be obtained from a central reporting office. More often, however, it is necessary for the investigator to obtain these data without this convenience. For example, in Uruguay, three retrospective surveys of all medical and surgical centers determined the number of hospital cases diagnosed annually during the years between 1962 and 1971.[211] The mean annual morbidity, whether expressed as the incidence of all hospital cases (20.7 cases per 100,000 population) or only new cases (17.7/100,000) gave Uruguay the highest echinococcosis national morbidity rate yet reported. In comparison, other high national figures were 12.9 cases per 100,000 in Cyprus,[174] 7.8 in Chile,[215] 7.5 to 8.3 in Greece,[171] 5.1 to 6.1 in Algeria,[201] and 3.7 in Yugoslavia.[290]

Infection rates expressed at the national level, however, often fail to reflect the true importance of the disease because all populations are not at equal risk. In most countries, hydatid disease is most prevalent in the rural areas. In Uruguay, for instance, the average annual incidence per 100,000 population was 123.0 for rural residents, but only 10.1 for urban and suburban residents.[211] In Argentina, the number of reported cases per year for the entire country varies between 1 and 2/100,000, but in several southern provinces the rate exceeds 150/100,000.[251] The same pattern is seen in many other countries in South America and elsewhere.

The use of diagnostic methods (radiology and serology) to detect asymptomatic cyst carriers indicates that symptomatic hospital cases represent only a tiny fraction of the total infections. For instance, in the province of Rio Negro, Argentina, where the annual incidence of hospital cases is 143/100,000, a mass miniature radiography survey of 15,000 persons demonstrated infection in 460/100,000. These included solely cyst infections, with pulmonary localization representing only one third or less of all infections.[253] Standardized radiologic diagnostic criteria permit an accuracy exceeding 90%.[211] Where mass miniature radiography surveys are carried out routinely at periodic intervals, they are useful for comparison of human prevalence over time and on a regional basis.

Immunodiagnostic methods are also potentially useful for estimating the true prevalence of human echinococcosis infection. The skin test and various serological procedures have been used for screening human populations in many different areas of the world.[19,43,112,141,143,153,170,214,253] However, little information of value could be concluded from most of these studies because the methods used were relatively nonspecific. In the few studies in which there was clinical follow-up, only a small proportion of persons with positive immunodiagnostic test results had evidence of active hydatid infection.[173,253] Recent advances in serologic methodology have provided epidemiologists with more specific techniques. Large numbers of serum samples can be screened with rapid, relatively simple techniques such as latex agglutination or indirect hemagglutination, and reactive serum specimens can then be tested for antibody to the echinococcosis-specific antigen 5.[309] The relatively specific arc-5 is particularly useful as a diagnostic criterion when results from different geographic areas are being compared, since indexes of serological prevalence thus obtained are not affected by the presence of other helminths, which cause cross-reactions in other serologic tests. Methods for measuring the prevalence of infection in dogs and animal intermediate hosts will be discussed in the section entitled "Diagnosis."

E. multilocularis

The geographic distribution of *E. multilocularis* has been reviewed by Rausch[221] and Lukashenko.[169] The map in Figure 8 represents the most recent knowledge concerning the approximate distribution of the organism. Apparently restricted by host requirements, *E. multilocularis* is limited to the Northern Hemisphere.[221] Its known range includes an endemic region in central Europe (central and southern Germany, western Austria, Switzerland, and southern France) and most of northern Eurasia, from Bulgaria and Turkey through the U.S.S.R., extending eastward to several of the Japanese islands (Rebun, Hokkaido, and Kuriles). In the U.S.S.R., the infection occurs in eastern and western Siberia, the upper and middle Volga districts, the Urals, the Caucasian republics (Azerbaijan S.S.R., Armenian S.S.R., and Georgian S.S.R.), Moldavian S.S.R., and the Central Asian republics (Kazakh S.S.R., Kirghiz S.S.R. and Uzbek S.S.R.). A recent report from northern Iran and India are the southernmost records of *E. multilocularis* in Asia.[3,188]

The distribution of this cestode in North America appears to be discontinuous. It is highly prevalent in the northern tundra zone, where its distribution corresponds closely to that of its most important definitive host, the arctic fox.[221] There is no present evidence that the cestode occurs in the zone of boreal forest, south of the tundra zone, but recent studies have demonstrated a large and increasing area of infection in south central Canada (Manitoba, Saskatchewan, and Alberta) and the north central U.S. (North Dakota, South Dakota, Minnesota, Iowa, Nebraska, Montana, and Wyoming).[164] The important sylvatic hosts in this region are red foxes, coyotes, deer mice, and field voles. The cestode may have been introduced to this region relatively recently by transport of infected dogs from Alaska,[221] or by southward migration of infected arctic foxes. The first human case definitely associated with the central North American focus was diagnosed in 1977 in Minnesota.[84] The availability of suitable hosts in adjacent areas presents a potential for further spread in North America.

E. multilocularis is not known to occur in the Southern Hemisphere. Reported cases of "alveolar hydatid disease" in Argentina and Uruguay[292,317] may have been atypical larval forms of *E. granulosus* or infection by *E. oligarthrus* or *E. vogeli*.

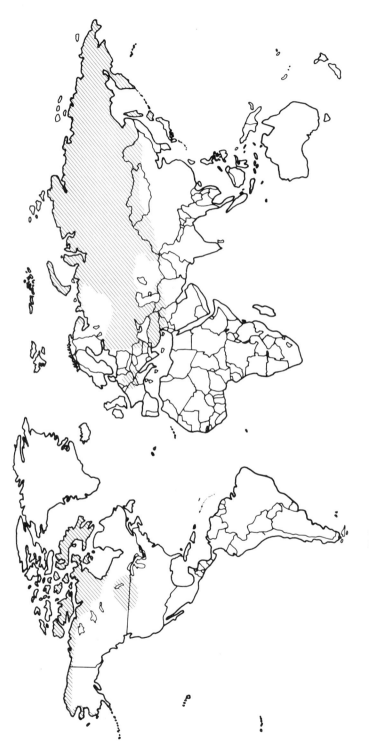

FIGURE 8.   World distribution of *Echinococcus multilocularis* infection.

Few data exist on the incidence and prevalence of human alveolar hydatid disease. Recent reviews indicate that cases occur frequently in parts of the U.S.S.R. (Yakutsk A.S.S.R.),[169] northern Japan,[36] western Alaska, and central Europe.[221] A recent report from Switzerland indicates that there was an annual mean incidence of autochthonous cases of 0.15/100,000 population between 1965 and 1969.[71] Prevalence rates are not reported from other endemic regions.

E. oligarthrus and E. vogeli

These species are indigenous to South America. They are sympatric over extensive regions of the continent and also in Central America, where ostensibly suitable hosts for both are present in humid tropical forest northward to about the Isthmus of Tehuantepec in southern Mexico (i.e., to circa latitude 18° N).[228] A recent report from Argentine Patagonia[252] indicates that *E. oligarthrus* also occurs in temperate regions.

Disease in Animals

E. granulosus

The establishment and survival of *E. granulosus* strobilae in the intestines of the canid definitive hosts are influenced by such host factors as sex and hormonal cycle, age, and immunity,[89,130,257] although little is known about the mechanisms involved. More than 50,000 worms may inhabit the duodenum and upper jejunum of infected dogs, and although individual worms are said to disrupt the intestinal mucosa,[281] such massive infections are well tolerated by the host. They rarely, if ever, produce clinical illness. Adult worms become senescent after 6 to 10 months,[7] and infections are lost spontaneously, although strobilae are occasionally retained for 2 years or longer.[39]

Hydatid cysts vary widely in their appearance in the different intermediate hosts, depending upon host-parasite adaptations.[50] In those hosts to which the sylvatic strain of the cestode is best adapted, such as the moose (*Alces alces* L.) and other cervids, cysts are unilocular and occur primarily in the lungs, with minimal host tissue reaction. By contrast, cysts in the liver and lungs of sheep, cattle, and swine may include unilocular, multilocular, or even multicystic forms, which sometimes provoke an intense host inflammatory response and degenerative changes, including calcification.[50,227,333] Occasionally, anomalous multicystic forms in cattle and humans have been confused with *E. multilocularis,* but careful observation will permit differentiation of the two species.[197]

Multiple, massive cystic infections are common in domestic animals, but infected ones rarely exhibit clinical signs. Anaphylaxis, a well-known potential cause of death in infected humans, can be produced experimentally in infected sheep[262] and may occasionally cause death in naturally infected sheep, although this has not yet been documented.

Economic losses due to *E. granulosus* in livestock are usually measured in terms of the value of condemned viscera. These losses may be considerable. In Chile during 1962 and 1963, they were estimated at about five million dollars.[194] Hydatidosis may interfere with animal growth and wool and milk production; however, alleged measurements of such losses[37,208,243] are unconvincing because of selection bias and methodology problems.

E. multilocularis

The number of worms in infected arctic foxes usually exceeds 100,000 to 200,000/animal, but they apparently cause no adverse effects.[215] Most worms are eliminated spontaneously 3 to 4 months after infection although some may remain for 7 or more months; however, these are senescent and can no longer produce eggs.[217]

Compared with cystic hydatid disease, larval *E. multilocularis* infection is more progressive and damaging to the hosts. In certain species of arvicoline rodents, focal hepatic lesions are visible macroscopically as early as 48 hr after infection.[217] After about 50 days, the weight of the liver can exceed that of the remainder of the animal. In heavy infections, death can occur in as quickly as 30 days; after 5 months, mortality is high. Susceptibility and growth characteristics vary widely between different species of natural and experimental intermediate hosts.[197] Tissue reactions evoked by the larval cestode are characterized as (1) progressive when the formation of granulation tissue in the process of encapsulation and organization of the lesion are involved, or (2) regressive in the response to chemical and mechanical effects of the parasites.[197] Primary larval foci appear almost invariably in the liver, but dissemination of tissue elements, including protoscolices, is common and results in the extension of the larval mass to serous surfaces and contiguous organs.

Disease in Man
E. granulosus

There are numerous descriptions of the diverse clinical manifestations of cystic hydatid disease in medical and surgical literature. Amir-Jahed et al.,[8] Grove et al.,[115] and Little[168] have recently written excellent reviews. It is apparent that many human infections remain asymptomatic. Hydatid cysts are frequently observed as incidental findings at autopsy at rates much higher than the reported local morbidity rates.[265] In other instances, the severity and nature of the signs and symptoms produced by larval cestodes are extremely variable and never pathognomonic. The particular manifestations are determined by the site of localization of the cysts, their size, and their condition.

The incubation period of human hydatid infections is highly variable and often prolonged for several years. Most infections are diagnosed in patients between the ages 10 and 50 years. It has been suggested that human *E. granulosus* infection is most often acquired in childhood,[270] a contention supported by observations in experimental animals[269] and by a study showing that the age-specific incidence of cerebral hydatid disease (which has a relatively short incubation period) is lower than that for other forms.[28] Nevertheless, age-specific incidence and prevalence rates increase gradually with age, suggesting that new infections continue to occur throughout the human life span.[253,265] Moreover, surgical incidence rates among persons aged 25 years or older declined significantly following successful interruption of parasite transmission in Australia and New Zealand.[26] These observations suggest that adults were relatively susceptible and that the latent period between infection and diagnosis in many cases is only a few years.

In most published reports of surgical case series, the most frequently reported site of localization of hydatid cysts is the liver (50 to 70%), followed by the lungs (20 to 30%), and less frequently, the spleen, kidneys, heart, bones, CNS, and elsewhere. The relative frequency of specific sites of localization often differs from one country to another because of differences in the availability and use of diagnostic technology. For example, pulmonary cysts are diagnosed relatively more often in areas where mass miniature radiography is employed in tuberculosis control programs. Cysts in multiple locations are detected more frequently where liver scans are performed routinely on patients with pulmonary cysts.[260] Cestode strain differences also affect sites of localization; larvae of the northern sylvatic strain localize predominantly in the lungs.[327]

The slowly growing hydatid cyst is well tolerated by the human host until it becomes large enough to cause dysfunction. Cyst rupture, often resulting from trauma, may cause a variety of immediate or delayed sequelae. Mild to severe anaphylactoid reactions (and, occasionally, death) may follow the sudden massive release of cyst fluid.[140] These shock reactions are largely a result of allergic reactions in sensitized hosts, but direct toxic properties of hydatid cyst fluid may also contribute.[262] Cyst fluid contains complement-activating factors which interact with complement to produce anaphyto-toxins.[119] In the lungs, ruptured cyst membranes may be evacuated entirely through the bronchi or retained to serve as a nidus for bacterial infection. Dissemination of protoscolices may result in multiple secondary disease; in one study of 106 patients the rate of postoperative recurrence within 3 years was 11%.[191]

Hydatid cysts of the liver may become relatively large before producing symptoms because of the large size of the organ and the distensible body area. Signs and symptoms presented may include hepatic enlargement with or without a palpable mass in the right upper quadrant, right epigastric pain, nausea, and vomiting. Rupture or leakage usually results in acute or intermittent allergic manifestations. Urgent complications, which existed at the time of initial presentation in 7% of Australian patients with hepatic cysts, include traumatic or spontaneous rupture, thoracobilia, and biliary fistula.[168] One fourth of patients with hepatic cysts also had cysts in their lungs.

Intact hydatid cysts in the lungs may cause no symptoms, but leakage or rupture causes chest pain, coughing, dyspnea, and hemoptysis.[331] Hydatid membranes may be coughed up sometimes resulting in spontaneous cure. Emergency complications, which existed in 20% of Australian patients at the time of initial presentation, included cyst rupture and secondary bacterial infection.[168] Nearly 40% of patients with pulmonary hydatidosis can be shown to have liver involvement as well.[168,260]

In most surgical series, 5 to 10% of the cases involve organs other than the lungs or liver. The first symptom of cerebral cysts may be raised intracranial pressure or focal epilepsy,[28] while kidney cysts may be manifested by loin pain or hematuria.[275] Bone cysts are often asymptomatic until pathologic fractures occur, and, because of a resemblance, they are often misdiagnosed as tuberculous lesions.[34] The prognosis for echinococcosis of the bone is poor, and amputation of the affected limb is frequently necessary. Cysts in the heart are especially dangerous because they may rupture and cause systemic dissemination of the protoscolices, anaphylaxis, or cardiac tamponade.[69]

Although infection prevalence and mortality rates due to hydatid disease may appear low in comparison with those for some other infectious diseases, the morbidity associated with each is considerable. Hydatid patients often require multiple surgical interventions. Extensive secondary hydatid disease often becomes inoperable, and involvement of the bones usually requires amputation. Economic losses to affected families include surgical and hospital expenses as well as loss of income. In Uruguay, it was shown that 60% of surgical patients were unable to return to normal activities for 4 months after leaving the hospital, and 40% were incapacitated for 6 months or longer.[247]

E. multilocularis

Alveolar hydatid disease in man is comparable to that in the natural intermediate hosts (viz., the primary larval lesion develops in the liver), but differs in that the larval mass is inhibited by the host from completing its development and remains in the proliferative stage indefinitely.[226] Thus it continues to invade and destroy the hepatic parenchyma, and retrogressive stages within the mass result in necrosis of the central portion.

Macroscopically, the hepatic lesion usually appears as one or more firm to solid whitish rounded masses slightly elevated above the surrounding tissue of the surface of the liver. When transected, it is seen to consist of a central cavity surrounded by dense, pale tissue that lacks a clearly defined border with respect to the adjacent hepatic tissue. In advanced cases, the cavity usually contains a turbid, yellowish to brown fluid with particles or fragments of necrotic tissue.[197]

Microscopically, there is evidence of a vigorous proliferation of fibrous tissue peripherally but also of regressive changes centrally (necrosis and cavity formation), indicating the strong reaction of the host in suppressing development of the larval cestodes. Cysts of various sizes are scattered or closely aggregated in the matrix of connective tissues. Only rarely are brood capsules and calcareous corpuscles present, usually focally. Metastasis by a hematogenous route is not uncommon, and secondary foci usually occur in the brain and lungs.

Most exposures are believed to occur in childhood, but the rate of growth of the larva is apparently so slow that clinical signs of the disease usually do not become evident until early adulthood or even middle age.

Initial symptoms in alveolar hydatid disease are generally vague. Mild upper quadrant and epigastric pain with hepatomegaly may progress to obstructive jaundice. Occasionally, the initial manifestations are related to metastasis to the lungs or brain.

Because alveolar hydatid disease is often not diagnosed until the disease is well advanced, the lesion is often inoperable. With or without surgery, the mortality ranges from about 50 to 75%.[329]

E. oligarthrus and E. vogeli

Cases of a polycystic form of human hydatid disease with lesion characteristics intermediate between cystic and alveolar hydatid disease have been described from Panama,[286] Ecuador,[339] Colombia,[297] and Venezuela. These had previously been considered to be caused by *E. oligarthrus* but live cysts from two Colombian patients were fed to dogs and strobilate *E. vogeli* was recovered.[65] Based on morphologic characteristics, including the length and shape of rostellar hooks, of other previously diagnosed polycystic hydatid infections (six Colombian, one Ecuadorian, and one Panamanian) it was concluded that all were also due to *E. vogeli*.[65]

In contrast to the larval *E. multilocularis,* the larval *E. vogeli* produces in man relatively large fluid-filled vesicles, brood capsules, and numerous protoscolices. Focal necrosis is commonly observed but large necrotic cavities have not been seen. The primary localization is the liver, but cysts may spread to contiguous sites. The disease appears less progressive than alveolar hydatid disease.

To date, no human infection caused by *E. oligarthrus* has been confirmed.

Mode of Spread

E. granulosus

The transmission of *Echinococcus* spp. from one host to another is an ecological phenomenon which *Echinococcus* spp. like other cestodes have mastered very well: transmission is effected from host to host through the conveyance of food[83] which harbors the infective stage of the parasite.

Dogs and other definitive hosts become infected upon ingesting organs of other animals which contain hydatid cysts or protoscolices released from recently ruptured cysts. Under natural conditions, such transmission is the result of a predator-prey relationship existing between hosts. However, transmission in a synanthropic cycle is considerably modified by human behavioral factors (to be discussed in greater detail later).

E. granulosus has remarkable biological potential. Arundel[15] reported that there may be as many as 40,000 worms in a heavily infected dog and that each worm sheds as many as 1000 eggs every 2 weeks. In areas where the prevalence of infection in the canine population is high, the environment may become contaminated with millions of eggs each day. Eggs contained in (or disrupted from) proglottids are passed in the feces of infected dogs. Through rhythmic muscular contractions, proglottids move away from fecal deposits and discharge most of the remaining eggs,[196] which are immediately infective. Further egg dispersal occurs through the intermediaries of wind, water, and arthropods. It has been shown that taeniid eggs may be dispersed throughout a pasture area of 20,000 m² within 10 days.[107]

Although inhalation of eggs might result in infection,[35] it is generally accepted that ingestion is the predominant mechanism of infection of intermediate hosts. Infection in lower animals commonly occurs when they ingest eggs in contaminated herbage. Much of our knowledge about the survival of taeniid eggs is a result of the study of eggs of various *Taenia* spp. rather than those of *Echinococcus* spp. Temperature and relative humidity are the most important factors affecting survival time of taeniid eggs in nature. However, other factors, including sunlight, soil type, wind dispersal, and vegetation cover, also affect the survival of eggs and their availability to potential hosts. Extremes of temperature (>60 and <−70°C) are instantly lethal to eggs;[55] however, within that range, survival is temperature dependent. Working with *Taenia pisiformis,* Coman[61] showed that high temperature (38°C) and, to a lesser extent, low humidity (33%) were quickly lethal to eggs, and few survived for more than 7 days. However, at 4°C and a relative humidity of 90%, some eggs may still be viable for as long as 300 days. In Kazakh S.S.R., eggs of *E. granulosus* were reported to survive and remain infective for 2 years or longer.[316]

Clumps of native grasses provide eggs with less protection from detrimental climatic factors than does the dense sward of improved grasses.[47] Additionally, highly porous soils allow eggs to be carried into the ground and thus become unavailable to grazing animals.[47]

Taeniid eggs deteriorate gradually over time, and some oncospheres that are still capable of invading the intermediate host are not fully capable of reorganizing to produce an infective metacestode.[62] Some have postulated that the ingestion of "senescent" eggs may produce an abortive infection and immunity against a subsequent infection,[107] which may explain why some animals are apparently immune to challenge infection in the absence of any evidence of previous infection. Gemmell and Johnstone[107] have reviewed current knowledge on extrinsic and intrinsic factors affecting the infective pattern and prevalence rates of *E. granulosus* and other taeniid cestodes in intermediate hosts.

E. multilocularis

Infection rates in the natural hosts, both intermediate and definitive, are influenced by the numerical densities of these mammals as well as by the kind of predator-prey relationship that exists between them.[221] In the northern tundra zone, a strongly defined predator-prey relationship exists between arctic foxes and microtine rodents. The arctic fox feeds almost exclusively on microtine rodents. In studies carried out during different years, infection rates in foxes and voles ranged from 40 to 100% and from 2 to 16%, respectively.[217] The variations seemed to correlate closely with fluctuations in the host populations. The parasites were least numerous when the hosts were also least abundant and most numerous when the host populations were in the high point of the cycle. In biotically more complex zones, foxes feed upon a greater variety of animals, and infection rates are usually lower than those observed in the tundra zone. Infection prevalence in these more complex zones is also dependent upon host density, but is additionally influenced by habitat and climatic season.[157,166]

Leiby and Nichol[163] have shown experimentally that deer mice can become infected with larval *E. multilocularis* by eating beetles previously exposed to fox feces. The insectivorous food habits of deer mice and their tendency to inhabit areas in and about abandoned carnivore dens increase the chances that this species will become infected.

E. oligarthrus and *E. vogeli*

The ecologic relationships between hosts and parasites have not been studied with these two species. It can be assumed that their life cycles depend upon predator-prey relationships existing between their respective hosts.

Epidemiology

E. granulosus

Local differences in prevalence and patterns of transmission are determined by a multiplicity of factors concerning the host, agent, environment, and human behavior.* One must understand these various factors in order to identify vulnerable points and develop practical intervention strategies to use against the infection.[270]

Numerous variables have been associated with echinococcosis transmission, including availability and abundance of suitable domestic and sylvatic animal hosts, cestode strains, climate, soil types, animal husbandry practices, and human behavior, i.e., cultural and religious practices, educational levels, and sanitation practices. The complexity of these multivariate factors has hindered the understanding of their interrelationships. One approach to the study of such systems is path analysis, which employs multiple regression techniques to construct biologically and statistically sound causal models of the systems under investigation. The models can then be tested and manipulated to allow the researcher to visualize and develop strategic preventive measures. Burridge et al.[47] have shown how this approach may be applied to the epidemiological study of echinococcosis in New Zealand. Harris et al.[120] used a deterministic model to compare various control strategies for *E. granulosus* and other parasites having two hosts.

The epidemiological significance of many factors related to animal hosts, the agent, and the environment was discussed in previous sections. Some human influences on *E. granulosus* transmission are discussed below.

Before the domestication of animals, and even today in some high-latitude regions, *E. granulosus* occurred in wolves and wild ungulates under conditions in which man only rarely became infected. By domesticating some of these hosts, man created nearly optimal conditions for the continued transmission of this cestode, its dispersal throughout the world, and, also, for their own entry into its life cycle. Common denominators in rural endemic areas of both advanced and developing countries are the widespread use of dogs for working livestock and the habit of feeding them on viscera of home-butchered sheep or other livestock. Thus an artificial system that is more efficient than the natural systems in perpetuating the life cycle has been created. Under such conditions, canine infection occurs repeatedly, producing high prevalence rates and environmental contamination with cestode eggs.

Human populations living under such conditions are frequently exposed, and the probability that any given individual will become infected depends, in part, upon other factors such as personal hygiene and cleanliness (which, in turn, are often a function of educational, socioeconomic, and cultural characteristics). Direct contact with infected dogs, particularly the characteristic playful and intimate contact between children and their pets would seem to be the most important source of human infection. Cestode eggs adhere to hairs around the infected dog's anus and may also be found on their muzzle and paws.[178,196] Indirect means of contact, via water and contaminated vegetables or through the intermediary of flies and other arthropods, may also result in human infections.

Socioeconomic and cultural characteristics are among the best-defined risk factors for human infection. A prevalence rate much greater than that of the local general population has been demonstrated for the Maori of New Zealand,[44] the Turkana of Kenya,[173,198] persons of Basque origin and Navajo and Zuni Indians in the U.S.,[260,261]

---

* Recent reviews on the epidemiology of cystic hydatid disease include those of Schwabe,[27] Rausch,[221] Gemmell,[95] Gemmell and Johnston,[107] Williams et al.,[324] and Schantz.[251]

and certain indigenous peoples of Argentina, Chile, and Peru.[251] In many instances, the higher infection rates appear to be related to lower levels of education, hygiene, and sanitation, but specific cultural practices often contribute directly to parasite transmission. For example, the greater intimacy of the Turkana with their dogs appears to account for the high disease prevalence in these people as compared with their neighboring nomadic tribes.[195,198] The Turkana tradiation of placing dead persons in open burial sites where they can be scavenged by wild dogs is thought to be an important mode of transmission in that region.[173]

In New Zealand, the prevalence among the Maori was six times as great as among persons of European origin.[44] Maori working dogs, which also serve as pets, may contribute to the higher risk of exposure of this group; non-Maoris in New Zealand usually differentiate between working dogs and pets.[44,45] A complicated Maori land-tenure system has reduced incentives to improve farming and dog management practices and may further contribute to opportunities for hydatid transmission.

In the U.S., the relatively high prevalence of infection in Navajo Indians[261] and persons of Basque origin[14] is related to the involvement of these groups in sheep raising and their practice of allowing dogs access to sheep offal and dead sheep. In Lebanon, Moslem beliefs concerning the uncleanliness of dogs appear to reduce this group's risk of exposure. Hydatid infection rates are much higher in Christian than in Moslem populations.[270]

Investigation of occupational factors is hindered by the relatively long periods between acquisition of infection and diagnosis (which may sometimes exceed 50 years),[289] during which period the patient may have changed occupations. The problem is further complicated in some areas by the lack of occupational specialization. In a rural area of southern Argentina, virtually all men had worked at some time during their lives with dogs and livestock (an obvious occupational risk factor); therefore, their occupational classification at the time of the interview had less significance.[253] Nevertheless, occupational risk factors were demonstrated in some other studies. Butchers and abattoir workers in many countries have higher infection rates than the general population because they carry home infected viscera to feed to their dogs. Higher infection rates in shoemakers were noted in Lebanon, an occurrence which may be related to a traditional custom of "bating" (tanning) leather in a mixture of dog feces and water.[270]

Although hydatid transmission is most intense in rural areas, considerable levels of transmission occur in most urban areas of some countries. In Arequipa, Peru, studies[193,247] that included only cases autochthonous to that city disclosed an annual surgical incidence of ten cases per 100,000 inhabitants. Retrospective studies traced most of these cases to the 11 city abattoirs, where hygienic conditions were completely inadequate. Dogs entered the abattoirs at will, and infected viscera that escaped sanitary inspection were removed from the premises for a variety of purposes, including for sale as dog food. In addition, in Peruvian cities and cities of many other countries, home slaughtering of animals brought from the country is not uncommon, particularly on festive occasions.

The epidemiological importance of sylvatic reservoirs of *E. granulosus* varies with the region. In extremely northern areas, cycles in wolves and wild ungulates represent a natural host-parasite association independent of domestic animals and man.[221] However, since the sylvatic strain of cestode is noninfective for domestic ungulates, the infection is of relatively less public health significance. In other areas, e.g., Australia, the pastoral strain of *E. granulosus* is established in certain native marsupial animals (kangaroos and wallabies) and dingoes in which it is maintained apparently independently of domestic animals but may represent a continuous reservoir of infection.[60,72] An independent cycle in deer and coyotes may also occur in California.[238] Currently employed control measures are aimed at interrupting the cycles of transmission between dogs and domestic livestock;[246] independent sylvatic cycles represent a significant potential obstacle to successful control.

In still other situations, a variety of local wild animals may become infected, but transmission to them depends upon the presence of infected dogs and/or livestock. This is the case in Argentina, where foxes and hares apparently become infected in areas where the disease occurs in domestic livestock.[248,255,257] Although these infected animals may contribute to the local perpetuation of the cestode, their epidemiological significance appears to be limited, and it is doubtful if the cestode would persist in the absence of a domestic animal reservoir.

E. multilocularis

Over most of its range, *E. multilocularis* is confined to sylvatic hosts and is thereby ecologically separated from man. Human exposure is determined by occupational and avocational factors. Hunters, trappers, and persons who work with fox fur are most frequently exposed.[169] Dogs that become infected by capturing and eating infected voles are even more important as a source of human infection. When infected voles exist in villages as commensal rodents (as they do, for example, in some Eskimo villages of the tundra zone in North America), the cycle of the cestode is readily completed and a hyperendemic focus is produced.[79,221,227] The poor sanitary conditions that usually exist in such villages permit extensive accumulation of dog feces and enhance the risk of human infection.

A potentially great human health problem would exist if an independent cycle of transmission were to develop in domestic cats and house mice. Domestic cats have been found naturally infected in Japan,[6] Canada,[329] the U.S., and Germany,[73] and infected house mice have been found in the U.S. on at least one occasion. In this case, a definite predator-prey relationship between domestic cats and house mice appeared to exist.[165] Should a synanthropic cycle of this nature become established, it would introduce the cestode into new geographical areas, including urban localities, and greatly increase potential for human exposure.

E. vogeli

Humans are incidental hosts to *E. vogeli*. In endemic areas, dogs are commonly fed viscera of paca, and human infections are probably acquired from the feces of infected hunting dogs. Bush dogs are rare and avoid human beings, and therefore, probably play little role in direct exposure of humans.[65]

E. oligarthrus

Human infections with *E. oligarthrus* have not yet been demonstrated. This species may not be highly infective to humans or the behavior of its felid definitive hosts may make potential human exposure very rare.

Diagnosis in Animals

E. granulosus

Necropsy examination of the intestine performed by an experienced person is the most reliable method for diagnosing echinococcosis in definitive hosts. More often, however, it is necessary to make a diagnosis in live dogs. Since all taeniid eggs are similar morphologically, it is impossible to make a specific diagnosis by demonstrating cestode eggs in stools. The alternative method is to demonstrate strobilae or portions thereof in the feces. The dog is first given a taeniafuge such as arecoline hydrobromide, which causes evacuation. The parasympathomimetic drug, arecoline hydrobromide, fails to induce purgation in approximately 20% of dogs,[95] and even when infected dogs are successfully purged, they do not always excrete strobilae.[21] These limitations can lead to an underestimation of the real prevalence of infection in dog populations examined.

Care must also be taken in identifying the cestodes. Because small strobilae are difficult to detect, particularly when there are only a few, adequate methods must be employed to separate the worms from the fecal material. Two techniques were developed and evaluated for this purpose.[93] The first—the salt flotation technique—was intended for making an immediate diagnosis in the field. The second—sieving under pressure—was designed for large-scale diagnostic operations in the laboratory. The importance of using adequate and standardized methods was made clear by the demonstration that it is possible to double or halve the apparent prevalence rate by varying the testing procedure. The use of arecoline hydrobromide for diagnosis and surveillance in dogs has been reviewed,[93,95,114] and a practical guide for using this drug has been published.[254]

Examination of livers and lungs at autopsy remains the only practical method of diagnosis of hydatid cysts in sheep and other intermediate hosts. Immunodiagnostic techniques, useful for diagnosis in man, are less sensitive in livestock and, at their present state of development, do not differentiate between *E. granulosus* infection and infection with some other common larval cestodes.[142,205,249,337] Affinity chromatography in combination with murine hybridoma antibody has been applied for the production of sensitive and species-specific immunodiagnostic antigens for serologic discrimination of larval cestode infections in sheep with partial success.[63]

For prevalence studies, the most practical method of data collection is to study animals slaughtered at commercial abattoirs. The latter usually handle only old sheep (6 years or older) and young lambs. To obtain information on intermediate age groups, special arrangements (such as purchasing representative samples) must often be made. Before commencing a survey, special attention must be given to the following factors: (1) identification and classification of parasitic lesions, (2) determination and recording of the age of the animals, and (3) identification and recording of the origin of the animals. These considerations are discussed in detail by Gemmell.[93]

E. multilocularis

Infection in foxes and other definitive hosts is usually diagnosed by the demonstration of cestodes at autopsy. The arecoline hydrobromide purge method is also effective. Larval *E. multilocularis* infections in rodents are also diagnosed by autopsy examination.

E. oligarthrus and E. vogeli

Strobilate forms recovered from carnivores at autopsy or by arecoline purging can be differentiated by their morphologic characteristics.[225]

E. oligarthrus and *E. vogeli* may use the same intermediate hosts species and the hydatid cysts may be grossly similar. However, Rausch and co-workers[228] have shown that it is possible to distinguish the two species by the dimensions of even a single fully developed protoscolex hook. The large and small hooks, respectively, of the two species were found to differ significantly in length as well as in relative proportions. Host-related variation in length of the rostellar hooks was not observed.

Diagnosis in Man

E. granulosus

Because of the diversity of clinical manifestations and the difficulty of demonstrating hydatid cysts, hydatid disease is often difficult to diagnose. An accurate history is often helpful in ruling out the disease in a patient who has not lived in or traveled to areas where echinococcosis is endemic. In areas with endemic disease, a history of occupational exposure to sheep and dogs or of other risk factors is useful in supporting the diagnosis.

Plain roentgenography permits the detection of hydatid cysts in the lungs, but usually only calcified cysts can be demonstrated in other sites.[17] Radioisotopic and ultrasonic scanning,[154] computerized axial tomography,[151,199,267] and angiography[86,118] are useful for visualizing the avascular cyst in many organs. Closed aspiration of hydatid cysts should not be attempted because accidental spilling of the contents could cause secondary spread or anaphylaxis. Cystic structures may sometimes be demonstrated in the sputum or bronchial washings,[5] in which case identification is facilitated by acid-fast staining of the hooklets.[139] An intravenous pyelogram is helpful in visualizing renal cysts.[275] Eosinophilia is present in one third or fewer of cyst carriers.[168]

Immunodiagnostic tests can be useful if factors that can influence the results are understood. First, negative test results do not rule out a diagnosis of echinococcosis because some cyst carriers do not have detectable antibody. The presence of a detectable immune response has been associated with the location, the integrity, and the "health" of the larval cyst. Cysts in the liver are more likely to elicit antibody than cysts in the lungs, and regardless of localization, tests are least sensitive for diagnosing intact hyaline cysts. Such health metacestodes produce a low level of antigenic stimulation,[304,306] and nearly 50% of carriers of this kind of cyst in the lungs may be serologically negative.[334] Fissuration or rupture of the cyst is followed by an abrupt stimulation of antibodies. Senescent or dead cysts apparently cease to stimulate the host, and such carriers may be seronegative. Differences in the host-parasite relationships between different strains of *E. granulosus* may also influence the immunodiagnostic results. For example, human infection with the northern sylvatic strain of *E. granulosus* is characterized by more frequent pulmonary localization, slower and more benign growth than the classic pastoral strain,[327] and may be associated with diminished antigenic stimulation. The possibility that subtle antigenic differences may also exist between strains of *E. granulosus* has not been sufficiently evaluated.

The current status of hydatid disease immunodiagnosis was reviewed comprehensively in recent articles by Matossian,[180] Rickard,[231] and Schantz and Kagan.[263] Circulating IgG, IgM, IgA, and IgE antibodies to *Echinococcus* antigens have been detected in the serum from infected individuals.[68,133,182,183] Although IgG, IgM, and IgE antibodies are commonly present during active infection, the IgM and IgE antibodies disappear soon after the cyst is removed or killed whereas IgG antibodies persist for several years.[68,182,183,204]

Virtually every immunodiagnostic technique ever devised has been evaluated for hydatid diagnosis,[142,144,145] often with considerable discrepancy in results. The results of different studies are rarely comparable because different patient populations vary in antibody reactivity and even slight variations in test methodology can cause large differences in sensitivity and specificity. The value of most tests is limited by varying degrees of nonspecificity[85,142,144,161,285,338] because some *Echinococcus* antigenic components are common to many helminths[31,53] and hydatid cyst fluid (the most common source of antigen) may contain proteins of host origin and other nonspecific antigens. Although results of most serodiagnostic tests agree well, sera from some patients are negative in one or more tests but positive in others. It is, therefore, usually suggested that more than one test be used to increase the sensitivity of immunodiagnosis. An important consideration, however, is that tests based on the detection of antibody to the *Echinococcus*-specific antigen 5 have the highest degree of specificity. All other tests developed thus far have a varying degree of nonspecificity. However, because antibody to antigen 5 is sometimes absent in the serum of hydatid cyst carriers who have antibodies reactive with other HCF antigens, serum specimens should be screened initially with one or more highly sensitive procedures and then tested for antibodies specific to antigen 5. Tests such as indirect hemagglutination, indirect immunofluorescence, latex agglutination, radioimmunoassay, and enzyme-linked immunosorbent assay are highly sensitive in detecting circulating antibody in serum from patients with hydatid disease (reviewed in Schantz and Kagan[263]). The IHA and LA tests are recommended for initial screening because they have been shown to be highly efficient for detecting sera with the arc 5, and they both are relatively simple procedures that can be performed in even the most minimlly equipped laboratory.[116,117,263,307-309]

Antigen 5 is one of ten or more distinct antigens of parasite origin present in hydatid cyst fluid and somatic tissues of the metacestode. Capron and co-workers,[52] using immunoelectrophoresis, showed that the presence of antibody to this in a patient's serum was diagnostic for echinococcosis. The diagnostic importance of the arc 5 has been confirmed and extended by numerous workers.[52,54,212,308,310,334-336] The presence of the arc 5 can be used to confirm a diagnosis of infection with *E. granulosus, E. multilocularis,* or *E. vogeli* in patients with compatible clinical signs. In published reports on more than 500 patients, not once was the arc 5 found in serum of a person without hydatid disease until Varela-Diaz and co-workers reported finding it in serum from a patient with cysticercosis (*Taenia solium*).[312] Since then we have found the arc 5 in approximately 5 to 10% of serum specimens we have tested from patients with cysticercosis.[264] The full impact of these findings on the diagnostic specificity of tests for arc 5 remain to be determined.

The immunoelectrophoresis test has been most widely used to detect antibody to antigen 5. Varela-Diaz, Coltorti, and co-workers at the Pan American Zoonosis Center (PAHO/WHO) modified the procedure to decrease the time and equipment needed for the test and thus made it more practical for use in laboratories in endemic areas.[58,310] Most recently, they described a double diffusion (DD5) test in which a control antiserum is used to recognize arc 5-positive sera by a reaction of identity.[59] Since the DD5 test is as specific as and more sensitive than the IEP test, it may provide an effective substitute for the IEP test. Other reported methods for the diagnostic demonstration of the arc 5 include a counterimmunoelectrophoresis (CEP 5) test in which a monospecific arc 5 antiserum is used to identify the arc 5 by a reaction of identity.[108,204,230] Coupling the CEP 5 test to enzyme-labeled antiimmunoglobulins raised sensitivity and permitted the immunoglobulin classes involved to be defined.[108]

The use of purified antigens may obviate the problem of nonspecificity in serologic tests for hydatid disease. The use of the purified antigen 5 in ELISA was highly specific in a study limited by small numbers of serum specimens;[38,76] however, other partially purified antigens used in various serologic tests have given somewhat disappointing results because they continued to produce cross-reactions with serum from persons with other parasitic diseases and were often less sensitive than whole HCF antigens.[33,70,135,162,192,209,308,325] Future work may be directed at characterizing all important and specific antigens involved in diagnostic systems. If these can be separated and purified, they might be prepared as a "pool" of diagnostic antigens.

The skin test is less specific, but when properly controlled, it compares favorably in sensitivity with most serologic tests.[142,335] Nevertheless, even with partially purified antigen solutions used at a low nitrogen concentration, high rates of false-positive reactions have been observed in persons with other parasitic diseases, as well as in some with nonparasitic pathologic conditions.[256,335]

Using a test for specific IgE antibody in combination with other serologic techniques would theoretically raise the sensitivity of laboratory diagnosis because the results would permit the detection of individuals with IgE responses as well as those with IgG or IgM responses. Results obtained with radioallergosorbent tests (RAST) show that the percentage of patients with significantly elevated specific IgE antibodies varies from 30 to 90%.[68,133,138,314,315] Demanding technical requirements and low sensitivity may limit the diagnostic possibilities for tests for specific IgE antibodies. The use of serologic and other diagnostic techniques for prevalence studies was discussed earlier.

In addition to their use for diagnosis, serologic tests have been used to evaluate surgical patients postoperatively for evidence of recurrence of disease. Todorov and Stojanov[302] showed that in patients without recurrence, serologic tests either became negative 6 months to 2 years after operation or remained positive during the entire postoperative period. In patients with recurring disease, titers either remained high (50%) or declined initially and then rose when the disease recurred. Certain tests have been reported more sensitive than others for measuring changes in antibody levels. The complement fixation test[181,182] and tests for specific IgE[29] revert to negative more rapidly than IHA and indirect immunofluorescent tests. Tests for arc 5 become negative between 6 months and 1 year following successful cyst removal.[54,212]

Hydatid cysts removed at surgery are frequently misidentified, particularly when protoscolices are lacking or the larva is otherwise degenerated or anomalous. Such lesions can be identified and differentiated from other larval cestodes (i.e., cysticerci or coenuri) and nonparasitic cysts by the characteristic appearance of the laminated membrane.[30,277]

E. multilocularis

Alveolar hydatid disease is typically observed in elderly persons and mimics hepatic carcinoma and cirrhosis, with which it is commonly confused.[227] Plain roentgenography shows hepatomegaly and characteristic scattered radiolucencies outlined by calcific rings (2 to 4 mm).[300]

Serologic tests usually show high titers of antibody, although it is unknown at what stage in the evolution of disease antibody becomes detectable. Although *E. granulosus* and *E. multilocularis* share common antigens and cross reactions occur with most tests, *E. multilocularis* infections could be distinguished from *E. granulosus* infections by their predominant homologous antibody activity in ELISA and CF tests.[80]

Needle biopsy confirms the diagnosis if larval elements can be demonstrated. Even in the absence of protoscolices, the larval membranes can be demonstrated using periodic acid-Schiff (PAS) stain, or the sterile larva can be reared to the adult stage after secondary passage in susceptible rodents.[226]

Exploratory laporatomy is often performed in order to diagnose and delineate the extent of the lesion. In Germany and other areas where both cystic and alveolar hydatid disease occur, the two can be distinguished by selective angiography. This procedure is also useful for delineating the lesion and its vascular supply.[118,240]

E. oligarthrus and E. vogeli

Little is known about the diagnostic aspects of human *E. oligarthrus* or *E. vogeli* infections. However, techniques that can demonstrate cystic or alveolar hydatid disease should also be useful for diagnosing infections with these cestodes. *E. vogeli* shares antigens with other *Echinococcus* spp. and immunodiagnostic tests are not useful at present for distinguishing the species.[311]

Prevention and Control

E. granulosus

Experiences with attempts to control hydatid disease have been reported from Iceland,[25,246] the U.S.S.R.,[16,175,210,244] New Zealand,[45,246] the Australian state of Tasmania,[39,40,187,246] and Cyprus.[207] The well-documented results of successful control programs in Iceland, New Zealand, Tasmania, and Cyprus have demonstrated that reducing the prevalence in all hosts is possible even though the means available to achieve control have been limited by the unavailability of effective drugs or vaccines.

In Iceland, which in the late 19th century had the highest human prevalence ever reported anywhere, an intensive health education program was begun in 1864. The effective education measures combined with a number of social and environmental factors peculiar to Iceland caused a rapid reduction in human prevalence and a gradual reduction in sheep. The infection is now believed to have been eradicated.[25] In both New Zealand and Tasmania, strong education programs were supported by a variety of technical and legislative measures which have resulted in marked reductions in prevalence. In Cyprus, virtual elimination of all stray and free-roaming dogs and strict control of sheep slaughtering have combined to greatly reduce opportunities for transmission.[207]

These areas share certain characteristics recognized as having contributed to their success: the highly developed nature of their pastoral economies, the nearly 100% literacy rates, and the fact that they are all relatively small islands. Many areas where the disease remains endemic are characterized by quite different conditions. Poor and largely illiterate rural populations, large and uncontrolled canine populations, vast continental geographic conditions, and large populations of potential sylvatic animal hosts for *E. granulosus* may create special problems for control. Can conventional control measures applied in these areas be expected to achieve the same results as in Iceland, New Zealand, and Tasmania? Pilot programs have been initiated in a number of countries to answer this question and to evolve different approaches if necessary. In many areas, the prospects for modifying or eliminating specific factors and human practices that facilitate echinococcosis transmission are largely dependent upon the prospects for broader changes in educational and socioeconomic conditions. The application of measures specifically directed against hydatid disease without concomitant programs to upgrade living conditions would have little chance of success. Gemmell[98] has recently reviewed the value and limitations of currently employed as well as new methods of control which, with further research, may provide a variety of options in a cost/benefit approach to control. Harris and co-workers[120] developed a deterministic model to compare various control strategies; the model indicated that maximum progress would be achieved with measures aimed at treating infection in both definitive and intermediate hosts.

The selection of specific control measures and their strategic implementation depend upon an adequate understanding of the local epidemiology, which must be obtained from preliminary epidemiological investigations.[250] Another objective of preliminary studies is to measure prevalence in important definitive and intermediate host species. Such baseline data are necessary so that future progress can be measured. Continued monitoring of prevalence indicators may indicate breakdowns in the control measures and thus alert authorities to the need for a change in control strategy.

It is generally agreed that the principal objectives of hydatid control are limitation of numbers and movement of dogs and reductions in parasite prevalence below levels necessary for continued transmission. Measures that have been employed in various circumstances include health education, control of livestock slaughtering in abattoirs and on farms, dog control, and periodic diagnostic testing of dogs.

Health Education

Hydatid disease control has been described as fundamentally a problem of health education.[23] The aim of such health education is to convince the population to change practices tending to perpetuate the transmission of the cestode. Health education activities that elicit community participation directed toward defined goals are the most effective. In New Zealand and Tasmania, the use of local citizens' committees has been an effective aspect of the educational campaign. The program should be broadly directed toward all segments of the population by using all available educational media. Educational materials should use language and images with which local audiences can readily identify.

Extensive experience has been obtained with a variety of educational techniques in hydatid control programs in several countries. The effectiveness of such programs in modifying behavior is not always clearly established. At the very least, they may induce enough awareness of the health problems to permit the introduction and acceptance of control measures. At best, they alone may be effective in reducing the disease in human populations. In both New Zealand and Tasmania after the initiation of health education measures the incidence of new cases began to decline perceptibly, even when the prevalence in dogs and sheep remained at high levels. This suggests that awareness of the risks may have been effective in reducing human exposure even in highly contaminated environments.[24]

Control of Livestock Slaughtering in Abattoirs and on Farms

From a hygienic viewpoint, the ideal situation would be the centralization of all slaughtering at modern abattoirs, with efficient veterinary inspection and proper disposal or adequate treatment of disease offal and carcasses. Hydatid control programs must aim to upgrade conditions at local abattoirs to approach the ideal.

In Cyprus, slaughtering is prohibited on individual farms. All slaughtering is performed in village abattoirs under the supervision of trained technicians. Slaughtering performed on each farm is more difficult to supervise. The problem has been approached in New Zealand and Tasmania by the construction of dog-proof killing facilities and adequate offal disposal pits or incinerators on farms. Methods of rendering infected offal safe to feed to dogs need to be developed. Boiling for at least 40 min[77] destroys cestode larvae. Freezing to $-20°C$ kills most cysts but an occasional one may survive. The impracticality of these and other recommendations reduces their effectiveness. For these reasons, the Tasmanian authorities completely prohibited the use of livestock viscera (cooked or uncooked) as dog food.[187]

Under cold winter conditions, such as those that exist in New Zealand[22] and Utah,[10] protoscolices within cysts in dead animals may retain infective for 3 weeks or longer. Therefore, carcasses should be removed promptly from the field to prevent infection in scavenging dogs.

Dog Control

When examining the situation in Iceland in 1864, Krabbe observed that the surest way to eliminate echinococcosis would be to eliminate dogs. Although it is generally agreed that dogs are necessary to help raise sheep and other livestock, it is often observed that the number of rural dogs far exceeds the working needs. Elimination of stray and surplus dogs and control of the movement of owned dogs are desirable objectives. Enforced registration of all dogs is useful, and registration fees may be used to help finance the control program.

Care should be taken to ensure that the control program is not labeled "anti-dog." Rather, the stated objectives should be to reduce the number of dogs to those necessary for working needs, to promote better care and feeding of those that remain, and to restrict their movement when they are not working. Compulsory spaying of bitches has been used in conjunction with dog population reduction in Cyprus.[207]

Periodic Diagnostic Testing of Dogs

Periodic dosing of entire populations or samples of dogs with arecoline hydrobromide has been an important feature of most control programs. Although surveys by the arecoline purge method tend to underestimate the true prevalence in dogs, the data have been used to monitor progress and to identify dog owners who are not complying with recommended preventive measures. Dogs that are repeatedly found to be infected may be treated at expense to their owner, quarantined until adequate home slaughtering facilities have been constructed, or destroyed.

Dog Treatment

The effectiveness of treating canine echinococcosis with drugs through hydatid control programs has not yet been demonstrated. In the long run, effective control and elimination of hydatid disease must be aimed at prevention, that is, breaking the cycle between dogs and sheep (or other locally important intermediate hosts). It has been argued that treating dogs through control campaigns may give a false sense of security to dog owners and promote the feeling that their personal responsibility regarding prevention ends there. On the other hand, treating dogs may be a useful interim measure to reduce environmental contamination with cestode eggs before the same objective can be achieved through education. This seems particularly necessary in those developing areas where conditions for effective health education appear minimal in the short run.

Until recently, the above arguments were a moot debate because of the lack of an effective drug; however, praziquantel, which is highly effective in a single oral or parenterally administered dose (see Treatment) appears particularly suitable for mass treatment. Results of preliminary experiments must be verified in controlled field trials, and the choice of a drug (or drugs) for use in a particular control program should take into consideration cost vs. benefit. Comprehensive treatment on a periodic basis requires a core of trained personnel supervised by veterinarians.

Immunization of Intermediate Hosts

Although laboratory experiments indicated that induction of immunity against larval cestodes in sheep is technically possible, the results of vaccination procedures tested in field trials[235] have shown that many details must be resolved before vaccination can be recommended as an adjunct to other control measures.

Legislation

It is impossible to legislate hydatid disease out of existence. Eventually, all control measures must become compulsory, but they must first be fully understood by the public. Best results are achieved when the first stage of the program is largely voluntary, using mass education and persuasion to effect compliance. Not all members of the community will comply, however, in a voluntary effort; as the program progresses, various degrees of compulsion are necessary to coerce resistant individuals. In Tasmania, surveillance of infections in dogs and, more recently, in sheep at slaughter[40] has been useful in identifying problem farms, which are then subjected to intensified education measures, quarantine, and fines.

E. multilocularis

Eliminating *E. multilocularis* from sylvatic animal hosts would be impractical under most circumstances. Personal preventive measures in areas where the infection is endemic include avoidance of contact with foxes and other potentially infected final hosts. Adequate control of pet dogs and cats in rural areas where *E. multilocularis* occurs is necessary to prevent the establishment of synanthropic cycles of the cestode. Patent infections in dogs and cats which are liable to eat infected rodents can be prevented by monthly treatments with praziquantel. Potentially exposed human populations should be educated about the dangers to promote better hygiene and sanitation.

Restricting movement of dogs from endemic areas may retard the geographic spread of this cestode. Such legislation was enacted in 1951 to prevent the spread from St. Lawrence Island to mainland Alaska[217] before it was realized that this movement had already taken place.

Treatment in Animals

E. granulosus

Until the late 1960s, the only drug available for treating *Echinococcus* infection in dogs was the purgative arecoline hydrobromide, a markedly inefficient anthelminthic. Even after successful purgation, many dogs retain some strobilae, and some require more than six consecutive treatments to eliminate all strobilae.[21] Increased attention to this problem, however, is yielding an increasing number of effective compounds, incuding bunamidine hydrochloride,[12,91,96,303,323] bithionol sulphoxide,[102] fospirate,[99,259] nitroscanate,[101,258] mebendazole,[100,104] and praziquantel.[9,103,105,239,294,298] Niclosamide, a compound that many consider to be the drug of choice for the larger tapeworms of dogs and humans, is not effective against *E. granulosus*.[81,155]

The efficacy of bunamidine hydrochloride is variable, depending upon whose study is consulted. Recent work in the U.S. demonstrated on 85.9 to 98.8% clearance of immature strobilae with single doses of 25 and 50 mg/kg of body weight; 100% clearance was obtained against mature strobilae.[12] However, workers in New Zealand showed that at a dose level of 50 mg/kg, three treatments may be required before tapeworms are expelled from a dog, a dosage level which may be lethal.[91] Bunamidine and most other drugs are less effective against immature than against mature worms. At least a partial explanation for this may be that the tiny immature strobilae, often located deep within the intervillous spaces, are protected from the action of the drug by the mucous secretions of the host.[82]

Nitroscanate, fospirate, and bithionol are highly echinococcocidal; however, when used at doses low enough to be well tolerated by the host, all require more than one treatment to completely eliminate the strobilae. A single dose of micronized particle (particle size: 55% less than 10 μm) formulation of mebendazole eliminated all strobilae (mature and immature);[100] however, in tablet formulations, the drug was less consistently effective.[104] Praziquantel appears to be the best echinococcocidal drug yet developed. A single oral or intramuscularly administered dose (5 mg/kg body weight) completely eliminates all juvenile and adult strobilae at doses well tolerated by the host.[9,103,105,239,294,298]

Attempts to immunize dogs against *E. granulosus* have given equivocal results. Experimental studies have shown reduced numbers and decreased size of worms, retarded sexual development, and suppressed egg production in immunized dogs.[89] However, the differences between immunized and control dogs have not been significant, and some dogs that developed resistance became susceptible again upon subsequent challenge. More recent studies using secretory antigens derived from adult tapeworms have demonstrated a highly significant suppression of cestode egg production in immunized dogs.[130] Further research may result in immunization techniques that will fill specific hydatid disease control needs.

To date, there is no practical and effective treatment for hydatidosis in intermediate hosts. Several of the benzimidazole-group compounds, particularly mebendazole, are partially effective in destroying larval cestodes, including *Echinococcus* spp.[51,74,125,126,129,146,158] Gemmell and co-workers[106] treated three groups of sheep (45 animals per group) with oral mebendazole (50 mg/kg/body weight) for 5 days, 1 or 3 months. Hydatid cysts in animals treated for 5 days appeared similar to those in non-treated control sheep. Observations on lethal effects from treatment for 1 month were equivocal, because although most cysts appeared damaged, some portions of the bladder wall were considered viable and some protoscolices were infective to dogs. All cysts in sheep treated for 3 months appeared degenerated, and remaining protoscolices were not infective to dogs. Nevertheless, many cysts were still structurally intact and some fluid was present even 4 months after the end of treatment. Further work may suggest practical chemotherapeutic approaches. Praziquantel killed larvae of *Taenia hydatigena* and *T. ovis* in sheep but was not active against hydatid cysts.[129,299]

The immunology of cestode infections, with special reference to problems of immunizing intermediate hosts, has been reviewed by Gemmell et al.[92,94,97,107] It has been shown that previous infection or the parenteral inoculation of oncospheres of a variety of taeniid cestodes produces partial or complete immunity to challenge infection.[90] Similarly, activated embryos within surgically implanted diffusion chambers or the inoculation of excretions and secretions of oncospheres grown in culture are capable of inducing complete immunity.[124,127,232,233,236] Further research, including isolation and characterization of the immunizing antigens,[234] may permit the development of practical immunization procedures. Once identified, the functional antigens might be mass produced using recombinant DNA technology.

E. multilocularis

Treatment of echinococcosis in sylvatic definitive and intermediate hosts has not been pursued because of its obvious impracticality. A single dose of praziquantel is highly effective in eliminating infections from domestic dogs and cats.[239]

Treatment and Prognosis in Man
E. granulosus

Surgical removal of the hydatid cyst remains the only treatment with proved effectiveness, although effective chemotherapy may soon be developed. Recent reviews of the surgical and medical management of human hydatid disease include those of Little[168] and Pissiotis et al.[206] for all sites; de Heredia and Sanz Sanz,[66] Papadimitriou and Mandrekas,[203] Saidi and Nazarian,[245] and Barros[18] for the liver; Wolcott et al.[331] and Lichter[167] for the lungs; and Booz,[34] Silber and Moyad,[275] and Dodek et al.[69] for other specific sites.

In cystic hydatid disease, the aim of surgery is to totally remove the cyst while avoiding the adverse consequences of spilling the cyst contents. The ideal result is enucleation of the total cyst followed by obliteration of the cavity, both of which are usually possible with intact, solitary, noncomplicated cysts. Surgical management of extremely large cysts or those complicated by infection or bronchus or biliary communication may require marsupialization, open drainage, segmental resection, or lobectomy. The possibility of anaphylaxis during surgical manipulation of the cyst can be minimized by packing off the area around the cyst and reducing the tension by careful aspiration of some of the cyst fluid. A device designed to completely isolate the evacuated cyst contents from the patient has been described.[245] Chemicals are often injected into the cyst prior to surgery to inactivate the protoscolices.[2,75] Formalin, widely used for this purpose, may diffuse out of the cyst and precipitate shock.[206] The use of cetrimide, a quaternary ammonium compound, for injection of cysts (5% solution) and for peritoneal lavage after solution (0.1 to 0.5% solution) has been associated with peritoneal adhesions[110] and methomeglobinemia.[20] Omentoplasty reduces the frequency of persistent fistulas and secondary bacterial infections.[203]

The early diagnosis of cystic hydatid disease before the cyst ruptures permits surgical removal of the lesion with a minimum risk of complications. Few viable cysts are found in patients older than 60 years; therefore, these patients may be managed conservatively to avoid the risk of surgical complications.[168] Conservative management rather than surgery is generally employed for pulmonary infection with the more benign, northern sylvatic strain of *E. granulosus*.[204] Patients infected with pastoral-strain *E.*

granulosus that develop symptoms are at high risk. Amir-Jahed and co-workers[8] in Iran reported death in 60% of 15 symptomatic hospital patients who were not operated. Of 27 Chinese patients with intrathoracic cysts, who refused surgery, 6 (22%) died of their disease an average of 2.9 years after discharge, 9 (33%) spontaneously eliminated their cysts with no radiologic evidence of recurrence after an average of 3.9 years, 5 (19%) returned for surgical treatment and the remaining 7 had survived with their cysts for an average follow-up period of 8.1 years.[340]

Surgery for cystic hydatid disease is not without risk. Recent reviews of case series have reported operative mortality rates ranging from 0.9 to 3.6%.[8,168,340] Operative risk depends upon case selection, operative technique and surgeon's skill among other things. Operative mortality for first, second, or third operation for hydatid disease was 2.6, 6.0 and 20.0%, respectively.[8]

The frequency of observed recurrent (secondary) hydatid disease following surgery for primary hydatid cysts has varied from 2 to 11% in different reports.[111,168,191,213,340] These rates vary greatly, in part because of difference in definition of recurrence. For example, Gilevich et al.[111] distinguished between true secondary recurrences (2.2%) from reinterventions for primary cysts that were apparently missed during the first operation (13.9%). Rupture of intra-abdominal cysts is more likely to result in secondary recurrence than those in the lung. There were only 2 recurrences (5.7%) among 35 cases in which rupture of primary intrathoracic cysts was known to occur.[342] In contrast, three of ten cases suffered recurrence within 1 to 3 years following known rupture or spillage of abdominal cysts.[268] More precise information is needed regarding the outcome of patients receiving alternative forms of management.

Hydatid disease has remained one of the few important helminth diseases for which there is no effective chemotherapy. However, experimental studies recently carried out in many laboratories have shown mebendazole to be the first drug capable of destroying larval cestodes, including hydatid cysts.[51,74,125,126,129,146,158] The drug has been used widely to treat human cases but the results have been unpredictable and adverse reactions have been reported.[27,29,152,264] When surgical removal of cysts is not possible because of the general condition of the patient and/or the extent or location of the cysts, mebendazole therapy may be of benefit. Pulmonary cysts seem to respond best, hepatic cysts less dramatically, and cysts in other locations, particularly brain, bone, and eye, poorly if at all. Doses of 50 to 150 mg/kg of body weight per day for 3 months is probably the minimal effective dose; many patients require repeated courses.[264]

Established hydatid cysts appear to be well protected from immunologic attack, and attempts to stimulate host immunity by injecting hydatid cyst fluid (a once-widespread practice) do not appear to be effective.[305] In contrast, injecting complement-rich serum from infected hosts directly into the cysts can kill them and has been recommended for the treatment of surgically nonresectable cysts.[148]

E. multilocularis

Resection of the entire larval mass is the aim of surgery for this otherwise progressive and fatal disease.[320] This usually requires removal of the entire affected lobe. When involvement is more extensive, wedge resections of the lesions may be attempted. Because alveolar hydatid disease is often not diagnosed until parasitic invasion is well advanced, the lesion is often inoperable, so partial resections and biliodigestive and hepatodigestive anastomoses are carried out as palliative measures, predominantly to ensure bile passage.[118] Alveolar hydatid disease is fatal in a large percentage of cases. The percentage of surgically resectable cases has varied in different case series from 26 to 58%.[147,190,273,328,329] Approximately 90% of the nonresectable cases die within 10 years. Even a proportion of those cases that appear entirely resectable at surgery have recurrence probably due to metacestode tissue unrecognized at surgery. Mosimann[190] believes that patients must be evaluated for 20 or 25 years before one can be certain that postoperative recurrence will not occur.

Effective chemotherapy would find wide application with this form of hydatid disease. Preliminary results with mebendazole for chemotherapy of cases of alveolar hydatid disease in Europe[4,152] and Alaska[328] have been reported. Although no evidence was obtained to indicate that the larval cestode had been killed by the drug, symptomatic improvement was observed in nearly all cases and larval lesions appeared to be inhibited or to regress.

E. vogeli

Little has been reported concerning clinical aspects of polycystic hydatid disease,[65] but management criteria similar to those for cystic and alveolar hydatid disease should apply.

REFERENCES

1. **Abuladze, K. I.,** K voprosu o klassifikatsii teniat, *Nauch. Konf. posviasheh.,* 40-let., Moskovsk. Vet. Akad., 1960, 66.
2. **Ahrari, H.,** L'emploi due cétremide dans la chirurgie des kystes hydatiques, *Bull. Soc. Pathol. Exot.,* 71, 90, 1978.
3. **Aikat, B. K., Bhusnurmath, S. R., Cadersa, M., Chuttani, P. N., and Mitra, S. K.,** *Echinococcus multilocularis* infection in India: first case report proved at autopsy, *Trans. R. Soc. Trop. Med. Hyg.,* 72, 619, 1978.
4. **Akovbiantz, A., Ammaan, R., and Eckert, J.,** Gibt es eine chemotherapie der echinokokkose des Menschen?, *Schweiz. Med. Wochenschr.,* 108, 1101, 1978.
5. **Allen, A. R. and Fullmer, C. D.,** Primary diagnosis of pulmonary echinococcosis by the cytologic technique, *Acta Cytol.,* 16, 212, 1972.
6. **Ambo, H., Ichikawa, K., Iida, H., and Abe, N.,** On *Echinococcus* alveolaris endemic parasitosis on Rebun Island, *Spec. Rep. Hokkaido Inst. Public Health,* 4, 1, 1954.
7. **Aminzhanov, M.,** Life span of *E. granulosus* in dogs (in Russian), *Veterinaria Moscow,* 12, 70, 1975; reprinted in *Vet. Bull. London,* 46, 2569, 1976.
8. **Amir-Jahed, A. K., Fardin, R., Farzad, A., and Bakshandeh, K.,** Clinical echinococcosis, *Ann. Surg. (Chicago),* 182, 541, 1975.
9. **Andersen, D. L., Conder, G. A., and Marsland, W. P.,** Efficacy of injectable and tablet formulations of praziquantel against mature *Echinococcus granulosus, Am. J. Vet. Res.,* 39, 1861, 1978.
10. **Andersen, F. L. and Loveless, R. M.,** Effect of temperature on survival of protoscolices of *Echinococcus granulosus, Proc. 3rd. Int. Congr. Parasitol.,* (Facta, Vienna), 1, 541, 1974.
11. **Andersen, F. L., Everett, J. R., Barbour, A. G., and Schoenfeld, F. J.,** Current studies on hydatid disease in Utah, *Proc. 78th Ann. Meet. U.S. Anim. Health Assoc.,* 78, 370, 1974.
12. **Andersen, F. L., Loveless, R. M., and Jensen, L. A.,** Efficacy of bunamidine hydrochloride against immature and mature stages of *Echinococcus granulosus, Am. J. Vet. Res.,* 36(5), 673, 1975.
13. **Annen, J. M., Kohler, P., and Eckert, J.,** Cytotoxicity of *Echinococcus granulosus* cyst fluid *in vitro, Z. Parasitenkunde,* 65, 79, 1981.
14. **Araujo, F. P., Schwabe, C. W., Sawyer, J. C., and Davis, W. G.,** Hydatid disease transmission in California. A study of the Basque connection, *Am. J. Epidemiol.,* 102, 291, 1975.
15. **Arundel, J. H.,** A review of cysticercoses of sheep and cattle in Australia, *Aust. Vet. J.,* 48, 140, 1972.
16. **Baidaliev, A. B.,** Experience in prophylaxis of echinococcosis in sheep (in Russian), *Veterinaria Moscow,* 7, 66, 1970.
17. **Balikian, J. P. and Mudarris, F. F.,** Hydatid disease of the lungs, a roentgenologic study of 50 cases, *Am. J. Roentgenol.,* 122, 692, 1974.
18. **Barros, J. L.,** Hydatid disease of the liver, *Am. J. Surg.,* 135, 597, 1978.
19. **Barbour, A. G., Everett, J. R., Andersen, F. L., Nichols, C. R., Fukushima, T., and Kagan, I. G.,** Hydatid disease screening: Sanpete County, Utah, 1971—1976, *Am. J. Trop. Med. Hyg.,* 27, 94, 1978.
20. **Baraka, A., Yamut, F., and Wakid, N.,** Cetrimide-induced methaemaglobinaemia after surgical excision of hydatid cyst, *Lancet,* 2, 88, 1980.

21. **Batham, E. J.,** Testing arecoline hydrobromide as an antihelminthic for hydatid worms in dogs, *Parasitology,* 37, 185, 1946.

22. **Batham, E. J.,** Notes on viability of hydatid cysts and eggs, *N.Z. Vet. J.,* 5, 74, 1957.

23. **Beard, T. C.,** Hydatid control, a problem in health education, *Med. J. Aust.,* 2, 456, 1969.

24. **Beard, T. C.,** Incidence in humans, in Symp. Recent Adv. Hydatid Dis., *Hamilton Veterinary Medical Association,* Hamilton, Victoria, Australia, Oct. 28 to 29, 1973.

25. **Beard, T. C.,** The elimination of echinococcosis from Iceland, *Bull. WHO,* 48, 653, 1973a.

26. **Beard, T. C.,** Evidence that a hydatid cyst is seldom "as old as the patient", *Lancet,* 2, 30, 1978.

27. **Beard, T. C., Rickard, M. D., and Goodman, H. T.,** Medical treatment for hydatids, *Med. J. Aust.,* 1, 633, 1978.

28. **Begg, N. C., Begg, A. C., and Robinson, R. G.,** Primary hydatid disease of the brain — its diagnosis, radiological investigation, treatment and prevention, *N.Z. Med. J.,* 56, 84, 1957.

29. **Bekhti, A., Schaaps, J-P., Capron, M., Dessaint, J-P., Santoro, F., and Capron, A.,** Treatment of hepatic hydatid disease with mebendazole: preliminary results in four cases, *Br. Med. J.,* 2, 1047, 1977.

30. **Benex, J.,** Evolution in vitro d'explants de membrane proligere d'*Echinococcus granulosus, Ann. Parasitol. Hum. Comp.,* 43, 573, 1968.

31. **Biguet, J., Capron, A., Tran Van Ky, P., and D'Haussy, R.,** Etude immunoélectrophorétique comparée des antigénes de divers helminthes, *C.R. Acad. Sci. (Paris),* 254, 3600, 1962.

32. **Blood, B. D. and Lelijveld, J. L.,** Studies on sylvatic echinococcosis in southern South America, *Z. Tropenmed. Parasitol.,* 20, 475, 1969.

33. **Bombardieri, S., Giordano, F., Ingrao, F., Ioppolo, A., Siracusano, A., and Vicari, G.,** An evaluation of an agar gel diffusion test with crude and purified antigens in the diagnosis of hydatid disease, *Bull. WHO,* 51, 525, 1974.

34. **Booz, M. K.,** The management of hydatid disease of bone and joint, *J. Bone Jt. Surg.,* 54, 698, 1972.

35. **Borrie, J., Gemmell, M. A., and Manktelow, B. W.,** An experimental approach to evaluate the potential risk of hydatid disease from inhalation of *Echinococcus* ova, *Br. J. Surg.,* 52, 876, 1965.

36. **Bortoletti, G. and Ferretti, G.,** Observations on the ultrastructure of the tegument in the larval forms of *Hydatigena (Taenia) taeniaeformis* and considerations on the development of the cyclophyllidean cestode larvae, *Rev. Parassitologia,* 32, 249, 1971.

37. **Bortoletti, G. and Ferretti, G.,** Investigation on larval forms of *Echinococcus granulosus* with electron (microscope), *Rev. Parassitologia,* 34, 89, 1973.

38. **Bout, D., Fruit, J., and Capron, A.,** Purification d'un antigéne spécifique de liquide hydatique, *Ann. Immunol. (Paris),* 125, 775, 1974.

39. **Bramble, A. J.,** Hydatid disease control 1964—74, *Tasmanian J. Agric.,* 45, 225, 1974.

40. **Bramble, A. J.,** Hydatid disease control in Tasmania . . . progress and new developments, *Tasmanian J. Agric.,* 46, 231, 1975.

41. **Brenes Madrigal, R., Monge Ocampo, E., Muñoz Montoya, G., and Rojas Herrera, G.,** Presencia en Costa Rica de *Echinococcus oligarthrus* Diesing 1863, colectado en el intestino delgado de *Felis concolor* costaricensis, *Rev. Biol. Trop.,* 21(1), 139, 1973.

42. **Bronzini, E. and Bertolino, P.,** Indagini sperimentali sulla specificita dell' *Echinococcus granulosus* allo stato adulto, *Boll. Zool.,* 21, 219, 1958.

43. **Buck, A. A., Anderson, R. I., Kawata, K., Abrahams, I. W., Ward, R. A., and Sasaki, T. T.,** *Health and Disease in Rural Afghanistan,* York Press, Baltimore, 1972, 131.

44. **Burridge, M. J. and Schwabe, C. W.,** Hydatid disease in New Zealand: an epidemiological study of transmission among Maoris, *Am. J. Trop. Med.,* 26, 258, 1977.

45. **Burridge, M. J. and Schwabe, C. W.,** Epidemiological analysis of factors influencing rate of progress in *Echinococcus granulosus* control in New Zealand, *J. Hyg.,* 78, 151, 1977.

46. **Burridge, M. J., Schwabe, C. W., and Fraser, J.,** Hydatid disease in New Zealand: changing patterns in human infection, 1872—1972, *N.Z. Med. J.,* 85, 173, 1977.

47. **Burridge, M. J., Schwabe, C. W., and Pullum, T. W.,** Path analysis: application in an epidemiological study of *Echinococcosis* in New Zealand, *J. Hyg.,* 78, 135, 1977.

48. **Cameron, W. M.,** Observations on the genus *Echinococcus* Rudolphi, 1801, *J. Helminthol.,* 4, 13, 1926.

49. **Cameron, T. W. M.,** The incidence and diagnosis of hydatid cysts in Canada: *Echinococcus granulosus* var. *canadensis, Parassitologia Rome,* 2, 381, 1960.

50. **Cameron, T. W. M. and Webster, G. A.,** The histogenesis of the hydatid cyst *(Echinococcus spp.), Can. J. Zool.,* 47, 1405, 1969.

51. **Campbell, W. C. and Blair, L. S.,** Treatment of the cystic stage of *Taenia crassiceps* and *Echinococcus multilocularis* in laboratory animals, *J. Parasitol.,* 60, 1053, 1974.

52. **Capron, A., Vernes, A., and Biguet, J.,** Le diagnostic immunoélectrophorétique de l'hydatidose, in *Le Kyste Hydatique du Foie,* SIMEP, Lyon, 1967, 27.

53. **Capron, A., Biguet, D., Vernes, A., and Afchain, D.,** Structure antigénique des helminthes. Aspects immunologiques des relations hôte-parasite, *Pathol. Biol.,* 16, 121, 1968.

54. **Capron, A., Yarzabal, L., Vernes, A., and Fruit, J.,** Le diagnostic immunologique de l'echinococcose humaine, *Pathol. Biol.,* 18, 357, 1970.

55. **Colli, C. W. and Williams, J. R.,** Influence of temperature on the infectivity of eggs of *Echinococcus granulosus* in laboratory rodents, *J. Parasitol.,* 58, 422, 1972.

56. **Coltorti, E. A. and Varela-Diaz, V. M.,** *Echinococcus granulosus:* penetration of macromolecules and their localization on the parasite membranes of cysts, *Exp. Parasitol.,* 35, 225, 1974.

57. **Coltorti, E. A. and Varela-Diaz, V. M.,** Penetration of host IgG molecules into hydatid cysts, *Z. Parasitol.,* 48, 47, 1975.

58. **Coltorti, E. A. and Varela-Diaz, V. M.,** Modification of the immunoelectrophoresis test for the immunodiagnosis of hydatidosis, *J. Parasitol.,* 61, 155, 1975b.

59. **Coltorti, E. A. and Varela-Diaz, V. M.,** Detection of antibodies against *Echinococcus granulosus* arc 5 antigens by double diffusion test, *Trans. R. Soc. Trop. Med. Hyg.,* 72, 226, 1978.

60. **Coman, B. J.,** A sylvatic cycle for the hydatid tapeworm (*Echinococcus granulosus*) in remote areas of eastern Victoria, *Aust. Vet. J.,* 48, 552, 1972.

61. **Coman, B. J.,** The survival of *Taenia pisiformis* eggs under laboratory conditions and in the field environment, *Aust. Vet. J.,* 51, 560, 1975.

62. **Coman, B. J., and Rickard, M. D.,** A comparison of *in vitro* and *in vivo* estimates of the viability of *Taenia pisiformis* eggs aged under controlled conditions, and their ability to immunize against a challenge infection, *Int. J. Parasitol.,* 7, 15, 1977.

63. **Craig, P. S., Mitchell, G. F., Cruise, K. M., and Rickard, M. D.,** Hybridoma antibody immunoassays for the detection of parasitic infection: attempts to produce an immunodiagnostic reagent for larval taeniid cestode infection, *Aust. J. Exp. Biol. Med. Sci.,* 58, 339, 1980.

64. **Dailey, M. D. and Seatman, G. K.,** The taxonomy of *Echinococcus granulosus* in the donkey and dromedary in Lebanon and Syria, *Ann. Trop. Med. Parasitol.,* 23, 267, 1965.

65. **D'Alessandro, A., Rausch, R. L., Cuello, C., and Aristizabal, N.,** First observation of *Echinococcus vogeli* in man, with a review of human cases of polycystic hydatid disease in Colombia and neighboring countries, *Am. J. Trop. Med. Hyg.,* 28, 303, 1979.

66. **de Heredia, J. B. and Sanz Sanz, T.,** The importance of biliary-cystic communications in surgery for hepatic hydatidosis, *Int. Surg.,* 53(6), 393, 1970.

67. **Deiana, S. and Arru, E.,** *Echinococcus granulosus* in *Vulpes vulpes* della sardegna, *Rev. Parassitologia,* 23, 267, 1962.

68. **Dessaint, J. P., Bout, D., Wattre, P., and Capron, A.,** Quantitative determination of specific IgE antibodies to *Echinococcus granulosus* and IgE levels in sera from patients with hydatid disease, *Immunology,* 29, 813, 1975.

69. **Dodek, A., deMots, H., Jr., Antonovic, J. A., and Hodam, R. P.,** *Echinococcus* of the heart, *Am. J. Cardiol.,* 30, 293, 1972.

70. **Dottorini, S. and Tassi, C.,** *Echinococcus granulosus:* characterization of the main antigenic component (arc 5) of hydatid fluid, *Exp. Parasitol.,* 43, 307, 1977.

71. **Drolshammer, I., Wiesmann, E., and Eckert, J.,** Echinokokkose beim Menschen in der Schweiz, 1956—1969, *Schweiz. Med. Wochenschr.,* 103, 1337, 1973.

72. **Durie, P. H. and Riek, R. F.,** The role of the dingo and wallaby in the infestation of cattle with hydatids (*Echinococcus granulosus* [Batsch, 1786] Rudolphi, 1805) in Queensland, *Aust. Vet. J.,* 28, 249, 1952.

73. **Eckert, J., Müller, B., and Partridge, A. J.,** The domestic cat and dog as natural definitive hosts of *Echinococcus (Alveococcus) multilocularis* in southern Federal Republic of Germany, *Tropenmed. Parasitol.,* 25, 334, 1974.

74. **Eckert, J. and Pohlenz, J.,** Zur wirkung von mebendazol auf metazestoden von *Mesocestoides corti* und *Echinococcus multilocularis, Tropenmed. Parasitol.,* 27, 247, 1976.

75. **Eslami, A., Ahrari, H., and Saadatzadeh, H.,** Brief communications: scolicidal effects of Cetrimide® on hydatid cyst *(Echinococcus granulosus), Trans. R. Soc. Trop. Med. Hyg.,* 72, 307, 1978.

76. **Farag, H., Bout, D., and Capron, A.,** Specific immunodiagnosis of human hydatidosis by the enzyme-linked immunosorbent assay (E.L.I.S.A.), *Biomedicine,* 23, 276, 1975.

77. **Fastier, L. B.,** The effect of physical agents on hydatid scolex viability, *Parasitology,* 39, 157, 1949.

78. **Fay, F. H.,** Development of larval *Echinococcus multilocularis* Leuckart in relation to maturation of the intermediate host, *J. Parasitol.,* 56, 175, 1970.

79. **Fay, F. H.,** The ecology of *Echinococcus multilocularis* Leuckart, 1863 (Cestoda: *Taeniidae*) on St. Lawrence Island, Alaska, *Ann. Parasitol. Hum. Comp.,* 48, 523, 1973.

80. **Felgner, P.,** Antibody activity in stick-ELISA as compared to other quantitative immunological tests in sera of echinococcosis cases, *Tropenmed. Parasitol.,* 29, 417, 1978.

81. **Forbes, L. S.,** The efficiency of N-(2'-chlor-4'-nitrophenyl)-5 chlorsalicylamid against *Taenia hydatigena* and *Echinococcus granulosus* infections in dogs, *Vet. Rec.,* 75, 321, 1963.

82. **Forbes, L. S.**, The efficiency of bunamidine hydrochloride against young *Echinococcus granulosus* infection in dogs, *Vet. Rec.*, 79, 306, 1966.

83. **Freeman, R. S.**, Ontogeny of cestodes and its bearing on their phylogeny and systematics, *Adv. Parasitol.*, 11, 481, 1973.

84. **Gamble, W. G., Segal, M., Schantz, P. M., and Rausch, R. L.**, Alveolar hydatid disease in Minnesota: first human case acquired in the contiguous United States, *JAMA*, 241(9), 904, 1979.

85. **Garabedian, G. A.**, Evaluation of the reactivity of hydatid whole-scolex antigen in hydatid disease serology, *Ann. Trop. Med. Parasitol.*, 65, 385, 1971.

86. **Garti, I. and Deutsch, V.**, The angiographic diagnosis of echinococosis of the liver and spleen, *Clin. Radiol.*, 22, 466, 1971.

87. **Gemmell, M. A.**, Hydatid disease in Australia. VI. Observations on the carnivora of New South Wales as definitive hosts of *Echinococcus granulosus* (Batsch, 1786) (Rudolphi, 1801), and their role in the spread of hydatidosis in domestic animals, *Aust. Vet. J.*, 35, 450, 1959.

88. **Gemmell, M. A.**, Advances in knowledge on the distribution and importance of hydatid disease as world health and economic problems during the decade 1950—1959, *Helminthol. Abstr.*, 29, 355, 1960.

89. **Gemmell, M. A.**, Natural and acquired immunity factors interfering with development during the rapid growth phase of *Echinococcus granulosus* in dogs, *Immunology*, 5, 496, 1962.

90. **Gemmell, M. A.**, Immunological responses of the mammalian host against tapeworm infections. IV. Species specificity of hexacanth embryos in protecting sheep against *Echinococcus granulosus*, *Immunology*, 11, 325, 1966.

91. **Gemmell, M. A. and Shearer, G. C.**, Bunamidine hydrochloride: its efficiency against *Echinococcus granulosus*, *Vet. Rec.*, 82, 252, 1968.

92. **Gemmell, M. A. and Soulsby, E. J. L.**, The development of acquired immunity to tapeworms and progress towards active immunization, with special reference to *Echinococcus* spp., *Bull. WHO*, 39, 45, 1968.

93. **Gemmell, M. A.**, The Styx field-trial. A study on the application of control measures against hydatid diseases caused by *Echinococcus granulosus*, *Bull. WHO*, 39, 73, 1968a.

94. **Gemmell, M. A. and MacNamara, F. N.**, Immune responses to tissue parasites, II, *Cestodes in Immunity to Animal Parasites*, 2, Soulsby, E. J. L., Ed., Academic Press, New York, 1972, 2, 236.

95. **Gemmell, M. A.**, Surveillance of *Echinococcus granulosus* in dogs with arecoline hydrobromide, *Bull. WHO*, 48, 649, 1973.

96. **Gemmell, M. A. and Oudemans, G.**, Treatment of *Echinococcus granulosus* and *Taenia hydatigena* in dogs with bunamidine hydroxynaphthoate in a prepared food, *Res. Vet. Sci.*, 16, 85, 1974.

97. **Gemmell, M. S.**, Immunological responses and regulation of the cestode zoonoses, in *Immunology of Human Parasitic Infections*, Cohen, S. and Sadun, E., Eds., Blackwell Scientific, Oxford, 1975, 334.

98. **Gemmell, M. A.**, Perspective on options for hydatidosis and cysticerdosis control, *Vet. Med. Rev.*, 1, 3, 1978.

99. **Gemmell, M. A. and Oudemans, G.**, The effect of fospirate of *Echinococcus granulosus* and *Taenia hydatigena* in dogs, *Res. Vet. Sci.*, 19, 216, 1975a.

100. **Gemmell, M. A., Johnstone, P. D., and Oudemans, G.**, The effect of mebendazole on *Echinococcus granulosus* and *Taenia hydatigena* infections in dogs, *Res. Vet. Sci.*, 19, 229, 1975a.

101. **Gemmell, M. A. and Oudemans, G.**, The effect of nitroscanate on *Echinococcus granulosus* and *Taenia hydatigena* infections in dogs, *Res. Vet. Sci.*, 19, 217, 1975b.

102. **Gemmell, M. A., Oudemans, G., and Sakamoto, T.**, The effect of bithionol sulfoxide on *Echinococcus granulosus* and *Taenia hydatigena* infections in dogs, *Res. Vet. Sci.*, 18, 109, 1975b.

103. **Gemmell, M. A., Johnstone, P. D., and Oudemans, G.**, The effect of EMBAY 8440 (Droncit) on *Echinococcus granulosus, Taenia hydatigena* and *T. ovis* in dogs, *Res. Vet. Sci.*, 23, 121, 1977.

104. **Gemmell, M. A., Johnstone, P. D., and Oudemans, G.**, The effect of mebendazole in food on *Echinococcus granulosus* and *Taenia hydatigena* infections in dogs, *Res. Vet. Sci.*, 25, 107, 1978.

105. **Gemmell, M. A., Johnstone, P. D., and Oudemans, G.**, The effect of route of administration on the efficacy of praziquantel against *Echinococcus granulosus* infections in dogs, *Res. Vet. Sci.*, 29, 131, 1980.

106. **Gemmell, M. A., Parmeter, S. N., Sutton, R. J., and Khan, N.**, Effect of mebendazole against *Echinococcus granulosus* and *Taenia hydatigema* infections in naturally infected sheep and its possible relevance to larval tapeworm infections in man, *Z. Parasitenkunde*, 64, 135, 1981.

107. **Gemmell, M. A. and Johnstone, P. D.**, Experimental epidemiology of hydatidosis and cysticercosis, *Adv. Parasitol.*, 15, 311, 1977.

108. **Gentilini, M. and Pinon, J. M.**, Value of electrosynerosis (or immuno-electro-diffusion) on a cellulose acetate membrane in hydatidosis diagnosis. Comparative study with other precipitation tests, *Ann. Med. Interne (Paris)*, 123, 883, 1972.

109. **Gil, H. S. and Rao, B. V.**, On the biology and morphology of *Echinococcus granulosus* of buffalo-dog origin, *Parasitology*, 57, 695, 1967.
110. **Gilchrist, D. S.**, Chemical peritonitis after cetrimide washout in hydatid-cyst surgery, *Lancet*, 2, 1374, 1979.
111. **Gilevich, I. S., Ataev, B. A., Vafin, A. Z., Gilevich, M. I., and Kardanov, V. Z.**, Relapses in echinococcosis disease, *Vestnick Khirugie (in Russian)*, 124, 39, 1980.
112. **Giunchi, G., Pauluzzi, S., and deRosa, F.**, Specificity of the indirect hemagglutination test for the diagnosis of human hydatid disease, *Boll. Ist. Sieroter. Milan.*, 51(2), 145, 1972.
113. **Gorina, N. S.**, The role of foxes in the epizootiology and epidemiology of *E. granulosus* (in Russian), *Sb. Nauchno Tekh. Inf. Vses. Inst. Gelmintol.*, 718, 21, 1961.
114. **Gregory, G. G. and McConnell, J. D.**, The toxicity and efficiency of arecoline hydrobromide in the Tasmanian hydatid control program, *Aust. Vet. J.*, 54, 193, 1978.
115. **Grove, D. I., Warren, K. S., and Mahmoud, A. A. F.**, Algorithms in the diagnosis and management of exotic diseases, *J. Infect. Dis.*, 133, 354, 1976.
116. **Guisantes, J. A. and Varela-Diaz, V. M.**, Las pruebas de aglutinacion del latex y doble difusion en gel en el immunodiagnostico de la hidatidosis humana, *Bol. Chil. Parasitol.*, 30, 54, 1975.
117. **Guisantes, J. A., Yarzábal, L. A., Varela-Diaz, V. M., Ricardes, M. I., and Coltorti, E. A.**, Standardization of the immunoelectrophoresis test with whole and purified hydatid cyst fluid antigens for the diagnosis of human hydatidosis, *Rev. Inst. Med. Trop. Sao Paulo*, 17, 69, 1975.
118. **Gutgemann, A., Kaufer, C., Prange, C. H., Raschke, E., Bucheler, E., and Biersack, H. J.**, Diagnostik und Chirurgie der Leberechinococcen, *Langenbecks Arch. Chir.*, 340, 285, 1976.
119. **Hammerberg, B., Musoke, A. J., and Williams, J. F.**, Activation of complement by hydatid cyst fluid of *Echinococcus granulosus*, *J. Parasitol.*, 63, 327, 1977.
120. **Harris, R. E., Revfeim, K. J. A., and Heath, D. D.**, Simulating control strategies for control of *Echinococcus granulosus*, *Taenia hydatigena* and *T. ovis*, *J. Hyg. Camb.*, 84, 389, 1980.
121. **Hatch, C. and Smyth, J. D.**, Attempted infection of sheep with *Echinococcus granulosus equinus*, *Res. Vet. Sci.*, 19, 340, 1975.
122. **Heath, D. D.**, The migration of oncospheres of *Taenia pisiformis*, *T. serialis* and *Echinococcus granulosus* within the intermediate host, *Int. J. Parasitol.*, 1, 145, 1971.
123. **Heath, D. D.**, The life cycle of *Echinococcus granulosus* — a review, in Symp. Recent Advances in Hydatid Disease, Hamilton Medical Veterinary Association, Hamilton, Victoria, Australia, 1973, 7.
124. **Heath, D. D.**, Immunization of neonatal lambs against the larvae of *Taenia hydatigena*, using viable eggs followed by chemotherapy, *Vet. Parasitol.*, 4, 11, 1978.
125. **Heath, D. D. and Chevis, R. A.**, Mebendazole and hydatid cysts (letter to the editor), *Lancet*, 2(874), 218, 1974.
126. **Heath, D. D., Christie, M. J., and Chevis, R. A. F.**, The lethal effect of mebendazole on secondary *Echinococcus granulosus*, cysticerci of *Taenia pisiformis* and tetrathyridia of *Mesocestoides corti*, *Parasitology*, 70, 273, 1975.
127. **Heath, D. D.**, Resistance to *Taenia pisiformis* larvae in rabbits: immunization against infection using non-living antigens from *in vitro* culture, *Int. J. Parasitol.*, 6, 19, 1976.
128. **Heath, D. D. and Lawrence, S. B.**, *Echinococcus granulosus*: development *in vitro* from oncosphere to immature hydatid cyst, *Parasitology*, 73, 417, 1976.
129. **Heath, D. D. and Lawrence, S. B.**, The effect of mebendazole and praziquantel on the cysts of *Echinococcus granulosus*, *Taenia hydatigena*, and *T. ovis* in sheep, *N.. Vet. J.*, 26, 11, 1978.
130. **Herd, R. P., Chappel, R. J., and Biddell, D. G.**, Immunization of dogs against *Echinococcus granulosus* using worm secretory antigens, *Int. J. Parasitol.*, 5, 395, 1975.
131. **Herd, R. P.**, The cestocidal effect of complement in normal and immune serum *in vitro*, *Parasitology*, 72, 325, 1976.
132. **Howkins, A. B., Gemmell, M. A., and Smyth, J. D.**, Experimental transmission of *Echinococcus* from horses to foxes, *Ann. Trop. Med. Parasitol.*, 59, 457, 1965.
133. **Huldt, G., Gunnar, S., Johansson, O., and Lantto, S.**, Echinococcosis in Northern Scandinavia, *Arch. Environ. Health*, 26, 36, 1973.
134. **Hustead, S. T. and Williams, J. F.**, Permeability studies on taeniid metacestodes. I. Uptake of proteins by larval stages of *Taenia taeniaeformis*, *T. crassiceps*, and *Echinococcus granulosus*, *J. Parasitol.*, 63, 314, 1977.
135. **Iacona, A., Pini, C., and Vicari, G.**, Enzyme-linked immunosorbent assay (ELISA) in the serodiagnosis of hydatid disease, *Am. J. Trop. Med. Hyg.*, 29, 95, 1980.
136. **Iida, H.**, Epidemiology of Multilocular Echinococcosis in Hokkaido, Japan, in *Multilocular Echinococcosis in Hokkaido, Japan*, Institute of Public Health, 1969, 5.
137. **Irgashev, I. K. and Sadikov, V. M.**, Effect of hydatid on meat production in pigs (in Russian), *Tr. Uzb. Nauchno Issled. Inst. Vet.*, 17, 109, 1965.

138. **Ito, K., Horiuchi, Y., Kumagai, M., Ueda, M., Nakamura, R., Kawanishi, N., and Kasai, Y.,** Evaluation of RAST as an immunological method for diagnosis of multilocular echinococcosis, *Clin. Exp. Immunol.,* 28, 407, 1977.

139. **Ishak, K. G.,** Acid-fast staining of hooklets of *Taenia echinococcus, Lancet,* 1, 556, 1972.

140. **Jakubowski, M. S. and Barnard, D. E.,** Anaphylactic shock during operation for hydatid disease, *Anesthesiology,* 34, 197, 1971.

141. **Jezek, Z., Rachkovsky, A., Mingir, G., and Galbadrakh, C.,** Casoni skin test survey in man in a limited area of the Mongolian Peoples' Republic, *J. Hyg. Epidemiol. Microbiol. Immunol.,* 17, 422, 1973.

142. **Kagan, I.,** A review of serological tests for the diagnosis of hydatid disease, *Bull. WHO,* 39, 25, 1968.

143. **Kagan, I. G. and Cahill, K. M.,** Parasitic serologic studies in Somaliland, *Am. J. Trop. Med. Hyg.,* 17(3), 392, 1968.

144. **Kagan, I.,** Advances in the immunodiagnosis of parasitic infections, *Z. Parasitenkd.,* 45, 163, 1974.

145. **Kagan, I. G.,** Serodiagnosis of hydatid disease, in *Imunology of Parasitic Diseases,* Cohen S. and Sadun, E., Eds., Blackwell Scientific, Oxford, 1976, 130.

146. **Kammerer, W. S. and Judge, D. M.,** Chemotherapy of hydatid disease (*Echinococcus granulosus*) in mice with mebendazole and bithionol, *Am. J. Trop. Med. Hyg.,* 25, 714, 1976.

147. **Kasai, Y., Koshino, I., Kawanishi, N., Sakamoto, H., Sasaki, E., and Kumagai, M.,** Alveolar echinococcosis of the liver, *Ann. Surg.,* 191, 145, 1980.

148. **Kassis, A. I. and Tanner, C. E.,** Novel approach to the treatment of hydatid disease, *Nature London,* 262, 588, 1976.

149. **Kassis, A. I. and Tanner, C. E.,** The role of complement in hydatid disease: *in vitro* studies, *Int. J. Parasitol.,* 6, 25, 1976.

150. **Kassis, A. I. and Tanner, C. E.,** Host serum proteins in *Echinococcus multilocularis:* complement activation via the classical pathway, *Immunology,* 33, 1, 1977.

151. **Kirschner, L. P., Ferris, R. A., Mero, J. H., and Moss, M. L.,** Case Report. Hydatid disease of the liver evaluated by computed tomography, *J. Comp. Assist. Tomog.,* 2, 229, 1978.

152. **Kern, P., Dietrich, M., and Volkmer, K. J.,** Chemotherapy of echinococcosis with mebendazole: clinical observations of 7 patients, *Tropenmed. Parasitol.,* 30, 65, 1979.

153. **Klock, L. E., Spruance, S. L., Andersen, F. L., Juranek, D. D., and Kagan, I. G.,** Detection of asymptomatic hydatid disease by a community screening program, *Am. J. Epidemiol.,* 97(1), 16, 1973.

154. **Kourias, B., Gyftaki, E., Peveretos, P., and Binopoulos, D.,** The value of pre- and post-operative scanning in liver echinococcosis, *Br. J. Surg.,* 57, 178, 1970.

155. **Kozakiewicz, B., Pawlowski, Z., and Zatonski, J.,** Efficacy of niclosamide and bunamidine in the treatment of echinococcosis in dogs (in Polish), *Med. Weter.,* 31, 460, 1975.

156. **Kozakiewicz, B.,** Studies on the infectivity of larval *Echinococcus granulosus* in pigs (in Polish), *Med. Weter.,* 31, 526, 1975, as reprinted in *Vet. Bull. London,* 46, 3132, 1976.

157. **Kritsky, D. C. and Leiby, P. D.,** Studies on sylvatic echinococcosis. V. Factors influencing prevalence of *Echinococcus multilocularis* Leuckart 1863, in red foxes from North Dakota, 1965—1972, *J. Parasitol.,* 64, 625, 1978.

158. **Krotov, A. I., Tchernaev, A. I., Kovalenko, F. P., Bajandina, D. G., Budanova, I. C., Kuznetsova, O. E., and Voskoboinik, L. V.,** Experimental therapy of alveococcosis. II. Effectivity of some defensive remedies against alveococcosis of laboratory animals (in Russian), *Med. Parzitol. Parazit. Bolezni,* 43, 314, 1974.

159. **Kuznetsov, M. I., Shubaderov, V. Y., and Tiltin, B. P.,** Biological morphological, and immunological features of *Echinococcus granulosus* sheep and pig in various regions of the U.S.S.R. (in Russian), in Antropozoogel'mintozy i Perspektivy ikh Likvidatsii: Vsesoyuznaya Akademiya Selskokhozyaistvennykh Nauk. im. V.I. Lenina VIGIS, Moscow 1975, 46; reprinted in *Helminthol. Abstr.,* 46, 2066, 1977.

160. **Lascano, E. F., Coltorti, E. A., and Varela-Diaz, V. M.,** Fine structure of the germinal membrane of *Echinococcus granulosus* cysts, *J. Parasitol.,* 61, 853, 1975.

161. **Lass, N., Laver, Z., and Lengy, J.,** The imunodiagnosis of hydatid disease: post-operative evaluation of the skin test and four serological tests, *Ann. Allergy,* 31, 430, 1973.

162. **Lauriola, L., Pinatelli, M., Pozzuoli, R., Arru, E., and Musiani, P.,** *Echinococcus granulosus:* preparation of monospecific antisera against antigens in sheep hydatid fluid, *Zentralbl. Bakteriol. Hyg. Abt. Orig. Reine A,* 240, 251, 1978.

163. **Leiby, P. D. and Nichol, M. P.,** Studies on sylvatic echinococcosis. Ground beetle transmission of *Echinococcus multilocularis* Leukart, 1863, to deer mice, *Peromyscus maniculatus* (Wagner), *J. Parasitol.,* 54, 536, 1968.

164. **Leiby, P. L., Carney, W. P., and Woods, C. E.,** Studies on sylvatic echinococcosis. III. Host occurrence and geographic distribution of *Echinococcus multilocularis* in the north central United States, *J. Parasitol.,* 56, 1141, 1970.

165. **Leiby, P. D. and Kritsky, D. C.,** *Echinococcus multilocularis:* a possible domestic life cycle in central North America and its public health implications, *J. Parasitol.,* 58, 1213, 1972.

166. **Leiby, P. D. and Kritsky, D. C.,** Studies on sylvatic echinococcosis. IV. Ecology of *Echinococcus multilocularis* in the intermediate host *Peromyscus maniculatus* in North Dakota, 1965—1972, *Am. J. Trop. Med. Hyg.,* 23, 667, 1974.

167. **Lichter, I.,** Surgery of pulmonary hydatid cyst — the Barrett technique, *Thorax,* 27, 529, 1972.

168. **Little, J. M.,** Hydatid disease at Royal Prince Alfred Hospital, 1964 to 1974, *Med. J. Aust.,* 1, 903, 1976.

169. **Lukashenko, N. P.,** Problems of epidemiology and prophylaxis of alveococcosis (multilocular echinococcosis): a general review — with particular reference to the U.S.S.R., *Int. J. Parastiol.,* 1, 125, 1971.

170. **Lupasco, G., Panaitesco, D., and Smolinski, M.,** Essais de délimitation des zones endémiques d'hydatidose en Roumanie à l'aide de l'intradermoréaction de Casoni, *Arch. Roum. Pathol. Exp. Microbiol.,* 26(1), 251, 1967.

171. **Maccas, M.,** El quiste hidatidico en Grecia, *Arch. Int. Hidatidosis,* 14, 130, 1955.

172. **Malczewski, A.,** The red fox *Vulpes vulpes* L. as the final host of the tapeworm *Echinococcus granulosus* (Batsch, 1786) in Poland, *Bull. Acad. Pol. Sci. Ser. Sci. Biol.,* 11, 295, 1963.

173. **Mann, I.,** The backround and outline of the research programme in echinococcosis (hydatidosis) in Kenya, *Proc. 3rd. Int. Congr. Parasitol. (Munich),* 1, 547, 1974.

174. **Marangos, G. N.,** International hydatid disease congress held in Algiers on May 20—24, 1951, and the lessons applicable to Cyprus, *Cyprus Med. J.,* 4, 668, 1951, as reprinted in *Helminthol. Abstr.,* 20, 720, 1951.

175. **Matchanov, N. M., Irgashev, I. K., Mirzayarov, M. K., and Oripov, A. O.,** Measures against coenurosis and echinococcosis (in Russian), *Veterinaria Moscow,* 49, 64, 1973.

176. **Matoff, K. N. and Tierarzt, J. J.,** Entwickelt sich *Echinococcus granulosus* normal in Darm des Fuchses (*Canis vulpes*)?, *F. Med. Vet.,* 26, 249, 1950.

177. **Matoff, K. N. and Jantscheff, J.,** Kann *Echinococcus granulosus* im Darm des Fuches (*Canis vulpes*) sich zur Geschlechtsreife entwickeln?, *Acta Vet. Hung.,* 4, 411, 1954.

178. **Matoff, K. and Kolev, G.,** The role of the hairs, muzzle, and paws of echinococcic dogs in the epidemiology of echinococcosis, *Z. Tropenmend. Parasitol.,* 15, 144, 1964.

179. **Matoff, K. and Yanchev, Y.,** The fox as definitive host of *Echinococcus granulosus, Acta Vet.*

180. **Matossian, R. M.,** The immunological diagnosis of human hydatid disease, *Trans. R. Soc. Trop. Med. Hyg.,* 71(2), 101, 1977.

181. **Matossian, R. M. and Araj, G. F.,** Serologic evidence of the postoperative persistence of hydatid cysts in man, *J. Hyg. (Cambridge),* 75, 333, 1975.

182. **Matossian, R. M., Kane, G. J., Chantler, S. N., Batty, I., and Sarhadian, H.,** The specific immunoglobulin in hydatid disease, *Immunology,* 22, 423, 1972.

183. **Matossian, R. M., Alami, S. Y., Salti, I., and Araj, G. F.,** Serum immunoglobulin levels in human hydatidosis, *I. J. P.,* 6, 367, 1976.

184. **Matossian, R. M., Rickard, M. D., and Smyth, J. D.,** Hydatidosis: a global problem of increasing importance, *Bull. WHO,* 55, 499, 1977.

185. **McManus, D. P. and Smyth, J. D.,** Differences in the chemical composition and carbohydrate metabolism of *Echinococcus granulosus* (horse and sheep strains) and *E. multilocularis, Parasitology,* 77, 103, 1978.

186. **McManus, D. P. and Smyth, J. D.,** Isoelectric focusing of some enzymes from *Echinococcus granulosus* (horse and sheep strains) and *E. multilocularsis, Trans. R. Soc. Trop. Med. Hyg.,* 73, 259, 1979.

187. **Meldrum, G. K. and McConnell, J. D.,** The control of hydatid disease in Tasmania, *Aust. Vet. J.,* 44, 212, 1968.

188. **Mobedi, I. and Sadighian, A.,** *Echinococcus multilocularis* Leuckart, 1863, in red foxes, *Vulpes vulpes* Linn., in Moghan, Azerbaijan Province, northwest of Iran, *J. Parasitol.,* 57, 493, 1971.

189. **Morseth, D. J.,** Fine structure of the hydatid cyst and protoscolex of *Echinococcus granulosus, J. Parasitol.,* 53, 312, 1967.

190. **Mosimann, F.,** Is alveolar hydatid disease of the liver incurable?, *Ann. Surg.,* 192, 118, 1980.

191. **Mottaghian, H. and Saidi, F.,** Postoperative recurrence of hydatid disease, *Br. J. Surg.,* 65, 237, 1978.

192. **Musiani, P., Piantelli, M., Arru, E., and Pozzuoli, R.,** A solid phase radioimmunoassay for the diagnosis of human hydatidosis, *J. Immunol.,* 112, 1674, 1974.

193. **Naquira, F., Montesinos, J., Cordova, E., and Valdivia, L.,** Observaciones epidemiologicas de la hidatidosis en Arequipa, Peru, *Arch. Int. Hidatidosis,* 24, 415, 1970.

194. **Neghme, A. and Silva, R.,** A hidatidose como problema medico, sanitario e social e esboco basico para sua profilaxis, *Rev. Asso. Med. Bras.,* 16, 279, 1970.

195. **Nelson, G. S. and Rausch, R. L.,** *Echinococcus* infections in man and animals in Kenya, *Ann. Trop. Med. Parasitol.,* 57, 136, 1963.

196. **Nosik, A. F.,** Epizootiology and epidemiology of hydatidosis (in Russian), *Sb. Tr. Khark. Vet. Inst.,* 21, 264, 1952; reprinted in *Helminthol. Abstr.,* 28, 1483, 1957.

197. **Ohbayashi, M., Rausch, R. L., and Ray, F. H.,** On the ecology and distribution of *Echinococcus* spp. (Cestoda: Taeniidae), and characteristics of their development in the intermediate host, *Jpn. J. Vet. Res.,* 19(3), 1, 1971.

198. **O'Leary, P.,** A five-year review of human hydatid cyst disease in Turkana District, Kenya, *E. Afr. Med. J.,* 53(9), 540, 1976.

199. **Owor, R. and Bitakaramire, P. K.,** Hydatid disease in Uganda, *E. Afr. Med. J.,* 52, 700, 1957.

200. **Özgen, T., Erbengi, A., Bertan, V., Saglam, S., Gürcay, Ö., and Pirnar, T.,** The use of computerized tomography in the diagnosis of cerebral hydatid cysts, *J. Neurosurg.,* 50, 339, 1979.

201. **Pampiglione, S.,** L'idatidosi dell'uomo in Algeria, *Parassitologia Rome,* 7, 135, 1965.

202. **Panday, V. S.,** Observations on the morphology and biology of *Echinococcus granulosus* (Batsch, 1786) of goat-dog origin, *Helminthology,* 46, 219, 1972.

203. **Papadimitriou, J. and Mandrekas, A.,** The surgical treatment of hydatid disease of the liver, *Br. J. Surg.,* 57(6), 431, 1970.

204. **Pinch, L. W. and Wilson, J. F.,** Non-surgical management of cystic hydatid disease in Alaska, *Ann. Surg.,* 176, 45, 1972.

205. **Pinon, J. M., Sulahian, A., Remy, G., and Dropsy, G.,** Immunological study of hydatidosis, *Am. J. Trop. Med. Hyg.,* 28(2), 318, 1979.

206. **Pissiotis, C. A., Wander, J. V., and Condon, R. E.,** Surgical treatment of hydatid disease, *Arch. Surg. (Chicago),* 104, 454, 1972.

207. **Polydorou, K.,** The anti-echinococcosis campaign in Cyprus, *Trop. Anim. Health Prod.,* 9, 141, 1977.

208. **Popov, A.,** Situation de l'echinococcose-hydatidose en Bulgarie et mesures de prophylaxie, *Off. Int. Epizoot. Bull.,* 62, 1023, 1964.

209. **Pozzuoli, R., Musiani, R., Arru, E., Patrono, C., and Piantelli, M.,** *Echinococcus granulosus:* evaluation of purified antigens' immunoreactivity, *Exp. Parasitol.,* 35, 52, 1974.

210. **Pukhev, V. I., Zinichenko, I. I., and Parharkov, A. G.,** Essential methods of elimination of coenurosis and echinococcosis of sheep (in Russian), *Veterinaria Moscow,* 4, 31, 1956.

211. **Purriel, P., Schantz, P. M., Beovide, H., and Mendoze, G.,** Human echinococcosis (hydatidosis) in Uruguay: a comparison of indices of morbidity and mortality, 1962—71, *Bull. WHO,* 49, 395, 1974.

212. **Quilici, M., Assadourian, Y., and Ranque, P.,** Le diagnostic immunologique de l'hydatidose, *Med. Trop. Marseille,* 31, 207, 1971.

213. **Quilici, M., Dumon, H., and Delmont, J.,** Les modalites de constitution des (recidives) postoperatoires de lechinococcose a *Echinococcus granulosus, Med. Malad. Infect.,* 6, 12, 1976.

214. **Ramirez, M., Macaya, J., Rojas, A., Scozia, A., Schenone, H., Rodriguez, F., Diag, L., and Hess, J. C.,** Encuesta epidemiologica sobre hidatidosis humana en un area de alta endemia hidatidica, *Bol. Chil. Parasitol.,* 26, 63, 1971.

215. **Ramirez, R.,** Algunos aspectos bioestadisticos de la hidatidosis humana en Chile durante los anos 1969—1970, *Bol. Chil. Parasitol.,* 26, 84, 1971.

216. **Rao, B. V.,** Experimental transmission of *Echinococcus* of buffalo origin to foxes (Vulpes bengalensis), *Vet. Rec.,* 83, 56, 1968.

217. **Rausch, R. and Schiller, E. L.,** Studies on the helminth fauna of Alaska, *Parasitology,* 46, 395, 1956.

218. **Rausch, R. L.,** Recent studies on hydatid disease in Alaska, *Parassitologia Rome,* 2, 391, 1960.

219. **Rausch, R. L.,** personal communication, 1972.

220. **Rausch, R. L. and Nelson, G. S.,** A review of the genus *Echinococcus* Rudolphi, 1801, *Ann. Trop. Med. Parasitol.,* 57, 127, 1963.

221. **Rausch, R. L.,** On the ecology and distribution of *Echinococcus* spp. (Cestoda:Taeniidae), and characteristics of their development in the intermediate host, *Ann. Parasitol. Hum. Comp.,* 42, 19, 1967.

222. **Rausch, R. L.,** A consideration of infraspecific categories in the genus *Echinococcus* Rudolphi, 1801, (Cestoda:Taeniidae), *J. Parasitol.,* 53, 484, 1967.

223. **Rausch, R. L.,** Taxonomic characters in the genus *Echinococcus* (Cestoda:Taeniidae), *Bull. WHO,* 39, 1, 1968.

224. **Rausch, R. L. and Richards, S. H.,** Observations of parasite-host relationships of *Echinococcus multilocularis* Leuckart, 1863, in North Dakota, *Can. J. Zool.,* 49, 1317, 1971.

225. **Rausch, R. L. and Bernstein, J. J.,** *Echinococcus vogeli* spp. n. (Cestoda:Taeniidae) from the bush dog, *Speothos venaticus* (Lund), *Tropenmed. Parasitol.,* 23, 25, 1972.

226. **Rausch, R. L. and Wilson, J. R.,** Rearing of the adult *Echinococcus multilocularis* Leuckart, 1863, from sterile larvae from man, *Am. J. Trop. Med. Hyg.,* 22, 357, 1973.

227. **Rausch, R. L.,** Taeniidae, in *Diseases Transmitted from Animals to Man*, Hubbert, W. T., Mc-Culloch, W. F., and Schnurrenberger, P. R., Eds., Charles C Thomas, Springfield, Ill., 1975, 678.

228. **Rausch, R. L., Rausch, V. R., and D'Alessandro, A.,** Discrimnation of the larval stages of *Echinococcus oligarthrus* (Diesing, 1863) and *E. vogeli* Rausch and Bernstein, 1972 (Cestoda:Taeniidae), *Am. J. Trop. Med. Hyg.*, 27, 1195, 1978.

229. **Reuben, J. M. and Tanner, C. E.,** Immunoprophylaxis with BCG of experimental *Echinococcus multilocularis* infections, *Aust. Vet. J.*, 55, 105, 1979.

230. **Richard-Lenoble, D., Smith, M. D., and Loisy, M.,** Human hydatidosis: evaluation of three serodiagnostic methods, the principal subclass of specific immunoglobulin and the detection of circulating immune complexes, *Ann. Trop. Med. Parasitol.*, 72, 553, 1978.

231. **Rickard, M. D.,** The immunological diagnosis of hydatid disease, *Aust. Vet. J.*, 55, 99, 1979.

232. **Rickard, M. D. and Bell, K. J.,** Immunity produced against *Taenia ovis* and *T. taeniaeformis* infection in lambs and rats following *in vivo* growth of their larvae in filtration membrane diffusion chambers, *J. Parasitol.*, 57, 571, 1971.

233. **Rickard, M. D. and Bell, K. J.,** Successful vaccination of lambs against infection with *Taenia ovis* using antigens produced during *in vitro* cultivation of the larval stages, *Res. Vet. Sci.*, 12, 401, 1971.

234. **Rickard, M. D. and Katiyar, J. C.,** Partial purification of antigens collected during *in vitro* cultivation of the larval stages of *Taenia pisiformis*, *Parasitology*, 72, 269, 1976.

235. **Rickard, M. D., White, J. B., and Boddington, E. B.,** Vaccination of lambs against infection with *Taenia ovis*, *Aust. Vet. J.*, 52, 209, 1976.

236. **Rickard, M. D. and Adolph, A. J.,** Vaccination of lambs against infection with *Taenia ovis* using antigens collected during short-term *in vitro* incubation of activated *T. ovis* oncospheres, *Parasitology*, 75, 183, 1977.

237. **Rickard, M. D., Mackinlay, L. M., Kane, G. J., Matossian, R. M., and Smyth,** Studies on the mechanism of lysis of *Echinococcus granulosus* protoscoleces incubated in normal serum, *J. Helminthol.*, 51, 221, 1977.

238. **Roman, M. N., Brunetti, O. A., Schwabe, C. W., and Rosen, M. N.,** Probable transmission of *Echinococcus granulosus* between deer and coyotes in California, *J. Wildl. Dis.*, 10, 225, 1974.

239. **Rommel, M., Grelck, H., and Horchner, F.,** The efficiency of praziquantel against tapeworms in experimentally infected dogs and cats (in German), *Berl. Muench. Tieraerztl. Wochenschr.*, 89, 255, 1976; reprinted in *Vet. Bull. London*, 46, 6579, 1976.

240. **Roneus, O.,** Prevalence of echinococcosis in reindeer (*Rangifer tarandus*) in Sweden, *Acta Vet. Scand.*, 15, 170, 1974.

241. **Rudofsky, G., Wolfert, W., and Rau, R. M.,** Angiographische darstellung der Leberarterien beim *Echinococcus alveolaris*, *Med. Klin. Munich*, 70, 1641, 1975.

242. **Sachs, R.,** Further studies on cysticercosis and echinococcosis of African game animals. Informal consultation on taeniasis/cysticercosis research, *Neuherberg*, 22, 1974.

243. **Sadikov, V. M.,** Effect of hydatidosis on beef production in the Uzbek SSR (in Russian), *Tr. Uzb. Nauchno Issled. Inst. Vet.*, 17, 205, 1965.

244. **Sadykov, V. M.,** Problems of echinococcosis prophylaxis in towns and cities (in Russian), *Med. Parazitol. Parazit. Bolezni*, 36, 168, 1967.

245. **Saidi, F. and Nazarian, I.,** Surgical treatment of hydatid cysts by freezing of cyst wall and instillation of 0.5 percent silver nitrate solution, *N. Engl. J. Med.*, 284, 1346, 1971.

246. **Schantz, P. M. and Schwabe, C. W.,** Worldwide status of hydatid disease control, *J. Am. Vet. Med. Assoc.*, 155, 2104, 1969.

247. **Schantz, P. M.,** Hidatidosis: magnitud del problema y perspectivas de control, *Bol. Of. Sanit. Panam.*, 74, 187, 1972.

248. **Schantz, P. M., Lord, R. D., and de Zavaleta, O.,** *Echinococcus* in the South American red fox (*Dusicyon culpaeus*) and the European hare (*Lepus europaeus*) in the province of Neuquen, Argentina, *Ann. Trop. Med. Parasitol.*, 66, 479, 1972.

249. **Schantz, P. M.,** Immunodiagnostic tests with *Echinococcus* antigens in sheep with homologous and heterologous larval cestode infections, *Rev. Inst. Med. Trop. Sao Paulo*, 15, 179, 1973.

250. **Schantz, P. M.,** La vigilancia epidemiologica de la hidatidosis, *Torax*, 22, 203, 1973.

251. **Schantz, P. M.,** Aspectos epidemiologicos de la hidatidosis quistica en America del Sur, *Torax*, 22, 222, 1973.

252. **Schantz, P. M. and Colli, C. W.,** *Echinococcus oligarthrus* (Diesing, 1863) from Geoffrey's cats (*Felis geoffroyi*, D'Orbigny and Gervais) in temperate South America, *J. Parsitol.*, 59, 1138, 1973.

253. **Schantz, P. M., Williams, J. F., and Riva Posse, C.,** The epidemiology of hydatid disease in southern Argentina. Comparison of morbidity indices, evaluation of immunodiagnostic tests and factors affecting transmission in southern Rio Negro Province, *Am. J. Trop. Med. Hyg.*, 22, 629, 1973.

254. **Schantz, P. M.,** Guia para el empleo de bromhidrato de arecolina en el diagnóstico de la infeccion por *Echinococcus granulosus* en el perro, *Bol. Chil. Parasitol.*, 28, 81, 1973.

255. **Schantz, P. M., Cruz-Reyes, A., Colli, C., and Lord, R. D.,** Sylvatic echinococcosis in Argentina. I. On the morphology and biology of strobilar *Echinococcus granulosus* (Batsch. 1786) from Argentine domestic and sylvatic animal hosts, *Tropenmed. Parasitol.,* 26, 334, 1975.

256. **Schantz, P. M., Ortiz-Valqui, R. E., and Lumbreras, H.,** Nonspecific reactions with the intradermal test for hydatidosis in persons with other helminth infections, *Am. J. Trop. Med. Hyg.,* 24, 849, 1975.

257. **Schantz, P. M., Colli, C., Cruz-Reyes, A., and Prezioso, U.,** Sylvatic echinococcosis in Argentina. II. Susceptibility of wild carnivores to *Echinococcus granulosus* (Batsch, 1786) and host-induced morphological variation, *Tropenmed. Parasitol.,* 27, 70, 1976.

258. **Schantz, P. M., Prezioso, U., and Marchevsky, N.,** The efficiency of divided doses of GS-23654 against immature *Echinococcus granulosus* in dogs, *Am. J. Vet. Res.,* 37, 621, 1976.

259. **Schantz, P. M. and Prezioso, U.,** The efficiency of divided doses of Fospirate against immature *Echinococcus granulosus* in dogs, *Am. J. Vet. Res.,* 37, 619, 1976.

260. **Schantz, P. M., Von Reyn, C. F., Welty, T., and Schultz, M. G.,** Echinococcosis in Arizona and New Mexico, survey of hospital records, 1969—1974, *Am. J. Trop. Med. Hyg.,* 25(2), 312, 1976.

261. **Schantz, P. M., Von Reyn, C. F., Welty, T., Andersen, F. L., Schultz, M. G., and Kagan, I. G.,** Epidemiologic investigation of echinococcosis in American Indians living in Arizona and New Mexico, *Am. J. Trop. Med. Hyg.,* 26(1), 121, 1977.

262. **Schantz, P. M.,** *Echinococcus granulosus:* acute systemic allergic reactions to hydatid cyst fluid in infected sheep, *Exp. Parasitol.,* 43, 268, 1977.

263. **Schantz, P. M. and Kagan, I. G.,** Immunological investigation of echinococcosis (hydatidosis), in *Immunologic Investigations of Tropical Parasitic Diseases,* Houba, V., Ed., Churchill Livingstone, Edinburgh, 1980, 104.

264. **Schantz, P. M., Shanks, D., and Wilson, M.,** Serologic cross-reactions with sera from patients with echinococcosis and cysticercosis, *Am. J. Trop. Med. Hyg.,* 29, 609, 1980.

265. **Schantz, P. M., Eckert, J., and van den Bossche, H.,** Mebendazole chemotherapy of hydatid disease: report of a workshop, *Z. Parasitenkd.,* in press.

266. **Schenone, H. and Reyes, H.,** Frecuencia de hidatidosis, cisticercosis y triquinosis en individuos fallecidos pro muerte violenta en Santiago de Chile (1947—1966), *Bol. Chil. Parasitol.,* 33, 62, 1971.

267. **Scherer, U., Weinzierl, M., Sturm, R., Schildberg, F., Zrenner, M., and Lissner, J.,** Computed tomography in hydatid disease of the liver: a report on 13 cases, *J. Comp. Assist. Tomog.,* 2, 612, 1978.

268. **Schiller, C. T.,** Complications of echinococcus cyst rupture: a study of 3 cases, *JAMA,* 195, 220, 1966.

269. **Schwabe, C. W., Schinazi, L. A., and Kilejian, A.,** Host-parasite relationships in echinococcosis. II. Age resistance to secondary echinococcosis in the white mouse, *Am. J. Trop. Med.,* 8, 29, 1959.

270. **Schwabe, C. W. and Daoud, K. A.,** Epidemiology of echinococcosis in the Middle East. I. Human infections in Lebanon, 1949—1959, *Am. J. Trop. Med. Hyg.,* 10, 374, 1961.

271. **Schwabe, C. W.,** Epidemiology of echinococcosis, *Bull. WHO,* 39, 131, 1968.

272. **Seddon, H. R.,** Helminth infestation, in Diseases of Domestic Animals in Australia, 2nd ed., Albiston, H. E., Ed., Department of Health, Canberra, 1967.

273. **Semenove, V. S., Pechen. O. R., and Papovodu,** Alveolianogo ekkinokokka, *Vestnik Khiruvgia Grekov,* 74, 20, 1954.

274. **Shumakovich, E. E. and Nikitin, V. F.,** Kornoruzheniiu *Echinococcus granulosus* (Batsch, 1786) u korsaka, *Biull. NauchoTekh. Inf. Vses. Inst. Gelmintol. im. K.I. Skriabina,* 5, 98, 1959.

275. **Silber, S. J. and Moyad, R. A.,** Renal echinococcus, *J. Urol.,* 108, 669, 1972.

276. **Simitch, T.,** Situation actuelle de l'échinococcose-hydatidose dans le monde, *Off. Int. Epizoot. Bull.,* 58, 747, 1962.

277. **Slãis, J.,** *The Morphology and Pathogenicity of the Bladder Worms Cysticercus cellulosae* and *Cysticercus bovis,* Junk, The Hague, 1970.

278. **Slãis, J.,** Functional morphology of cestode larva, *Adv. Parasitol.,* 11, 395, 1973.

279. **Smyth, J. D.,** The biology of the hydatid organisms, *Adv. Parasitol.,* 2, 169, 1964.

280. **Smyth, J. D. and Smyth, M. M.,** Natural and experimental hosts of *Echinococcus granulosus* and *E. multilocularis,* with comments on the genetics of speciation in the genus, *Echinococcus, Parasitology,* 54, 493, 1964.

281. **Smyth, J. D.,** The biology of the hydatid organisms, *Adv. Parasitol.,* 6, 327, 1968.

282. **Smyth, I. D.,** *In vitro* studies and host specificity in *Echinococcus, Bull. WHO,* 39, 5, 1968.

283. **Smyth, J. D. and Davies, Z.,** Occurrence of physiological strains of *Echinococcus granulosus* demonstrated by *in vitro* culture of protoscoleces from sheep and horse hydatid cysts, *Int. J. Parasitol.,* 4, 443, 1974.

284. **Smyth, J. D.,** Strain differences in *Echinococcus granulosus,* with special reference to the status of equine hydatidosis in the United Kingdom, *Trans. R. Soc. Trop. Med. Hyg.,* 71, 93, 1976.

285. Sorice, F., Pauluzzi, S., Castagnari, L., and Tolu, A., La fissazione del complemento per l'idatidosi, *Boll. Ist. Sieroter. Milan.*, 44(1 and 2), 22, 1965.

286. Sousa, O. E. and Lombardo Ayala, J. E., Informe de un caso de hidatidosis en sujeto nativo panameño; primer caso autoctono, *Arch. Med. Panam.*, 14, 79.

287. Sousa, O. E. and Thatcher, V. E., Observations on the life-cycle of *Echinococcus oligarthrus* (Diesing, 1863) in the Republic of Panama, *Ann. Trop. Med. Parasitol.*, 63, 165, 1969.

288. Sousa, O. E., Development of adult *Echinococcus oligarthrus* from hydatids of naturally infected agoutis, *J. Parasitol.*, 56, 197, 1970.

289. Spruance, S. L., Latent period of 53 years in a case of hydatid cyst disease, *Arch. Intern. Med.*, 134, 741, 1974.

290. Sweatman, G. K. and Williams, R. J., Comparative studies on the biology and morphology of *Echinococcus granulosus* from domestic livestock, moose and reindeer, *Parasitology*, 53, 339, 1963.

291. Suic, M., L'échinococcose humaine en Yougoslavie, *Arch. Int. Hidatidosis*, 16, 51, 1957a.

292. Szidat, L., Studien über den erreger del alveolaren echinococcenkrankheit des menschen in Sudamerika, *Z. Parasitenkd.*, 23, 80, 1963.

293. Szidat, L., *Echinococcus pampeanus*, una nueva especie de la Argentina, parasito de *Felis colocolo pajeros* Desmarest, 1916 (Cestoda), *Neotropica*, 13, 90, 1967.

294. Thakur, A. S., Prezioso, U., and Marchevsky, N., Efficacy of droncit against *Echinococcus granulosus* infection in dogs, *Am. J. Vet. Res.*, 39, 859, 1978.

295. Thatcher, V. E. and Sousa, O. E., *Echinococcus oligarthrus* Diesing, 1863, in Panama and a comparison with a recent human hydatid, *Ann. Trop. Med. Parasitol.*, 60, 405, 1966.

296. Thatcher, V. E. and Sousa, O. E., *Echinococcus oligarthrus* (Diesing, 1863) from a Panamanian jaguar (*Felis onca* L.), *J. Parasitol.*, 53, 1040, 1967.

297. Thatcher, V. E., Neotropical echinococcosis in Colombia, *Ann. Trop. Med. Parasitol.*, 66, 99, 1972.

298. Thomas, H. and Gönnert, R., The efficacy of praziquantel against cestodes in cats, dogs, and sheep, *Res. Vet. Sci.*, 24, 20, 1978.

299. Thomas, H. and Gönnert, R., Zur wirksamkeit von praziquantel bei der experimentellen cysticercose and hydatidose, *Z. Parasitol.*, 55, 165, 1978.

300. Thompson, W. M., Chisholm, D. P., and Tank, R., Plain film roentgenographic findings in alveolar hydatid disease — *Echinococcus multilocularis, Am. J. Roentgenol.*, 116, 345, 1972.

301. Thompson, R. C. A. and Smyth, J. D., Equine hydatidosis: a review of the current status in Great Britain and the results of an epidemiological survey, *Vet. Parasitol.*, 1, 107, 1975.

302. Todorov, T. and Stojanov, G., Circulating antibodies in human echinococcosis before and after surgical treatment, *Bull. WHO*, 57, 751, 1979.

303. Trejos, A., Szyfres. B., and Marchevsky, N., Comparative value of arecoline hydrobromide and bunamidine hydrochloride for the treatment of *Echinococcus granulosus* in dogs, *Res. Vet. Sci.*, 19, 212, 1975.

304. Varela-Diaz, V. M. and Coltorti, E. A., Further evidence of the passage of host immunoglobulins into hydatid cysts, *J. Parasitol.*, 58, 1015, 1972.

305. Varela-Diaz, V. M. and Marchevsky, N., Aspectos immunologicos del tratamiento biológico de la hidatidosis, *Zoonosis (Buenos Aires)*, 15, 20, 1973.

306. Varela-Diaz, V. M., Williams, J. F., Coltorti, E. A., and Williams, C. S. F., Survival of cysts of *Echinococcus granulosus* after transplant into homologous and heterologous hosts, *J. Parasitol.*, 60, 608, 1974.

307. Varela-Diaz, V. M., Lopez-Lemes, M. H., Prezioso, U., Coltorti, E. A., and Yarzábal, L. A., Evaluation of four variants of the indirect hemagglutination test for human hydatidosis, *Am. J. Trop. Med. Hyg.*, 24, 304, 1975.

308. Varela-Diaz, V. M., Coltorti, E. A., Prezioso, U., Lopez-Lemes, M. H., Guisantes, J. A., and Yarzábal, L. A., Evaluation of three immunodiagnostic tests for human hydatid disease, *Am. J. Trop. Med. Hyg.*, 24, 312, 1975.

309. Varela-Diaz, V. M., Coltorti, E. A., Ricardes, M. I., Prezioso, U., Schantz, P. M., and Garcia, R., Evaluation of immunodiagnostic techniques for the detection of human hydatid cyst carriers in field studies, *Am. J. Trop. Med. Hyg.*, 25, 617, 1976.

310. Varela-Diaz, V. M. and Coltorti, E. A., Tecnicas immunodiagnosticas para la hidatidosis humana, Centro Panamericano de Zoonosis, Oficina Sanitaria Panamericana, *Ser. Monograf.*, 7, 48, 1976.

311. Varela-Diaz, V. M., Eckert, J., Rausch, R. L., Coltorti, E. A., and Hess, U., Detection of the *Echinococcus granulosus* diagnostic arc 5 in sera from patients with surgically confirmed *E. multilocularis* infection, *Z. Parasitol.*, 53, 183, 1977.

312. Varela-Diaz, V. M., Coltorti, E. A., and D'Alessandro, A., Immunoelectrophoresis tests showing *Echinococcus granulosus* arc 5 in human cases of *Echinococcus vogeli* and cysticercosis-multiple myeloma, *Am. J. Trop. Med. Hyg.*, 27, 554, 1978.

313. Verster, A. J. M., Review of *Echinococcus* species in South Africa, *Onderstepoort J. Vet. Res.*, 32, 7, 1965.

314. Vervloet, D., Dumon, H., Quilici, M., and Charpin, J., Les IgE spécifiques dans l'hydatidose, *Rev. Fr. Allergol.*, 16, 73, 1976a.

315. Vervloet, D., Dumon, H., Quilici, M., and Charpin, J., Hydatidose pulmonaire dosage des IgE spécifiques répondant aux antigénes solubles et figurés du *Taenia* échinocoque, *Rev. Fr. Mal. Respir.*, 4, 975, 1976.

316. Vibe, P. P., Survival of *Echinococcus* eggs in the environment, *Vestn. Skh. Nauki Alma Ata*, 7, 75, 1968, as reprinted in *Helminthol. Abstr.*, 38, 1969.

317. Viñas, M., Echinococcosis alveolar humana en la Republica Argentina, *Accion Med. (Buenos Aires)*, 3, 535, 1932.

318. Vogel, H., Über den *Echinococcus multilocularis* Süddeutschlands. I. Das Bandwurmstadium von Stammen menschlicher und tierischer Herkunft, *Tropenmed. Parasitol.*, 8, 404, 1957.

319. Vogel, H., Über den *Echinococcus multilocularis* Süddeutschlands, II. Entwicklung der larvenstadien und histopathologische reaktion in der feldmaus *Microtus arvalis*, *Tropenmed. Parasitol.*, 28, 409, 1977.

320. West, J. D., Hillman, F. J., and Rausch, R. L., Alveolar hydatid disease of the liver: rationale and technics of surgical treatment, *Ann. Surg.*, 157, 548, 1963.

321. Wheeling, C. H., Carney, W. P., Cross, J. H., Purnomo, R., Sudomo, M., and Simandjuntah, G., A review of *Echinococcus ganulosus* in Southeast Asia and a report on a natural infection from Sulawesi, Indonesia, *Proc. 3rd. Int. Congr. Parasitol. (Facta, Vienna)*, 1, 552, 1974.

322. Williams, J. F., Recent advances in the immunology of cestode infections, *J. Parasitol.*, 65, 337, 1979.

323. Williams, J. F. and Trejos, A., The influence of gelatin capsules upon the activity of bunamidine hydrochloride against *Echinococcus* in dogs, *Res. Vet. Sci.*, 2(4), 392, 1970.

324. Williams, J. F., Adaros, H. L., and Trejos, A., Current prevalence and distribution of hydatidosis, with special reference to the Americas, *Am. J. Trop. Med. Hyg.*, 20, 224, 1971.

325. Williams, J. F., Perez Esandi, M. V., and Oriol, R., Evaluation of purified lipoprotein antigens of *Echinococcus granulosus* in the immunodiagnosis of human infection, *Am. J. Trop. Med. Hyg.*, 20, 575, 1971.

326. Williams, R. J. and Sweatman, G. K., On the transmission, biology and morphology of *Echinococcus granulosus equinus*, a new subspecies of hydatid tapeworm in horses in Great Britain, *Parasitology*, 53, 391, 1963.

327. Wilson, J. F., Diddams, A. C., and Rausch, R. L., Cystic hydatid disease in Alaska. A review of 101 autochthonous cases of *Echinococcus granulosus* infection, *Am. Rev. Respir. Dis.*, 98, 1, 1968.

328. Wilson, J. F., Davidson, M., and Rausch, R. L., A clinical trial of mebendazole in the treatment of alveolar hydatid disease, *Am. Rev. Resp. Dis.*, 118, 747, 1978.

329. Wilson, J. F. and Rausch, R. L., Alveolar hydatid disease. A review of clinical features of 33 indigenous cases of *Echinococcus multilocularis* infection in Alaskan Eskimos, *Am. J. Trop. Med. Hyg.*, 29, 1340, 1980.

330. Wobeser, G., The occurrence of *Echinococcus multilocularis* (Leuckart, 1863) in cats near Saskatoon, Saskatchewan, *Can. Vet. J.*, 12, 65, 1971.

331. Wolcott, M. W., Harris, S. H., and Briggs, J. N., Hydatid disease of the lungs, *J. Thorac. Cardiovasc. Surg.*, 62, 465, 1971.

332. Xanthakis, D., Efthimiadis, M., Papadakis, G., Primikirios, N., Chassapakis, G., Roussaki, A., Veranis, N., Akrivakis, A., and Aligizakis, C. J., Hydatid disease of the chest, *Thorax*, 27, 517, 1972.

333. Yamashita, J., Ohbayashi, M., and Konno, S., Studies on echinococcosis. V. Experimental infection of the sheep, *Jpn. J. Vet. Res.*, 5, 43, 1957.

334. Yarzabal, L. A., Leiton, J., and Lopez-Lemes, M. H., The diagnosis of human pulmonary hydatidosis by the immunoelectrophoresis test, *Am. J. Trop. Med. Hyg.*, 23, 662, 1974.

335. Yarzabal, L. A., Schantz, P. M., and Lopez-Lemes, M. H., Comparative sensitivity and specificity of the intradermal and immunoelectrophoresis tests for hydatid disease, *Am. J. Trop. Med. Hyg.*, 24, 843, 1975.

336. Yarzabal, L. A., Bout, D. T., Naquira, F. R., and Capron, A. R., Further observations on the specificity of antigen 5 of *Echinococcus granulosus*, *J. Parasitol.*, 63, 495, 1977.

337. Yong, W. K., Heath, D. D., and Parmeter, S. N., *Echinococcus granulosus, Taenia hydatigena, T. ovis:* evaluation of cyst fluids as antigen for serodiagnosis of larval cestodes in sheep, *N. Z. Vet. J.*, 26, 231, 1978.

338. Zanussi, C., Sorice, F., and Castagnari, L., Studio parellelo di diverse tecniche sierologiche nella diagnosi dell'idatidosi umana, *Boll. Ist. Sieroter. Milan.*, 45, 102, 1966.

339. Zerega Pendola, F., Hidatidosis alveolar, *Rev. Ecuatiana Higiene Med. Trop.*, 22, 115, 1965.

340. Zenkov, A. V., Some biological differences of *E. granulosus* from pigs and sheep (in Russian), *Tr. Vses. Inst. Gelmintol.*, 18, 89, 1971, as reprinted in *Helminthol. Abstr.*, 44, 474, 1975.

341. **Zhongxi, O., Shuyuan, G., Guoxue, T., Ruilin, L., Mingbai, W., Jun, Q., and Kurban,** Immediate and long-term results of surgical treatment of intrathoracic hydatid cysts, *Chin. Med. J.,* 93, 569, 1980.

342. **Zhongxi, O., Shuyuan, G., Guoxue, T., Ruilin, L., Mingbai, W., Jun, Q., and Kurban,** Evaluation of Barrett's technique in 167 cases of pulmonary hydatid cyst, *Chin. Med. J.,* 93(74), 577, 1980.

HYMENOLEPIS DIMINUTA INFECTION

Nonette L. Jueco

Common Synonyms

Rat tapeworm disease, hymenolepiasis diminuta.

Etiologic Agent

Hymenolepis diminuta (Rudolphi, 1819) Blanchard, 1891 (synonyms: *Taenia diminuta* Rudolphi, 1819; *H. flavopunctata* Weinland, 1858; *T. flavomaculata* Leuckart, 1863).[5,25] The "rat tapeworm."

H. diminuta is a common tapeworm of rats; the length varies from 100 to 600 mm depending upon the species of host, size of the small intestines, and other physical features of the intra-intestinal environment.[15] The proglottids number 800 to 1300. The scolex is globular with four cup-like suckers; the rudimentary rostellum is unarmed. The segments are wider than long, the maximum width of the gravid proglottids being 1.3 to 3.1 mm. Genital pores are usually unilateral. Normally there are three testes in each mature segment — one poral and two aporal — arranged more or less in a straight line across the segment separated by the ovary. Occasionally this arrangement is reversed. The ovary is bilobed. In the gravid segment the uterus hollows out sending diverticula to all directions; and in the fully developed state it has the appearance of a sac incompletely divided by partitions into egg capsules occupying nearly the entire space within the segment. Mature eggs are spherical or slightly oval. The outermost shell is thick, faintly striated, and yellowish brown in color; a thinner membrane often with two polar projections envelope the oncosphere. There is an intermediate layer between the outer shell and inner membrane composed of albuminous substance which has a granular appearance.[25]

True and Alternate Hosts

H. diminuta is found in the small intestines of rats, mice, man, and hamsters; it was once recovered from a dog.[5,16,21]

Insects which serve as obligatory intermediate hosts for this tapeworm include beetles (*Akis spinosa, Scaurus striatus, Tenebrio molitor, Dermestes peruvianus, Gootrupes, stercosus, Tribolium castaneum, T. confusum, Ulosonia parvicornis, Aphodius distinctus,* and *Stegobium paniccum);* cockroaches *(Blatta orientalis and Blatella germinica);* earwigs (*Anisolabis annulipes*); fleas (*Xenopsylla cheopis, Nosopsyllus fasciatus, Orchopeas wickhami, Ctenopsyllus musculi, Ctenocephalides canis* and *Pulex irritans*); lepidopterans (*Tinea granella, T. pollionella, Aglossa dimidiata, Aphornia gularis, Asopia farinalis*); mealworm (*Anisopia farinalis*); and the myriapods (*Fontaria virginiensis* and *Julius* sp.).

Eggs ingested by these various arthropods develop and metamorphose into a cysticercoid larva in the hemocoel.

Distribution

This common tapeworm of rats was first reported in man by Weinland in 1958. Since then, a number of human infections have been reported from different parts of the world. Countries which have reported human hymenolepiasis diminuta infections include Africa, Central Africa (3 cases), Argentina, Belgium, Brazil (1 case), Burma, Chile (11 cases), China, Colombia, Cuba, Ecuador, Granada, India, Indonesia (6 cases), Iran (0.33 to 1.1% prevalence), Italy, Japan, Martinique, Mexico (0.2 to 1.9%

prevalence in 6 to 15 years old), Nicaragua, Philippines (5 human cases and 64% prevalence in rats), Rhodesia (3 cases), U.S., U.S.S.R., and Venezuela.[3-12,14,18-23,25]

Disease in Animals

This common parasite of rats apparently does not produce any symptom or pathology. The parasite inhabits the small intestines of the host, specifically the duodenum. It has a motor system specifically coordinated to overcome the peristalsis and can recognize a specific region of the intestines.[2] The presence of this tapeworm lowers the intestinal pH to about 6.9 in the anterior half of the intestines. This is believed to be due to the acid secretion of the worm.[13] *H. diminuta* seems to live as long as the rat host and remains young in the sense that a high growth rate is maintained for an indefinite period.[16] By successive surgical transplantation it has even been shown to live for 14 years showing that its potential life span is long, far exceeding its rodent host. The tapeworm utilizes carbohydrates from the host's diet and the size of the worm is affected by the quality of carbohydrate eaten by the host. Starch is the most important carbohydrate needed by the parasite and the competition for the utilization of this carbohydrate is the limiting factor involved in determining the size of individual tapeworms in infections of varying intensity. The presence of other species of worms in the intestines also affects the size of the worm.[16] Although a competition for this carbohydrate has been shown between tapeworms of the same species and between worms of different species, it does not seem to compete with the host in the utilization of carbohydrates.[16]

Rats get infected by ingestion of the various arthropod intermediate hosts containing the cysticercoid larva. Eggs in rat feces which are ingested by the arthropod vectors develop into cysticercoid larvae in 7 to 8 days.[24] The prepatent period in rats is usually between 19 to 21 days.[15]

Disease in Man

Infection in man does not cause any serious pathology except for the absorption of the metabolic waste products of the parasite into the human host's system. Multiple infection in man is rare.

General Mode of Spread

Ingestion of the arthropod vectors harboring the cysticercoid larva causes infection of the definitive host. These arthropods, such as grain beetles, cockroaches and fleas, usually live in close association with rats and mice, the animal reservoir hosts. Rat droppings containing *H. diminuta* eggs are found in stored grains which in turn infect the grain beetles. Man gets infected by accidental ingestion of infected arthropod intermediate hosts.

Epidemiology

In nature, the epidemiological cycle is usually rat-insect-rat. Rats are more ideal definitive hosts than mice. The faster intestinal emptying time in mice affects the establishment of *H. diminuta* cysticercoid larvae in these animals which explains why *H. diminuta* only rarely occurs in house mice.[15] Infection in man is rare, usually less than 1 to 2% in countries where human cases have been reported.

Diagnosis

Diagnosis is by stool examination for *H. diminuta* eggs. The worm may at times be expelled spontaneously and diagnosis is based on the morphologic identification of the scolex, gravid segments, and eggs.

Prevention and Control

Preventive and control measures consist of elimination of rats and mice in houses; destruction of beetles, cockroaches, and other insects that act as intermediate hosts; protection of foods from insects; proper disposal of stools of infected persons; and treatment of human cases.

Treatment

Thelmesan® (dymanthine hydrochloride), Yomesan® (niclosamide), and quina-crine have been found effective in the treatment of *H. diminuta* infection.[1,5]

REFERENCES

1. **Alterio, O. L.**, Treatment of *Hymenolepis* infection with dymanthine hydrochoride, *Rev. Dras. Med.*, 25, 341, 1968.
2. **Braten, T. and Hopkins, C. A.**, The migration of *H. diminuta* in the rat intestines during normal development and following surgical transplantation, *Parasitology*, 59, 891, 1969.
3. **Chandler, A. C.**, The distribution of *Hymenolepis* infections in India with a discussion of its epidemiological significance, *Indian J. Med. Res.*, 14, 973, 1927.
4. **Cross, J. H., Gunawan, S., Gaba, A., Watten, R. H., and Sulianti, J.**, Survey for human intestinal and blood parasites in Bojolale, Central Java, Indonesia, *S.E. Asian J. Trop. Med. Pub. Health*, 1, 354, 1970.
5. **Faust, E. C., Russell, P. F., and Jung, R. C.**, *Craig and Faust's Clinical Parasitology*, 8th ed., Lea & Febiger, Philadelphia, 1970.
6. **Ghadirian, E. and Arfaa, F.**, Human infection with *Hymenolepis diminuta* in villages of Minok, southern Iran, *Int. J. Parasitol.*, 2, 481, 1972.
7. **Goldsmid, J. M.**, A note on the occurrence of *H. diminuta* (Rudolphi, 1819) Blanchard, 1891 (Cestoda) in Rhodesia, *Central Afr. J. Med.*, 19, 51, 1973.
8. **Jueco, N. L.**, personal communication, Dept. of Parasitology, Institute of Public Health, University of the Philippines, Manila, 1976.
9. **Lima, D. F., Froes, O. M., and Zingano, A. G.**, Intestinal helminth infections in the municipality of Campo Bon in the state of Rio Grande de Sul, Brazil, *Hospital Rio de Janeiro*, 78, 313, 1970.
10. **MacDonald, F. and Goldsmid, J. M.**, Intestinal helminth infection in the Burma Valley area of Rhodesia, *Cent. Afr. J. Med.*, 19, 113, 1973.
11. **McMillan, B., Kelly, Z., and Walker, J. C.**, Prevalence of *H. diminuta* infection in man in the New Guinea Highlands, *Trop. Geogr. Med.*, 23, 390, 1971.
12. **Meggit, K. and Subramanian, K.**, The tapeworms of rodents of the sub-family Murinae with special reference to those occurring in Rangoon, *J. Burma Res. Soc.*, 17, 189, 1927.
13. **Mettrick, D. F.**, *Hymenolepis diminuta*: pH changes in rat intestinal contents and worm migration, *Exp. Parasitol.*, 29, 386, 1971.
14. **Ransom, B. H.**, An account of the tapeworms of the genus Hymenolepis parasitic in man, *U.S. Publ. Health Mar. Hosp. Scrv. Hyg. Lab. Bull.*, 18, 1, 1904.
15. **Read, C. P. and Voge, M.**, The size attained by *H. diminuta* in different host species, *J. Parasitol.*, 40, 88, 1954.
16. **Read, C. P.**, The role of carbohydrates in the biology of Cestodes. VIII. Some conclusions and hypotheses, *Exp. Parasitol.*, 8, 365, 1959.
17. **Read, C. P.**, Longevity of the tapeworm, *Hymenolepis diminuta*, *J. Parasitol.*, 53, 1055, 1967.
18. **Reyes, H., Insunza, E., and Lloren, G.**, Frequency of human infection by *H. diminuta* in Santiago, Chile, 1957—71, *Bol. Chil. Parasitol.*, 27, 29, 1972.
19. **Riley, W. A. and Shannon, W. R.**, The rat tapeworm, *Hymenolepis diminuta*, in man, *J. Parasitol.*, 8, 109, 1922.
20. **Schwartz, B. and Tubangui, M.**, Uncommon intestinal parasites of man in the Philippine Islands, *Phil. J. Sci.*, 20, 611, 1922.
21. **Spindler, L. A.**, On the occurrence of the rat tapeworm (*H. diminuta*) and the dwarf tapeworm (*H. nana*) in man in Southwest Virginia, *J. Parasitol.*, 16, 38, 1929.
22. **Stiles, C. W. and Hassall, A.**, Key-catalogue of the worms reported for man, *U.S. Publ. Health Serv. Hyg. Lab. Bull.*, 142, 69, 1926.

23. **Vargas-Mena, J., Vasquez, J., and Montes, E.,** Frequency of intestinal parasites in the state of Nuevo Leon, Mexico. III. Stool examinations performed in 14 districts of the west of the state, *Rev. Lat. Am. Microbiol.,* 13, 213, 1971.

24. **Voge, M. and Heyneman, D.,** Development of *Hymenolepis nana* and *Hymenolepis diminuta* (Cestoda: Hymenolepididae) in the intermediate host *Tribolium confusum, Univ. Calif. Publ. Zool.,* 59, 549, 1957.

25. **Tubangui, M.,** Worm parasites of the brown rat (*Mus norvegicus*) in the Philippine Islands, with special reference to those forms that may be transmitted to human beings, *Phil. J. Sci.,* 46, 537, 1931.

HYMENOLEPIS NANA INFECTION

Nonette L. Jueco

Common Synonyms
Dwarf tapeworm disease, hymenolepiasis nana.

Etiologic Agent
Hymenolepis nana (v. Siebold, 1852) Blanchard, 1891. (Synonyms: *Taenia murina* Dujardin, 1845, *T. nana* v. Siebold, 1852; *H. fraterna* Stiles, 1906). The "dwarf tapeworm."

This tapeworm measures 5 to 90 mm long, often shorter, the size and length inversely proportional to the number of worms in the host. The minute scolex has four cup-like suckers; the short rostellum is armed with a ring of 20 to 30 spines. The maximum size of the proglottids is 0.15 to 0.3 mm in length by 0.8 to 1 mm in breadth. There is a single set of reproductive organs. In the mature segment, the distinguishing feature is the three testes, one on the left and two on the right side of the median line arranged in a more or less straight transverse line at the posterior portion of the proglottids. In the gravid segment, the uterus elongates, hollows out, and becomes completely filled up with eggs. The male reproductive organs disappear. The eggs are globular or oval, hyaline, measure 30 to 47 μm in diameter and contain an oncosphere enclosed in an inner envelope with two polar thickenings from which arise 4 to 8 polar filaments.[15,48]

True and Alternate Hosts
The definitive hosts are mice, rats, and, occasionally, man. There is experimental evidence to indicate that *H. nana* and *H. fraterna* differ physiologically but not morphologically. Some considered the occurrence of two strains: the human and the rat strains. The human strain probably is acquired from rodents just as the rat strain is derived from the mouse strain; but, after a generation or more in man, the worms probably become more infective for man than those directly from rats.[36]

Although *H. nana* normally has a direct life cycle in which the eggs are already infective to the next host, insects occasionally may serve as an intermediate host. The insect intermediate hosts include: *Ctenocephalides canis, Xenopsylla cheopis, Pulex irritans, Menephilus cylindricus, Spleophorus piceus, Tribolium confusum,* and *Tenebrio molitor*[13,14,44] The larva and the imago of *Tribolium* sp. can be infected with the gravid strobila *H. nana* and the cysticercoids develop in these insects to the infective stage.[27] Cockroaches (*B. germanica*) have also been found to support the development of the cysticercoid larvae when fed with *H. nana* eggs, the development being faster at temperatures 30 to 37°C.[17]

Distribution
H. nana is cosmopolitan in distribution and is just as common in cold as well as in warm countries. The prevalence of infection depends on the sanitary conditions of the environment and is higher in places where the sanitary conditions are poor or where there is over-crowding, such as in children's homes, orphanages, and other similar institutions. The countries where human infection has been reported are: Algeria (20% in children), Argentina (7 to 9% in children and 0.7 to 2.7% in adults), Brazil (5.9%),[3] Borneo (found in man but not in rats and mice),[36] Canada,[11] Chile (0.17%), Colombia (0.38%), Costa Rica (1.38% in children), Cuba (0.07%), Ecuador (6.94 to 30.0% in children),[30] Egypt (7 to 12% in children and infants),[12] Formosa (40% in children), Greece (16.6% in children and 1.16% in adults), Haiti (0.16%), India (3.2 to

20.0%),[10,35] Iran (4 to 27%, higher in children than in adults),[18,19,42] Italy (11.7%, incidence higher in urban than rural areas),[16,40] Japan,[33] Korea (12.9% in hospital patients, also present among Korean forces in South Vietnam),[23,24] Mexico (0.62 to 16.2%), Netherlands (in children),[26,46] New Guinea (one case in a child), Nicaragua (7.0%), Peru (3.17%), Philippines (found in children, 1.7% in rats),[21] Poland (in children),[38] Puerto Rico (0.10%), Rio de Janeiro,[6] Russia (3.8%, 16.3 to 58.3% in orphans), Sardinia (12.6% in children),[31,37] Senegal (8.9% in rural areas and 2.7% in urban areas, higher in children),[22] Sikkim (less than 1%),[32] Spain (12.9% in children), South Vietnam (less than 1%),[7] Sicily (34.5%), U.S. (1% in children), Venezuela (2.5%),[29] West Pakistan (in children),[5] and Yemen Arab Republic (13.0%).[15,34,41,45,47,49]

Disease in Animals

H. nana infection in mice and rats apparently do not cause any serious pathology or produce significant symptoms. The parasite consumes carbohydrate from the host's intestines but the amount needed by the parasite is not as much as to compete with the host's requirements. It may however compete with the host for other kinds of nutritional substances such as amino acids and vitamins.[39]

Disease in Man

The symptomatology of *H. nana* infection depends on the number of worms in the body. Metabolic wastes of the worms absorbed into the host's system may produce generalized toxemia. Large numbers of worms in the small intestines produce considerable irritation of the intestinal mucosa.[15] Ectopic localization of *H. nana* in man has been reported in Japan. A 19 mm long tapeworm was found in a tumor removed from the chest wall of a 75-year-old woman.[33] The potential for extra-intestinal migration and development of the larval stages was shown in animals other than the definitive hosts. Larval development occurred when eggs were inoculated in subcutaneous or intramuscular sites, and that intestinal enzymes were not necessary for hatching.[9,50] The development from egg to adult worm takes about 2 weeks. The infection may last for about 25 to 60 days after which the worm dies.[14] The persistence of infection in the host is due to autoinfection. In 26% of cases, infection persists for as long as 22 months.[5]

Mode of Spread

The eggs are already infective when passed out with the feces. When ingested, the eggs develop to the cysticercoid stage in the villi of the small intestines and become adults in about 2 weeks time. Indirect infection may take place when insects, such as fleas, grain beetles, mealworms, and cockroaches, ingest the eggs and develop into cysticercoid larvae in the insect's body. Infection may result from accidental ingestion of infected insects.

Epidemiology

H. nana of man is said to differ physiologically from *H. nana* var. *fraterna* of mice. But other investigators believe that the human and murine strains are identical as evidenced by the experiment where children were infected with eggs from murine sources and mice were infected with eggs from human sources.[25,52] The prevalence of human infection varies from place to place depending upon the sanitary conditions of the environment. Infection rates are higher in children than in adults, and more common in institutions such as children's homes and orphanages. Eggs of *H. nana* are infective immediately upon being laid; but they are quickly killed under natural conditions, thus suggesting that transmission is hand-to-mouth rather than through a rodent reservoir.[3]

Eggs do not survive long outside the body so that transmission is effected from person-to-person where gross contamination occurs between infected and noninfected. Young mice are more resistant to infection than mice 2 to 3 months old. The resistance of younger mice is due to the short length of its intestines as compared to older mice which expel the eggs before the cysticercoids can develop.[28] *H. nana* equally has the ability to elicit host resistance in as brief as 12 hr after ingestion of eggs lasting for 163 days. A local rapidly mobilized antibody reaction by the affected immediate cells could be responsible for the immune response.[20] Autoinfection is responsible for the persistence of the infection in the murine and human hosts. In an infected child, *H. nana* eggs, in varying degrees of development, and cercocysts may be present in the villi of the ileum suggesting that *H. nana* could perpetuate itself in the intestines of the same host.[47]

Diagnosis

Gravid segments rupture while still inside the intestines so that it is very rare to see the passage of gravid proglottids. Fecal concentration methods such as brine flotation, Kato, zinc sulfate flotation, and formalin-ether concentration, can be used for diagnosis.

Prevention and Control

Human infection is caused by ingestion of *H. nana* eggs or infected intermediate hosts such as fleas, beetles, mealworms, or cockroaches. Personal hygiene is important. Foods should be kept out of the reach of rats and mice, especially foods that are eaten raw, or, after cooking, are kept for some time before being eaten. Stored grains or cereals should be protected from grain beetle infestations. Rats and mice in domestic dwellings should be eliminated to prevent the possibility of human infection from murine sources. Proper human excreta disposal is important.

Treatment

The different drugs used for the treatment of this infection are: Yomesan® (niclosamide), reported to have a cure rate of 91 to 100%;[1,29] Acranil, 96% effective;[8] Thelmesan, has a cure rate of 81% but with side effects of nausea and vomiting in some children;[45] Emetine hydrochloride, cures the infection in man, 100% effective in mice but too risky to use in man;[11,43] Paromomycin sulfate (Humatin), cure rate up to 92%;[43] and Jonit, which has a cure rate of 67 to 95%.[35]

It must be remembered however that, due to autoinfection, the treatment of patients using current anticestode drugs may be effective under conditions of successive influence on new generations; that is, it must be for long terms and the intervals between treatment should not exceed 7 days.[4] In the presence of adult *H. nana*, the emergence and rate of development of subsequent generations are inhibited considerably. The appearance of new *H. nana* in patients after treatment is due to the emergence of new generations of cysticercoids from the villi of the small intestines.

REFERENCES

1. **Ahkami, S. and Hajian, A.,** Radical treatment of *H. nana* with niclosamide, *Am. J. Trop. Med. Hyg.,* 73, 258, 1970.
2. **Alonzo Fiel, R., Sotolongo, F., Jaime, A., Soto Travieso, R., Perello, A., and Quintana, S.,** Findings in the contents of the terminal ileum obtained by Miller-Abbott found in human case of *H. nana* infection, *Rev. Cub. Med. Trop.,* 18, 47, 1966.

3. **Artigas, P. T., Perez, M. D., Otsuko, J. M., and Mishimori, G.,** Parasitological studies, in particular of *S. mansoni* infection, in the cities of Itanhaem and Mongagua (southern coast of the state of Sao Paulo, Brazil), *Rev. Saude Pub.,* 4, 35, 1970.

4. **Bayandina, D. G.,** On the problem of causes of relapses in *Hymenolepis* infections (Russian with English summary), *Medskaya Parazitol.,* 40, 137, 1971.

5. **Buscher, H. N. and Haley, A. S.,** Epidemiology of *H. nana* infection of Puyabi Villagers in West Pakistan, *Am. J. Trop. Med. Hyg.,* 21, 42, 1972.

6. **Camillo-Coura, L., Soli, A. V., de Carvalho, H. T., and Rodriguez de Silva, J.,** Treatment of taeniasis (*H. nana*) with a derivate of salicylamide, *Hospital Rio de Janeiro,* 69, 93, 1966.

7. **Colwell, E. J., Welsh, J. D., Bome, S. C., and Legters, L. J.,** Intestinal parasitism in residents of the Mekong delta of Vietnam, *S.E. Asian J. Trop. Med. Pub. Health,* 2, 25, 1971.

8. **Del Trono, L.,** *Hymenolepis nana* and its mass treatment, *Geoin. di Malatti Infect. Parasittol.,* 13, 126, 1961.

9. **Di Conza, J. J.,** Hatching requirements of dwarf tapeworm eggs (*H. nana*) in relation to extraintestinal development of larval stages in man, *Z. Parasitkd.,* 31, 276, 1968.

10. **Dikshit, S. K. and Lalit, O. P.,** Hymenolepiasis in childhood and its treatment by indigenous drugs, *Indian J. Med. Res.,* 58, 616, 1970.

11. **Eaton, R. D. P.,** Emetine in hymenlepiasis nana, *Trans. R. Soc. Trop. Med. Hyg.,* 63, 153, 1969.

12. **El Gholmy, A., Khalifa, A. S., Rifaat, M., Salem, S., and Moustafa, S.,** Parasitic infestation in Egyptian infants and children, *Am. J. Trop. Med. Hyg.,* 71, 216, 1968.

13. **El-Refaii, A. H., Hieppe, T., Nickel, S., and Ribbeck, R.,** A new potential intermediate host for tapeworm *H. nana* Siebold, 1853, *Acta Parasitol. Pol.,* 21, 263, 1973.

14. **Farris, E. J. and Griffith, J. Q., Jr.,** *The Rat in Laboratory Investigation,* 2nd ed., J. B. Lippincott, Philadelphia 1949.

15. **Faust, E. C., Russell, P. F., and Jung, R. C.,** *Clinical Parasitology,* 8th ed., Lea & Febiger, Philadelphia, 1970.

16. **Foresi, C. and Equi, A.,** Investigations on the epidemiology of hymenolepiasis. Second report. Spread of *H. nana* in animals in the urban zone of Piza, *Arch. Ital. Sci. Med. Trop. Parassitol.,* 49, 43, 1968.

17. **Furukawa, T.,** German cockroaches (*Blattella germanica*) as an intermediate host of *Hymenolepis nana, Jpn. J. Parasitol.,* 19, 482, 1970.

18. **Ghadirian, E., Arfaa, F., and Joussefi, A.,** Studies on intestinal helminthiasis in the south of Iran. I. The Bandar Abbas and Minab areas, *Iran J. Pub. Health,* 1, 50, 1972.

19. **Ghadirian, E. and Missaghian, G. H.,** Studies on intestinal helminthiasis in the south of Iran. II. The areas of Kazeroun, Borazjan and Bandar Bushehr, *Iran J. Pub. Health,* 1, 126, 1973.

20. **Heyneman, D., Studies of helminth immunity.** V. Rapid onset of resistance by the white mouse against a challenging infection with eggs of *H. nana* (Cestoda: Hymenolepididae), *J. Immunol.,* 88, 217, 1962.

21. **Jueco, N. L.,** personal observation, Department of Parasitology, Institute of Public Health, University of the Philippines, Manila, 1976.

22. **Juminer, B., Diallo, S., and Laurens, D.,** Parasitological survey in a community in the Sine Valley, Senegal, *Bull. Soc. Pathol. Exot.,* 64, 901, 1971.

23. **Kim, G. S.,** An epidemiological analysis on parasite infection among the patients of Chonnam National University Hospital, *Korean J. Pub. Health,* 6, 325, 1969.

24. **Kim, J. H., Yoon, J. J., Lie, S. H., and Seo, B. S.,** Parasitological studies of Korean forces in South Vietnam. II. A comparative study on the incidences of intestinal parasites, *Korean J. Parasitol.,* 8, 30, 1970.

25. **Kiribayashi, S.,** Studies on the growth of *Hymenolepis nana* with special reference to the possibility of differentiation of *H. nana* var. *fraterna, Taiwan Igakkai Zasski,* 32, 1175, 1933.

26. **Kleewans, J. W. L. and Lee Haas, R. A.,** A case of *H. nana* in Netherlands New Guinea, *Trop. Geogr. Med. Amsterdam,* 11, 376, 1959.

27. **Lang, N. N. and Berezhnaya, V. G.,** On the role of intermediate hosts in the epidemiology of *Hymenolepis* infections (Russian with English summary), *Medskaya Parazitol.,* 37, 85, 1968.

28. **Larsh, J. E., Jr.,** The relationship between the intestinal size of young mice and their susceptibility to infection with the cestode, *H. nana* var. *fraterna, J. Parasitol.,* 29, 61, 1943.

29. **Latuff, H., Yamin, G., and Gonzalez, R.,** The treatment of *H. nana* infections in children with Yomesan®, *Arch. Venezolanos Puericult. Pediatr.,* 26, 368, 1963.

30. **Lopez Ortiz, R.,** Incidence of intestinal parasites in Bahia de Caraquez and surrounding areas of the Province of Manabi, *Rev. Ecuat. Hig. Med. Trop.,* 26, 133, 1969.

31. **Masia, C., Maida, A., and Muresu, E.,** Investigations into the prevalence of intestinal parasites in subjects aged 0 to 14 years permanently resident in institutions in the town of Sassari, Sardinia, *Muovi Ann. Ig. Microbiol.,* 22, 262, 1971.

RAILLIETINA INFECTION

Nonette L. Jueco

Common Synonym
Raillietiniasis.

Etiologic Agent
Raillietina infection could be caused by any of the several species of tapeworms belonging to the genus *Raillietina* Fuhrmann, 1920. Several species have been involved in human infections.[5]

Raillietina celebensis (Janicki, 1902) Fuhrmann, 1920 (Synonyms: *Davainea formosana* Akashi, 1916; *Davainea celebensis* Janicki, 1902); *R. dermerariensis* (Daniels, 1895) Dollfus, 1939—1940 (Synonyms: *Taenia demerariensis* Daniels, 1895; *Davainea madagascariensis* of Davila, 1922; *R. quitensis* L. A. Leon, 1935; *R. luisaleoni* Dollfus, 1939; *R. equatoriensis* Dollfus, 1939; *R. leoni* Dollfus, 1939); *R. asiatica* (v. Lonstow, 1901) Stiles and Hassall, 1926; *R. garrisoni* Tubanqui, 1913 [Synonym: *Davainea madagascariensis* (Davaine) of Garrison, 1911]; and *R. siriraji* Chandler and Pradatsundarasar, 1957 (Synonym: *T. madagascariensis* Davaine, 1870).

Tapeworms of the genus *Raillietina* are common intestinal cestodes of rodents and monkeys. The worm measures about 60 cm long; the scolex is very tiny, subglobular with four suckers. The rostellum is armed with hammer-shaped hooks arranged in two alternating rows. The number of hooks varies from 80 to 82 or 90 to 140 depending on the species. The rostellum is also surrounded by several rows of comma-shaped spines, while the four suckers may or may not be armed with several rows of minute spines. The segments are broader than long, except at the posterior end where the gravid proglottids are longer than wide. Genital pores are normally unilateral and dextral, situated near the anterior extremity of the lateral border of the segments. Testes number about 36 to 54. The fully gravid segments are about 2 mm in length and contain 200 to 400 egg capsules. Each egg capsule in turn contains 1 to 4 elongated or spindle-shaped eggs. The gravid segments detach from the rest of the strobila by apolysis and may be passed out with the feces of infected individuals. The segments are opaque white in color, and appear like grains of rice.[4,13]

True and Alternate Hosts
The usual definitive hosts are rodents (viz., rats, squirrels, cotton rats, etc.) and howler monkeys; man is only an accidental host.[4,5,13] The life cycle of the various *Raillietina* species that have been reported to cause infection in man has not been thoroughly studied. It is suspected that household insects, such as cockroaches and beetles *Tribolium confusum*, may serve as intermediate hosts.[2,10]

Distribution
Countries where human cases of *Raillietina* infections have been reported include: Southeast Africa, Australia (1 case of *R. celebensis*), Batavia, British Guiana (1 case), Cuba (3 cases of *R. demerariensis*), Ecuador (5% of patients with *R. demerariensis*), Formosa (1 case of R. celebensis), North Iran (1 case of *R. asiatica*), Japan (1 case of *R. celebensis*), Madagascar region (Comeres Island, Mauritius Island — 2 cases), Philippines (20 cases of *R. garrisoni*), Russian Turkestan, and Thailand (11 cases of *R. siriraji*).[1-6,8,11,12,13]

Disease in Animals
The disease in animals has not been described.

Disease in Man

The majority of reported human cases have been confined to young children 5 years old and below. The tapeworms are usually spontaneously expelled without drug administration.[4,8] Two cases were admitted to the hospital with chief complaints of diarrhea and passage of "cucumber-like seeds" in the stools.[2] The incubation period is not known. Man is only an accidental host of *Raillietina* sp. This may serve to explain the spontaneous expulsion even without treatment of this parasite from its human host presumably because it is not biologically adapted to man.

Mode of Spread

Unknown.

Epidemiology

Raillietinae are common tapeworms of rodents, especially the rat *Rattus norwegicus*. Since the life cycle of these tapeworms has not been adequately studied, it is not known definitely how man acquires the infection. Attempts have been made to study the life cycle by feeding gravid segments to cockroaches.[2] Flour beetles have been fed with gravid segments of *R. garrisoni* obtained from rats. Cysticercoid larvae developed in these infected beetles in 2 to 3 weeks.[10] Rats probably acquire the infection by ingestion of the arthropod vectors harboring the cysticercoid.

Diagnosis

Diagnosis is made by the finding of gravid segments or strobila passed with the feces. The segments appear like "cucumber seeds" or "rice grains". The segments are about 2 mm in length and contain from 200 to 400 egg capsules. Each egg capsule contains 1 to 4 spindle-shaped or elongated eggs.

Prevention and Control

No definite preventive measure can be adopted except the destruction of rats, mice, and household insect pests, proper disposal of stools, and the practice of all-around hygiene.

Treatment

Dithiazanine iodide has been tried and found effective against *Raillietina* infection. Atabrine and bithionol have been used successfully in the treatment of *R. garrisoni.*[9]

REFERENCES

1. **Africa, C. H. and Garcia, E. Y.,** A rat tapeworm (*R. garrisoni*) transmissible to man, *Phil. J. Pub. Health*, 1, 44, 1935.
2. **Arrekul, S. and Radomyos, P.,** Preliminary report of *Raillietina* sp. infection in man and rats in Thailand, *S.E. Asian J. Trop. Med. Pub. Health*, 1, 559, 1970.
3. **Baer, J. G. and Sandars, E. E.,** The first record of *R. celebensis* (Janicki, 1902), (Cestoda) in man from Australia, with a critical survey of previous cases, *J. Helminthol.*, 30, 173, 1956.
4. **Chandler, A. C. and Pradatsundarasar, A.,** Two cases of *Raillietina* infection in infants in Thailand, with a discussion of the taxonomy of the species of Raillietina (Cestoda) in man, rodents and monkey, *J. Parasitol.*, 43, 81, 1957.
5. **Faust, E. C., Russell, P. F., and Jung, R. C.,** *Craig and Faust's Clinical Parasitology*, 8th ed., Lea & Febiger, Philadelphia, 1970.
6. **Garrison, P. E.,** Davainea madagascariensis (Davaine) in the Philippine Islands, *Philipp. J. Sci.*, 6, 165, 1911.

7. **Hsieh, H., Maa, Y., and Chen, T.,** The treatment of *Raillietina madagascariensis* with dithiazanine iodide, *J. Formosan Med. Assoc.,* 55, 258, 1959.

8. **Jueco, N. L.,** *Raillietina* (a rat tapeworm) infection in young children in the Philippines, *Acta Med. Philipp.,* 11, 49, 1975.

9. **Jueco, N. L.,** Zoonosis Associated with Rodents, unpublished.

10. **Jueco, N. L. and Cruzada, S. F.,** The role of certain arthropods in the transmission of *Raillietina garrisoni,* research in progress.

11. **Pradatsundarasar, A.,** Nine cases of *Raillietina* infection in Bangkok, *J. Med. Assoc. Thailand,* 43, 56, 1960.

12. **Stransky, E. and Lorenzo, A. S.,** On raillietiniasis in the Philippines, *Acta Tropica,* 17, 80, 1960.

13. **Tubangui, M. A.,** Worm parasites of the brown rat (*Mus norvegicus*) in the Philippine Islands, with special reference to those forms that may be transmitted to human beings, *Philipp. J. Sci.,* 46, 537, 1931.

SPARGANOSIS

James J. Daly

Common Synonyms
Sparganosis, Plerocercoidosis, Ligulosis.

Etiologic Agents
Dubium erinacei-europaei (Rudolphi, 1819), genotype, *erinacei-europaei, Bothriocephalis felis* (Creplin, 1825; Southwell, 1928), *B. maculatus* (Leuckart, 1848), *Dibothrium decipiens* (Diesing, 1850), *D. serratum* (Diesing, 1850), *Ligula reptans* (Diesing, 1850), *Sparganum reptans* (Diesing, 1854), *S. affine* (Diesing, 1854), *S. erinacei-europaei* (Diesing, 1854), *L. ranarum* (Gastaldi, 1854), *Bothriocephalus sulcatus* (Molin, 1858), *S. ellipticum* (Molin, 1858), *L. pancerii* (Polonio, 1860), *B. decipiens* (Railliet, 1866), *L. mansoni* (Cobbold, 1882), *B. liguloides* (Leuckart, 1886), *B. mansoni* (Blanchard, 1888), *D. mansoni* (Ariola, 1900), *S. mansoni* (Stiles and Taylor, 1902), *Plerocercoides prolifer* (Ijima, 1905), *S. proliferum* (Stiles, 1906),[184] *S. baxteri* (Sambon, 1907),[3] *Gatesius proliferum* (Stiles, 1908),[184] *P. mansoni* (Guiart, 1910), *S. raillieti* (Ratz, 1912), *S. philippinensis* (Tubangui, 1924), *S. canis* (Fernandez and Vogelsang, 1935),[58] *S. okapiae* (Fain, 1948),[55] *S. ameiva* (Vogelsang and Gallo, 1949),[195] *S. fernandezi* (Vogelsang and Gallo, 1949),[195] and *S. cuniculi* (Lizcano Herrera, 1958).[111]

Diphyllobothrium decipiens (Gedoelst, 1911), *D. raillieti* (Ratz, 1913), *D. longicolle* (Parodi and Widakowich, 1917), *D. tangalongi* (MacCallum, 1921), *D. reptans* (Meggitt, 1924), *D. ranarum* (Meggitt, 1925), *D. bresslauei* (Baer, 1927), *D. gracile* (Baer, 1927), *D. mansoni* (Joyeux and Houdemer, 1927), *D. felis* (Southwell, 1928), *D. houghtoni* (Faust, Campbell, and Kellog, 1929), *D. erinacei* (Faust, Campbell, and Kellog, 1929), *D. okumurai* (Faust, Campbell, and Kellog, 1929), *D. fausti* (Vialli, 1931), *D. serpentis* (Yamaguti, 1935), *D. Mansonoides* (Mueller, 1935), *D. urichi* (Cameron, 1936), *D. parvum* (Fain, 1947),[54] *Lueheella pretoriensis* (Baer, 1924),[6] *Spirometra janickii* (Furmaga, 1953,[61] and *Spirometra theileri* (Opuni and Muller, 1974; n. comb. from *D. theileri,* Baer, 1925).[147] (Unless specifically cited, refer to References 196, 202).

Sparganosis is an infection of the tissues of vertebrates by the plerocercoid stage of certain pseudophyllidean tapeworms. The adult forms of these tapeworms are generally found in the intestinal lumen of domestic, feral, or wild canids and felids. The infective plerocercoid is called a sparganum, a term originally used to describe any unknown pseudophyllidean larva. Spargana do not have adequate morphological characteristics for differentiation, therefore they must be fed to a definitive host (dog or cat) to grow to adult tapeworms which have morphological differences that can be used for taxonomic separation. Unfortunately, the variability in adult morphology as well as lack of communication and agreement among investigators, has led to confusion about the classification of this group of tapeworms. This has resulted in a large number of generic and specific synonyms for the etiologic agent of sparganosis in different parts of the world. To clarify this variety of synonyms the following summary is presented.

The first sparganum found in vertebrate tissue was observed by Rudolphi in 1815 and was found in the European hedgehog, *Erinaceus europeus.* Thereafter, generic names such as *Dubium, Sparganum, Ligula,* and *Plerocercoides,* indicative of larval forms, were used to describe tissue phases found in other vertebrates. Early in the 20th century the adult forms from carnivores were being described as *Diphyllobothrium* spp. with associations being made with spargana as part of the life cycle of these worms. Several workers thereafter experimentally infected definitive hosts with spargana and described the resulting adult forms.

In 1937, Mueller erected the genus *Spirometra*, (a term used earlier by Faust and co-workers)[56] which he separated from *Diphyllobothrium* primarily by the relationships of the cirrus, vagina, and genital atrium in adult proglottids.[129] *Spirometra* has become the most commonly used descriptor for this group of tapeworms in the present literature. However, it has been pointed out that the correct taxonomic usage is that of the genus *Lueheella* used by Baer in 1924 for an African tapeworm with similar characteristics to Mueller's *Spirometra*.[6,162] Recently, a plea has been made to overrule the code of The International Commission on Zoological Nomenclature in favor of *Spirometra*, presumably because of its overwhelming usage relative to other generic names.[180] Two major sources for tapeworm taxonomy have used *Spirometra*[196,202] and this review shall refer to these worms as such. Nevertheless, because of this disorder *Spirometra*, *Diphyllobothrium*, and infrequently *Lueheella* can all be found in the recent sparganosis literature to describe essentially the same group of organisms.

A large number of spirometrid species have been described from adult forms. As with generic classification, speciation is also uncertain because the morphological characteristics used to separate these organisms have been found to be quite variable.[62] In earlier reports, weight was attached to geographic area as well as definitive and intermediate host uniqueness. These are probably not valid since certain forms (*Spirometra mansoni* and *S. mansonoides*) are sometimes found in the same geographic regions[138] and, insofar as hosts are concerned, spargana are notoriously unselective when invading vertebrate tissue while adults can be raised in different host species. In recent years, investigators have pragmatically tended to ascribe the etiologic agent of human and animal sparganosis to only a few spirometrid species. In the vast majority of these cases only the sparganum form is known and an opinion as to species is usually based on the general nature of the plerocercoid, knowledge of adult forms in hosts from that area, or previously reported sparganosis cases from that area. The most commonly used names have been *Spirometra mansoni*, *S. mansonoides*, *S. theileri*, and *S. erinacei-europaei*.

Morphology

Spargana are flat, slender, white worms that are long and ribbon-like (Figure 1). The anterior end (scolex) ranges from being slightly enlarged with dimpling to being bulbous with a cup-shaped groove on the crown. Invaginations are sometimes seen representing the bothria of the adult tapeworm. Transverse striations on the sparganum surface may be present giving a false impression of segmentation (pseudosegmentation). The general appearance of spargana may vary. Forms obtained in the Far East are more massive but much more fragile than spargana from other geographic areas. Longitudinal splitting of the body may sometimes occur resulting in bi- or triradiate forms which nevertheless develop into normal tapeworms when fed to a definitive host.[134]

There is a rare proliferating form of sparganum (*Sparganum proliferum*) in which the larvae reproduce in the intermediate host by uncontrolled division and metastasize to almost every tissue. These spargana are very irregular in symmetry and lack a scolex. Histological examination shows a loss of ordered growth as evidenced by poor development and lack of differentiation of the two sets of internal muscles.[130]

Spargana develop from procercoids measuring approximately 70 to 300 μm in length and can be found in vertebrate tissue as short as a few millimeters. Most usually they are found as elongate forms ranging from 1 to 36 cm in length and several millimeters in width. Spargana as long as 80 cm have been reared in laboratory mice[134] and spargana from human infections have been reported to be as long as 25 to 36 cm.[19] As a

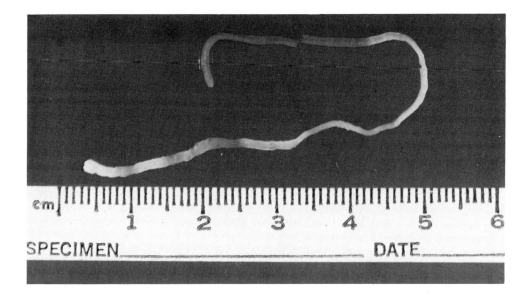

FIGURE 1.   Sparganum taken from a nodule removed from the right thigh of a patient in Little Rock, Arkansas.

rule, spargana 4 to 10 cm by 1 to 3 mm appear to be average size for most worms removed from vertebrate tissue. Some representative lengths of spargana from various vertebrates are: frog, 8.5 cm;[120] snake, 6 cm;[160] marsupial mouse, 20 cm;[118] okapi, 15 cm;[55] pig, 5 to 8 cm;[5] baboon, 1 to 31 cm;[105] and green monkey, 2.5 to 13 cm.[124] Proliferating spargana from a human have been descibed as 3 to 12 mm in length and lacking a scolex.[84]

In the definitive host adult spirometrids are small to medium sized pseudophyllidean tapeworms. They range in body length from the small *S. gracile* (7 to 8 cm) to the larger *S. mansonoides* specimens (1.5 m — exceptional) and *S. Janickii* (1 m).[7,61,135,196] Usually the length ranges from 25 cm (*S. mansonoides*) to 100 to 115 cm (*S. ranarum, S. reptans,* and *S. serpentis*).[120,121,201] Proglottid width varies from 1 to 12 mm with the length to width ratio differing among the various species. Adult spirometrids can be differentiated from other pseudophyllids by the morphology of the proglottids. The vagina and cirrus openings are independent rather than meeting in a common sinus. A general recognition feature is the uterus being organized as a spiral of closely compressed coils unlike the rosette-type uterus seen in *Diphyllobothrium* spp. The spirometrid scolex is elongate, spoon- or finger-shaped with bothrial lips attenuated along the free margin. The bothrial slits are broad and shallow.

The eggs of spirometrids are typically pseudophyllidean, having a single shell with an inconspicuous operculum at one end. Most spirometrid eggs have measured 55 to 66 μm in length to 27 to 41 μm in width (averages) with the smallest dimensions (40 × 20 μm) recorded for *S. tangalongi*.[114] The eggs tend to be elongate ovals with somewhat pointed ends helping to differentiate them from *Diphyllobothrium* ova which are slightly larger and more round. The eggs are yellow to brownish in color. Recovery and examination of proglottids and ova from the definitive host should identify the tapeworm as *Spirometra* sp.

Life Cycle

The adult tapeworms live in the intestine of a cat, dog, or similar carnivore and produce operculated eggs which pass out with the feces (Figure 2). Upon contact with

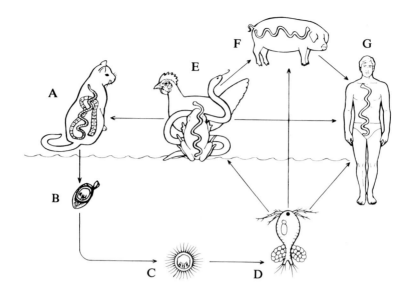

FIGURE 2.   The life cycle of *Spirometra* sp. illustrating the variety of infectious routes to human and animal hosts. (A) Definitive host, a cat or other suitable carnivore. (B) Operculated ovum. (C) Free-swimming coracidium. (D) Procercoid in first intermediate host *(Cyclops* sp.). (E) Second intermediate hosts. (F) Pig, or other omnivore, as a second intermediate or paratenic host. (G) Human infection acquired from ingestion of a procercoid, a plerocercoid, or from wound exposure to animal flesh infected with plerocercoids. (Modified from Mueller.[135])

water ciliated coracidia hatch from the eggs and the free-swimming larvae are eaten by the first intermediate host, a copepod crustacean, usually a *Cyclops* sp. The ingested coracidium invades the hemocoel of the copepod and grows into a vermiform procercoid. The procercoid matures and the copepod is swallowed by the drinking activity of a vertebrate intermediate host. Intermediate hosts have been found to include large numbers of species of amphibians, reptiles, and mammals, both small and large, as well as birds. The procercoid penetrates the intestinal villi of the second intermediate host and is carried to adipose, connective, or subcutaneous tissue to become the long, slender plerocercoid. If the tissue containing the plerocercoid is eaten by other than a definitive host, the plerocercoid penetrates the intestine and reestablishes itself in the tissues of the new paratenic host. The cycle is complete when the plerocercoid is consumed by a definitive host to develop into an adult tapeworm.

The first life cycle of a spirometrid was completed in 1919 and since that time there has been an increasing experimental interest in this group of tapeworms. Although speciation of this group of tapeworms is clouded, there are probably different species with minor differences regarding their life cycles. Nevertheless, certain generalities can be made about the group as a whole. Maturation of eggs is dependent upon temperature with the ova embryonating faster at warmer (37°C) than lower temperatures.[108] At ambient laboratory temperatures hatching time ranges from 7 to 120 days with 10 to 21 days appearing average.[10,131 134,187] Eggs from older infections appear less viable and slower to hatch. Free-swimming coracidia can survive 1 to 2 days and their infection of the copepod seems due to the feeding habits of the host since infection rate appears to be related to density of the coracidium population.[108,134] The nauplii and young adults of *Cyclops* are more susceptible than the older forms.[131] *Cyclops* are capable of ingesting numerous coracidia (up to 40 to 60) but average 3 to 4 per copepod without severely affecting the viability of the host. Penetration of the oncosphere into the hemocoel cavity of *Cyclops* occurs within 25 to 240 min.[108,145] The infective procercoid then takes 3 to 21 days (temperature dependent) to develop, growing to a length of about 200 to 300 μm.[10,108,131,145,147] Laboratory animals develop plerocercoid (spargana) infections when they are orally fed infected *Cyclops.* Frogs, tadpoles and mice are favored experimental second intermediate hosts because of their susceptibility. Spargana can be found as early as 5 to 7 days in the body cavity or tissues of these animals but are usually found from 12 to 22 days after procercoids are ingested.[65,108,131,177,187,207] Infection rates vary based on the number of ingested procercoids but 80 to 100% infectivity has been obtained by intraperitoneal injection rather than *per os.*[148] Infection through unbroken skin of mice by procercoids has been demonstrated but is in dispute.[108,134]

Procercoids penetrate the intestine and break out to the abdominal cavity and become spargana (sparganules) when about 1 mm long. Some, however, fail to penetrate the visceral peritoneum and instead form cysts in the gut wall. From the body cavity the spargana migrate to the subcutaneous tissues and increase in size. Migration to internal organs is rare but extensive liver invasion has been noted in tadpoles and frogs.[130] Growth of spargana in tissue is at a steady arithmetic rate with *S. theileri* in mice increasing its length 27 mm/week for 8 weeks.[147] Spargana can survive for long periods in host tissue with some human infections observed for 8 to 12 years.[186] Spargana surviving 16 years of transfers in experimental hosts have produced normal adult tapeworms.[136] The scolex of the sparganum is necessary to successfully transfer the infection to a paratenic or definitive host.

Plerocercoids are infective to a definitive host after as little as 4½ days in the second intermediate host.[135] When fed to the definitive host the sparganum establishes itself in the small intestine with the site dependent upon age of the host. The anterior portion near the pyloric valve is favored in kittens and the middle third is preferred in older cats.[134] Although small (young) spargana are capable of producing adult worms, patency with these forms is longer with eggs being found after 17 to 26 days as compared to 11 days when hosts are fed older, larger spargana.[134] Up to ten adult tapeworms have been established experimentally in a single cat. These worms show a crowding effect by their smaller size.[134] In nature, 1 to 2 adults per host seems average although up to 200 have been found in one host.[85] Adult spirometrids are shorter-lived than spargana with the maximum survival date noted with *S. mansonoides* in cats as 3 years 7 months.[135]

Duality of host can occur with potential definitive hosts also serving as intermediate hosts. This has been observed in cats, dogs, hyenas, raccoon dogs, foxes, civet cats, and raccoons. Sparganosis has experimentally been established in cats by feeding them procercoids but only adult tapeworms will develop when cats are fed plerocercoids. Dogs, however, have been shown to develop sparganosis when fed either procercoids or plerocercoids, as well as developing adult tapeworms when fed plerocercoids.[38] The reason for the duality in dogs is not clear but it has been suggested that plerocercoids in gut tissue may migrate back out to the intestinal lumen to become tapeworms.[38]

True and Alternate Hosts
First Intermediate Host

The first successful experimental infection of a copepod (*Cyclops leuckarti*) with spirometrid-type coracidia was reported in Japan by Okumura in 1919.[145] Since then a number of *Cyclops* species have been shown capable of serving as the initial copepod host for these worms. Infection of local cyclops with native *Spirometra* has been demonstrated with *Cyclops leukarti, C. viridis, C. bicuspidatus,* and *C. vernalis* in the U.S.,[131,134] in nine *Cyclops* species in Japan,[205] eight in China,[107] two in Indochina,[92] one in Indonesia,[67] several species in the Philippines,[1] and five species in Australia including the genera *Mesocyclops, Leptocyclops,* and *Pachycyclops.*[9,10,177]

Second Intermediate and Paratenic Hosts

Spargana are ubiquitous parasites that are world-wide in distribution and have been observed many times in the tissues of wild and domestic animals. Infections have been found in hosts representing most vertebrate classes with fish being a possible exception. The following is a generalized list of these hosts, both natural and experimental (excluding man) grouped by host geographic area.

1.   North America: black bear; raccoon; opposum; pig; gray, silver, black, and red foxes; white-footed field mouse; otter; domestic rabbit; mice; alligator; and 8 species of snakes[13,37,41,75,117,128,131,133,190]

2.   South America: goat; raccoon; crab-eating fox; opposum; dog; South American fox; grison; river otter; hog-nosed skunk; Argentine field mouse; Norwegian rat; brown rat; thick-tailed opposum; cuckoo (*Aves*); seven species of snake; jungle-runner lizard; and nest-building frog[45,74,113,170,195,200]

3.   Europe: hedgehog; rabbit; pig; common shrew; 2 species of white-toothed shrews; water shrew; Norwegian rat; 2 species of field mice (*Apodemus* sp.); European polecat; crow; frog; watersnake; and four species of zoo snakes imported from Thailand[51,69,111,144,171]

4.   Africa: green monkey; vervet; baboon; lemur; buffalo; zebra; eland; waterbuck; wildebeest; hartebeest; topi; warthog; antelope; spotted hyena; okapi; serval; pig; genet; Sykes monkey; swamp rat; mynah bird and domestic hen[24,63,70,83,95,105,142,143,173]

5.   Asia: (India, Burma, Ceylon) mongoose; watersnake; and frog;[119,120,160] (Korea) hedgehog; mink; marten; raccoon dog; red fox; wolf; pig; 11 snake species; and frogs[29,100,102,198] (China) hedgehog; hamster; raccoon dog; cat; leopard; rat; snakes; and frogs;[23,79] (Japan) pig; rabbit; mouse; muskrat; Japanese weasel; Siberian weasel; hen; pigeon; frog; toad; and 4 species of snake;[87,89,103] (Southeast Asia) large Indian civet; small Indian civet; mouse; rat; guinea pig; macaque; numerous species of birds including red jungle fowl, guinea-fowl, rock dove, starling, robin magpie, barn owl, shrike, thrush, goshawk, crow, king-crow, woodpecker, magpie (*Pica* sp.), hoopoe, and silver pheasant; frogs; lizard; toad; turtle and 7 species of snake;[64,77,93,159] (Taiwan) 4 species of amphibians, 23 species of reptiles, 3 species of birds, and 6 species of mammals[104]

6.   Australopacific: (Australia) tadpole; frog; pig; rabbit; rat; mouse; marsupial mouse; fox; marsupial cat; tasmanian tiger cat; lizard; frogs; and 10 species of snake;[9,10,73,118,157,177] (Indonesia) pig; monkey; shrew; frog and toad;[15,16,122] (Philippines) mice; rabbit; monkey; rat; bittern; 6 species of reptiles and frog;[104,207] (North Borneo) 5 species of reptiles, 3 species of birds.[104]

Definitive Hosts

The domestic dog (*Canis familiaris*) and the domestic cat (*Felis domesticus*) have an almost cosmopolitan distribution as definitive hosts for *Spirometra*.[9,10,15,23,33,34,161,48,66,82,85,91,93,98,99,101,103,115,121,122,125,127,146,152,153,154,156,163,165,175,176,178,181,182,191,194,197,200,207] Other related carnivores found as hosts for spirometrid tapeworms are listed below

1.   Europe: fox; arctic fox; jaguar (zoo)[18,158,165]
2.   North America: raccoon; bobcat; arctic fox; and sledge dog[75,112,117,202]
3.   South America: crab-eating fox; jaguar; jaguarundi; South American wild cats and foxes; ocelet; crab-eating raccoon; and grison[21,45,74,169,195,200]
4.   Africa: lion; hyena; jackal; leopard; bat-eared fox; wildcat and serval[54,83,142,166,173]

5. Asia: wildcat; tiger; red fox; wolf; amur leopard; raccoon dog; snake; clouded leopard; himalayan palm civet; and Indian lion[76,93,101,125,174,182,201]

6. Australopacific: civet; fox and dingo[34,72,91,114,156] In rare instances humans have been definitive hosts for spirometrids with cases reported from China and Japan.[56,90,192]

Distribution

Spirometrid tapeworms and their corresponding spargana are world-wide in distribution. They have been reported from all continents with the exception of Antarctica. Definitive and intermediate animal hosts have been found in the following countries: Europe: Russia, Spain, Italy, Yugoslavia, Bulgaria, Poland, and Hungary; Africa: Belgian Congo, Kenya, Tanzania, Ethiopia, South Africa, and Madagascar; Asia: China, Taiwan, Korea, Japan, Southeast Asia, India, Iran, and Burma; Australopacific: Australia, Tasmania, Philippines, Indonesia, and Borneo; South America, Central America and Caribbean: Venezeula, Argentina, Chile, Brazil, Uruguay, Guatemala, Trinidad, Surinam, Dutch Antilles, Puerto Rico, and Cuba. In the continental U.S. infected animals have been found in Florida, North Carolina, South Carolina, Louisiana, Alabama, Georgia, Southeastern U.S. (unspecified), New York, New Jersey, and Texas, as well as in the Pacific state of Hawaii.

Human sparganosis is reported infrequently from most geographic areas of the world. Human infections are rare in Australia (four cases),[178] the Philippines (four cases),[68] Indonesia (two cases),[16] Europe (Holland, Italy, Russia; five cases),[14,123,155,168] and South America (Columbia, Uruguay, Brazil, Venezuela, Ecuador, Argentina, and British Guiana; nine cases).[45,167] This disease is more commonly found in Africa and North America. Thirty cases of sparganosis have been reported from Uganda, Mozambique, Liberia, South Africa, Kenya, Ruanda-Urundi, French Equatorial Africa, Gabon, Tanzania, and Madagascar.[20,143,179] In the U.S., 56 cases have been reported with 1 case each from Alabama, Georgia, Michigan, Missouri, Pennsylvania, Oklahoma, Tennessee, Virginia, and Wisconsin; 2 each from California, North Carolina, and South Carolina, 3 from Mississippi; 5 each from Arkansas, Florida, and Texas; 4 from New York and 16 from Louisiana.[27,36,42,59,116,139,186] Two cases were also from the Arkansas-Texas, Arkansas-Louisiana borders.[186] Two of these sparganosis cases (California and Michigan) were probably not autochthonous to the U.S.[22,185] Three cases were also found near the U.S. in British Honduras,[186] Canada,[2] and Puerto Rico.[186]

Most human sparganosis has been found in the Orient. By 1975, 213 cases had been reported in Japan and additional cases have been seen since.[203] In Korea, 63 cases were reported between 1917 and 1975.[28] Approximately 23 cases have been documented from China with 8 from Formosa,[26,110] 2 from Hong Kong[81] and the rest representing primarily the older literature regarding mainland China.[23,80] Additionally 12 cases have been from Thailand,[708] as well as numerous cases reported by French workers in Southeast Asia especially regarding ocular sparganosis.[12,32,39,63,77,78,97,126,151]

Interestingly, no human sparganosis has appeared to have been noted in two major areas of human population, the Indian subcontinent, and the Middle East.

Endemicity

The level of endemicity in animals appears to vary greatly for either spargana or the adult tapeworm. High incidence would appear to be dependent upon definitive hosts with suitable eating habits associated with an aquatic environment containing the appropriate copepods. In North America (and Hawaii) an important definitive host appears to be the domestic cat with 1 to 10% infection rates reported.[109,135,146,161] Raccoons, which may play an important role in sylvatic sparganosis, have shown 1 to 16% infection rates from selected areas of the southeastern U.S.[75] The watersnake, *Natrix* sp., appears to be the most significant second intermediate host with an incidence of 18% in Louisiana and 90% in Florida.[37,128] In Europe few surveys have been done but incidence is high (73 to 89%) in cats, dogs, and foxes from the Soviet Union,[172] and 57% of pigs in Yugoslavia were infected with spargana.[171] Paucity of host surveys and reports of few human infections may indicate that spirometrid infections in Europe are not common. There seems to be a correlation between the number of human cases of sparganosis and high incidence in animals. In India the incidence of *Spirometra* sp. in dogs and cats from five surveys is low, from 0.5 to 3.0%.[25,115,176,181] In contrast, Japan which has reported many human sparganosis cases, has reported very high rates of infection in cats (23 to 95%) but somewhat lower rate in dogs (1 to 11%).[4,85,103]

Snakes are believed to play a significant host role in Korea, as in the U.S., and have a 41% infection rate with spargana.[30] Frogs are believed to be important second intermediate hosts in many parts of the world and reports range from few infections reported for the U.S. to 3.9 to 11% (Korea),[100] 12% (Philippines),[197] 33% (Burma),[121] 50% (Uruguay),[45] 51% (Indonesia),[122] 60% (Vietnam),[64] and 67% (Japan).[103] Host incidence in South America and Africa is difficult to estimate due to lack of data. Only 1 of 429 cats in the Dutch Antilles was found infected (none in Surinam),[164] whereas 10 of 20 dogs were found infected in Venezuela.[58] In Africa the hyena (70% rate) appears to be a major definitive host.[143] Vervet monkeys from Tanzania show little infection with spargana (0.8%) whereas baboons were heavily infected (42%) which probably reflects dietary differences between the two primates.[105] In Australia the incidence of sparganosis in feral pigs is as high as 43 to 100%.[8] Foxes (8.6 to 19.7%), feral dogs, and dingoes (7%) are believed important definitive hosts in a rural cycle involving the feral pigs.[5,34,35,46,52] Cats, both domestic and feral, are also an important definitive host with infection rates of 16, 21, and 50% reported from four surveys in Australia.[8,11,98]

Disease in Animals

Adult tapeworms do not appear to cause much discomfort or disease in the definitive host although some mild physical manifestations have been reported in the cat. Spargana, although invasive, appear to be relatively well adapted and benign parasites. Sparganosis would most likely be diagnosed at post-mortem and it is not considered a serious veterinary problem. However, spargana can cause serious illness or death especially if they occur in large numbers in a single host, if invasion of internal organs occurs, or if they invade a critical area impairing movement or sensual function.

Experimental infections of intermediate hosts (primarily frogs, mice, and monkeys) have resulted in detailed descriptions of the pathological processes produced by spargana. Initial invasion of the intestine by large numbers of procercoids in a monkey caused extensive hemorrhage and tissue damage in the submucosa. In the muscle layer there was edema and hemorrhage along with macrophage, polymorphonuclear leucocyte, and lymphocyte infiltration.[148] In mice, heavy infection with procercoids caused death through hemorrhagic ascites and acute peritonitis. Plerocercoids apparently invade the gut of a paratenic host much faster and with less tissue reaction than do procercoids. In mice there is much less inflammatory reaction noted with plerocercoids.[148] In hamsters plerocercoid scolices can penetrate to the peritoneum in 45 min, creating a large hole in the intestinal wall but with little or no accompanying peritonitis.[57]

Upon reaching the muscle or subcutaneous areas the spargana tunnel through this tissue causing edema, subcutaneous abscesses, and cellular infiltration. In some instances, the spargana will become encapsulated by a membrane produced by the host and undergo degenerative changes. Host response to this phase includes accumulation of eosinophils, neutrophils, macrophages, and lymphocytes as well as fibroblasts, resulting in a chronic granulomatous inflammatory reaction at the site of infection. Also, blood vessels near the worm show an Arthus-like response. The cyst resulting from these reactions eventually contains the dead worm surrounded by pus cells within a highly vascularized two-layered fibrous structure.[148] In infections with numerous spargana the edema can be severe enough to produce an elephantiasis-like condition with the skin of the animal thrown into loose-folds filled with a gelatinous-like fluid.[130]

Sparganosis has been divided into an early acute phase (approximately 4 to 6 weeks) following penetration and migration of the larvae and a later chronic phase in which the host reaction to the worm has lessened.[130,148] During the acute phase an interesting physical finding in mice is the development of hemorrhagic skin lesions and joint swelling which may be due to an allergic response to sparganum toxic products.[148] Circulating antibodies (complement fixation and precipitating) can be detected near the end of the acute phase. Eosinophilia also occurs toward the end of the acute phase and declines during the chronic phase.[130,148] A peculiar effect on certain young, growing mammals (mice and hamsters) during the chronic phase of sparganosis is the stimulation of host growth by an endocrine-like substance (sparganum growth factor) released by the worm.[135] This substance is, however, not produced by all spirometrid plerocercoids.[149]

Disease in Man

The first human case of sparganosis was found in 1882 by Manson in a patient from South China.[31] Spargana were removed at autopsy from the subperitoneal fascia behind the kidneys. Credit has also been given to Scheube who recovered a sparganum from the urethra of a patient in Japan in 1881 but this case was not reported until 1886.[205] Reports of this disease were rare until the early 20th century with scattered cases noted from Australia (1892),[183] Africa (1907),[179] U.S. (1908),[184] Europe (1910),[168] South America (1910),[44] and Indochina (1911).[151] Following Ijima's report in 1905 on proliferative sparganosis in Japan,[84] numerous sparganum infections were reported from the Far East and the disease became known as one found primarily in the Orient. In the U.S. sparganosis was considered extremely rare until the 1950s after which numerous cases were reported. This has been attributed to improvements in rural health care and concern about early cancer detection regarding subcutaneous nodules rather than a natural increase in incidence.[42,186] Human sparganosis is probably more prevalent in most countries than actually reported due to its relatively benign nature in most infections.

Sparganosis usually occurs as a painful, inflamed, subcutaneous nodule which may have a history of migration, disappearing, and reappearing due to movements of the worm. One report from Japan claims nodular migration in breast tissue for 30 years.[203] Nodules may contain a living or degenerating plerocercoid and the histopathology is similar to that seen in experimental animals. Plerocercoids have been inoculated subdermally into human volunteers and in one case intense inflammatory and allergic reactions ensued.[137] Eosinophilia may or may not be present in natural infections but was found to range from slight to marked in patients and volunteers.[22,137] In other cases, erythematous areas and acneform pustules have been found on the skin and are associated with the plerocercoids' presence.[23] As a rule, only one nodule is found but in some cases more nodules may appear and in a few cases heavy, multiple infections have been seen.[3] Usually only one worm is present but six to eight or more have been removed from a single site of infection.[60]

Although most common in the subcutaneous tissue, spargana have been found in the eye, brain, lung, epididymus, urethra, jejunum, colon, scrotum, and free in the peritoneum. Tansurat has clinically divided sparganosis lesions into (1) ocular, (2) subcutaneous, (3) visceral, and (4) lymphatic.[188] Numerous cases of ocular sparganosis have been reported from Southeast Asia due to the practice of using plerocercoid-infected frog poultices around the eye. The spargana migrate from the poultice into human tissue forming a localized encapsulated lesion. Pronounced periorbital edema, pruritis, and pain can be found with ocular infections and consequences range from a slight blepharitis to severe panopthalmitis with loss of the globe.[106,185]

A rare, unusual, and mysterious form of this disease in man is proliferating sparganosis where the plerocercoids multiply and invade every tissue except bone. Only nine cases have been reported from man[110] and perhaps one in an animal host,[105] although the latter is disputed on histological evidence.[140] Extensive invasion produces the pronounced edema and elephantiasis-like symptoms mentioned earlier. Nothing is known of the etiology of this disease but it is believed that these organisms are aberrant forms of known spirometrids. It has been suggested that oncological factors, such as the C-type virus-like particles found associated with sparganum excretory ducts,[140] may play a role in the loss or disarray of the growth-regulating mechanisms of proliferating spargana. However, such C-type particles are found in the ducts of both normal and proliferating spargana and further evidence for a viral nature of these particles is lacking.[43,50,141] Other mutagenic factors, as well as an interaction of the immune state of the host, has also been suggested by a recent case of disseminated sparganosis in a patient with Hodgkin's disease who had been treated with cobalt irradiation and cyclophosphamide.[36]

Mode of Spread

Sparganosis in animals is acquired through ingestion of copepods infected with procercoids or ingestion of a second intermediate (or paratenic) host containing a plerocercoid. Such animals as frogs and tadpoles obtain their infections ingesting infected copepods and serve as sources for larger carnivores and omnivores to become paratenic hosts. Large herbivores, such as those described from Africa, must obviously obtain their infections from a drinking source. Cats and dogs can obtain the adult tapeworm by ingestion of plerocercoids through eating infected meat.

Human sparganosis is also obtained through drinking water contaminated with infected copepods or through eating poorly cooked or raw meat containing plerocercoids. A unique third route in humans is application sparganosis. Use of infected frog or other animal meat as a poultice allows the sparganum to transfer hosts by invading human tissue.

Epidemiology

Successful maintenance of sparganosis in nature requires that the eating and defecation habits of the definitive host coincide with the presence of suitable first and second intermediate hosts. The suitability of a host may not be the same for different strains or species of spirometrids. The degree of susceptibility to infection and development of procercoids in various species of *Cyclops* may differ depending on the geographic origin of the worms. *Cyclops vernalis* is a suitable host for *S. mansonoides* of North American origin, but not for the larger, more robust, *S. mansoni* from the Orient.[134] However, *C. vernalis* collected in England serves as an accommodating host for *S. theileri* from Africa.[147]

The second intermediate host that ingests the infected copepod is also a sensitive link in the life cycle. Not all small amphibians, reptiles, and mammals appear to be equally suited for such a role and the significant second intermediate host may differ from area to area. In southeast Asia *Rana tigrina*, the leopard frog, has been shown to be an important initial vertebrate host as suggested by observation of natural infections.[93] Experiments in Indochina and Indonesia indicated that adult frogs may obtain the majority of their infections as tadpoles because of active ingestion of infected copepods by the larval stages.[67] Several investigators have reported difficulty in infecting adult frogs with procercoids,[65,130] whereas others have not.[10,65] In other geographic areas frogs may not be as important as second intermediate hosts. A study in the southeastern U.S. showed a very low incidence of plerocercoid infection in amphibia collcted in the same vicinity where watersnakes showed a much greater infection rate.[37] Watersnakes (*Natrix* sp.) may be the primary initial vertebrate host in North America although raccoons and opposum may also be significant in that role. It has been suggested that watersnakes may obtain their infections by ingesting fish stuffed with infected copepods.[134] Although laboratory mice are easily infected with procercoids, field observations tend to discount wild rodents as major initial vertebrate hosts which may be due to their not frequenting water sources where copepods are plentiful. Animals that share common watering holes with definitive hosts can become infected such as the herbivores reported with sparganosis from the African savannah.[147]

Plerocercoids of *Spirometra* are highly infectious and can invade a large variety of vertebrates. They also have the capacity (under laboratory conditions) to outlive the host. Spargana can thus provide an important long term reservoir of infection in nature. The most significant paratenic hosts, however, are those most likely to be eaten by the definitive host. In Australia a connection with adult tapeworms in wild canids has been made with a high incidence of sparganosis in feral pigs captured from the same localities.[5]

High incidence of sparganosis in humans is due to eating, drinking, or sociological habits that lend themselves to infection. Previous mention has been made of split-frog poultices related to sparganosis in southeast Asia. The nomadic Masai of East Africa apparently acquire sparganosis by ingesting infected *Cyclops* from drinking water since their main dietary source is the milk and blood of their cattle.[179] The Masai may then act as unusual obligatory human intermediate hosts since they practice leaving their dead unburied to be eaten by potential definitive hosts, such as hyenas.[143,199] In Korea a strong relationship has been established between the ingestion of raw snake meat (for nutritive and medicinal purposes) and sparganosis.[198] In the U.S. ingestion of procercoids with drinking water has been implicated as a source of infection in rural areas.[40,134] Open dug wells often contain copepods and are easily accessible to definitive hosts which may contaminate the water through defecation.[42] Poorly cooked pork, chicken, tadpoles, frogs, and game have also been suggested as potential sources for human sparganosis in the U.S., Africa, Japan, Indonesia, and Southeast Asia.[37,49,78,81,205]

Diagnosis

Diagnosis of sparganosis is made by finding the plerocercoid in a tumerous nodule or free in the tissue. From a nodule the living plerocercoid can be expressed and identified as a whitish, ribbon-like worm with little morphological differentiation. Histological examination of a nodule will reveal the larva possessing an outer eosinophilic "cuticle" with an underlying row of subcuticular muscle fibers and the nuclei of tegument cells (Figures 3, 4). Within the worm there is a loose fibrillar network within which are thin-walled vascular (osmoregulatory) canals. Concentric basophilic staining calcareous corpuscles can also be found in the fibrillar network. These structures are characteristic of cestodes. Surrounding the worm will usually be necrotic debris, cellular infiltration, and peripheral fibrotic elements.[42] Charcot-Leyden crystals have also been noted in nodules associated with chronic infections.[132,198]

In humans the sensation of a moving larva has been felt in the infected area.[179] Although circulating antibodies and skin testing have been demonstrated with experimental hosts, immunological testing has had little clinical use since most cases of sparganosis are not suspected until the worm is found, in which case the diagnosis is estab-

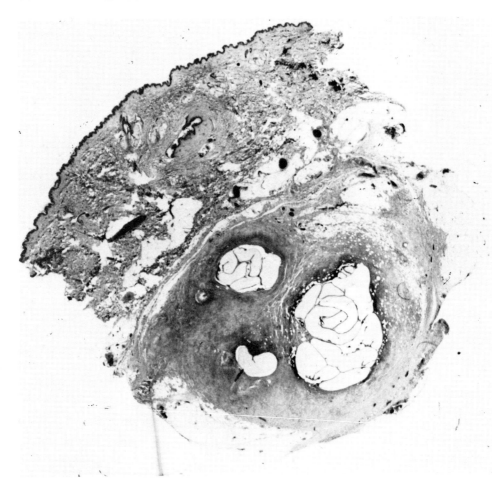

FIGURE 3.   Cross section of a sparganum-containing nodule removed from the chest wall of a patient from Arkansas. Three areas with coiled sparganum can be seen.

lished. The indirect flourescent antibody test has been studied in Japan as a potential diagnostic tool to detect sparganosis.[86]

Infections with the adult tapeworm in definitive hosts, such as cats and dogs, can be made by finding spirometrid-like ova in the stool and the recovery of the characteristic proglottids (Figure 5).

Prevention and Control

Control of sparganosis in wild animal populations is not feasible since a primary source of infection is drinking water containing copepods that are an important part of the normal environmental fauna. The ubiquity of infection in paratenic hosts and feeding habits of potential definitive hosts would also make control difficult.

Prevention of sparganosis and adult tapeworm infections in domestic animals depends upon control of drinking water and food supply to minimize the possibility of infection. Dogs and cats can be treated for adult tapeworms with the usual cestocidal agents niclosamide (Yomesan) or dichlorophen.[17]

Prevention of infection in man can be accomplished by not ingesting poorly-cooked meat, especially pork and flesh from such game animals as raccoon and bear. Potentially contaminated untreated drinking water such as that from lakes, streams, ponds,

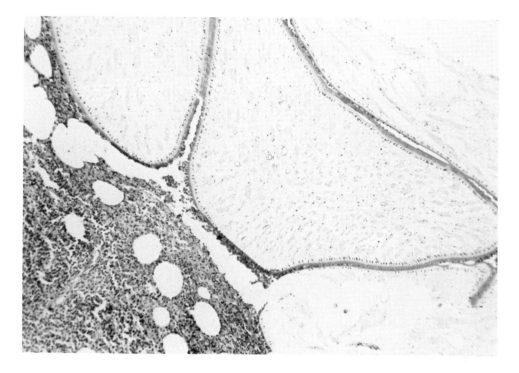

FIGURE 4. Higher magnification of the sparganum seen in Figure 3. The nuclei of tegument cells are noticeable under the dense outer cuticle of the tapeworm larva. Within the worm is a loose fibrillar network containing thin-walled osmoregulatory canals and scattered muscle fibers.

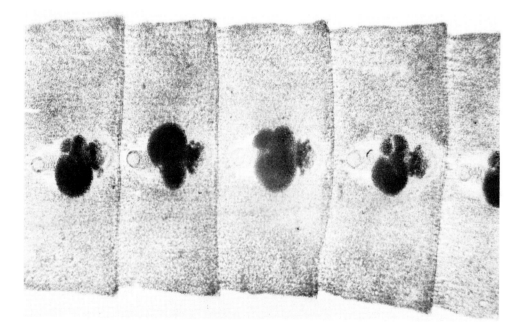

FIGURE 5. Proglottids of a *Spirometra* sp. from an Arkansas bobcat *(Lynx rufus).* The median genital pore can be seen adjacent to the darkly staining compact uterus.

etc. should be avoided. Dug wells should be properly covered to prevent entry of *Spirometra* ova through defecation of definitive hosts.

Excision of the nodule or extirpation of the worm is the only practical treatment in man. More detailed surgical procedures are described for removal of spargana from sensitive areas such as in ocular sparganosis.[106]

REFERENCES

1. **Africa, C. M.**, Studies on experimental infections of Philippine *Cyclops* with coracidia of *Diphyllobothrium mansoni* Cobbold, 1882, *Philipp. J. Publ. Health*, 1, 27, 1934.
2. **Ali-Kahn, Z., Irving, R. T., Wignall, N., and Bowmer, E. J.**, Imported sparganosis in Canada, *Can. Med. Assoc. J.*, 108, 590, 1973.
3. **Alves, W. D., Gelfand, M., and Weinberg, R.**, A case of sparganosis in an african from Portuguese East Africa, *Trans. R. Soc. Trop. Med. Hyg.*, 48, 87, 1954.
4. **Ando, A.**, Considerations relating to the history of the development of *Sparganum mansoni*, especially of its *Dibothriocephalus decipiens, Trans. 6th Congr. Far Eastern Assoc. Trop. Med. Tokyo*, 1, 421, 1925.
5. **Appleton, P. L. and Norton, J. H.**, Sparganosis: a parasitic problem in feral pigs, *Queensl. Agri. J.*, 102, 339, 1976.
6. **Baer, J. G.**, Contribution a la faune helminthologique Sud-Africaine, *Ann. Parasitol.*, 2, 239, 1924.
7. **Baer, J. G.**, Die cestoden der säugetiere Brasiliens, *Abh. Senkenb. Naturforsch. Ges.*, 40, 377, 1927.
8. **Baldock, F. C. and Hopkins, T. J.**, *Spirometra erinacei* in cats and dogs in Australia, *Aust. Vet. Assoc. 53rd Ann. Conf. Proc.*, 1976, 87.
9. **Bearup, A. J.**, Observations on the life cycle of *Diphyllobothrium (Spirometra) erinacei* in Australia (*Cestoda*: Diphyllobothriidae), *Aust. J. Sci.*, 10, 183, 1948.
10. **Bearup, A. J.**, Life history of a spirometrid tapeworm, causing sparganosis in feral pigs, *Aust. Vet. J.*, 29, 217, 1953.
11. **Bearup, A. J.**, Parasitic infections in cats in Sydney with special reference to the occurrence of *Ollulanus tricuspis, Aust. Vet. J.*, 36, 352, 1960.
12. **Beauchamp, F. and Fontan, R.**, Sur quelques helminthiasis oculaires observees au Laos, *Med. Trop.*, 36, 225, 1976.
13. **Becklund, W. W.**, Occurrence of a larval trematode (*Diplostomidae*) in a larval cestode (Diphyllobothriidae) from *Sus scrofa* in Florida, *J. Parasitol.*, 48, 286, 1962.
14. **Berdonosova, T. I., Miretski, O. Ya., and Skryabin, A. J.**, A case of human sparganosis in the U.S.S.R., *Med. Parazitol. Parazit. Bolezni (Moskva)*, 37, 739, 1968.
15. **Bonne, C.**, Researches on sparganosis in the Netherlands East Indies, *Am. J. Trop. Med.*, 22, 643, 1942.
16. **Bonne, C. and Joe, L. K.**, Darmwandhelminthiasis teweeggebracht door spargana, *Geneesk. Tijdushr. Nederl. Indie*, 80, 2788, 1940.
17. **Brander, G. C. and Pugh, D. M.**, *Veterinary Applied Pharmacology and Therapeutics*, 3rd ed., Lea & Febiger, Philadelphia, 1977.
18. **Brglez, J., Rakovec, R., and Mrzel, I.**, *Spirometra felis* — a tapeworm found in the Jaguar (*Felis onca* L.) in a zoological garden, in Verhandlungsbericht des 19th Int. Symp. uber die erkrankungen der zootiere, Budapest, 6 to 10 Mai, 1970, Matthias, D., Ed., Berlin Akademic-Verlag Deutsche Akademic der Wissenschaften, 1970, 291.
19. **Bruijning, C. F. A. and deJongh, R. T.**, A case of human sparganosis in Liberia, *Trop. Geogr. Med.*, 12, 356, 1960.
20. **Brygoo, E. R. and Catala, P.**, Premier cas de sparganose humaine a Madagascar, *Arch. Inst. Pasteur. Madagascar*, 29, 75, 1961.
21. **Cameron, T. W. M.**, Studies on the endoparasitic fauna of Trinidad. III. Some parasites of Trinadad carnivores, *Can. J. Res.*, 14, 25, 1936.
22. **Campbell, E. W. and Beals, C.**, Striking eosinophilia in sparganosis, *Postgrad. Med.*, 62, 138, 1977.
23. **Campbell, H. E., Webster, J. L. A., and Li, S. Y.**, Human sparganosis in the Foochow area, *Chin. Med. J.*, 1, 423, 1936.
24. **Capron, A. and Brygoo, E. R.**, Sparganose experimentale de *Lemur fulvus* Geoffr., *Arch. Instit. Pasteur Madagascar*, 28, 189, 1960.
25. **Chandler, A. C.**, The helminthic parasites of cats in Calcutta and the relation of cats to human helminthic infections, *Indian. J. Med. Res.*, 13, 213, 1925.
26. **Chen, T. Y. and Cross, J. H.**, Subcutaneous sparganosis — a case report, *J. Formosan Med. Assoc.*, 74, 515, 1975.

27. Cho, C. and Patel, S. P., Human sparganosis in the northern United States, *N.Y. State J. Med.*, Aug., 1456, 1978.

28. Cho, S. Y., Bae, J., and Seo, B-S., Some aspects of human sparganosis in Korea, *Korean J. Parasitol.*, 13, 60, 1975.

29. Cho, S. Y. and Seo, B. S., Sparganum in the Korean terrestrial snakes, *Korean J. Parasitol.*, 10(Suppl.), 122, 1972.

30. Cho, S. Y., Hwang, K. I., and Seo, B. S., On the *Sparganum mansoni* infection in some Korean terrestrial snakes, *Korean J. Parasitol.*, 11, 87, 1973.

31. Cobbold, T. S., Description of *Ligula mansoni*, a new human cestode, *J. Linnean Soc. Lond. Zool.*, 17, 78, 1883.

32. Collin, M., La sparganose oculaire en Annam, *Bull. Mem. Soc. Franc. Opthalmol.*, 43, 395, 1930.

33. Coman, B. J., A survey of the gastro-intestinal parasites of the feral cat in Victoria, *Aust. Vet. J.*, 48, 133, 1972.

34. Coman, B. J., Helminth parasites of the dingo and feral dog in Victoria with some notes on the diet of the host, *Aust. Vet. J.*, 48, 456, 1972.

35. Coman, B. J., Helminth parasites of the fox (*Vulpes vulpes*) in Victoria, *Aust. Vet. J.*, 49, 378, 1973.

36. Connor, D. H., Sparks, A. K., Strano, A. J., Neafie, R. C., and Juvelier, B., Disseminated parasitosis in an immunosuppressed patient: possibly a mutated sparganum, *Arch. Pathol. Lab. Med.*, 100, 65, 1976.

37. Corkum, K. C., Sparganosis in some vertebrates of Louisiana and observations on a human infection, *J. Parasitol.*, 52, 444, 1966.

38. Corkum, K. C., The duality of host function in spirometrid tapeworm infections, *Proc. La. Acad. Sci.*, 36, 64, 1973.

39. Cornet, E., Essai de traitment de la sparganose retrobulbaire. Deux cas det deux succès, *Bull. Soc. Med. Chir. Indochin.*, 11, 452, 1933.

40. Cross, J. H., Sparganosis in two members of an Arkansas family, *J. Parasitol.*, 49, 154, 1963.

41. Crum, J. M., Nettles, V. F., and Davidson, W. R., Studies on endoparasites of the black bear (*Ursus americanus*) in the Southeastern United States, *J. Wildl. Dis.*, 14, 178, 1978.

42. Daly, J. J., Baker, G. F., and Johnson, B. R., Human sparganosis in Arkansas, *J. Ark. Med. Soc.*, 71, 397, 1975.

43. Daly, J. J., Sun, C. N., Barron, A. L., and White, H. J., C-type virus-like particles in a non-proliferating sparganum of human host origin, *J. Parasitol.*, 61, 775, 1975.

44. Daniels, C. W., *Tropical Medicine and Hygiene*, 2nd ed., Vol. 2, W. Wood and Co., New York, 1914.

45. Dei-Cas, E., Rodriguez, N., Botto, C., and Osimani, J. J., Plerocercoid larvae of *Spirometra* (Dibothriocephalidae) in man and wild animals from Uruguay, *Rev. Instit. Med. Trop. Sao Paulo*, 18, 165, 1976.

46. Dent, C. H. R. and Kelly, J. D., Cestode parasites of the fox in the central tablelands of New South Wales, *Aust. Vet. J.*, 50, 176, 1974.

47. Deschiens, R., Ceccaldi, J., Lamy, L., and Ravisse, M., Sur un nouveau cas africain de sparganose humaine, *Bull. Soc. Pathol. Exot.*, 46, 958, 1953.

48. Dikmans, G., (Abstr.) *J. Parasitol.*, 18, 47, 1931.

49. Dinnik, J. A. and Sachs, R., Zystizerkose, echinokokkose und sparganose bei wildiebenden herbivoren in Ostafrica, *Vet. Med. Nachrichten*, 2, 112, 1969.

50. Dougherty, R. M., DiStefano, H., Feller, L. I., and Mueller, J. F., On the nature of particles lining the excretory ducts of pseudophyllidean cestodes, *J. Parasitol.*, 61, 1006, 1975.

51. Dubinina, M. N., Biology and distribution of *Diphyllobothrium erinacei-europei* (Rudolphi, 1819) Iwata, 1933, *Zool. Zurn.*, 30, 421, 1951.

52. Durie, P. H. and Riek, R. F., The role of the dingo and wallaby in the infestation of cattle with hydatids (*Echinococcus granulosus* [Batsch, 1786] Rudolphi, 1805) in Queensland, *Aust. Vet. J.*, 28, 249, 1952.

53. Evanno, Sur la sparganose oculaire, *Bull. Acad. Vet. France*, 6, 355, 1933.

54. Fain, A., Un cas de spargonose chez l'homme deux cas de sparganose chez le serval et un cas de diphyllobothriose (*D. parvum*) chez le chacal au Congo Belge, *Ann. Soc. Belg. Med. Trop.*, 27, 65, 1947.

55. Fain, A., Vers nouveaux de l'okapi, *Rev. Zool. Botan. Afr.*, 41, 222, 1948.

56. Faust, E. C., Campbell, H. E., and Kellogg, C. R., Morphological and biological studies on the species of *Diphyllobothrium* in China, *Am. J. Hyg.*, 9, 560, 1929.

57. Feng, L. C. and Hoeppli, R., Sparganum of *Diphyllobothrium erinacei* as carrier of bacteria and the problem of its bactericide action, *Chin. Med. J.*, 50, 1457, 1936.

58. Fernandez, A. J. and Vogelsang, E. G., Contribucion al estudio de la parasitologia animal en Venezuela. III. Formas larvales de cestodos, *Rev. Policlin. (Carcacas)*, 5, 1472, 1935.

59. **Fischman, N. H., Blalock, J. B., and Carrera, G. M.,** Human sparganosis in Louisiana: a case report, *J. La. State Med. Soc.,* 129, 215, 1977.

60. **Foster, R., Birch, N. H., and Urasa, J.,** A case of sparganosis from Tanzania (Tanganyika), *East Afr. Med. J.,* 42, 74, 1965.

61. **Furmaga, S.,** *Spirometra Janickii* sp. n. (Diphyllobothriidae), *Acta Parasitol. Polonica,* 1, 29, 1953.

62. **Furukawa, T.,** Morphological variations in *Diphyllobothrium erinacei, Jpn. J. Parasitol.,* 18, 553, 1969.

63. **Gaide, L. and Rongier,** De la sparganose oculaire en Annam, *Bull. Soc. Med. Chi. Indochin.,* 6, 93, 1915.

64. **Galliard, H.,** Infestation naturelle des batraciens et reptiles par les larves plérocercoides de *Diphyllobothrium mansoni* au Tonkin, *Ann. Parasitol. Hum. Comp.,* 23, 23, 1948.

65. **Galliard, H. and Ngu, D. V.,** Particularités du cycle évolutif de *Diphyllobothrium mansoni* au Tonkin, *Ann. Parasitol. Hum. Comp.,* 21, 246, 1946.

66. **Galli-Valerio, B.,** *Bothriocephalus latus.* Brems. chez le chat, *Centralbl. Bakt. I. Abt.,* 32, 285, 1902.

67. **Gan, K. H.,** Research on the life history of *Diphyllobothrium ranarum, Doc. Neerland. Indonesia. Mor. Trop.,* 1, 90, 1949.

68. **Garcia, O. P. and Reyes, A. I.,** Sparganosis in filipinos with a review of reported cases in the Philippines, *J. Philipp. Med. Assoc.,* 38, 608, 1962.

69. **Genov, T.,** Natural infestation of vertebrates with plerocercoids of *Spirometra erinacei-europaei* (Cestoda: Diphyllobothriidae), *Izv. Tsent. Khelmint. Lab. Sofia.,* 13, 197, 1969.

70. **Geoffroy and Poisson,** Sparganose du porc à Madagascar, *Rec. Med. Vet. Exot.,* 1, 21, 1932.

71. **Gordon, H. McL.,** The occurrence of *Diphyllobothrium latum,* the broad fish tapeworm in dogs in Australia, *Aust. Vet. J.,* 15, 256, 1939.

72. **Gordon, H. McL.,** The occurrence of the broad fish tapeworm of man and carnivores in dogs in Australia, *Med. J. Aust.,* 1, 47, 1940.

73. **Gordon, H. McL., Forsyth, B. A., and Robinson, M.,** Sparganosis in feral pigs in New South Wales, *Aust. Vet. J.,* 30, 135, 1954.

74. **Guttierres, V. C., Froes, O. M., and Amato, J. F. R.,** Identification of an intermediate host of *Spirometra mansonoides* in the Porto Alegre region, Rio Grande do Sul, Brazil, *Rev. Brasil. Biol.,* 37, 131, 1977.

75. **Harkema, R. and Miller, G. C.,** Helminth parasites of the raccoon, *Procyon lotor,* in the Southeastern United States, *J. Parasitol.,* 50, 60, 1964.

76. **Hiregoudar, L. S.,** *Spirometra* and *Schistosoma* infection among lions of Gir Forest in India, *Curr. Res.,* 4, 134, 1975.

77. **Houdemer, E., Dodero, L., and Cornet, E.,** Les sparganoses animales et la sparganose oculaire en Indochine, *Bull. Soc. Med. Chir. Indochin.,* 11, 425, 1933.

78. **Houdemer, E., Dodero, L., and Cornet, E.,** Les sparganoses animales oculaires en Indochine et la sparganose, *Ann. Oculistique,* 171, 311, 1934.

79. **Hsu, H. F.,** Contribution à l'etude des cestodes de Chine, *Rev. Suisse Zool.,* 42, 477, 1935.

80. **Hsu, P. C.,** Ocular sparganosis, *Chin. Med. J.,* 62, 107, 1944.

81. **Huang, C. T. and Kirk, R.,** Human sparganosis in Hong Kong, *J. Trop. Med. Hyg.,* 65, 133, 1962.

82. **Huang, Y. Y., Ikeuchi, H., and Yuda, K.,** A human case with *Sparganum mansoni.* Distribution of *Diphyllobothrium erinacei* in cats and dogs in Miyagi Prefecture, *Igaku To Seibut. Med. Biol.,* 80, 121, 1970.

83. **Hudson, J. R.,** A list of cestodes known to occur in East Africa mammals, birds, and reptiles, *J. East. Afr. Uganda Nat. His. Soc.,* Nos. 49—50, 205, 1933.

84. **Ijima, I.,** On a new cestode larva (*Plerocercoides prolifer*) in man, *J. Coll. Sci. Imp. Univ. Tokyo,* 20, 1, 1905.

85. **Iseki, M., Tanabe, K., Uni, S., and Sano, R.,** A survey on *Toxoplasma* and other protozoal and helminthic parasites of adult stray cats in Osaka area, *Jpn. J. Parasitol.,* 23, 317, 1974.

86. **Ishii, A.,** Indirect fluorescent antibody test in human sparganosis, *Jpn. J. Parasitol.,* 22, 75, 1973.

87. **Isobe, C.,** New second intermediate hosts of *Diphyllobothrium mansoni* in Miyazaki Prefecture, *Med. Biol. Tokyo,* 57, 150, 1960.

88. **Iwata, S.,** Some experimental and morphological studies on the post embryonal development of Manson's tapeworm, *Diphyllobothrium erinacei* (Rudolphi), *Jpn. J. Parasitol.,* 5, 209, 1933.

89. **Iwata, S.,** Some experimental studies on the regeneration of the plerocercoid of Manson's tapeworm, *Diphyllobothrium erinacei* (Rudolphi) with special reference with *Sparganum proliferum* Ijima, *Jpn. J. Parasitol.,* 6, 139, 1934.

90. **Iwata, S., Kaida, K., and Kifune, T.,** The second case of human infection with the adult of *Diphyllobothrium erinacei, Kur. Igakki Zasshi.,* 34, 291, 1971.

91. **Jackson, P. J. and Arundel, J. H.,** The incidence of tapeworms in rural dogs in Victoria, *Aust. Vet. J.,* 47, 46, 1971.

92. Joyeux, C. and Baer, J. G., Sur quelques larves de bothriocephales, *Bull. Soc. Pathol. Exot.*, 20, 921, 1927.

93. Joyeux, C. and Houdemer, E., Recherches sur la faune helminthologique de l'Indochine (Cestodes et Trematodes), *Ann. Parasitol.*, 6, 27, 1928.

94. Joyeux, C., Houdemer, E., and Baer, J., Recherches sur la biologie des *Sparganum* et l'etiologie de la sparganose oculaire, *Bull. Soc. Pathol. Exot.*, 27, 70, 1934.

95. Joyeux, C., Baer, J. G., and Gaud, J., Recherches sur des cestodes d'Indochine et sur quelques *Diphyllobothrium* (Bothriocephales). *Bull. Soc. Pathol. Exot.*, 43, 482, 1950.

96. Joyeux, C., Houdemer, E., and Baer, J. G., Etiologie de la sparganose oculaire, *Marseille Med.*, 69, 405, 1932.

97. Joyeux, B., Truong-Cam-Cong, and Nguyen-Xuan-Nguyen, Nouvelles contributions a l'étude de la sparganose oculaire au Tonkin, *Rev. Med. Fran. Ext. Orient.*, 17, 27, 1939.

98. Kelly, J. D., Anthropozoonotic helminthiasis in Australia: the role of animals in disease transmission. I. Meat and offal-borne anthropozoonoses, *Int. J. Zoon.*, 1, 1, 1974.

99. Kelly, J. D., Anthropozoonotic helminthiasis in Australia: the role of animals in disease transmission. II. Anthropozoonoses associated with domesticated vertebrates, *Int. J. Zoon.*, 1, 13, 1974.

100. Kim, C. H. and Shin, D. W., Pevalence of sparganum of frogs (*Rana nigromaculata*) in Dae-Jeon area, Chung-Nam, Korea, *Korean J. Parasitol.*, 13, 159, 1975.

101. Kobayashi, H., On the animal parasites in Korea, *Jpn. Med. World*, 5, 9, 1925.

102. Kobayashi, H., On the animal parasites in Chosen (Korea). Second report, *Acta Med. Keijo.*, 5, 109, 1928.

103. Kobayashi, H., Studies on the development of *Diphyllobothrium mansoni* cobbold 1882 (Joyeux, 1927). Sixth report. Development in the second intermediate host and plerocercoid in natural infection of frogs and musk-rat (*Crocidura murina*), *J. Formosa Med. Assoc.*, 30, 363, 1931.

104. Kuntz, R. E., Sparganosis (*Spirometra*) in vertebrates of Taiwan (Republic of China), North Borneo (Malaysia) and Palawan (Republic of the Philippines), in *H.D. Srivastava Commem.*, Singh, K. S. and Tandan, B. K., Eds., Indian Veterinary Research Institute, 1970, 477.

105. Kuntz, R. E., Meyers, B. J., and Katzberg, A. A., Sparganosis and "proliferative" spargana in vervets (*Cercopithecus aethiops*) and Baboons (*Papio* sp.) from East Africa, *J. Parasitol.*, 56, 196, 1970.

106. LaPierre, J., Sparganose, *Encycloped. Med Chir.*, Paris, 1966.

107. Li, C-H. and Faust, E. C., Infection of *Cyclops* with coracidium of oriental diphyllobothrids and their development to mature procercoid stage, *Proc. Soc. Exp. Biol. Med.*, 26, 250, 1928.

108. Li, H. C., The life histories of *Diphyllobothrium decipiens* and *D. erinacei*, *Am. J. Hyg.*, 10, 527, 1929.

109. Lillis, W. G. and Burrows, R. B., Natural infections of *Spirometra mansonoides* in New Jersey cats, *J. Parasitol.*, 50, 680, 1964.

110. Lin, T. P., Su, I. J., Lu, S. C., and Yang, S. P., Pulmonary proliferating sparganosis, *J. Formosan Med. Assoc.*, 77, 467, 1978.

111. Lizcano Herrera, J., Hallazgo de unas formas de *Sparganus* en un conejo de Granada, *Rev. Iberica Parasitol.*, 18, 227, 1958.

112. Lofftin, H., An annotated check-list of trematodes and cestodes and their vertebrate hosts from Northwest Florida, *Q. J. Fla. Acad. Sci.*, 23, 302, 1960.

113. Lopez-Neyra, C. R. and Diaz-Ungria, C., Cestodes de Venezuela V. Cestodes de vertebrados Venezolanos, *Noved. Cient. Mus. Hist. Nat. LaSalla Zool.*, 23, 1, 1958.

114. MacCallum, G. A., Studies in helminthology, *Zoopathologica*, 1, 216, 1921.

115. Maplestone, P. A. and Bhaduri, N. V., The helminth parasites of dogs in Calcutta and their bearing on human parasitology, *Indian J. Med. Res.*, 28, 595, 1940.

116. Markell, E. and Haber, S. L., A case of human sparganosis from California, *Am. J. Med.*, 37, 491, 1964.

117. McIntosh, A., New host records for *Diphyllobothrium mansonoides* Mueller, 1935, *J. Parasitol.*, 23, 315, 1937.

118. McMillan, B. and Walker, J. C., The marsupial mouse, *Antechinus stuartii*, as an intermediate host of *Spirometra erinacei* (Cestoda: Diphyllobothriidae). *Aust. J. Sci.*, 32, 207, 1969.

119. Meggitt, F. J., On two species of Cestoda from a mongoose, *Parasitology*, 16, 48, 1924.

120. Meggitt, F. J., On the occurrence of *Ligula ranarum* in a frog, *Ann. Mag. Nat. Hist.*, 13, 216, 1924.

121. Meggitt, F. J., On the life history of a reptilian tapeworm (*Sparganum reptans*), *Ann. Trop. Med. Parasitol.*, 18, 195, 1925.

122. Meijer, W. C. P. and Sahar, Over een lintworm van den hond, *Diphyllobothrium raillieti*, Rátz en het bijbehoorende plerocercoid *Sparganum raillieti* Rátz van het varken, *Neder. Ind. Blad. Diergeneesk. Dierent.*, 46, 1, 1934.

123. Monolo, L., Pantiggia, M., Tarfani, A., and Dorizzi, A., A case of cerebral sparganosis, *Acta Neurochir.*, 38, 146, 1977.

124. **Morton, H. L.**, Sparganosis in African green monkeys. (*Cercopithecus aethiops*), *Lab. Anim. Care,* 19, 253, 1969.

125. **Mudaliar, S. V. and Alwar, V. S.**, A check-list of parasites, (Classes-Trematoda and Cestoda) in the Department of Parasitology, Madras Veterinary College laboratory, *Indian Vet. J.,* 23, 423, 1947.

126. **Motais, F.**, La sparganose oculaire en Annam, *Bull. Soc. Pathol. Exot.,* 13, 215, 1920.

127. **Mueller, J. F.**, A *Diphyllobothrium* from cats and dogs in the Syracuse region, *J. Parasitol.,* 21, 114, 1935.

128. **Mueller, J. F.**, Spargana in *Natrix, Science,* 85, 519, 1937.

129. **Mueller, J. F.**, A repartition of the genus *Diphyllobothrium, J. Parasitol.,* 23, 308, 1937.

130. **Mueller, J. F.**, Studies on *Sparganum mansonoides* and *Sparganum proliferum, Am. J. Trop. Med.,* 18, 303, 1938.

131. **Mueller, J. F.**, The life history of *Diphyllobothrium mansonoides* Mueller, 1935, and some considerations with regards to sparganosis in the United States, *Am. J. Trop. Med.,* 18, 41, 1938.

132. **Mueller, J. F.**, The occurrence of Charcot-Leyden crystals in the lesions of sparganosis, *J. Parasitol.,* 26(Suppl.), 23, 1940.

133. **Mueller, J. F.**, Spargana from the Florida alligator, *J. Parasitol.,* 37, 317, 1951.

134. **Mueller, J. F.**, Host-parasite relationships as illustrated by the cestode *Spirometra mansonoides,* in *Host-Parasite Relationships,* McCauley, J. F., Ed., 26th Biology Colloquium, Oregon State University Press, Corvalis, 1966, 15.

135. **Mueller, J. F.**, The biology of *Spirometra, J. Parasitol.,* 60, 3, 1974.

136. **Mueller, J. F.**, Potential longevity of life history stages of *Spirometra* spp., *J. Parasitol.,* 60, 376, 1974.

137. **Mueller, J. F. and Coulston, F.**, Experimental human infection with the sparganum larva of *Spirometra mansonoides* (Mueller, 1935), *Am. J. Trop. Med.,* 21, 399, 1941.

138. **Mueller, J. F., Frões, O. M., and Fernández, T. R.**, On the occrrence of *Spirometra mansonoides* in South America, *J. Parasitol.,* 61, 774, 1975.

139. **Mueller, J. F., Hart, E. P., and Walsh, W. P.**, Human sparganosis in the United States, *J. Parasitol.,* 49, 294, 1963.

140. **Mueller, J. F. and Strano, A. J.**, *Sparganum proliferum,* a sparganum infected with a virus?, *J. Parasitol.,* 60, 15, 1974.

141. **Mueller, J. F. and Strano, A. J.**, The ubiquity of type-C viruses in spargana of *Spirometra* spp., *J. Parasitol.,* 60, 398, 1974.

142. **Muller, R. L. and Opuni, E. K.**, Studies on the biology of *Spirometra theileri,* a pseudophylid tapeworm from East Africa, *Proc. 3rd Int. Congr. Parasitol.,* 1, 384, 1974.

143. **Nelson, G. S., Pester, F. R. N., and Rickman, R.**, The significance of wild animals in the transmission of cestodes of medical importance in Kenya, *Trans. R. Soc. Trop. Med. Hyg.,* 59, 507, 1965.

144. **Odening, K. and Bockhardt, I.**, Plerozercoid-befall bei thailandischen reptilien aus dem Tierpark Berlin, *Angew. Parasitol.,* 17, 9, 1976.

145. **Okumura, T.**, An experimental study on the life history of *Sparganum mansoni* Cobbold, *Kitsato Arch. Exp. Med.,* 3, 190, 1919.

146. **Olsen, O. W. and Haas, W. R.**, A new record of *Spirometra mansoni,* a zoonotic tapeworm, from naturally infected cats and dogs in Hawaii, *Hawaii Med. J.,* 35, 261, 1976.

147. **Opuni, E. K. and Muller, R. L.**, Studies on *Spirometra theileri* (Baer 1925) n. comb. I. Identification and biology in the laboratory, *J. Helminthol.,* 48, 15, 1974.

148. **Opuni, E. K. and Muller, R. L.**, Studies on *Spirometra theileri* (Baer 1925) n. comb. II. Pathology of experimental plerocercoid infections, *J. Helminthol.,* 49, 121, 1975.

149. **Opuni, E. K., Muller, R., and Mueller, J. F.**, Absence of sparganum growth factor in African *Spirometra* spp., *J. Parasitol.,* 60, 375, 1974.

150. **Osimani, J. J. and Dei Cas, E. V.**, Experimental studies on *Spirometra* sp., *Neotropica,* 20, 57, 1974.

151. **Paucot**, Note sur une tumeur lacrymale due à un bothriocéphale, *Bull. Soc. Med. Chir. Indochin.,* 2, 328, 1911.

152. **Pérez Vigueras, I.**, Sobre la presencia en Cuba de *Diphyllobothrium mansoni* (Cobbold), *Mem. Soc. Cubana Hist. Nat.,* 8, 351, 1934.

153. **Power, L. A.**, Contribucion al conocimiento de los helmintos parasitos del gato (*Felis domesticus*) de Maracay y sus alrededores (Venezuela), *Rev. Med. Vet. Parasitol.,* 20, 99, 1964.

154. **Prockopic, J. and Hernandez, L.**, Helmintofauna de *Canis familiaris* y *Felis catus* en Cuba, *Poeyana,* 92, 1, 1971.

155. **Pujatti, D.**, Un caso di sparganosi umana, *Riv. Parassitol.,* 14, 213, 1953.

156. **Pullar, E. M.**, The control of internal parasites in dogs, *Aust. Vet. J.,* 22, 204, 1946.

157. **Pullar, E. M. and McLennan, G. C.**, Sparganosis in a victorian pig, *Aust. Vet. J.,* 25, 302, 1949.

158. **Raffaele, G.**, Su alcuni cestodi rinvenuti in una pantera, *Boll. Zool.,* 3, 299, 1932.

159. **Railliet, A. and Henry, A.**, Helminthes du porc recueillis par M. Bauche en Annam, *Bull. Soc. Pathol. Exot.,* 4, 693, 1911.

160. Raju, P. R., On the sparganum (plerocercoid) of *Spirometra* sp. (Pseudophyllidea: Diphyllobothriidae) from *Tropidonotus piscator* Wall, *Curr. Sci.*, 43, 193, 1974.

161. Read, C. P., *Spirometra* from Texas cats, *J. Parasitol.*, 38, 71, 1948.

162. Rego, A. A., Sôbre a validez do gênero *Lüheela* Baer, 1924 (Cestoda, Diphyllobothriidae), *Rev. Bras. Biol.*, 21, 155, 1961.

163. Rep, B. H., Intestinal helminths in dogs and cats on the antillian islands Aruba, Caracao, and Bonaire, *Trop. Geogr. Med.*, 27, 317, 1975.

164. Rep, B. H. and Heinnemann, D. W., Changes in hookworm distribution in Surinam, *Trop. Geogr. Med.*, 28, 104, 1976.

165. Rizhenko, G. F., Definitive hosts of *Spirometra erinacei-europaei, Byull. Vses. Inst. Gelmintol. K. I. Skryabina,* 2, 88, 1969.

166. Rodgers, W. A., Weights, measurements, and parasitic infestation of six lions from Southern Tanzania, *East. Afr. Wildl. J.*, 12, 157, 1974.

167. Rolon, P. A., Sparganose humaine. Presentation et de ses filiales, *Bull. Soc. Pathol. Exot.*, 69, 351, 1976.

168. von Römer, L. S., Uber einen fall von *Sparganum mansoni, Arch. Schiffs. Trop. Hyg.,* 14, 289, 1910.

169. Romero, E. A., Contribución al estudio de las técnicas de coloracion y montaje de platelmintos con referencia especial de un cestode encontrado por primera vez en el Estado Zulia, *Cien. Vet.*, 4, 253, 1974

170. Rosales, L. F., Primer caso de esparganosis en mapaches (*Procyon lotor*) de Guatemala, *Rev. Fac. Med. Vet. Zootec. Univ. San Carlos,* 3, 71, 1971.

171. Rukavina, J., Džumurov, N., and Delic, S., Larvae of *Diphyllobothrium erinacei-europaei* in pigs, *Vet. Sarajevo,* 6, 46, 1957.

172. Ryzhenko, G. F., Experimental determination of the reservoir hosts of *Spirometra erinacei-europaei, Tr. Vses. Inst. Gelmintol.,* 15, 252, 1969.

173. Sachs, R. and Sachs, C., A survey of parasitic infestation of wild herbivores in the Serengeti region in Northern Tanzania and the Lake Rukwa region in Southern Tanzania, *Bull. Epizoot. Dis. Afr.,* 16, 455, 1968.

174. Sadighian, A., Helminths of wildcats in the Shahsavar area, Caspian region, Iran, *J. Parasitol.,* 56, 270, 1970.

175. Sahasrabudhe, V. K. and Shah, H. L., On the pseudophyllidean genus *Spirometra*, Mueller, 1937 in Indian dogs, *Indian J. Helminthol.,* 19, 87, 1968.

176. Sahasrabudhe, V. K., Dubey, J. P., and Srivastav, H. O. P., Helminth parasites of dogs in Madhya Pradesh and their public health significance, *Indian J. Med. Res.,* 57, 56, 1969.

177. Sandars, D. F., A study of Diphyllobothriidae (Cestoda) from Australian hosts, *Proc. R. Soc. Queensl.,* 63, 65, 1953.

178. Sandars, D. F., A sparganum from a Queensland woman, *Med. J. Aust.,* 2, 817, 1954.

179. Schmid, H. and Watschinger, H., Sparganosis in the Masailand, *Acta Trop. Basel,* 29, 218, 1972.

180. Schmidt, G. D., The taxonomic states of *Spirometra* Faust, Campbell, and Kellog, 1929 (Cestodea:Diphyllobothriidae), *J. Helminthol.,* 48, 175, 1974.

181. Shah, H. L. and Pandit, C. N., A survey of helminth parasites of domesticated animals in Madhya Pradesh. I., *J. Vet. Anim. Husb. Res. (India),* 4, 1, 1959.

182. Southwell, T., Cestoda, in *The Fauna of British India, Including Ceylon and Burma,* Vol. 1, Taylor and Francis, London., 1930.

183. Spencer, W. W., *Bothriocephalus liguloides,* the cause of certain abdominal tumours, Intercolonial Med. Congr. Australasia Trans. 3rd Session 1892, 1893, 433.

184. Stiles, C. W., The occurrence of a proliferating cestode larva (*Sparganum proliferum*) in man in Florida, *Hyg. Lab. Bull.,* 40, 7, 1908.

185. Strauss, W. G. and Manwaring, J. H., Sparganosis: a new case in the United States and review of the literature, *Dermatol. Trop.,* 3, 73, 1964.

186. Swartzwelder, J. C., Beaver, P. C., and Hood, M. W., Sparganosis in Southern United States, *Am. J. Trop. Med. Hyg.,* 13, 43, 1964.

187. Takahashi, T., Studies on *Diphyllobothrium mansoni*, I. Life cycle and host specificity, *Jpn. J. Parasitol.,* 8, 567, 1959.

188. Tansurat, P., Sparganosis, in *Pathology of Protozoal and Helminthic Diseases,* Marcial-Rojas, R. A., Ed., Williams & Wilkens, 1971, 585.

189. Tashiro, K., Clinical-anatomical and experimental studies on "*Plerocercoides prolifer* Ijima (1905)", "*Spaganum proliferum* stiles (1906)," *Mitt. Med. Fak. Univ. Kyushu Fukuoka,* 9, 1, 1924.

190. Thomas, L. S., A new source of *Diphyllobothrium* infection, *Science,* 85, 119, 1937.

191. Thorson, R. E. and Jordan, E. M., A pseudophyllidean tapeworm from a dog in Southeastern United States, *Proc. Helminthol. Soc. Wash.,* 21, 123, 1954.

192. **T'u, C. T., Ch'iu, M. H., and Chou, Y. C.**, Adult *Spirometra mansoni* infection, a case report, *Chin. Med. J.*, 11, 691, 1973.

193. **Tubangui, M. A.**, Pseudophyllidean cestodes occurring in the Philippines, *Libro Jubilar Prof. Travassos*, 489, 1938.

194. **Vogelsang, E. G.**, Contribucion al estudio animal en Venezuela. XVI. Ecto y endoparasitos en animales domesticos y salvajes de la Guayana Venezolana, *Rev. Med. Vet. Parasitol.*, 7, 145, 1948.

195. **Vogelsang, E. G. and Gallo, P.**, Contribucion al estudio de la parasitologia animal en Venezuela. XVII. Dos huevos sparganum, *Rev. Med. Vet. Parasitol. Caracas*, 8, 79, 1949.

196. **Wardle, R. A. and McLeod**, *The Zoology of Tapeworms*, Hafner Publ., New York, 1968, (reprint 1952 ed.)

197. **Wharton, L. D.**, The intestinal worms of dogs in the Philippine islands, *J. Parasitol.*, 4, 80, 1917.

198. **Weinstein, P. P., Krawczyk, H. J., and Peers, J. H.**, Sparganosis in Korea, *Am. J. Trop. Med. Hyg.*, 3, 112, 1954.

199. **Widmer, E. A.**, Cultural factors in the transmission of echinococcosis and sparganosis in the Masai of East Africa, *Med. Arts Sci.*, 28, 29, 1974.

200. **Wolffhugel, K.**, Es autóctono el *Diphyllobothrium* en Chile?, *Bol. Soc. Biol. Concepcion (Chile)*, 24, 85, 1949.

201. **Yamaguti, S.**, Studies on the helminth fauna of Japan, VII. Cestodes of mammals and snakes, *Jpn. J. Zool.*, 6, 233, 1935.

202. **Yamaguti, S.**, *Systema Helminthum. The Cestodes of Vertebrates*, Vol. 2, Interscience, New York, 1959.

203. **Yamane, Y., Okada, N., and Takihara, M.**, On a case of long term migration of *Spirometra erinacei* larva in the breast of a woman, *Yonaga Acta Med.*, 19, 207, 1975.

204. **Yokogawa, S.**, Report on experiments with *Sparganum mansoni*, undertaken in an endeavor to clarify the nature of *Sparganum proliferum*, *Taiwan Igakei Zasshi*, 32, 1013, 1933.

205. **Yokogawa, S. and Kobayashi, H.**, On the species of *Diphyllobothrium mansoni* sensu lato, and on the infectious mode of human sparganosis. Trans. 8th Congr. Far East Assoc. Trop. Med., 1932, 215.

206. **Yoshida, S.**, The occurrence of *Bothriocephalus liguloides* Leuckart, with especial reference to its development, *J. Parasitol.*, 3, 171, 1917.

207. **Yutuc, L. M.**, Observations on Manson's tapeworm, *Diphyllobothrium erinacei* Rudolphi, 1819, in the Philippines, *Philipp. J. Sci.*, 80, 33, 1951.

208. **Khamboonruang, C., Premasathian, D., and Little, M. D.**, A case of intra-abdominal sparganosis in Chiang Mai Thailand, *Am. J. Trop. Med. Hyg.*, 23, 538, 1974.

TAENIASIS AND CYSTICERCOSIS

Zbigniew S. Pawłowski

INTRODUCTION

The latest taxonomic revision of the genus *Taenia* done by Verster[1] presents a good review of different species belonging to the genus *Taenia*. She accepted as valid only 30 species out of 70 described and concluded that the generic name *Taeniarhynchus* Weinland 1858, as suggested by Abuladze[2] for *T. saginata*, is unwarranted and confusing. Only two species: *Taenia solium* Linnaeus, 1758 and *Taenia saginata* Goeze, 1782 are found in man as their definitive host. Man can act as an intermediate host for at least four species: *T. solium* Linnaeus, 1758, *T. saginata* Goeze, 1782, *T. multiceps* Leske, 1780, and *T. hydatigena* Pallas, 1766. Only *T. saginata* and *T. solium* are the subject of this review; because of their obligatory association with man and cattle or pigs, they are unique zoonoses and have therefore been classified as perfect or "Euzoonoses" by Garnham.[3]

The 19th World Veterinary Congress held in Mexico City in 1971 fully recognized the pressing urgency of the taeniasis-cysticercosis problem which affects both human and animal welfare. Some examples illustrate the situation. In Mexico human cysticercosis occupied the ninth place as a cause of death.[4] More than 2500 cases of human cysticercosis described in some 200 papers published in two decades presents the world range of the problem.[5] As much as $50,000, which may be the cost of the social service in a single case of human cysticercosis, could not save the life of many patients with cerebral localization of the parasite. The debilitating effect of *T. saginata* tapeworm on populations living on a protein deficient diet and already loaded with other parasites is a grave drain on human resources which cannot be assessed in figures.[6] In East Africa extensive *T. saginata* cysticercosis is taking a heavy toll on the meat industry estimated at nearly ten million dollars annually and inhibits the economic development of that area.[6]

In many countries in Europe *T. saginata* infection is a progressive zoonosis.[7]

Although taeniasis has been known since ancient times and although a great deal is known about the infection, there are still many gaps in our knowledge of the biology of the parasite, the clinical aspects of the disease, and the epidemiology of the infection; that is why the measures taken to control the infection are often ineffective.

TAENIA SAGINATA INFECTION

Disease

Taenia saginata taeniasis is a nonfatal intestinal infection in man, caused by the adult beef tapeworm, *Taenia saginata*.

Taenia saginata cysticercosis is an infection in cattle with the larval stage, cysticercus, localized mainly in the muscle tissue of the animals.

Etiological Agent

Taenia saginata has four different stages in its life cycle: (1) adult worm, an intestinal parasite of man; (2) eggs, disseminated in external environment and invasive for cattle; (3) oncospherae, penetrating bovine tissues, and (4) cysticercus, a bladder worm, muscle tissue parasite, invasive for man.

The Adult Form

The adult form is a flat tapeworm consisting of a head *scolex*, a neck *collum* and a

Table 1

DIAGNOSTIC CHARACTERS OF *T. SOLIUM* AND
T. SAGINATA ADULT FORMS[13]

	T. solium	T. saginata
Entire body		
Length m	1.5—8	4—12
Maximal breadth mm	7—10	12—14
Number of proglottids	700—1000	Ca. 2000
Scolex		
Diameter mm	0.6—1	1.5—2
Suckers: number	4	4
Diameter mm	0.4—0.5	0.7—0.8
Rostellum	Present	Absent
Hooks: number	22—32	Absent
Large length μm	159—173	
Small length μm	93—127	
Mature proglottids		
Testes number	375—575	800—1200
Confluent posterior to the vitellarium	Yes	No
Cirrus pouch extend the excretory vessels	Yes	No
Ovary	3 lobes	2 lobes
Vaginal sphincter	Absent	Present
Gravid proglottids		
Uterus branches:		
Number each side	7—12[16]	[15] 18—32
Pattern	Dendritic	Dichotomic
Way of leaving host	In groups and passively	Single and spontaneously

From Pawłowski, Z. S., and Schultz, M. G., *Advances in Parasitology*, Dawes, Ben, Ed., Academic Press, New York, 1972, 10. With permission.

chain of about 2000 proglottids *strobila* (Table 1, Figure 1). The length of the adult tapeworm is between 4 and 12 m and it depends much on the degree of relaxation of proglottids. Scolex is quadrangular in shape and less than 2 mm in diameter (Figure 2). It has four strong suckers, hemispherical, 0.7 to 0.8 mm in diameter, and frequently pigmented. The process of strobilization occurs at the distal part of the neck, which is much more narrow than the head but few times longer. The strobila consists of immature, mature, and gravid proglottids. The mature proglottids are filled with female and male genital organs and a parenchymatous tissue; the nervous and excretory systems occupy little space. After the cross-fertilization, when the proglottids become gravid, the uterus filled with eggs develops 18 to 32 lateral extensions each side (Figure 3). The last gravid proglottids, about 20 mm long and 5 to 7 mm broad, single detached from the strobila, leave the host, usually spontaneously.

T. saginata adult forms show a strong tendency to morphological abnormalities. They refer to the entire strobila (tri-, tetra-, penta-radiation, pigmentation, or bifurcation), to one or several proglottids (bifurcation, fenestration, fusion, variations in segmentation supernumerary, or intercalary proglottids) or to the variations in structure of reproductive organs only. These abnormalities have caused many taxonomic confusions in the past and resulted in different synonyms for one species.[1,2]

The existence of ''crowding effect'' in multiple infections with human tapeworm shows that the host capacity in terms of available space and/or nutritional substances

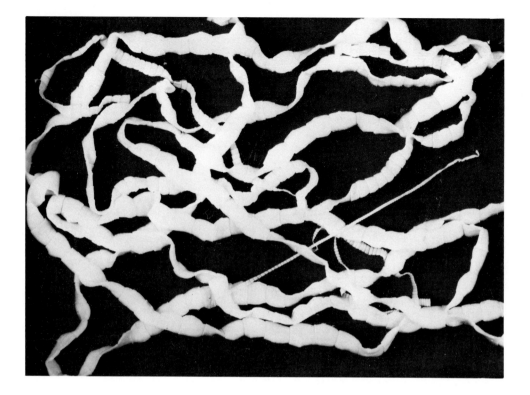

FIGURE 1.   *Taenia saginata*. Adult worm.

is limited. In one patient infected with 16 *T. saginata*, the tapeworms were only 50 to 80 cm long.[8] The multiple infections, however, are uncommon; in Poland they occur approximately in 1:200 *T. saginata* carriers.[9] In some endemic foci, e.g., in Azerbaijan and Armenia (U.S.S.R.), they are as frequent as 67% of all the cases.[10] This is because a successful superinfection with *T. saginata* cysticerci is possible.[11] There are also numerous reports of the coexistence of *T. saginata* and *T. solium*. Multiple and mixed infections strongly speak against the widely held misconception that adult *Taeniidae* in man are usually solitary.

The common localization of *T. saginata* scolex is the jejunum, about 40 to 50 cm below the duodenojejunal flexure.[12] The strobila might extend down to the terminal ileum where its thicker parts might occasionally be seen during a radiological examination. Very rarely have the tapeworms been found in the gallbladder, appendix, and nasopharynx.[13]

Localization of *T. saginata* in human jejunum exposes the tapeworm surface to the action of intestinal digestive enzymes of the host. They are alive — they resist digestion, but when the tapeworm is killed by a drug the digestion of a part or even the whole of the strobila may happen within a relatively short time.

The studies on ultrastructural morphology of the tegument of adult cestodes helped to understand some physiological functions of the tegument and integration of inner parasite environment and its physiological activity with the external environment.[14,15] The tegument of *T. saginata* is not an inert citicule but an active digestive-absorptive structure showing some morphological and functional similarities to the luminal mucosal structures of the vertebrates. Very little is known about the uptake of nutritional substances by *T. saginata*, but the observations of Read[16] in *H. diminuta* showed that a contact digestion plays an important role in adult forms of cestodes. A large absorp-

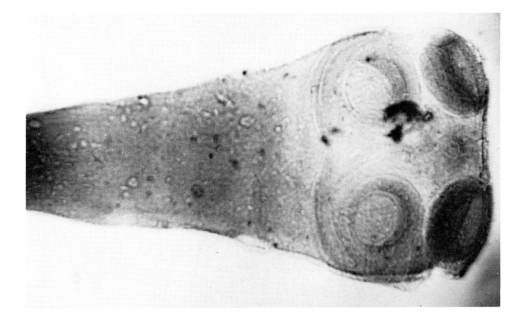

FIGURE 2.   *Taenia saginata.* Scolex.

tive area of the tegument and plenty of available food accelerate the processes of growth and segmentation, as well as differentiation of sexual organs and cells, eggs production, and regeneration.

A rapid development of new proglottids results in the production of 6 to 9 gravid proglottides, i.e., 12 to 27 cm of *T. saginata* strobila per day. After an unsuccessful treatment strobila regenerates within 3 to 3½ months. *T. saginata* adult worm has a relatively long lifespan in man which may be 30 to 40 years.

Eggs

T. saginata proglottids produce about 80,000 eggs each.[17] The uterine eggs have an outer shell with two characteristic filaments (Figure 4). But this outer shell is very delicate and what is usually seen outside the uterus (in the feces, or the anal swabs) is an embryophore containing a more or less developed oncosphere but not the complete egg itself. Since the embryophores of *T. saginata* and *T. solium* as well as of some other *Taeniidae*, are practically identical in their morphology, this makes their identification impossible. The thick and globular embryophore, 31 to 43 μm in diameter, consists of many prismatic elements cemented by a substance easily digested by pepsin and trypsin.

There is uneven maturation of oncospheres in the eggs present in the last 30 to 50 proglottides. About 50% of *T. saginata* embryophores leaving the proglottids contain fully developed and invasive oncospheres.[18] The immature ones may develop to maturity outside the host.

The majority of *T. saginata* eggs leave the proglottids shortly after their detachment from the strobila through an opening (*proctosoma*) which develops by a disruption of a bundle of uterine branches (*thysanus*) situated close to the anterior margin of the proglottis.[19] At the time of extrusion the pressure of the masses of eggs filling up the uterus and the active movement of the proglottid are responsible for the active expulsion of eggs within a short time after their detachment from the strobila. Some several hundreds or thousands of eggs only are released by maceration of the proglottids.[19,20]

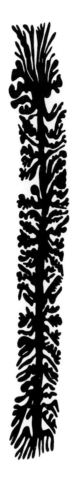

FIGURE 3. *Taenia saginata.* Gravid proglottid.
(From Verster, A., *Z. Parasitkd.,* 29, 313, 1967.
With permission.)

T. saginata proglottids migrate actively through the anus and are excreted not only at the time of defecation. All these facts explain the easy and wide distribution of invasive embryophores in the surroundings.

Oncosphere

The oncosphere is 30 μm large, has a globular body, with 6 embryonic hooklets, a pair of penetration glands, and some hundreds of cells including those of the muscle and excretory system. There are two steps in getting the oncosphere ready to invade the immediate host: disintegration of the embryophore and activation of the oncosphere itself. The penetration of the host mucosa by a free oncosphere is accomplished by its hooks, secretion of penetrating glands, and active movements of its body. After 1 or 2 hr the oncosphere enters the blood or lymphatic vessels in submucosa, but its further fate is largely unknown, although there is some evidence that the oncosphere actively penetrates the lymphatic vessels in the muscles.[21]

Cysticercus

The most important steps in the development of *T. saginata* cysticercus from an oncosphere are described next.[22] On day 11 after infection the first cysticerci can be found by the naked eye, having the size of 0.1 × 0.13 mm and 2 × 3 mm together with

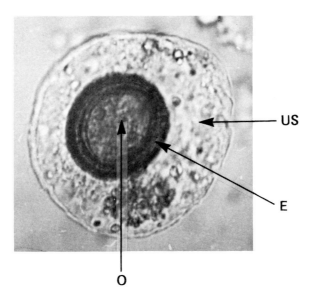

FIGURE 4.   *Taenia saginata.* Uterine egg. US — uterine shell, E—
embryophore, O — oncosphere.

the surrounding connective tissue; 3 weeks after infection a cavity and immature scolex
are formed. At the 5th and 6th weeks the scolex is fully developed and at the 10th
week an invaginated neck can be found. Ten to twelve weeks old cysticerci are the
youngest stage invasive for man.

The developed cysticercus consists of an invaginated scolex in the vesicle filled with
an opalescent fluid. The size of this ovoid bladder larva is 7 to 10 mm by 4 to 6 mm.
The structure of the wall of *T. saginata* cysticercus vesicle proved to be a very complicated one; the external tissue consists of hairlike processes situated on the peripheral
collagenous-fibrous layer below which some groups of oval cells, muscle bundles, a
duct system, some flame cells, and fine fibers have been identified; the internal tissue
fold has a peripheral fibrous layer, two muscle layers and peripheral cells, calcareous
corpuscules, flame cells, and a duct system embedded in a loose fibrous net, an a
central band of muscles.[21,23] Based on this morphological observation an analogy has
been suggested between the bladder of cysticercus and the trophoblast, i.e., between a
parasite larva and a mammalian embryo, both developing in another macroorganism
and at its expense.[21]

The primary localization of developing cysticerci are the dilated lymphatic spaces in
the skeletal muscles or the heart (including endocardium).[21] In atypical organs such as
liver and lung, cysticerci degenerate as early as 20 days after infection. The same is
partly true for the heart muscle.

The longevity of cysticerci varies in various experiments from 9 months[24] to 3
years.[25] This might be attributable at least to different strains of *T. saginata*, various
strains of cattle, different infective dose, and host immunity. It was found that the
life span of primary cysticerci has been shortened by secondary exposure.[26]

Hosts

Man is the only definitive *T. saginata* host known. An extensive search for *T. saginata* adults performed in 271 wild African primates and 143 carnivores did not reveal
T. saginata in any of them.[27] The attempts failed to induce *T. saginata* infection in
baboons and monkeys by experimentally feeding them with *T. saginata* cysticerci.[28]

The typical intermediate hosts for *T. saginata* are domestic *Bovidae (Bos taurus, B.*

bufellus, B. indicus, B. grunniens). In 1960 the reindeer (*Rangifer tarandus*) has proved to be a common intermediate host for *T. saginata* in northern Siberia, U.S.S.R.[29] There was a suggestion that wild goats might serve as intermediate hosts for *T. saginata* in a remote mountainous area in Taiwan where there were human *T. saginata* carriers but no cattle.[30] That suggestion as well as sporadic findings of unhooked cysticerci in llamas, proghorn, oryx and oribi antelopes, bushbucks, Dorcas and redfronted gazellas, wildebeests, giraffes, and lemurs need experimental confirmation; e.g., in experiments gazella Thomsoni was found resistant to the infection with *T. saginata* eggs.[31] Experimental infection of African dwarf goats was also unsuccessful.[32] In sheep and goats in Poland infected experimentally *T. saginata* cysticerci were found to degenerate before the invasive stage had been reached.[32]

The question as to whether man can be an intermediate host for *T. saginata* has not been satisfactorily answered.[13] There is no doubt that cysticerci with hookless scolices have been found in the human body. In some cases they have been numerous; in others they were found accompanying intestinal *T. saginata* infection.[13] Unfortunately, the majority of cases lack sufficient documentation. In any event the phenomenon is of extremely rare occurrence.

Distribution

The *T. saginata* taeniasis and cysticercosis is widespread in most cattle breeding countries in the world. The knowledge about the prevalence of infection in man and animals is defective because of the lack of sources of objective and comparable epidemiological data. There are three sources of data on human tapeworm infection: mass helminthological surveys in selected groups of population, laboratory and hospital records, and analyses of reported cases.

There are a few countries in which mass helminthological surveys are performed regularly; these give some notion about the prevalence of human tapeworm infection. In the U.S.S.R., the mean prevalence of *T. saginata* taeniasis was 0.6% in 1950 as based on 14.2 million stool examinations and 0.3% in 1960 in 46.4 million examined people.[33,34] The distribution of *T. saginata*, however, is very uneven; up to 1% in the western republics (Russian SFSR, Ukrainian, Latvian, Estonian, Lithuanian, and Belorussian SSR) and between 8 and 45% in the Caucasian area (southern Dagestan ASSR, western Azerbaijan, northern Armenian, eastern Georgian SSR) and in the south-central Asian republics (Uzbek, Kirghiz and Kazakh SSR).[13,33,34]

Although the data taken from laboratories and hospitals are selected, they give a better index of the actual situation in the population. The available hospital and laboratory records from Kenya are high (up to 50%), while mass-helminthological surveys reveal much lower infection rates, mainly due to the inadequacy of the methods of examination of feces.

A few countries have introduced the compulsory notification of human *T. saginata* infections. A survey in the city of Poznan showed that 10 years after the introduction of the compulsory notification as many as 20% of *T. saginata* cases diagnosed had not been formally registered, although the specialized parasitological service is well organized and active.[35] In other countries the notification seems to be even less effective.

The *T. saginata* incidence in man can roughly be classified into three groups: (1) countries or regions which are highly endemic with the incidence in human population exceeding 10%, (2) those with moderate infection rates, and (3) those with very low prevalence, below 0.1% or even free from *T. saginata*.

The highly endemic areas are Central and East African countries (Ethiopia, Kenya, Zair), Caucasian and south-central Asian U.S.S.R. republics (Dagestan ASSR, Azerbaijan, Armenian, Georgian, Uzbek, Kirghiz, Kazakh SSR), Near-East countries (Syria, Lebanon) and small areas in Yugoslavia (Bosnia, Montenegro).

Europe belongs to the region with moderate infections, so also do Southeast Asia (Thailand, India, Vietnam, the Philippines, and Japan) and South America (Brazil, Argentina, Ecuador, Guatemala, and Cuba).

Low incidence of *T. saginata* is in the U.S., Canada, Australia, and some Western Pacific countries.

The incidence of *T. saginata* in cattle roughly corresponds to that of taeniasis. FAO/WHO/OIE[36] register 37 countries with a widespread bovine cysticercosis: Morocco, Algeria, Libyan Arab Republic, Chad, Niger, Upper Volta, Mauritania, Senegal, Gambia, Portuguese Guinea, Guinea, Sierra Leone, Ivory Coast, Dahomey, Nigeria, Cameroon, Central African Republic, Ethiopia, Kenya, Tanzania, Uganda, Rwanda, Burundi, Botswana, South Africa, Swaziland, Argentina, Chile, Peru, Nicaragua, Sweden, Albania, Turkey, Afghanistan, Burma, Laos, and New Zealand. Bovine cysticercosis has not been recorded in: Liberia, Mauritius, Guyana, Bermuda, Bahamas, Iceland, Saudi Arabia, Malaysia, Brunei, Fiji, New Hebrides, New Caledonia, Western Samoa, and Papua, New Guinea.

The prevalence of *T. saginata* taeniasis and cysticercosis has been changing, e.g., in Germany before the introduction of the official meat inspection at the end of the 19th century the prevalence of human taeniasis was about 5% and that of cysticercosis more than 5%; the meat inspection reduced the percentage of bovine cysticercosis down to 0.37% in 1910 and for 40 years its prevalence was maintained at 0.3%; since the early 1950s it has increased nearly ten times exceeding 2% in the 1960s. It was reported as high as 7% and 7.32% from Halle[37] and Frankfurt/Oder[38] in 1962 and 1969, respectively. *T. saginata* taeniasis and cysticercosis were rarely diagnosed in England before World War II, but in 1955 the prevalence of cysticercosis was estimated between 0.81 to 3.47%.[39] An analysis of 85 publications on taeniasis-cysticercosis from various European countries after 1945 showed that *T. saginata* became common in the U.K., Denmark, and Holland in the late 1940s; in Belgium, Germany, Italy, Yugoslavia, Czechoslovakia and Poland in the 1950s; and in Sweden, Hungary, Romania, and Bulgaria in the 1960s.[7] The statistics from various slaughterhouses clearly illustrate this point:[13] Prague 0.32% (1945) — 1.6% (1955) — 3.1% (1964); Berlin: about 1% (1945—1959) — 5.5% (1965); Genoa: 3.4% (1951) — 8% (1953); St. Polten: 0.6% (1954) — 2.3% (1960); Poznań: 0.5% (1955) — 2,3% (1962).

The transmission of *T. saginata* in a highly developed country such as the U.S. has its unique character.[40] In general, the incidence of cysticercosis in federally inspected cattle persists at a very low level; 0.14% in 1912, 0.37% in 1930, 0.6% in 1942[41] and 0.09 to 0.12% in 1948 to 1954,[42] and 0.04 to 0.08% in 1959 to 1967.[40] There is an evident concentration of bovine cysticercosis in California (72.6% of all cases in 1967), and some concentration in Texas, Colorado, and Arizona (5.4%; 2.3% and 2.2%, respectively). The intensity of infection is rather low; about 0.8% of measled carcasses were condemned.

The exact prevalence of human taeniasis in the U.S. is not known. The fact that in the years 1963 to 1967 stool sample examinations done in State Health Department laboratories revealed 429 cases of *Taenia* infection, and another 211 cases were diagnosed in 16 hospital institutions, indicates the continuing transmission of *T. saginata* in the U.S. Human infections are frequent in New York City, California, and Florida and especially in the affluent and most travelled part of the population. A special epidemiological problem is the introduction of *T. saginata* from Mexico.[43,44]

The epidemiological situation in the developed countries, like the U.S., greatly favors the creation of sporadic epizootic foci of bovine cysticercosis. On the contrary, the enzootic *T. saginata* cysticercosis and endemic taeniasis is characteristic of pastoral or nomadic communities living close to the cattle herds as in southern republics of the U.S.S.R. and in cattle breeding Africa.

Bovine Cysticercosis

Light or moderate cysticercosis in cattle is usually not associated with any defined clinical picture. But very heavy infection, e.g., those induced experimentally by one million of *T. saginata* eggs or more, may give rise to symptoms (fever, weakness, profuse salivation, anorexia, higher temperature) and may cause death between 14 to 16 days due to a degenerative myocarditis.[45] Pericarditis and coronary embolism were reported in an oryx antelope kept in a zoo and infected with *T. saginata.*[46]

The course of cysticercosis depends on the immunological processes. There are at least four immunological mechanisms directed against different stages of *T. saginata* in an intermediate host. IgA antibodies in the immune animals may be responsible for the disturbances in hatching of oncospheres. A little is known about the immunological reactions against *T. saginata* oncospheres invading the intestinal mucosa, but the existence of an immunological intestinal barrier has been suggested.[47] The intestinal barrier seems to depend on the level of circulating antibodies as well as on a general nonspecific protective mechanism. Experiments with the parenteral injection of *T. saginata* oncospheres gave inconclusive results as to the possibility of establishing an infection in the immune cattle by by-passing the intestinal barrier.[48,49] Very little is known about the immunological reactions directed against the migrating and reorganizing oncospheres, and later of developing cysticerci. As in *T. pisiformis* the liver may filter migrating oncospheres.

As far as the serology and resistance to bovine cysticercosis are concerned, the direct relation between the titres of hemagglutinating and precipitating antibodies and resistance has not been confirmed.[50,51] Those authors suggested that serologically demonstrable antibodies are not to be involved in the resistance to infection. They found that calves repeatedly infected with small doses of *T. saginata* eggs developed a strong resistance to challenge infection after a year but those infected with a single dose failed to become resistant, although in both of the groups the titers of hemagglutination antibodies were similar.

The living cysticerci in a natural host provoke a slight cellular reaction, but in the immune cattle or unspecific host (sheep, goats)[32] the young cysticerci provoke an extensive host reaction and soon undergo a degeneration.

T. Saginata Taeniasis

Human *T. saginata* infection may very much differ in symptomatology and clinical pathology in individual cases.[13] Of *T. saginata* carriers, 98% feel some sensation in the perianal area during the discharging proglottids.[52] The other symptoms were registered in 79% of women and 75% of men in a study on symptomatology of 2200 cases of *T. saginata* taeniasis.[13,53] The most common were abdominal pain (35%) and nausea (32%); less frequent were weakness (18%) and loss of body weight (15%), followed by increased (13%) or decreased (13%) appetite and headache (13%). Much less frequent were constipation (7%) or diarrhoea (5%), salivation (5%) and vomiting (5%), irritability (4%) and dizziness (4%), quite uncommon increase of body weight (2%), pruritus ani (1%), urticaria (0.5%), and syncope (0.5%). A cross correlation of the various symptoms, as evaluated by dendrite statistical analysis, showed four different groups of symptoms: the first (statistically most separate) one consisted of the cases with increased appetite and increased body weight; the second group included some allergic symptoms (pruritus ani, urticaria) and neurotic conditions (irritability, pruritus ani); the third group was characterized by lowered appetite, loss of body weight, and a general weakness including dizziness syndrome; and finally the fourth most numerous group consisted of intestinal symptoms (abdominal pains, nausea, vomiting, discomfort, diarrhea or constipation).[54] Some symptoms are of a psychological nature because they have been realized shortly after the patients become conscious of the tapeworm infection, i.e., after the first discharge of proglottids or strobila, which usually happens 3 months after infection. The infants and children usually react to the infection worse than the adult carriers. The infected women report slightly higher frequency of symptoms; the sensation of a lump in the throat (globus hystericus) was registered only in women.[13,53]

There is a considerable number of reports on complications of *T. saginata* taeniasis as appendicitis and cholecystitis caused by stray *T. saginata* proglottids.[13,55,56] The introduction of niclosamid has resulted in a diminished frequency of *T. saginata* complications.

The few clinical pathological studies performed in uncomplicated cases of *T. saginata* infection revealed some morphological and functional changes. The examination of intestinal mucosa taken by biopsy in a number of cases showed a slight subacute inflammatory change,[57,58] which was interpreted as the reaction of small intestine mucosa to the presence of the tapeworm.

There are well documented data concerning the lowered gastric secretion both in volume and in acidity in taeniasis. This phenomenon was observed in man,[11,59] and confirmed experimentally.[60] The impaired secretion may be responsible for some symptoms as well as for increased susceptibility to other parasitic or bacterial infections.

Moderate eosinophilia has been reported in from 5[61] to 46%[62] of *T. saginata* carriers. A higher level of eosinophilia, 36 to 53% was observed sporadically.[63] Eosinophilia up to 16.5% can be provoked in man by injections of extracts of *T. saginata*.[64]

An increased level of serum immunoglobulin E in some patients infected with *T. saginata* was found by Nepote et al.[65] This is the first step towards better understanding of some immunological consequences of *T. saginata* parasitism and some allergic reactions observed in *T. saginata* taeniasis.

General Mode of Spread

The general mode of transmission is presented in Figure 5.

Epidemiology

Man, as the definitive host of *T. saginata* tapeworm, is the only disseminator of eggs of the parasite. The mean daily production is 6 to 9 proglottids and 480,000 to 720,000 eggs.[17]

The direct transmission of eggs is uncommon and can be realized on occasion when a human carrier is handling or feeding calves or cattle with his contaminated hands.[66,67] The *T. saginata* eggs can be easily spread out in the close environment of the carriers. There is an observation that a temporary worker of Mexican origin was the source of cysticercosis for 743 cattle in a feedlot in Texas.[43]

In the indirect transmission of infection from man to animals the main steps are the contamination of external environment, store and spread of *T. saginata* eggs in it, and contamination of animal food and water.

In developed countries the migration of people in the form of camping and tourism or occupational purposes brings closer the urban population, the potential *T. saginata* carriers, to cattle breeding rural areas.[68] The uncontrolled defecation and inadequate elimination of viable *Taenia* eggs in sewage play an important role in spreading *T. saginata* infection.[13] Most of the conventional sewage treatment is only partly effective, mainly because of the overloaded systems and the interference with natural purification processes due to high concentration of chemicals.[69,70] The *Taenia* eggs were found 32 km below the sewage outlet into Moskwa river[71] and 250 m out in the Caspian Sea at Baku.[72] Epizootic *T. saginata* infections attributed to sewage have been described in the U.S.[40] and in Germany.[73,74] In Poznań region (Poland) the evident concentration of bovine cysticercosis was found along the rivers, railway tracks, and roads.[68,75]

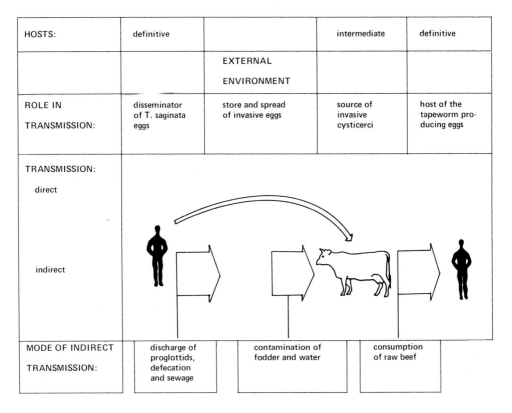

HOSTS:	definitive		intermediate	definitive
		EXTERNAL ENVIRONMENT		
ROLE IN TRANSMISSION:	disseminator of T. saginata eggs	store and spread of invasive eggs	source of invasive cysticerci	host of the tapeworm pro- ducing eggs
TRANSMISSION: direct indirect				
MODE OF INDIRECT TRANSMISSION:	discharge of proglottids, defecation and sewage	contamination of fodder and water	consumption of raw beef	

FIGURE 5.   *Taenia saginata.* Mode of spread.

The field experiments done in New Zealand with *T. ovis* revealed that the taeniid eggs can be widely dispersed from one place on a 20,000 m² pasture within a 10 day period.[76] The ecological factors responsible for so effective a dispersion of eggs in the natural conditions are only partly known. Both birds and invertebrate animals may play a role in spreading *T. saginata* eggs in the environment. Blackheaded gulls (*Larus ridibundus*) and common gulls (*L. canus*) were found to disseminate *T. saginata* eggs in Denmark[77] and in the Liverpool area.[78,79] *Taenia* eggs are also able to pass the intestinal tract of young chickens,[80] sparrows, and crows.[81] The transmission of *T. saginata* eggs by some flies has been confirmed in Uzbek SSR,[82] Azerbaijan SSR,[83] and in Kenya.[84] Recent experiments with coprophagic beetles (*Aphodius fimetarius, A. fossor* and *Sphaeridium scarabacoides*) and earthworm (*Eisenia foetida, Allolobophora caliginosa,* and *Lumbricus terrestris*) showed that these invertebrates may effectively transport *T. saginata* eggs on the ground.[85]

The eggs present in the external environment vary in their age and invasiveness. They are juvenile, mature, and senescent. Some eggs passing out from proglottids are juvenile and are not invasive unless they become mature within a few days or weeks. This transition as well as the survival time of mature eggs depends much on temperature and moisture. The taeniid eggs are rather resistant to unfavorable external conditions including chemicals.[86,87] The optimum temperature for survival of *T. saginata* eggs is −4°C.[88] The temperature above 59°C[89] and desiccation[86] rapidly kill the taeniid eggs. *T. saginata* eggs in hay or grass silage loss their infectivity after 70 to 90 days.[90] Under natural conditions *T. saginata* eggs survive better several months in cold winter than in a few weeks in a hot and dry summer.[88] The *T. saginata* eggs were found to survive half a year in Denmark,[91] 100 to 337 days in the Ukraine,[92] and 1 year in the highlands of Kenya.[93] The similar conditions which are responsible for the survival of taeniid eggs influence their aging processes. The "senescent" eggs, stored for a longer time in the environment, are supposed to have a lowered invasiveness.

The transmission from the external environment to the cattle is realized by contamination of their pastures, food, and water. The contamination of the water used for watering the cattle is of special epizootic importance.[39,68,94] The way of *T. saginata* infection in cattle is mainly peroral. Prenatal infection by the intrauterine route seems to be rather frequent in Kenya,[66,95,96] but has not been experimentally confirmed in Europe.[97]

In cattle the invasive cysticerci develop within 10 to 12 weeks after the consumption of *T. saginata* eggs and remain viable for months or years.

The transmission of *T. saginata* infection between animal and man depends much on the human habit of eating raw or semiraw beef dishes like beef tartar shashlik in the U.S.S.R.,[98] basterma in the Near East,[99] Sikh Khabab and biriyani in India,[100] larb in Thailand,[101] or pieces of meat simply roasted against the open fire in Central and East Africa.[102] There is also the chance of being infected by tasting meat during cooking.[11] Within 3 months after consumption of an invasive cysticercus man who is rather susceptible for the primary as well as for the further infections, starts to discharge *T. saginata* proglottids. If not treated man may remain a *T. saginata* carrier to the end of his life.

Diagnosis

Human T. Saginata Taeniasis

There are usually three steps in the specific diagnosis of taeniasis: (1) justified suspicion based on the questioning of a patient about a discharge of proglottids or a defect of contrast in the radiological examination of ileum; (2) genus diagnosis by finding *Taenia* eggs in feces or on an anal swab; (3) final species diagnosis based on an examination of the scolex or the gravid proglottids by counting uterine branches or, when doubtful, by using Verster's taxonomic criteria.[103] A differential diagnosis of *T. saginata* and *T. solium* is important for clinical (treatment, prognosis) and epidemiological (danger of cysticercosis) reasons.

The laboratory methods in the order of their decreasing effectiveness are: examination of proglottides, anal swab, thick fecal smear, concentration of flotation techniques, and thin fecal smear.[104-107]

The important clinical problem to be solved is the finding of an effectual method of diagnosing *T. saginata* infection before the strobila is fully developed, eggs excreted, and proglottids discharged. Improved serological techniques are required because routine serological tests performed with various antigens are not useful in the diagnosis of human taeniasis.

Bovine Cysticercosis

The problem of intravital diagnosis of bovine cysticercosis has not been solved by intradermal reactions nor by serological tests because of unsatisfactory levels of specificity and sensitivity of the tests and a weak immunological response of the host in natural light infections.

The development of serological tests for the diagnosis of bovine cysticercosis have been directed towards the adaptation of the most effective, specific, and simple tests which can be performed on the spot in slaughterhouses. So far, the hemagglutination test is the most promising serological method for diagnosing bovine cysticercosis.[50,51,108] Studies on 3-months-old calves experimentally infected produce evidence of hemagglutinating antibodies as early as 4 to 5 weeks after infection with a sharp rise of the titers during the following 3 months; the highest titers were around the 6th month and positive titers were still evident at 10 months.[51] The hemagglutination tests show a great range of titers. The test depends on individual reactions of the host, their age, and the time of their first exposure. When older cattle are first exposed to infection the antibody response develops well and serological diagnosis is successful.[109] But when calves are infected early in their lives, as usually happens in East Africa, their weak serological response makes serological diagnosis in the field difficult.[50]

Precipitating antibodies as examined in micro-gel-diffusion test according to Crowle were detected in experimentally infected calves at 2 weeks following the infection and remained relatively strong only 3 to 6 months.[50,110] This test does not have a practical value in diagnosis of natural light infections. There are also some difficulties in adapting the enzyme-linked immunoabsorbent assay (ELISA) to mass diagnosis of bovine cysticercosis.

The post-mortem meat inspection is so far the only practically applied diagnostic method for bovine cysticercosis. The question of "predilection sites" for *T. saginata* cysticerci has a long history and many papers have been published on the subject.[13] The opinions are still controversial in some details but there is agreement in general that the masseters, heart and tongue as well as the shoulder muscles (*triceps brachii*),[111,112] are the ones that should be examined. Other authors insist on a thorough examination of the diaphragm, esophagus, and lungs. The breed of cattle, their age and activity of a particular muscle group[113] as well as the age and intensity of infection may influence the localization of cysticerci and the effectiveness of meat inspection.

Prevention and Control

There are at least two examples which show the possibility of success in the control of *T. saginata*: the eradication program for human *T. saginata* carriers in the U.S.S.R. has significantly reduced *T. saginata* incidence,[33,34] and the changing sanitary and economic conditions in modern Israel have virtually eliminated *T. saginata* from that country.[114]

The better prevention of taeniasis and cysticercosis has three goals: development of new drugs against both adult and larval stages, improvement of meat inspection, and vaccination against bovine cysticercosis. But they should not lessen the importance of sanitary education, and sanitation and improvement of general social and economic conditions in reducing the transmission of *Taenia saginata*.[13,115,116]

Chemotherapy of Taeniasis and Cysticercosis

The most important advance made in the treatment of human *T. saginata* taeniasis was the introduction of niclosamide (Yomesan®) in 1960. The efficacy of niclosamide is between 85 to 95%.[117] There are usually no strict contraindications to the treatment with niclosamide, but it is not, as a rule, indicated in the first trimester of pregnancy unless uncontrollable vomiting is present. The side effects during the treatment with niclosamide are slight and uncommon, but some cases of syncope have been reported.[118-120] The mode of action of niclosamide is not very clear; the drug inhibits the uptake of oxygen and glucose and increases the decomposition of glycogen[121] which may result in a kind of energetic paralysis of the parasite. The drug is rapidly excreted with the feces (70 to 75%) or in the urine (25%) in the form of metabolites.[121] For this reason niclosamide is well tolerated and has a high degree of safety.

Other drugs proposed or used in the last two decades including dichlorophen, hypertonic solutions of magnesium sulfate, extracts of pumpkin seeds, synthetic chemicals related to extracts of male fern, bithionol, paromomycine and mebendazole, have not been accepted for routine use either because of their low efficacy or high toxicity. Alternative drugs include tin compounds which are widely used in Europe after the sometime successful experience of Cuban, French, and German investigators.[13] The tin compounds differ in formula and form as well as in efficacy and tolerance.[117,122] Their use is contraindicated in pregnancy[123] and severe gastrointestinal, liver, and renal diseases. The effect of tin compounds consists in the interference with the mechanism which keeps the tapeworm resistant to digestion. The average number of treatments required for a successful dehelminthtization dropped from 1.9 in 1953—56 (treatment with pumpkin seeds, mepacrine, and male fern) to 1.1 in 1966—68 due to introduction of niclosamide and tin compounds.[124]

A new schistosomicide praziquantel is going to be a new drug of choice in human taeniasis. In *T. saginata* taeniasis the cure rate following a single 5mg/kg dose of 96.6% in 141 patients out of 146 and with a single 10 mg/kg dose it was 95.9% or 256 out of 267 patients treated. The tolerance to a single dose of praziquantel is excellent; side effects are mostly mild with some transient abdominal pain and in some cases soft stools or diarrhea may occur; headache, dizziness, and skin rashes are rare. During the treatment with praziquantel the strobila usually disintegrate and only some distal parts, if any, are discharged.[194]

Recently two drugs: mebendazole and praziquatel have been suggested as effective against *T. saginata* cysticercosis in cattle. If the preliminary reports are confirmed and the drugs are economic, the mass chemotherapy of cattle may be the most effective method of preventing the *T. saginata* transmission from animals to men.

Improvement of Meat Inspection

Although meat inspection may not be an absolute safeguard in the control of *T. saginata* it is in many countries the only measure that is applied routinely. There is no doubt that meat inspection has played and still plays a positive role in preventing heavily infected carcasses from being consumed, but it becomes less efficient as the infections become more industralized. The importance of predilected localization of cysticerci in the musculature and the selection of cuts test for effective meat inspection were overestimated in the past. The individual skill and conscientious work of inspectors and the conditions in which they do their work, including light, humidity, and speed of conveyers influence the effectiveness of their meat inspection.

There is an opinion that the extensive examination or repeated inspection are required when the meat is intended for consumption raw.

The intravital diagnosis of cysticercosis, e.g., by highly authomatized ELISA test as in trichinellosis might change much of the procedure of traditional meat inspection but this problem is still under laboratory investigations.

The destruction of cysticerci in carcasses is an important problem which is not being solved to the satisfaction of meat hygienists and economists. As a rule only heavily infected cattle carcasses are condemned. Other carcasses are either subjected to freezing or boiled. Freezing of meat at −10°C (15°F) for 10 days or at −18°C (0°F) for 5 days effectively kills cysticerci.[125,126] Investigations on gamma irradiation showed that the inactivation of *T. saginata* cysticerci in carcasses requires high doses of irradiation.[127]

Vaccination Against Bovine Cysticercosis

As early as 1936 a strong resistance to reinfection with *T. saginata* was found in cattle[128] and confirmed later.[129,130] Soulsby[131] showed that calves younger than 4 months might reveal an immunological tolerance. Gallie and Sewell[51] found that 3-months-old calves displayed only a partial protection against a challenge infection 10 months later.

Theoretically, the best way of developing a vaccine is through isolation and characterization of the functional antigens inducing protection against, e.g., *T. saginata* cysticerci, and understanding the mode of the action of antigens. As the knowledge of *T.*

saginata functional antigens is limited, living or attenuated *T. saginata* eggs or larval stages have been used in the experiments performed on vaccination. Urquhart et al.[129] used *T. saginata* eggs irradiated with Kr 40; these were not able to induce cysticercosis in calves but only a partial resistance; the calves with challenge infection of 1,000 to 40,000 *T. saginata* eggs produced 7 to 20 times fewer living cysticerci 34 to 42 days after vaccination than the unvaccinated ones. Apart from the fact that the acquired resistance was only a partial one, there are two potential difficulties associated with the practical use of this type of vaccine; the difficulty consists in obtaining *T. saginata* eggs from human sources and in protecting the calves against an infection in the time between the vaccination and the development of the resistance.[129] Froyd and Round[48] and Froyd[130,132] showed that when hatched *T. saginata* oncospheres were introduced artificially into the muscles of calves they develop *in situ*. This led Wikerhauser and his group[133] to perform a series of experiments on the value of intramuscular vaccination with *T. saginata* hatched oncospheres. A dose of 10,000 hatched and activated oncospheres given intramuscularly to a number of calves provoked an absolute resistance in some of them and in some others a high degree of resistance by challenge 2 to 18 weeks later; experiments with injected *T. saginata* eggs or activated oncospheres given subcutaneously and with heterologous vaccination with *T. hydatigena* oncospheres did not give as satisfactory results.[133] Passive immunization offers some protection against cysticercosis and accelerates the degeneration of the remaining cysts but it needs a great amount of immune bovine serum.[134]

Any success in the control of taeniasis and cysticercosis will finally depend on the promotion of adequate research, better cooperation between workers in the veterinary and medical professions in both the field and the laboratory, and the acceptance and understanding of control measures by meat-eating peoples and by authorities deciding matters of economic importance.[13]

TAENIA SOLIUM INFECTION

Disease

Taenia solium taeniasis is a nonfatal intestinal infection in man, caused by the adult pork tapeworm, *T. solium*.

T. solium cysticercosis is an infection with the larval stage, cysticercus. *T. solium* cysticercosis in man is a serious and chronic disease, often fatal because of the frequent cerebral location. In pigs cysticerci localized in various tissues, mainly in the muscles, rarely causing an apparent disease.

Etiological Agent

T. solium is similar to *T. saginata* in many aspects but its structure and biology is less studied. For that reason the best presentation of *T. solium* is four stages: adult form, egg, oncosphere, and cysticercus, is by description of differences between these two species of tapeworms.

The Adult Form

The morphological features of *T. solium* that differ from *T. saginata* compiled from the works by du Noyer and Baer,[135] Brumpt,[136] Abuladze[2] and Verster[1] are presented in Table 1 and Figures 2, 3, 6, 7, 8, and 9.

Verster[103] stresses that for taxonomic differentiation between *T. solium* and *T. saginata* adult worm only three critria are essential: (1) the presence or absence of an armed rostellum (Figure 6), (2) the number of ovarian lobes (Figure 7), and (3) the presence or absence of a vaginal sphincter (Figure 8). The value of these criteria was confirmed by Proctor.[137]

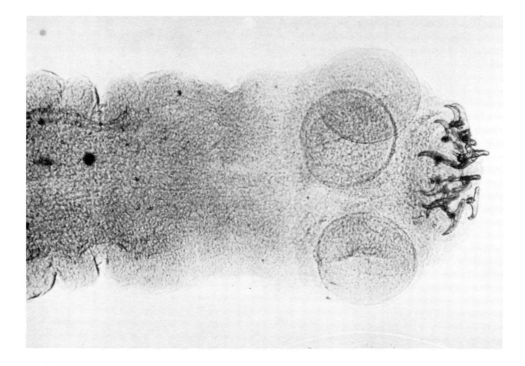

FIGURE 6.   *Taenia solium.* Scolex.

In general, *T. solium* is smaller and more delicate than *T. saginata*. The strobila needs only 62 to 72 days to be fully developed.[138] the gravid proglottids (Figure 9) are not as active as those of *T. saginata*; they are detached from the strobila in groups of 3 to 5 and are usually expelled passively with feces.

Eggs

The uterine eggs of *T. solium* differ from those of *T. saginata* in an ovoid shape and lack of two filaments which are characteristic for *T. saginata* eggs. Outside the uterus the delicate outer shell of *T. solium* egg is most often lost and the embryophore is practically identical with the embryophores of some other *Taeniidae*. There were also no differences found under the electron microscopic examination.[20,139] Brygoo et al.[140] and Capron and Rose[141] claimed that the embryophores could be differentiated by staining with Ziehl-Nelson stain; those of *T. saginata* stain positive, but those of *T. solium* remain negative, probably due to acid-alcohol resistance of the egg membranes. This observation has not been confirmed by other authors.

There are usually less than 50,000 eggs in a single *T. solium* proglottid. The average number was 40,436 eggs per one gravid proglottid in Yoshino's studies.[142] A part of the eggs is released from the anterior branches of the uterus, being opened by detachment of a proglottid from the strobila. The majority of invasive embryophores is liberated after maceration of the proglottids outside the host. This accounts for the common massive *T. solium* cysticercosis in pigs which are frequently infected by consuming the whole proglottids.

Oncosphere

The major interest in this stage of *T. solium* was in connection with the possible development of human cysticercosis as a result of an internal autoinfection. This last was suggested by Leukart in 1856 and cited by many other authors, but it is probably

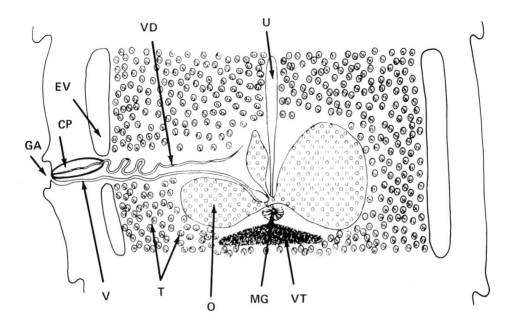

FIGURE 7.   *Taenia solium.* Mature proglottid. CP — cirrus pouch, EV — excretory vessel, GA — genital atrium, MG — Mehlis glands, O — ovary, T — testes, U — uterus, V — vagina, VD — vas deferens, VT — vitellaria. (From Verster, A., *Z. Parasitkd.,* 29, 313, 1967. With permission.)

not a frequent phenomenon.[143,144] It was experimentally proved that at least a short peptic digestion is necessary for disintegration of the embryophore,[144-146] which is the first step in making the oncosphere ready for invasion. It is rather unlikely that *T. solium* eggs or the gravid proglottids enter the stomach by vomiting or reverse peristalsis. Vomiting is exceptional in the course of medication with niclosamide or tin compounds, but it may happen when atebrine or magnesium sulfate are used[118] or during anesthesia. Only on that rare occasion when the invasive eggs may be subjected to peptic digestion may they eventually cause an internal autoinfection.

The migration of the invasive oncospheres was studied experimentally in pigs by Yoshino[147] with a conclusion that the larvae are evenly scattered in liver, brain, muscle tissue, and myocardium. However, the way to the final site through the intestinal, hepatic and/or lymphatic barriers remains unknown.

Cysticercus

T. solium cysticercus develops in a cavity lined by tall epitheloid cells, which originate from a vascular wall.[148] Sixty to seventy days after infection the cysticerci reach the size 5.6 to 8.5 mm by 3.1 to 6.5 mm and are mature; at that time the invaginated scolex measures 2.5 to 4.5 mm in length (Figure 10). On the scolex there are double, concentric circular rows of 22 to 28 hooks, larger and smaller ones situated alternately.[147] The size of the hooks is important taxonomically.[1,149]

In general *T. solium* cysticerci are bigger than those of *T. saginata* (5 to 20 mm in diameters vs. 3 to 16 mm of *T. saginata*), the bladder is more transparent, the fluid thinner, and invaginated scolex smaller, and the suckers more delicate and less frequently pigmented. According to Šlais[21] the differential diagnosis between *T. saginata* and *T. solium* is possible by an analysis of the histological structure of the wall when the scolex is not available. In *T. solium* cysticercus the bladder wall has wartlike processes (rugae in *T. saginata*) with protuberances 27 to 38 μm at the base and 15 to 27 μm in height (50 to 70 μm and 23 to 27 μm in *T. saginata*, respectively) and the superficial hairlike processes not exceeding 2.5 μm (3 to 6 μm in *T. saginata*) (Table 2).

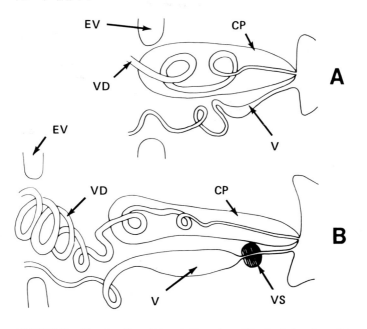

FIGURE 8.   *Taenia solium* (A) and *T. saginata* (B). Genital atrium. CP — cirrus pouch, EV — excretory vessel, V — vagina, VD — vas deferens, VS — vaginal sphincter. (From Verster, A., *Z. Parasitkd.,* 29, 313, 1967. With permission.)

The problem of predilection of *T. solium* cysticerci to the central nervous system is still obscure. *T. solium* cysticerci were observed in the brain of 60% of heavily infected pigs.[111] Hsieh[150] showed that *T. solium* cysticerci were distributed throughout the body of an experimentally infected monkey (*Macacus cyclopis*) roughly in proportion to the weight of the organs. The comparison of the data from autopsy and surgery,[151] biopsy,[148] and radiology[152] indicates a rather frequent location of *T. solium* cysticerci in human muscles, heart, and lung. Not uncommon are the reports on massive human muscle invasion without any evident involvement of the central nervous system.[153]

The subcutaneous location of *T. solium* is frequently reported, but Thomas et al.[148] suggest that cysticerci originating in muscle tissue may easily project into the loose, soft, and noncontractile subcutaneous tissue, giving an erroneous impression of being primarily of subcutaneous location.

Hosts

The list of hosts for *Taenia solium* is far from being complete. *T. solium* adult and larval form is less host specific than *T. saginata* is. Man is the only natural definitive host but *T. solium* taeniasis may also be established in the lar gibbon (*Hylobates lar*),[154] chacma baboon (*Papio ursinus*),[155] and golden hamster (*Mesocricetus auratus*).[156,157] The experimental infection of *Macaca radiata* with 20 *T. solium* cysticerci was not successful.[158]

The essential intermediate host for *T. solium* is the pig, but *T. solium* cysticerci are not uncommon in man and have been recorded in various mammals including monkeys (*Ateles geoffroyi, Cercopithecus cephus, C. patas, C. aethiops, Macacus inuus, M. cyclopis* and *Macaca mulatta*), wild boars, bushbabies, bushpigs, camels, rabbits, hares, rock hyraxes, brown bears, dogs as well as cats, foxes, polecats, coatis, rats, and mice.[1,2,159] The identity of these cysticerci has not always been confirmed. The existence of varieties or subspecies has been suggested to explain the different size of hooks of *T. solium* cysticerci found in pigs, cats, baboons, dogs, and man[149] or differences in the immunoelectrophoretic pattern of cysts.

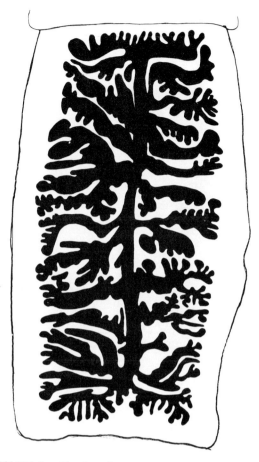

FIGURE 9.   *Taenia solium.* Gravid proglottid. (From
Verster, A., *Z. Parasitkd.,* 29, 313, 1967. With permission.)

The bladder worms recorded from man as *Cysticercus cellulosae* may represent more
than one species. It has been suggested that cysticerci in man in Africa may be due to
other species of *Taenia* that are prevalent in wild carnivora.[27] Still controversial is the
problem of so called *C. racemosus.*[160,161] *C. racemosus* is a lobulated or ramifying,
thin-walled, translucent large vesicle, having no scolex and usually located in subarachnoid space or in ventricles (Figures 11, 12). There are suggestions that it is a larval
stage of *T. multiceps*[162] or some other *Taenia*[160] but its microscopical structure rather
suggests a hypothesis that it is a *T. solium* cysticercus degenerated or grown unob-
structed by the surrounding tissue.[161]

Distribution

While *T. saginata* taeniasis and cysticercosis is found in both highly developed and
undeveloped countries, *T. solium* infection is prevalent in poor communities. While
T. saginata infection often occurs in urban populations eating sophisticated raw beef
dishes, *T. solium* taeniasis is prevalent in the rural population eating raw or semiraw
pork of occasion of a pig slaughter. The FAO/WHO/OIE[36] records the regions endemic for *T. solium* in Central and South America, Central and South Africa, Southeast Asia, and South and East Europe.

The data collected from 21 countries of Latin America by Schenone and Letonja[163]
revealed seven countries in which swine cysticercosis was registered in over 1% of pigs
slaughtered: Brazil, Honduras, Guatemala, Costa Rica, Nicaragua, Peru, El Salvador.

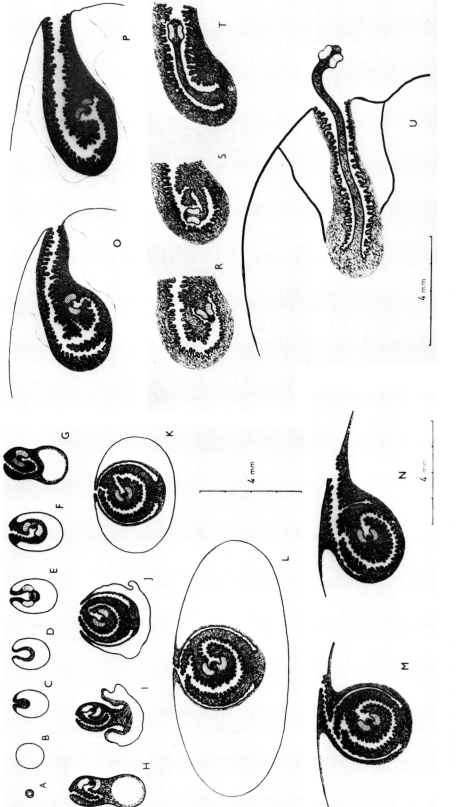

FIGURE 10. *Taenia solium.* Development of cysticercus. A—L — development in muscle tissue; M—P — development in human cerebrum; R—U — over-age forms in human cerebrum. (From Šlais,[97] With permission.)

Table 2
DIAGNOSTIC CHARACTERS OF SOME CESTODE LARVAE WHICH MAY BE FOUND IN MAN[a]

Larva	*Taenia so-lium* Cysticercus	*Taenia sa-ginata* Cysticercus	*Tacnia mul-ticeps* Coenurus	*Echinococcus granulosus* Echinococcus
Scolex				
Number	One	One	Several	Many
Hooks	Present	Absent	Present	Present
Bladder[a]				
Surface	Cuticle	Cuticle	Cuticle	Stratified hyaloidine membrane
Superficial hairlike cuticular extensions in μm	<1—2.5	3—6	1—2	
Subcuticular groups of muscles	Present	Absent	Absent	Absent
Make-up of wall	Wartlike processes	Rugae	Smooth and also rugose	Smooth
Base of superficial protuberances in μm	27—38	50—70	28—46	
Height of superficial protuberances in μm	15—27	23—27	15—22	

[a]   See Reference 21.

In Mexico the very unsatisfactory situation[4] has been improved and in 1973 only 0.85% of pigs were infected with cysticerci.[163] Altogether in 1973 in 21 countries of Latin America 1,539,926 pigs were found infected with *T. solium* out of 58,964,000 examined.[163]

In Central and South Africa both human and pig infections are reported as common from the South African Republic, Zimbabwe, Gambia, Guinea, Togo, Rwanda, Burundi, Malawi, Swaziland, Madagascar, and Zaire.

There are regions in Southeast Asia with prevalent human or pig cysticercosis as India, Thailand, Taiwan, and Korea. During the period of 6 months, 13 cases of human cysticercosis were diagnosed in the area of the Wissel Lakes, West Irian (Indonesia).[164] In Cheju Do Island (South Korea) 7.35% of 979 pigs were infected with *T. solium.*[165]

T. solium taeniasis and cysticercosis have been eliminated in most of West and Central Europe. It is slowly disappearing from East and South Europe; in the U.S.S.R. cysticercosis was found in 0.16% of pigs in 1961 and in 0.02% in 1971.[166] In Hungary the incidence was 0.48% in 1927 and 0.0002% in 1967.[167]

Porcine Cysticercosis

The pig as a typical intermediate host usually tolerates the living cysticerci well. Round a cysticercus there is a cavity coated with tall epithelioid cells, originated from a distended wall of the lymphatics. Between the cellular coating and the most external proliferating fibrous connective tissue there is a zone of plasma cells, lymphocytes, monophages, and eosinophils. These cells as well as the process of vascularization around the cysticercus are evidence of a slight chronic inflammatory cell response of

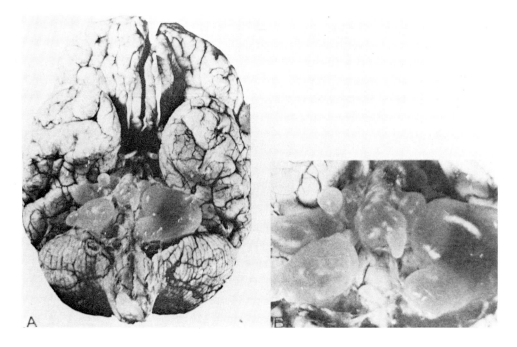

FIGURE 11.   *Taenia solium.* (A) Racemose form of cysticercosis at the base of the brain. (B) Close-up view of the same case. (From Márquez-Monter, H., Cysticercosis, in *Pathology of Protozoal and Helminthic Diseases,* Marcial-Rojas, R. A., Ed., Williams & Wilkins, Baltimore, 1971. With permission.)

the host. The reaction is frequently more pronounced at the opening of the invaginated scolex.[148] The exact mechanism which provokes an acute host cellular reaction, a development of caseous necrosis or autolysis of the cysticercus, intensive resorptive processes, and finally fibrous scarring or calcification is not well understood. It is probable that the dying cysticercus is a trigger, but undoubtedly the immunological mechanisms of the host are involved in destroying the developing or developed cysticerci, e.g., in an atypical intermediate host and in heavily infected or previously immunized animals.

The light or moderate cysticercosis does not usually cause any clinical picture. Sows infected experimentally with 200,000 *T. solium* embryophores showed anorexia, fever, accelerated pulse and respiration, vomiting, and diarrhea.[168] An infection 14 days before birth may cause abortion.[168] In pigs the cysticerci seem to show predilection to the central nervous system. In a group of naturally infected pigs the cerebral localization was found in 50% of the animals with one to three cysticerci present in the anconeus muscle and in 100% of those animals with seven or more cysticerci in the anconeus muscle.[169] But in 60 pigs with neuro-cysticercosis, cysticerci were occasionally seen in ventricles and never in the cerebellum.[169] That is why the neurologic signs in infected pigs are infrequent and may be related to the absence of the complications like hydrocephalus, intracranial hypertension, and disequilibrium. Another reason is that the pigs are usually slaughtered before the neurological symptoms develop.

Taenia Solium Taeniasis and Human Cysticercosis

The clinical course of *T. solium* taeniasis is mild and similar to that of *T. saginata* infection; only the excretion of proglottids is different as passive. From the experiments in four human volunteers it is known that the first excretion of *T. solium* proglottids takes place between 62 to 72 days after infection.[138] At that time the tapeworms were 218 and 223 cm long. After the unsuccessful treatment *T. solium* proglottids reappeared within 57 to 61 days.[170] *T. solium* adult forms live many years.

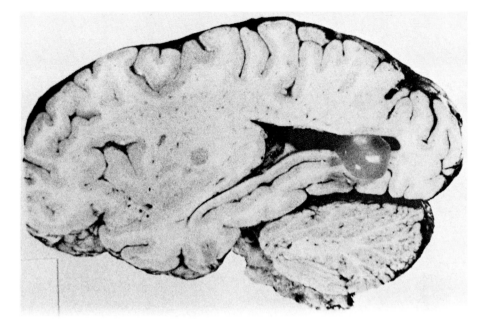

FIGURE 12. *Taenia solium.* Ventricular form of racemose cysticercosis. A large cyst protrudes from a lateral ventricle. (From Márquez-Monter, H., Cysticercosis, in *Pathology of Protozoa, and Helminthic Diseases,* Marcial-Rojas, R. A., Ed., Williams & Wilkins, Baltimore, 1971. With permission.)

The clinical picture of human cysticercosis is rather varied according to the location, number and stage of parasites, and individual reactivity of the patient. The number of cysticerci in a human body is from one to thousands.[171] Although the parasites are found in various human tissues the most frequent locations diagnosed by surgery and autopsy are the central nervous system (74.3% of all the diagnosed cases) and eyes (31.1%).[171]

Among 104 cases of cysticercosis and epilepsy summarized by Arseni and Cristescu[172] the location of cysticerci was hemispheric (74 cases), basal (5), ventricular (8), and generalized (17). In the group of 93 cases presented by Briceno et al.[173] the location of cysticerci was the following: brain (48 cases), subarachnoid space at the base (46), ventricles (12), brain stem (6), cerebellum (6), spinal cord (3), and pituitary (1). In about 50% of the cases of cerebral cysticercosis there are one or two cysticerci present, but they were as numerous as 1234 in one patient.[174] Nieto[175] and Escobar[176] described four essential forms of cerebral cysticercosis: (1) meningeal-producing chronic meningitis, seldom acute meningitis or meningoencephalitis or slight pathological changes only; (2) ventricular-provoking ependymitis granulosus, (3) parenchymatous with round cell infiltration in the grey or white substance, and (4) mixed form. The meningeal and ventricular form are predominant (Figures 13,14,15).

The clinical analysis of cerebral cysticercosis based on 132 cases was presented by Stępień.[5] He used the classification into three groups based on pathological changes and the clinical picture proposed by Stępień and Choróbski.[177] The first group of patients (41.7%), mostly with a single cysticercus, had the symptoms of slowly progressing intracranial tumor with focal neurological deficits, epileptic seizures, and increased intracranial pressure. In the second group of 25.7% of the patients, mainly children with an intensive infection, the clinical course was stormy with a rapid development of increased intracranial pressure, loss of vision, and organic mental syndrome. The third group consisted of 32.6% of the patients with cysticerci localized mainly at the base of the brain and they had a rather chronic course with symptoms of leptomenin-

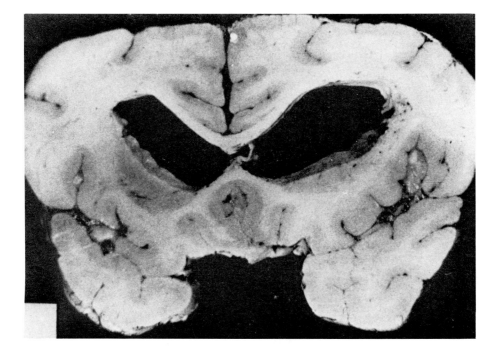

FIGURE 13.   *Taenia solium.* Hydrocephalus due to basal cysticercus meningitis. (From Márquez-Monter, H., Cysticercosis, in *Pathology of Protozoal and Helminthic Diseases,* Marcial-Rojas, R. A., Ed., Williams & Wilkins, Baltimore, 1971. With permission.)

gitis, ependymitis, and internal hydrocephalus (Figure 13). Surgical intervention resulted in recovery in 35.5% of the first group of patients only, improvement in 40%, 53%, and 28% of patients in I, II, and III groups, respectively, but death in 24%, 33%, and 67% of patients in respective groups.

The most obvious sign of cerebral cysticercosis is epilepsy.[172,178,179] Epilepsy was found in 60% of 181 cases of cerebral cysticercosis described by Arseni and Cristescu,[172] and in 36.5% of 132 cases described by Stępień.[5] On the other side, among 200 adult Bantu mine workers with epilepsy, 31 had cysticercosis.[179] The variability and polymorphism of epileptic manifestations, predominantly focal, is generally considered as characteristic of cerebral cysticercosis.[172] Cerebral cysticercosis is an important cause of morbidity and death in endemic areas.[4] The mean mortality rate in spite of surgery in 132 cases presented by Stępień[5] was 40.1%. Not rarely, cerebral cysticercosis causes a sudden death.[180]

Ocular cysticercosis is the next serious and common clinical form of infection. In 299 cases described by de Almeida and Oliveira[181] the most common was location in vitreous humor (147 cases) and subretinal (90 cases), but cysticerci may invade other tissues, including the anterior chamber and conjunctiva. The range of pathological changes varies greatly from a minimal reaction round the parasite to a severe inflammatory process and complications such as retinal detachment or atrophy, iridocyclitis, chorioiditis, and cloudiness of vitreous fluid occur.

Myocardial cysticercosis is frequently found in massive infection but seldom causes clinical signs.[182] Similarly, skin and muscle tissue location of cysticerci, which is so common, is usually of negligible clinical importance. A good example of asymptomatic infection is the case of a generalized muscle cysticercosis in an athlete, a winner of several medals for running and jumping described by Evans.[153]

General Mode of Spread

The general mode of *T. solium* transmission is presented in Figure 16. The internal

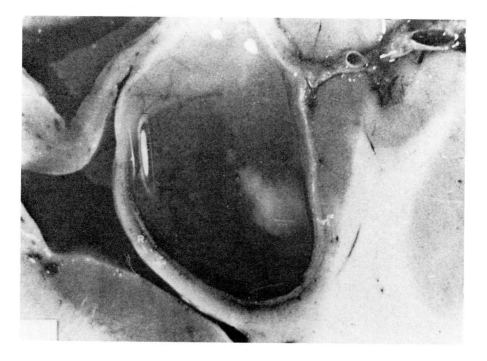

FIGURE 14.   *Taenia solium*. Parenchymatous form of cysticercosis. (From Márquez-Monter, H., Cysticercosis in *Pathology of Protozoal and Helminthic Diseases,* Marcial-Rojas, R. A., Ed., Williams & Wilkins, Baltimore, 1971. With permission.)

and external autoinfection of the human host is not included in the diagram because it has nothing to do with the spread of infection in the populations not being cannibal.

Epidemiology

The *T. solium* infected man is the disseminator of invasive eggs and the potential source of infection for himself, other people, and pigs. The production of *T. solium* eggs by one human carrier is about 250,000 daily, assuming that five proglottids are expelled per day.

The frequent coexistence of intestinal infection and cysticercosis which is between 4 and 26%[172,174,183] suggests that autoinfection is not a rare phenomenon. In such cases the external autoinfection with eggs transmitted from anus to mouth or through dirty hands or contaminated food seems to be a more probable way of contracting *T. solium* cysticercosis than internal autoinfection.[143] The last depends on a rare occasion, when gravid proglottids or eggs are passively translocated by reverse intestinal peristalsis or vomiting, e.g., during the tapeworm treatment.[184] Nevertheless the autoinfection or at least a close contact with the source of infection is the most probable cause of human generalized cysticercosis, in which the infective dose must be of several thousands eggs. In primitive societies, e.g., Bantu people, the massive invasion may also be caused by using local medicine prepared of tapeworm proglottids.[179] The tapeworm proglottid is a frequent source of infection for pigs, as the generalized cysticercosis is common in pigs and most important cause of the condemnation of pig carcasses.[111,151,169]

Little is known about the survival and spread of invasive *T. solium* eggs in the external environment. In general the spread of *T. solium* is less wide than the spread of *T. saginata* and causes mostly focal distribution of infection. The limiting factors are the smaller number of human carriers recruiting mainly among rural populations, smaller range of migration of both human hosts and pigs, and more frequent private unin-

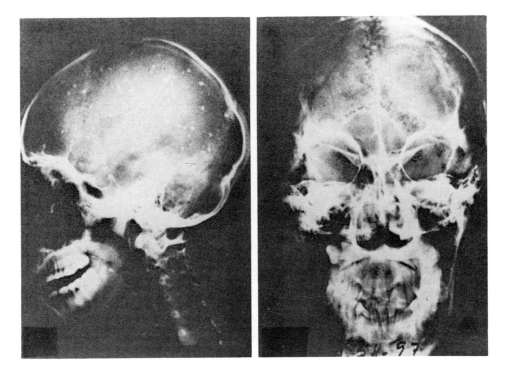

FIGURE 15. *Taenia solium*. Simple X-ray picture of the skull showing multiple calcified cysticerci. (From Márquez-Monter, H., Cysticercosis, in *Pathology of Protozoal and Helminthic Diseases,* Macial-Rojas, R. A., Ed., Williams & Wilkins, Baltimore, 1971. With permission.)

spected slaughter of pigs and local consumption of most of the pork. This view is supported by the following examples. In Guatemala 42% of *T. solium* infected patients came from rural areas; most of the others had at some time lived in a rural environment.[151] Only about 15% of the pig carcasses in Central American countries are subject to veterinary inspection.[151]

In developed societies raw pork is less frequently eaten than raw beef. There is a ritual prohibition of pork consumption in Moslem and orthodox Jewish communities. But aborigines in West Irain, Indonesia used to eat semiraw pork cooked between hot stones and leaves.[185] In Southeast Asia dog meat used as food may be a source of infection also. The close contact between the people living in a low standard of personal and housing hygiene with the pigs kept in the same building and used to grouting freely around greatly increases the transmission of infection. Therefore a high standard of general sanitation, including animal hygiene and effective veterinary inspection are the most important factors deciding upon *T. solium* transmission.

Diagnosis
Human T. Solium Taeniasis

T. solium intestinal infection can be diagnosed exclusively by examination of scolex or proglottids of the tapeworm. Finding *Taenia* eggs during a coproscopic examination or on an anal swab makes the species diagnosis impossible. The questioning of a patient about eating raw pork or expulsion of proglottids has limited practical value.

Elsdon-Dew and Proctor,[186] discussing the discrepancy between the high incidence of cysticercosis in pigs and low incidence of *T. solium* taeniasis in man in South Africa, paid attention to the possibility of a misidentification of *T. solium* and *T. saginata* infection when only gravid proglottids are diagnosed. Following this line Verster[1,103] denied the diagnostic value of the number of lateral uterine branches in the gravid

HOSTS:	definitive		intermediate	definitive
		EXTERNAL ENVIRONMENT		
ROLE IN TRANSMISSION:	disseminator of T. solium eggs	store and spread of invasive eggs	source of invasive cysticerci	host of the tapeworm producing eggs
TRANSMISSION: direct indirect				
MODE OF INDIRECT TRANSMISSION:	defecation and sewage	contamination of fodder and water	consumption of raw pork	

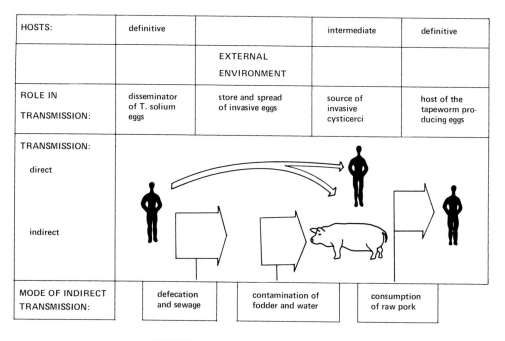

FIGURE 16. *Taenia solium.* Mode of spread.

proglottids, although counting these has been a routine method of species identification in the medical laboratories for more than a 100 years. At this point the taxonomic requirements conflict with the practical routine laboratory procedures. In the medical practice nowadays a scolex can hardly be found after a treatment with niclosamide or tin compounds which usually cause a disintegration of the anterior part of strobila. The identification of the ovary lobes or vaginal sphincter makes necessary the preparation of stained permanent slides. This complex procedure which needs a considerable helminthological experience might be important in doubtful cases somewhere in Africa, but is not necessary in the area where *T. solium* is practically absent and *T. saginata* common, and in the cases when the number of uterine branches by examination of unfixed proglottids clearly exceeds 20 branches on one side. The differentiation of taeniid cestodes by enzyme electrophoresis is possible but it is still a matter of research rather than a general practice.[195]

Human Cysticercosis

Heinz and Klinworth[179] examined 200 adult Bantu males for cysticercosis and found positive serological results in 25 cases, radiological signs of calcified cysticerci in 9 cases (Figure 15), and palpable subcutaneous cysts in 4 cases. Twenty of these people had Taenia eggs in their feces. The computerized tomography of the brain is now widely used to visualize the location and size of most of the cysticerci in the central nervous system as well as some of the complications of cysticercosis.

The indirect hemagglutination and immunofluorescence tests are the most specific and responsive[187-190] and helpful both in field and clinical diagnosis. Intradermal tests with acid soluble protein fractions of cestode antigens are reported as useful.[191] The immunology of human and animal cysticercosis has recently been reviewed by Flisser et al.[198]

However, the final diagnosis of *Taenia* species in postoperative or autopsy material is possible by examining of hooks, if present, and/or microscopic structure of the bladder wall (Table 2).[21]

Porcine Cysticercosis

So far meat inspection is the only routine method used for diagnosis of porcine cysticercosis. It mostly consists of examination of some cuts in masseters, aconeus muscle, and myocardium. The meat inspection for *T. solium* is more effective than that for *T. saginata* because *T. solium* cysticerci are larger and the infection frequently massive.

The serological tests as indirect hemagglutination and immunofluorescent tests and precipitin reactions as well as intradermal reactions are not specific and sensitive enough in lightly infected animals.

Prevention and Control

In the second half of the 19th century in Central Europe, especially in Germany where the people were fond of raw pork products and sausages, both *Trichinella spiralis* and *Taenia solium* were prevalent. In 1860 Virchow estimated human cerebral cysticercosis rate as high as 2% at autopsy examination. After the introduction of meat inspection the incidence of *T. solium* dropped, e.g., in a Berlin slaughterhouse from 0.58% in the years 1883—1890 to 0.002 to 0.008% in 1925—1930.[111] But it is unlikely that meat inspection alone was responsible for complete eradication of *T. solium* infection in most of Europe; much of the credit must be due to the changes in socioeconomic conditions, mainly a higher level of general sanitation and animal hygiene, the change from individual pig rearing to indoor industralized pig farming.

Therefore the following preventive measures are essential in control of *T. solium* infection in endemic areas: (1) free and effective treatment of human carriers diagnosed by individual examination or during a mass survey; (2) improvement of general sanitation and animal hygiene; (3) adequate and effective veterinary meat inspection; and (4) the health education of the public in individual prevention and social control measures.

T. solium intestinal infection is more easily cured than that of *T. saginata*; the drug of choice is niclosamide (Yomesan®). Praziquantel is going to be another drug of choice in *T. solium* taeniasis; a single dose of 10 mg/kg was effective in all 27 patients and a single dose of 5 mg/kg cured all but one of 26 patients (96%).[196] The drug provoking vomiting, i.e., atebrine, magnesium sulfate should not be used because of the danger of human cysticercosis.[143] Immediate treatment of *T. solium* human carriers is essential to minimize the risk of human cysticercosis. For that reason human *T. solium* carriers should be isolated until treated.[192] Some drugs, i.e., mebendazol and praziquantel, have been reported as lethal to taeniidae cysticerci. This is a good prospect for the chemotherapy of human larval *T. solium* infections.

The man-pig transmission of *T. solium* eggs is fecal and restricted mostly to rural areas. Therefore the use of adequate latrines instead of uncontrolled defecation and keeping pigs indoors or in enclosures are both of great importance. The meat inspection of pork should be a required procedure, easily available. It is usually more effective than those of beef because *T. solium* cysticerci are larger and more numerous in infected carcasses. The infected carcasses should be condemned or boiled until the whole carcass changes the color into grey. Freezing of infective meat is not always effective in destroying the cysticerci.

Human cysticercosis is often an exotic disease contracted during a visit in the tropics.[183] Therefore the visitors to endemic areas should respect the individual preventive hygienic measures.

There are some plans concerning control of *T. solium* in endemic regions.[4,116] They will not be successful without the changes in the sanitary, social, and economic situation of the afflicted human population. The history of *T. solium* in Europe is a good example of the radical disappearance of infection without the intended human intervention except the meat inspection.

A new problem is that due to the migration of people *T. solium* may be introduced into regions that were free of infection for many years.[193]

EDITORIAL COMMENT*

James H. Steele

Swine Cysticercosis in Colorado

Beginning in October 1977 and continuing through March 1978, *Taenia solium* cysticercosis was detected by the U.S. Department of Agriculture veterinary inspectors in 3.3% of 427 hogs sent to slaughter from a single swine feedlot in southern Colorado. The infected animals were culled breeder sows that were among the original stock acquired 4 years prior to the investigation. Subsequently, no infection was found in 858 butchered hogs that had been farrowed and raised on the feedlot premises during the 35 weeks prior to the investigation, which suggested that transmission was not continuing. It was impossible to determine, retrospectively, the original source of infection; however, taeniid eggs could have become available to the sows through several possible mechanisms. Direct fecal contamination of the pig pen by an infected worker appeared to be the most likely source because the infections were massive and occurred in only a few (less than 4%) of the older animals. The coprophagic habits of swine often result in the ingestion of large numbers of eggs by a few aggressive animals. In contrast, egg contamination by most other mechanisms would have resulted in a dilution effect resulting in a higher attack rate but fewer cysts per infected animal.

The public health threat posed by *T. solium* is great because cysticercosis in humans is a serious disease; cerebral cysticercosis is fatal in 25 to 65% of cases. Although taeniasis/cysticercosis caused by *T. solium* occurs world-wide, particularly in developing countries, local transmission between swine and humans is believed to be rare in the U.S. In 1974—1976, according to U.S. Department of Agriculture data, infection was found in an annual average of 6 carcasses of approximately 70,000,000 examined per year. Factors that limit the potential for transmission of this parasite in the U.S. include modern swine husbandry methods, which keep swine enclosed, thus preventing their scavenging on human fecal waste, widespread use of indoor toilets, and the preference of most American consumers for well-cooked pork (to prevent trichinosis).

However, conditions in swine feedlots create the potential for explosive spread if the parasite is introduced by an infected worker. Taeniasis caused by *T. solium* is widely prevalent in Mexico, and, although none of 28 feedlot employees examined at the time of the investigation were found to have tapeworm infection, it was noted that 13% of the employees had visited Mexico within the past year and the majority of these individuals were previous residents of Mexico. It may be assumed that infection is brought into the U.S. occasionally from Mexico and other endemic regions by emigrants and returning tourists.

Recommendations to control the problem included education of management and employees about *T. solium* transmission and how to prevent it, parasitologic examination of prospective employees and periodic examination of all employees, and installation of additional toilets and adequate maintenance of all toilet facilities.

---

* Source: John K. Emerson, DVM, Colorado State Dept. of Health, Denver, Colorado; Parasitic Diseases Division, Bureau of Epidemiology, CDC, Morbidity and Mortality Reports.

REFERENCES

1. **Verster, A.,** A taxonomic revision of the genus *Taenia* Linnaeus, 1758, *Onderstepoort J. Vet. Res.,* 36, 3, 1969.
2. **Abuladze, K. I.,** *Principles of Cestology, Taeniata,* Vol. 4, Izd. Nauka, Moscow, 1964.
3. **Garnham, P. C. C.,** Zoonoses or infections common to man and animals, *J. Trop. Med. Hyg.,* 61, 92, 1958.
4. **Chavarria, M. and Enriquez, A.,** Promotion for the combat of the cysticercosis produced by *Cysticercus, Helmintologia,* 8, 1, 1967.
5. **Stępień, L.,** Cerebral cysticercosis in Poland, *J. Neurosurgery,* p. 505, 1962.
6. **Mann, I.,** The eradication of cysticercosis/taeniasis — a challenge to the veterinary profession, 19th World Vet. Congr., Mexico City, 1971.
7. **Pawłowski, Z. S.,** Taeniarhynchosis, a progressive zoonosis in Europe, C. R. 1st Multicolloq. Europeen de Parasitol., Rennes, 1971, 35.
8. **Altmann, G. and Bubis, J. J.,** A case of multiple infection with *Taenia saginata, Isr. Med. J.,* 18, 35, 1959.
9. **Pawłowski, Z. S. and Rydzewski, A.,** Observations on taenia-rhynchosis in the Poznań province, *Wiad. Parazyt.* 4, 509, 1958.
10. **Podyapolskaya, V. P. and Kapustin, V. T.,** *Helminthic Diseases of Man,* 3rd ed., Medgiz, Moscow, 1958.
11. **Hornbostel, H.,** *Bandwurmprobleme in neuer Sicht,* Ferdinand Enk-Verlag, Stuttgart, 1959.
12. **Prévot, R., Hornbostel, H., and Dorken, H.,** Lokalisations-studien bei *Taenia saginata, Klin. Wochenschr.,* 30, 78, 1952.
13. **Pawlowski, Z. S. and Schultz, M. G.,** Taeniasis and Cysticercosis *Taenia saginata,* in *Advances in Parasitology,* Dawes, Ben, Ed., Academic Press, New York, 1972, 10.
14. **Lumsden, R. D., Oakes, J. A., and Dike, S. C.,** Cytoarchitectural and cytochemical features of tapeworm surfaces, *J. Parasitol.,* 56, 217, 1970.
15. **Arme, C. and Read, C. P.,** A surface enzyme in *Hymenolepis diminuta* Cestoda, *J. Parasitol.,* 56, 514, 1970.
16. **Read, C. P.,** Contact digestion in tapeworm, *J. Parasitol.,* 59, 672, 1973.
17. **Penfold, W. J., Penfold, H. B., and Phillips, M.,** The criteria of life and viability of mature *Taenia saginata* ova, *Med. J. Aust.,* 24, 2, 1937.
18. **Silverman, P. H.,** Studies on the biology of some tapeworms of the genus *Taenia.* The morphology and development of the taeniid hexacanth embryo and its enclosing membranes, with some notes on the state of development and propagation of gravid segments, *Ann. Trop. Med. Parasitol.,* 48, 356, 1954b.
19. **Rijpstra, A. C., Smit, A. M., and Swellengrebel, N. H.,** How and where to search for the ova of *Taenia saginata, Trop. Geogr. Med.* 13, 160, 1961.
20. **Gönnert, R., Meister, G., and Thomas, H.,** Das Freiwerden der Eier aus Taenia-Proglottiden, *Z. Parasitenkd.,* 31, 282, 1968.
21. **Šlais, J.,** *The Morphology and Pathogenicity of the Bladder Worms: Cysticercus cellulosae* and *Cysticercus bovis,* Academia, Prague, 1970.
22. **McIntosh, A. and Miller, D.,** Bovine cysticercosis with special reference to the early development stages of *Taenia saginata, Am. J. Vet. Res.,* 21, 169, 1960.
23. **Voge, M.,** Observations on the structure of cysticerci of *Taenia solium* and *Taenia saginata (Cestoda: Taeniidae), J. Parasitol.,* 49, 85, 1963.
24. **Penfold, W. J., Penfold, H. B., and Phillips, M.,** *Taenia saginata:* its growth and propagation, *J. Helminthol.,* 15, 41, 1937b.
25. **van den Heever, L. W.,** On the longevity of *Cysticercus bovis* in various organs in a bovine, *J. Parasitol.,* 53, 6, 1967.
26. **Leikina, E. S., Moskvin, S. N., Sokolovskaya, O. M., and Poletaeva, O. G.,** Life span of *Cysticercus bovis* and development of immunity in cysticerciasis, *Medskaya Parazit.,* 33, 694, 1964.
27. **Nelson, G. S., Pester, F. R. N., and Rickman, R.,** The significance of wild animals in the transmission of cestodes of medical importance in Kenya, *Trans. R. Soc. Trop. Med. Hyg.,* 59, 507, 1965.
28. **Clarenburg, A.,** Onderzoekingen over de levensvatbaarheid van *Cysticercus inermis, Tijdschr. Diergeneeskd.,* 59, 1, 1932.
29. **Safronow, M. G.,** O gelmintofaunie olenej w Tomponskom i Olenjekskom rajonach Jakutskoj ASSR (in Russian), in *Tr. Jakutsk. Nauchno-Issled. Inst. Selsk. Hoz Wa.,* 3, 1960.
30. **Huang, S. W.,** Studies on *Taenia species* prevalent among the aborigines in Wulai District, Taiwan, *Bull. Inst. Zool. Acad. Sin.,* 6, 29, 1967.

31. **Fay, L. D.**, Exposure of Thomson's gazelle to experimental infection with *Cysticercus bovis* (correspondence), *Vet. Rec.*, 90, 34, 1972.

32. **Boczoń, K., Gustowska, L., Hadaś, E., Jarczewska, K., Kotlińska, B., Kozakiewicz, B., Pawłowski, Z., Rydzewski, A., and Wiśniewska, M.**, Experimental *Taenia saginata* cysticercosis in goats and sheep, Proc. 3rd Int. Congr. Parasitol. Munchen, 1974, 581.

33. **Prokopenko, L. I.**, Taeniasis and its control in U.S.S.R., *Medskaya Parazit.*, 35, 652, 1966.

34. **Prokopenko, L. I.**, Approaches and methods of taeniarhynchosis eradication in the U.S.S.R., 8th Int. Congr. Trop. Med. Malar., Teheran, 233, 1968.

35. **Pawłowski, Z. S.**, Tasiemczyce człowieka, *Wiad. Parazyt.*, 20, 359, 1974.

36. **FAO/WHO/OIE Animal Health Yearbook for 1973**, Food and Agriculture Organization, Italy, 1974.

37. **Ockert, G.**, Über die Verbreitung einiger Darmparasiten unter die Bevölkerung des Bezirkes Halle, *Z. Arztl. Fortbild.*, 59, 850, 1965.

38. **Mielke, D.**, Ein Beitrag zum Taeniose-Zystizerkose-Problem, *Dtsch. Gesundheitswes.*, 24, 470, 1969.

39. **Silvermann, P. H.**, Bovine cysticercosis in Great Britain from July 1950 to December 1953, with some notes on meat inspection and the incidence of *Taenia saginata* in man, *Ann. Trop. Med. Parasitol.*, 49, 429, 1955.

40. **Schultz, M. G., Hermos, J. A., and Steele, J. H.**, Epidemiology of beef tapeworm infection in the United States, *Publ. Health Rep.*, 85, 169, 1970.

41. **Marx, G. W.**, Sewage disposal in relation to the beef tapeworm problem in Arizona, *Publ. Health News*, 35, 1, 1942.

42. **Schwartz, B.**, Parasites that attack animals and man, *Yearbook of Agriculture. Animal Diseases*, U.S. Government Printing Office, Washington, D.C., 1956.

43. **Schultz, M. G., Halterman, L. G., Rich, A. B., and Martin, G. A.**, An epizootic of bovine cysticercosis, *J. Am. Vet. Med. Assoc.*, 155, 1708, 1969.

44. **Schultz, M. G.**, Parasitic diseases along the Mexican-USA frontier, *Helminthol. Abstr.*, 41, 309, 1971.

45. **Soulsby, E. J. L.**, Helminths, in *Textbook of Veterinary Clinical Parasitology*, Vol. 1, Blackwell Scientific, Oxford, 1965, 1059.

46. **Taylor, D. C.**, Cysticercosis in an oryx (clinical note), *Vet. Rec.*, 70, 1207, 1958.

47. **Leonard, A. B. and Leonard, A. E.**, The intestinal phase of the resistance of rabbits to the larvae of *Taenia pisiformis*, *J. Parasitol.*, 27, 375, 1941.

48. **Froyd, G. and Round, M. C.**, The artificial infection of adult cattle with *Cysticercus bovis*, *Res. Vet. Sci.*, 1, 275, 1960.

49. **Urquhart, G. M.**, Parenteral production of cysticercosis, *J. Parasitol.*, 51, 544, 1965.

50. **Gallie, G. J. and Sewell, M. M. H.**, The serological response of calves infected neonatally with *Taenia saginata (Cysticercus bovis)*, *Trop. Anim. Health Prod.*, 6, 173, 1974.

51. **Gallie, G. J. and Sewell, M. M. H.**, The serological response of three month old calves to infection with *Taenia saginata (Cysticercus bovis)* and their resistance to reinfection, *Trop. Anim. Health Prod.*, 6, 163, 1974.

52. **Belyaev, A. E. and Monisov, A. A.**, Excretion of *Taenia saginata* proglottides in the early stages of infection, *Medskaya Parazit.*, 36, 487, 1967.

53. **Pawłowski, Z. S., Chwirot, E., and Sikora, B.**, Symptomatologia inwazji *Taenia saginata*, Materialy naukowe VI Zjazdu Polskiego Towarzystwa Epidemiologow i Lekarzy Chorob Zakaznych, 1972, 285.

54. **Pawłowski, Z. S.**, *Taenia saginata* taeniasis; infection and disease, Proc. 6th Int. Congr. Infectious Parasitic Dis., Warsaw, 1974, 424.

55. **Berry, L. R. and Burrows, R. B.**, Appendicitis mit Cestodes, *Arch. Pathol.*, 59, 587, 1955.

56. **Upton, A. C.**, Taenial proglottides in the appendix. Possible association with appendicitis. Report of cases, *Am. J. Clin. Pathol.*, 20, 1117, 1950.

57. **Gasparov, A., Šmircič, P., and Filipovič, B.**, Morphological changes in the mucosa of the small intestine in Taeniasis, *Med. Pregl.*, 15, 451, 1962.

58. **Kubicki, S. and Karlińska, A.**, Zmiany histopatologiczne błony śluzowej jelita cienkiego w niektórych chorobach pasozytniczych przewodu pokarmowego, *Wiad. Parazytol.*, 13, 1, 1967.

59. **Chodera, L., Chwirot, E., and Antoniewicz, K.**, Secretory activity of the mucous membrane of the stomach in cases of infections with *Taeniarhynchus saginatus*, *Acta Parasitol. Pol.*, 14, 301, 1967.

60. **Todorov, R. D.**, Study of quantitative deviation of gastrointestinal enzymes in taeniid infections, *Izv. Tsentr. khelmintol. Lab. Bulg. Akad. Nauk.*, 11, 173, 1966.

61. **Bacigalupo d'A., A.,** Clinica de la teniasis humana por *Taenia saginata, Prensa Méd. Argent.,* 43, 1520, 1956.

62. **Adonajło, A. and Bończak, J.,** Zakazenia tasiemcami w świetle materiałów z poradni schorzeń jelitowych Warszawa-Praga Połnoc, *Przegl. Epidem. (Warsaw),* 15, 425, 1961.

63. **Lapierre, J.,** Un cas d'éosinophilie exceptionnellement élevée au cours d'un taeniasis à *Taenia saginata, Ann. Parasitol. Hum. Comp.,* 28, 126, 1953.

64. **Talyzin, F. F.,** *The Effect of Parasitic Worms on the Function of the Digestive Tract,* Medgiz, Moscow, 1949.

65. **Nepote, K. H., Pawlowski, Z. S., and Soulsby, E. J. L.,** Immunoglobulin levels in patients infected with *Taenia saginata,* in *Parasitic Zoonoses. Clinical and Experimental Studies,* Soulsby, E. J. L., Ed., Academic Press, New York, 1974, 241.

66. **Urquhart, G. M.,** Epizootiological and experimental studies on bovine cysticercosis in East Africa, *J. Parasitol.,* 47, 857, 1961.

67. **Goulart, E. G., Da Silva, W. R. K., Faraco, B. F. C., and de Morales, D. S.,** Presquisa de cistos e ovos de entero-parasitos do homem no depósito subunqueal, *Rev. Bras. Med.,* 23, 465, 1966.

68. **Adonajlo, A., Kozakiewicz, B., Pawłowski, Z. S., and Rokossowski, H.,** Transmission of *Taenia saginata* in rural areas, *Wiad. Parazytol.,* 22, 499, 1976.

69. **Greenberg, A. E. and Dean, B. H.,** The beef tapeworm, measly beef and sewage — a review, *Sewage Ind. Wastes,* 30, 262, 1958.

70. **Liebman, H.,** Untersuchungen über die Bedeutung der verschiedenen Systeme der mechanischen und biologischen Abwasserreinigung für die Bekämpfung der Cysticercose des Rindes, *Proc. 17th Int. Vet. Congr., Hanover, 1963,* 2, 861, 1963.

71. **Vasilkova, Z. G.,** The problem of purification of the water of the River Moskva from the eggs of helminths, *Medskaya Parazit.,* 13, 11, 1944.

72. **Amirov, R. O. and Salamov, D. A.,** Sanitary and helminthological evaluation of the use of sewage water for field irrigation in the climate of the Apsheronsk Pennisula, *Gig. Sanit.,* 31, 104, 1967.

73. **Sinnecker, H.,** Über die Bedeutung städtlicher Abwasser für die Verbreitung von Infektionsmöglichkeiten. II. Die ausseren Infektketten von *Taenia saginata* (Goeze, 1782) vom Menschen zum Rind im Kreis Cottbus, *Wiss. Z. Naturwiss. Reihe,* 4, 325, 1955.

74. **Denecke, K.,** Starker Rückgang der Verwurmung im Müsterland und seine Ursachen, *Arch. Hyg. Bakt.,* 150, 558, 1966.

75. **Pawłowski, Z. S.,** Epidemiologia tasiemczycy i wagrzycy *Taenia saginata* (in Polish). *Wiad. Parazytol.,* 26, 539, 1980.

76. **Gemmell, M. A. and Johnstone, P. D.,** Experimental epidemiology of hydatidosis and cysticercosis, *Advances in Parasitology,* Dawes, B., Ed., 15, 311, 1977.

77. **Guildal, J. A.,** Mogers betydning som spredere af baendelormeaeg, *Nord. Vet. Med.,* 8, 727, 1956.

78. **Crewe, S. M.,** Worm eggs found in gull droppings, *Ann. Trop. Med. Parasitol.,* 61, 358, 1967.

79. **Crewe, W. and Crewe, S. M.,** Possible transmission of bovine cysticercosis by gulls (Demonstration), *Trans. R. Soc. Trop. Med. Hyg.,* 63, 17, 1969.

80. **Silverman, P. H. and Griffiths, R. B.,** A review of methods of sewage disposal in Great Britain, with special reference to the epizootiology of *Cysticercus bovis, Ann. Trop. Med. Parasitol.,* 49, 436, 1955b.

81. **Gladkov, G. N.,** Wild birds as possible vectors of *Taenia saginata* oncospheres (in Russian), *Probl. Parazitol.,* 1, 69, 1969.

82. **Sycevskaya, V. L. and Petrova, T. A.,** Rol'much w rasprastrenenii jaic gelmintov v Uzbekistanie, *Zool. Zh. Moskva,* 37, 563, 1958.

83. **Nadzhafov, I. G.,** The role of different species of flies in dissemination of onchospheres of *Taenia saginata, Medskaya Parazit.,* 36, 144, 1967.

84. **Round, M. C.,** Observations on the possible role of filth flies in the epizootiology of bovine cysticercosis in Kenya, *J. Hyg.,* 59, 505, 1961.

85. **Lonc, E.,** The possible role of soil fauna in the epizootiology of cysticercosis in cattle. Parts 1 and 2. *Angew. Parasitol.* 21, 133, 1980.

86. **Laws, G. F.,** Physical factors influencing survival of taeniid eggs, *Exp. Parasitol.,* 22, 227, 1968.

87. **Mackie, A. and Parnell, I. W.,** Some observations on Taeniid ovicides: the effect of some organic compounds and pesticides on activity and hatching, *J. Helminthol.,* 41, 167, 1967.

88. **Suvorov, V. Y.,** Viability of *Taenia saginata* oncospheres, *Medskaya Parazit.,* 34, 98, 1965.

89. **Silverman, P. H.,** The longevity of eggs of *Taenia pisiformis* and *T. saginata* under various conditions, *Trans. R. Soc. Trop. Med. Hyg.,* 50, 8, 1956b.

90. **Enigk, K., Stoye, M., and Zimmer, E.,** Die Lebensdauer von Taenieneiern in Gärfutter, *Dtsch. Tierarztl. Wochenschr.,* 76, 421, 1969.

91. **Jepsen, A. and Roth, H.,** Epizootiology of *Cysticercus bovis* — resistance of the eggs of *Taenia saginata*, *Proc. 14th Int. Vet. Congr. London*, 2, 43, 1952.

92. **Gladkov, G. N.,** Survival of *Taenia saginata* oncospheres under laboratory conditions and on the soil surface in Kiev, *Probl. Parazit.*, 1, 71, 1969.

93. **Duthy, B. L. and van Someren, V. D.,** The survival of *T. saginata* eggs on open pasture, *E. Afr. Agric. J.*, 13, 147, 1948.

94. **Guilhon, J.,** Le role de la pollution hydrique dans l'étiologie et l'épidemiologie de la cysticercose bovine et du téniasis humain, *Rec. Méd. Vet. École d'Alfort*, 151, 39, 1975.

95. **McManus, D.,** Prenatal infection of calves with *Cysticercus bovis*, *Vet. Rec.*, 72, 847, 1960.

96. **Urquhart, G. M.,** Bovine cysticercosis, *Proc. 1st Int. Congr. Parasitol. 1st Rome*, 2, 829, 1966.

97. **Kozakiewicz, B.,** Examinations on the possibility of penetration of *Taenia saginata* to foetuses following the experimental infection of cows, *Med. Wet.*, 31, 334, 1975.

98. **Abdullaev, A. M.,** Survival of cysticercus of beef tapeworm in veal dishes prepared in the Buryal ASSR, *Medskaya Parazit.*, 37, 108, 1968.

99. **Nagaty, H. F.,** Is measled beef cured as "basterma" fit for human consumption?, *J. R. Egypt. Med. Assoc.*, 29, 128, 1946.

100. **Anantaraman, M.,** The prevalence and transmission of human taeniasis in India, *Proc. 3rd Int. Congr. Parasit. Munich*, 1, 394, 1974.

101. **Chularerk, P., Rasameeprabha, K., Papasarathorn, T., and Chularerk, U.,** Some aspects of epidemiology and mass treatment of taeniasis in Ban Tard, Udorn Thani, *J. Med. Assoc. Thai*, 50, 666, 1967.

102. **Carmichael, J.,** Animal-man relationship in tropical diseases in Africa, *Trans. R. Soc. Trop. Med. Hyg.*, 46, 385, 1952.

103. **Verster, A.,** Redescription of *Taenia solium* Linnaeus, 1758 and *Taenia saginata* Goeze, 1782, *Z. Parasitkd.*, 29, 313, 1967.

104. **Menschig, G.,** Vergleichende koprologische Untersuchungen zur Ermittlung der optimalen Nachweismethode von Eiern des *Taeniarhynchus saginatus* (Goeze 1782), *Z. Med. Labortech.*, 13, 130, 1972.

105. **Thornton, H. and Goldsmid, J. M.,** Cellophane tape as an aid to the detection of *Taenia saginata* eggs, *Cent. Afr. J. Med.*, 19, 149, 1973.

106. **Farahmandian, L., Sahba, G. H., Arfaa, E., and Movafagh, K.,** A comparison of stool examination and mass treatment for indication of the prevalence of *Taenia saginata*, *Trop. Geogr. Med.*, 25, 171, 1973.

107. **Frolova, A. A. and Dzhumaev, M. D.,** Laboratory diagnosis of *Taenia saginata* infections, *Medskaya Parazit.*, 41, 404, 1972.

108. **Walther, M. and Grossklaus, D.,** Untersuchungen zur Frage der Diagnose der Rinderzystizerkose mit Hilfe der indirekten Hämagglutination, *Zentralbl. Veterinaermed. Reihe B*, 19, 309, 1972.

109. **Dewhirst, L. W., Cramer, J. D., and Sheldon, J. J.,** An analysis of current inspection procedures for detecting bovine cysticercosis, *J. Am. Vet. Med. Assoc.*, 150, 412, 1967.

110. **Grossklaus, D. and Walther, M.,** Zur Serodiagnose der Zystizerkose des Rindes, *Zentrabl. Veterindermed. Reihe B*, 17, 828, 1970.

111. **Viljoen, N. F.,** Cysticercosis in swine and bovines, with special reference to South African conditions, *Onderstepoort J. Vet. Res.*, 9, 337, 1937.

112. **van den Heever, L. W. and Reinecke, R. K.,** The significance of the shoulder incision in the routine inspection of food animals for cysticercosis, *Int. Vet. Congr. (17th), Hanover, Proc.*, 2, 909, 1963.

113. **Kearney, A.,** *Cysticercus bovis* — some factors which may influence cyst distribution, *J. Parasitol.*, 56, 183, 1970.

114. **Witenberg, G. G.,** Helminth fauna in man and domestic animals in Israel, *Isr. J. Med. Sci.*, 4, 1069, 1968.

115. **Schwabe, U. W.,** *Veterinary Medicine and Human Health*, Williams & Wilkins, Baltimore, 1963.

116. **Rukavina, J. and Delić, S.,** Problem organizacije i mjera u suzbijanju cisticerkoze goveda i svinja i tenijaza ljudi, *Acta Parasitol. Jug.*, 3, 5, 1972.

117. **Pawłowski, Z. S.,** Inorganic tin compounds as the alternative drug in human taeniarhynchosis, *J. Parasitol.*, 56, 261, 1970a.

118. **Pawłowski, Z. S. and Chwirot, E.,** Nebenwirkungen bei der Behandlung von Taeniarhynchosen. I. Beobachtungen bei 2014 ambulanten Patienten, *5th Int. Congr. Infect. Diseases Vienna*, 46, 277, 1970.

119. **Beier, A.,** Die *Taenia saginata* Infektion und ihre Behandlung mit Acranil und Yomesan, *Münch. Med. Wochenschr.*, 105, 2075, 1963.

120. **Beier, A.,** Terapeutische Erfahrungen mit Yomesan bei menschlichen Bandwurminfektionen, *Z. Tropenmed. Parasitol.*, 17, 50, 1966.

121. **Gönnert, R.,** Experimental and clinical experiences with Yomesan, *8th Int. Congr. Trop. Med. Malar., Teheran*, 1968, 1088.

122. **Chodera, L., Chwirot, E., and Pawłowski, Z.**, Nebenwirkungen bei der Behandlung von Taeniarhynchosen. II. Beobachtungen bei 856 hospitalisierten Kranken, *Int. Congr. Infect. Dis. 5th, Vienna,* 1970, 281.

123. **Notter, A., Robert, J., and Boudenes, G.**, Agénésie de la main droite chez un nouveau-né a terme. Role étiologique possible d'un taenifuge à base d'étain métalique absorbé par le niere au deuxieme mois de la gestation, *Sem. Hop. (Paris),* 39, 2701, 1963.

124. **Kalawski, K. and Pawłowski, Z. S.**, Inwazje tasiemca nieuzbrojonego *Taeniarhynchus saginatus* na terenie miasta Poznania w latach 1954—1968, *Przegl. Epidemiol.,* 24, 377, 1970.

125. **Hajduk, F., Müller, K. H., Saalbreiter, R., and Eymmer, H. J.**, The occurrence distribution and control of taeniasis and cysticercosis, *Z. Arztl. Fortbild.,* 63, 1146, 1969.

126. **Kozakiewicz, B.**, personal communication, 1976.

127. **van Kocy, J. G. and Robijns, K. G.**, Gamma irradiation elimination of *Cysticercus bovis* in meat, in *Panel Proceedings Series "Elimination of Harmful Organism from Food and Feed by Irradiation",* International Atomic Energy Agency, Vienna, 1968.

128. **Penfold, W. J. and Penfold, H. B.**, Cysticercosis bovis and its prevention, *J. Helminthiol.,* 15, 37, 1937.

129. **Urquhart, G. M., McIntyre, W. I. M., Mulligan, W., Jarett, W. F. H., and Sharp, N. C. C.**, Vaccination against helminth disease, *Int. Vet. Congr. (17th) Hanover Proc.,* 1, 769, 1963.

130. **Froyd, G.**, The artificial oral infection of cattle with *Taenia saginata* eggs, *Res. Vet. Sci.,* 5, 434, 1964.

131. **Soulsby, E. J. L.**, Immunological unresponsiveness to helminth infections in animals, *Int. Vet. Congr. (17th) Hanover Proc.,* 1, 761, 1963.

132. **Froyd, G.**, The artificial infection of calves with oncospheres of *Taenia saginata, Res. Vet. Sci.,* 2, 243, 1961.

133. **Wikerhauser, T., Zukowić, M., and Dzakula, N.**, *Taenia saginata* and *T. hydatigena:* intramuscular vaccination of calves with oncospheres, *Exp. Parasitol.,* 30, 36, 1971.

134. **Lloyd, S. and Soulsby, E. J. L.**, Passive transfer of immunity to metacestodes of *Taenia saginata,* Proc. 3rd Int. Congr. Parasitol., Munich, August 25-31, 1974, 583.

135. **du Noyer, M. R. and Baer, J. G.**, Etude comparee du *Taenia saginata* et du *Taenia solium, Bull. Sci. Pharmacol.,* 35, 209, 1928.

136. **Brumpt, E.**, *Précis de Parasitologie,* 6th ed., Masson, Paris, 1949.

137. **Proctor, E. M.**, Identification of tapeworms, *S. Afr. Med. J.,* 46, 234, 1972.

138. **Yoshino, K.**, On the subjective symptoms caused by the parasitism of *Taenia solium* and its development in man, *Taiwan Igakkai Zasshi,* 33, 183, 1934.

139. **Morseth, D. J.**, Ultrastructure of developing taeniid embryophores and associated structures, *Exp. Parasitol.,* 16, 207, 1965.

140. **Brygoo, E. R., Capron, A., and Randriamalala, J. Ch.**, Sur quelques méthodes de coloration sélective des coques d'oeufs d'helminthes parasites de l'homme, *Bull. Soc. Pathol. Exot.,* 52, 655, 1959.

141. **Capron, A. and Rose, F.**, Sur la constitution des oeufs d'helminthes. II. L'alcoolo-acido-résistance chez les cestodes. Différence de colorabilité par le Ziehl des embryophores de *Taenia saginata* et *Taenia solium, Bull. Soc. Pathol. Exot.,* 55, 765, 1962.

142. **Yoshino, K.**, On the evacuation of eggs from the detached gravid proglottids of *Taenia solium* and on the structure of its eggs, *Taiwan Igakkai Zasshi,* 33, 47, 1934.

143. **Webbe, G.**, The hatching and activation of taeniid ova in relation to the development of cysticercosis in man, *Z. Tropenmed. Parasitol.,* 18, 354, 1967.

144. **Gönnert, R., Meister, G., Strufe, R., and Webbe, G.**, Biologische Probleme bei *Taenia solium, Z. Tropenmed. Prasitol.,* 18, 76, 1967.

145. **Silverman, P. H.**, Studies on the biology of some tapeworm of the genus *Taenia.* I. Factors affecting hatching and activation of taeniid ova and some criteria of their viability, *Ann. Trop. Med. Parasitol.,* 48, 207, 1954.

146. **Gönnert, R. and Thomas, H.**, Einfluss von Verdauungssaften auf die Eihülen von *Taenia*-eiern, *Z. Parasitenkd.,* 32, 237, 1969.

147. **Yoshino, K.**, Studies on the post-embryonal development of *Taenia solium.* Parts I, II, III, *Taiwan Igakkai Zasshi,* 32, 1392, 1569, 1717, 1933.

148. **Thomas, J. A., Kothare, S. N., and Baptist, S. J.**, Cysticercus cellulosae, *J. Trop. Med. Hyg.,* 76, 106, 1973.

149. **Heinz, H. J. and Aron, L.**, Studies on *Cysticercus cellulosae, S. Afr. J. Med. Sci.,* 31, 61, 1966.

150. **Hsieh, H. C.**, Experimental transmission of *Cysticercus cellulosae* in Taiwan monkey, *Macaccus cyclopis* (Swinhoe, 1862), *Formosan Sci.,* 14, 66, 1960.

151. **Acha, P. N. and Aguilar, F. J.**, Studies on cysticercosis in Central America and Panama, *Am. J. Trop. Med. Hyg.,* 13, 48, 1964.

152. **Gelfand, M. and Jeffrey, C.**, Cerebral cysticercosis in Rhodesia, *J. Trop. Med. Hyg.,* 76, 4, 1973.

153. Evans, R. R., Cysticercosis in an athlete, *Trans. R. Soc. Trop. Med. Hyg.*, 32, 549, 1939.

154. Cadigan, F. C., Stanton, J. S., Tanticharoenyos, P., and Chaicumpa, V., The lar gibbon as definitive and intermediate host of *Taenia solium, J. Parasitol.*, 53, 844, 1967.

155. Verster, A., *Taenia solium* Lin. 1758 in the chacma baboon, *Papio ursinus* (Kerr 1792), *J. S. Afr. Vet. Med. Assoc.*, 36, 580, 1967.

156. Gnezdilov, V. G., The golden hamster *Mesocricetus auratus* (Waterhouse) as a potential definitive host of the tapeworm *Taenia solium, Zool. Zh.*, 36, 1770, 1957.

157. Verster, A., The golden hamster as a definitive host of *Taenia solium* and *Taenia saginata, Onderstepoort J. Vet. Res.*, 41, 23, 1974.

158. Anantaraman, M., personal communication, 1973.

159. Mazzotti, L. Davalos, A., and Martinez-Maranon, R., Natural and experimental infection of different mammal species by *Cysticercus cellulosae, Rev. Inst. Salubr. Enferm. Trop. Mexico City*, 25, 151, 1965.

160. Biagi, F. F., Briceno, C. E., and Martinez, B., Diferencias entre *Cysticercus cellulosae* y *C. racemosus, Rev. Biol. Trop.*, 9, 141, 1961.

161. Dixon, H. B. F. and Lipscomb, F. M., Cysticercosis. An Analysis and Follow-Up of 450 Cases, Med. Res. Council Spec. Rep. Ser. Her Majesty's Stationery Office, London, 299, 1961.

162. Abuladze, K. I. and Sadykov, V. M., A recent notion about the pathogenic role of larval stages of taeniids, Proc. 4th Int. Conf. Wld. Ass. Advmt. Vet. Parasit., 1971.

163. Schenone, H. and Letonja, T., Cisticercosis porcina y bovina en Latinoamerica, *Bol. Chil. Parasitol.*, 29, 90, 1974.

164. Tumada, L. R. and Margono, S. S., Cysticercosis in the area of the Wissel Lakes, West Irian, *S.E. Asian J. Trop. Med. Publ. Health*, 4, 371, 1973.

165. Han, H. R., A survey on *Cysticercus cellulosae* infection in swine of Cheju-Do, *Korean J. Publ. Health*, 6, 23, 1969.

166. Bessonov, A. S., Perspectives of eradication of several helminthozoonetic diseases in the U.S.S.R., 6th Int. Conf. Wld. Ass. Advmt. Vet. Parasitol., 1973.

167. Bodrossy, L., A parazitozisok husginiona jelentösege hazankban, *Magy. Allatorv, Lapja*, 27, 401, 1972.

168. Tyshkevich, L. S., Experimental cysticercosis *Cysticercus cellulosae* in sows at different stages of pregnancy, *Sb. Nauchn. Tr. Mosk. Vet. Akademiya im. K.I. Skryabina*, 65, 190, 1973.

169. Hernández-Jáuregui, P. A., Márquez-Monter, H., and Sastré-Ortiz, S., Cysticercosis of the central nervous system in hogs, *Am. J. Vet. Res.*, 34, 451, 1973.

170. Asada, J., Otagaki, H., Kaji, F., Aokage, K., and Ochi, G., On the longevity and the development of the pork and beef tapeworms in human hosts, *Tokyo Iji Shinshi*, 73, 153, 1956.

171. Schenone, H., Ramirez, R., and Rojas, A., Aspectos epidemiológicos de la neurocisticercosis en América Latina, *Bol. Chil. Parasitol.*, 28, 61, 1973.

172. Arseni, C. and Cristescu, A., Epilepsy due to cerebral cysticercosis, *Epilepsia*, 13, 253, 1972.

173. Briceno, C. E., Biagi, F., and Martinez, B., Cisticercosis. Observaciones sobre 97 casos de autopsia, *Prensa Med. Mex.*, 26, 193, 1961.

174. Márquez-Monter, H., *Cysticercosis in Pathology of Protozoal and Helminthic Diseases*, Marcial-Rojas, R. A., Ed., Williams & Wilkins, Baltimore, 1971.

175. Nieto, D., Sobre la histopatologia de la cisticercosis cerebral, *Bol. Inst. Est. Med. Biol.*, 2, 73, 1943.

176. Escobar, A. I., Cysticercosis cerebral con el studio de 20 casos, Part I, II, *Arch. Mex. Neurol. Psiquiatr.*, 1, 149, 1962 and 1, 171, 1963.

177. Stepień, L. and Chorobski, J., Cysticercosis cerebri and its operative treatment, *Arch. Neurol. Psychiatry*, 61, 499, 1949.

178. Powell, S. J., Proctor, E. M., Wilmot, A. J., and MacLoed, I. N., Cysticercosis and epilepsy in Africans: a clinical and serological study, *Ann. Trop. Med. Parasitol.*, 60, 152, 1966.

179. Heinz, H. J. and Klinworth, G. K., Cysticercosis in the aetiology of epilepsy, *S. Afr. Med. Sci.*, 30, 32, 1965.

180. Bhaskaran, C. S., Cerebral cysticerciasis as a cause of unnatural deaths, *Indian J. Med. Sci.*, 27, 545, 1973.

181. de Almeida, A. A. and de Oliveira, J. E. B., Cisticercose ocular, *Rev. Inst. Med. Trop. S. Paulo*, 13, 1, 1971.

182. Ibarra-Perez, C., Fernandez-Diez, J., and Rodriguez-Trujillo, F., Myocardial cysticercosis: report of two causes with coexisting heart disease, *South. Med. J.*, 65, 484, 1972.

183. Dixon, H. B. F. and Hargreaves, W. H., Cysticercosis *Taenia solium.* A further ten years clinical study covering 284 cases, *Q. J. Med.*, 13, 107, 1944.

184. Mody, V. R., Treatment of tapeworm infections, *Br. Med. J.*, Suppl. 1, 1184, 1964.

185. Holz, Z., personal communication, 1976.

186. Elsdon-Dew, R. and Proctor, E. M., Distinction between *Taeniarhynchus saginatus* and *Taenia solium, S. Afr. J. Sci.*, 61, 215, 1965.

187. **Proctor, R. M., Powell, S. J., and Elsdon-Dew, R.,** The serological diagnosis of cysticercosis, *Ann. Trop. Med. Parasitol.,* 60, 146, 1966.

188. **Dao, C., Arnaud, J. P., Petithory, J., and Brumpt, L.,** Apport de la technique de fluorescence indirecte au diagnostic immunologique de la cysticercose humaine, *Ann. Parasitol. Hum. Comp.,* 48, 23, 1973.

189. **Konovalova, L. M.,** Search for and use of new methods for immunodiagnosis of human cysticercosis, *Medskaya Parazit.,* 42, 536, 1973.

190. **Rydzewski, A. K., Chisholm, E. S., and Kagan, I. G.,** Comparison of serologic tests for human cysticercosis by indirect immunofluorescent antibody, and agar gel precipitin test, *J. Parasitol.,* 61, 154, 1975.

191. **Zapart, W., Slusarski, W., and Ptasiński, J.,** Intradermal tests with acid soluble protein fractions of cestode antigens in the diagnosis of cerebral cysticercosis in man, in *Parasitic Zoonoses. Clinical and Experimental Studies,* Soulsby, E. J. L., Ed., Academic Press, New York, 1974, 223.

192. **Benenson, A. S.,** *Control of Communicable Diseases in Man,* American Public Health Association, Washington, D.C., 1975.

193. **Wyburn-Mason, R. and Shaikh, M. A.,** Disseminating cysticercosis in England, *Br. Med. J.,* 20, 173, 1973.

194. **Groll, E.,** Praziquantel for cestode infections in man, *Acta Trop.,* 37(3): 293-296, 1980.

195. **Le Riche P. D. and Sewell, M. M. H.,** Differentiation of *Taeniid* cestodes by enzyme electrophoresis, *Int. J. Parasitol.,* 8, 479, 1978.

196. **Rim, H. J., Park, S. B., Lee, J. S., and Joo, K. S.,** Therapeutic effects of praziquantel (Embay 8440) against *Taenia solium* infection, *Korean J. Parasitol.,* 17, 67, 1979.

197. **Šlais, J.,** Die Morphologie und histologische Diagnostik des Parasiten bei der Gehirncysticerkose. *Acta Neuropath.,* 10, 295, 1968.

198. **Flisser, A., Pérez-Montfort, R. and Larralde, C.,** The immunology of human and animal cysticercosis: a review. *Bull. World Health Organization,* 57, 839, 1979.

INDEX

INDEX